December 1, 2010

BIOPSY INTERPRETATION SERIES

BIOPSY INTERPRETATION OF SOFT TISSUE TUMORS

BIOPSY INTERPRETATION SERIES

Series Editor: Jonathan I. Epstein, MD

Interpretation of Breast Biopsies, 4/e
Darryl Carter, 2002

Prostate Biopsy Interpretation, 3/e
Jonathan I. Epstein, Ximing J. Yang, 2002

Bladder Biopsy Interpretation
Jonathan I. Epstein, Mahul B. Amin, and Victor E. Reuter, 2004

Biopsy Interpretation of the Gastrointestinal Tract Mucosa
Elizabeth A. Montgomery, 2005

Biopsy Interpretation of the Upper Aerodigestive Tract and Ear
Edward B. Stelow and Stacey E. Mills, 2007

Biopsy Interpretation of the Prostate, 4/e
Jonathan I. Epstein and George Netto, 2007

Biopsy Interpretation of the Breast
Stuart J. Schnitt and Laura C. Collins, 2008

Biopsy Interpretation of the Liver, 2/e
Stephen A. Geller and Lydia M. Petrovic, 2009

Biopsy Interpretation of the Uterine Cervix and Corpus
Anais Malpica, Michael T. Deavers and, Elizabeth D. Euscher, 2009

Biopsy Interpretation: The Frozen Section
Jerome B. Taxy, Aliya N. Hussain, and Anthony G. Montag, 2009

Biopsy Interpretation of the Skin
A. Neil Crowson, Cynthia M. Magro, and Martin C. Mihm, 2009

Biopsy Interpretation of the Thyroid
Scott L. Boerner and Sylvia L. Asa, 2009

Biopsy Interpretation of Soft Tissue Tumors
Cyril Fisher, Elizabeth A. Montgomery, and Khin Thway 2010

Biopsy Interpretation of the Bladder, 2/e
Jonathan I. Epstein, Mahul B. Amin, and Victor E. Reuter, 2010

Biopsy Interpretation of the Lung
Saul Suster and Cesar Moran, 2011

Biopsy Interpretation of the Central Nervous System
Daniel J. Brat and Matthew J. Schniederjan, 2011

BIOPSY INTERPRETATION SERIES

BIOPSY INTERPRETATION OF SOFT TISSUE TUMORS

Cyril Fisher, MD, DSc, FRCPath
Department of Histopathology
Royal Marsden Hospital
London, United Kingdom

Elizabeth A. Montgomery, MD
Department of Pathology
Johns Hopkins Hospital
Baltimore, Maryland

Khin Thway, BSc, MBBS, FRCPath
Department of Histopathology
Royal Marsden Hospital
London, United Kingdom

Wolters Kluwer | Lippincott Williams & Wilkins
Health
Philadelphia • Baltimore • New York • London
Buenos Aires • Hong Kong • Sydney • Tokyo

Senior Executive Editor: Jonathan W. Pine, Jr.
Product Manager: Marian A. Bellus
Vendor manager: Bridgett Dougherty
Senior Marketing Manager: Angela Panetta
Senior Manufacturing Manager: Benjamin Rivera
Creative Director: Doug Smock
Production Service: SPi Technologies

530 Walnut Street
Philadelphia, PA 19106 USA
LWW.com

Printed in the People's Republic of China

Library of Congress Cataloging-in-Publication Data
Fisher, Cyril.
Biopsy interpretation of soft tissue tumors / Cyril Fisher, Elizabeth A. Montgomery.–1st ed.
p. ; cm.–(Biopsy interpretation series)
Includes bibliographical references and index.
ISBN 978-0-7817-9559-3 (alk. paper)
1. Soft tissue tumors–Pathophysiology. 2. Soft tissue tumors–Diagnosis. 3. Biopsy.
I. Montgomery, Elizabeth (Elizabeth A.), 1958- II. Title. III. Series: Biopsy interpretation series.
[DNLM: 1. Soft Tissue Neoplasms–diagnosis. 2. Soft Tissue Neoplasms–pathology.
3. Biopsy–methods. 4. Diagnosis, Differential. WD 375 F533b 2011]

RC280.S66F57 2011
616.99'4–dc22

2010025303

---

10 9 8 7 6 5 4 3 2 1

RRS1009

CONTENTS

PREFACE

There are more than two hundred types of soft tissue tumors, including many variant patterns. In most textbooks, they are organized by differentiation or diagnostic subtype in line with the World Health Organization classification scheme. Detailed information is available – for those who already know the approximate diagnosis. However, in limited material, especially core needle biopsy, soft tissue tumors first appear to the pathologist as one of a number of microscopic patterns in which the line of differentiation is not always obvious or in which there is a wide differential diagnosis.

This book, intended as a practical guide for the diagnostic surgical pathologist, additionally approaches diagnosis by cytomorphologic pattern – spindle, epithelioid, pleomorphic, small round cell, or plexiform. Other chapters deal with those in which the line of differentiation is apparent (adipose, vascular, nerve sheath, smooth muscle) but which in core biopsies are sometimes hard to categorize or evaluate for malignant potential; tumors that favor specific anatomical locations such as skin and retroperitoneum; and those in which stromal changes are the predominant feature. The latter, such as myxoid lesions, are relatively common and often difficult to distinguish. Some tumor types are discussed in more than one chapter, but this is essential as they are approached from different angles.

The key features of specific tumors and tumor-like lesions are detailed within each category, using morphologic, immunohistochemical, ultrastructural, and genetic data. This parallels and complements the normal diagnostic process. In addition to color photomicrographs, the book includes numerous tables for differential diagnosis within each category. Relevant clinical data that inform the pathologic diagnosis, and subsequent implications for therapy, are included. Sampling techniques, specimen handling, application of ancillary diagnostic modalities, sarcoma grading and staging, and reporting are discussed in the introductory chapter.

Sarcomas and many benign soft tissue tumors are rare and present a real challenge to those who encounter them infrequently. We hope this book will be of value to all pathologists faced with diagnosis and assessment of likely behavior in a soft tissue tumor biopsy.

Cyril Fisher
Elizabeth A. Montgomery
Khin Thway

1

BIOPSY TECHNIQUES, DIAGNOSTIC METHODS, AND REPORTING

INTRODUCTION

Soft tissue tumors comprise a group of entities showing mesenchymal differentiation which can be located in skin, subcutis, or deep soft tissue. The latter includes subfascial limb and limb girdle tumors, and those located in head and neck, abdomen, retroperitoneum (including paratestis), pelvis, and thoracic and intracranial cavities. Similar lesions can also involve viscera. Typically, soft tissue tumors are classified by the type of differentiation which they display,[1] and the principal objectives of the surgical pathologist are to identify the lineage of the lesional cells and assess their malignant potential. Nonmesenchymal lesions such as carcinoma or melanoma can also present as soft tissue neoplasms.

In many cases, the tumor is seen initially as a spindle cell, epithelioid cell, small round cell, or pleomorphic lesion which needs to be characterized further with the aid of ancillary techniques including immunohistochemistry, electron microscopy, and genetic analysis. Lesions with adipose, osteochondroid, or vascular space formation can readily be identified morphologically but often present difficulties in precise subcategorization and in assessment of malignancy. This book is, therefore, organized into chapters representing the main morphologic categories as they present to the surgical pathologist. Each entry includes relevant clinical data, morphologic features, and information from ancillary techniques wherever appropriate. The differential diagnosis within each category is presented in detailed tabular form. It is hoped that this approach will reflect the diagnostic process as practiced by the pathologist and will facilitate diagnosis and provision of relevant information to the clinician in this rare and difficult group of neoplasms. Necessarily, some entities appear in more than one category with the main entry corresponding to the most common pattern or location in each case.

BIOPSY

Most superficial tumors and those <5 cm in diameter can be excised in their entirety, but deep tumors often grow to a large size and require diagnosis by biopsy for optimal management. Interpretation can be difficult because a biopsy represents only a very small proportion of the tumor and the appearances in sarcomas can be heterogeneous and modified by myxoid, fibrous, or inflammatory stromal changes. Accurate diagnosis involves two major decision-making steps: Is the lesion malignant? If so, what sort of a sarcoma is it? Tumor grade should also be assessed when possible. Because of the rarity of soft tissue tumors, a patient with a soft tissue mass should ideally be referred to a specialized center for evaluation, biopsy (or review of pathology if carried out elsewhere), and, if necessary, treatment by a multidisciplinary team which includes an experienced pathologist.

Biopsy Techniques

Biopsy of a soft tissue tumor can be excisional, open incisional, or closed.

1. *Excisional biopsy* aims to remove the whole lesion for both diagnostic and therapeutic purposes and is usually indicated for superficial lesions and those <5 cm in diameter. The excision should include a margin of normal tissue, though microscopic examination might later reveal tumor at the margin, indicating further excision. This applies especially to lesions that are “shelled” out as they are generally removed through the false capsule within which tumor remains.
2. *Open incisional biopsy* involves surgical opening of skin and subcutaneous tissues and direct sampling of the tumor, from which a wedge can be removed. This approach results in a larger sample for diagnosis but has the potential complications of a formal surgical procedure, including wound dehiscence and infection, and compromise of subsequent definitive surgery or radiation therapy. It can also facilitate spread of tumor from the main lesion into adjacent or overlying tissues. In addition, an open procedure also requires more resources and is therefore less cost-effective than closed methods.
3. *Closed biopsies* can be carried out as office procedures carry minimal risk of infection or seeding of the wound with tumor and provide adequate material for all investigative modalities. They are simple and relatively inexpensive procedures that are readily repeated if more material is required. Techniques include *core needle biopsy* (CNB) and *fine needle aspiration cytology* (FNAC).
   (a) CNBs are usually taken with a Trucut needle, which can be inserted through a tiny skin incision and angled to sample different parts of the tumor. Several studies of cutting needle biopsies for soft tissue tumors have demonstrated that the larger the needle, the more optimal the specimen. Ultrasound- or computerized axial tomography–guided biopsy can be performed for less accessible lesions such as those deep in body cavities, although they usually yield thinner cores because of the use of a smaller

gauge needle. The use of CNB has become more widespread in recent years, and practiced operators can achieve a very high proportion of adequate biopsies. An experienced pathologist can differentiate benign from malignant tumors with a sensitivity of 99.4%, a specificity of 98.7%, a positive predictive value of 99.4%, and a negative predictive value 98.7%.[2] Ninety-five percent accuracy can be obtained in subtyping, and 85% in grading of soft tissue neoplasms on needle biopsies. Grading is less accurate than histologic typing, usually because a higher grade area is identified in the excised specimen. However an "at least" grade, or an indication of low- or high-grade malignancy, can be given. For some pediatric tumors, grading, classification, and prognostic categorization have specific issues that may limit the utility of core needle biopsies.

(b) FNAC is used for initial diagnosis of soft tissue tumors in some large centers and gives good results in expert hands.[3] However, tumor architecture and mitotic index cannot be assessed and it is less effective in determining histologic subtype and grade. Compared with CNB, FNAC has limitations in the areas of adipose, myxoid, and fibrous neoplasms.[4] For these reasons, one group with a very large experience of FNAC has advocated a combined NCB and FNA approach to diagnosis.[5] FNAC alone can have a role, however, in identifying recurrent or metastatic tumors.

Following prior biopsy diagnosis, frozen section is rarely indicated for immediate management, as margins are better assessed on the excised specimen. Intraoperative pathologic examination is, however, sometimes required at open biopsy, either for diagnosis or to confirm that adequate viable tissue is available.

SPECIMEN COLLECTION AND HANDLING

Core Biopsies

A minimum of three needle biopsy cores is optimal for morphology, immunohistochemistry, electron microscopy, touch imprints, molecular genetic analysis (which may be done on paraffin sections), cytogenetics, and storage of frozen tissue for future molecular studies. Specimen adequacy can be evaluated with touch imprints or frozen section at the time of the biopsy procedure. Touch imprints are useful for a variety of possible genetic and cell marker studies, and some experts have advocated performing touch imprints until the pathologist is comfortable with the adequacy of the entire specimen. This is not, however, usually necessary in routine use. If required, one core can be used for frozen section examination and a portion can be placed in glutaraldehyde for possible ultrastructural studies. The remainder of the cores should be submitted in formalin.

Core needle biopsies should be counted and measured. If the cores are not fragmented, and resources allow, it is preferable to separate and embed them in more than one cassette to allow maximal use of the available material.

Open Biopsies

These should also be submitted in formalin, but if the specimen is large enough, a small portion can be frozen in liquid nitrogen and stored at –80°C.

Resection Specimens

Surgical excision specimens should be sent to the laboratory directly after removal from the patient, without formalin, to allow orientation and sampling of fresh tissue for genetic studies. The latter might include freezing a suitable portion in liquid nitrogen and storage at –80°C in an appropriate facility. All likely investigative options should be considered at the time that fresh tissue arrives in the laboratory to maximize potential diagnostic and prognostic information.

After the specimen is weighed, orientated, and measured, its surface should be painted completely with specimen-marking ink and the ink allowed to dry. Alternatively, for large specimens and to prevent spillage of ink on to the cut surface, ink can be dabbed at the surface where the block is to be taken (e.g., the closest resection margin). One color is generally sufficient unless there is a particular clinical need to identify different aspects of the specimen. Intraabdominal and retroperitoneal sarcomas do not usually require surface marking unless locally required by the surgeon. The specimen should then be sliced transversely at 1-cm intervals. After small portions of tumor are removed for freezing, the specimen is placed in formalin in an adequately sized container and allowed to fix for 24 to 48 hours. After fixation, a suitable portion of the specimen should be photographed (this can also be done with the fresh specimen).

Resection specimens should be measured in three dimensions, and the closest distance of each margin from the edge of the tumor noted, including the deep aspect for subcutaneous or intramuscular sarcomas. The tissue plane(s) in which the tumor is located is recorded. Color, consistency, presence of cysts, hemorrhage, and necrosis are noted. The amount of necrosis is assessed as a percentage of the whole tumor. Blocks should be taken to include the nearest resection edge and the deep margin where appropriate. It is not necessary to take a resection margin which is more than 3 cm from the main tumor with the exceptions of some superficial sarcomas, such as low-grade myxofibrosarcoma[6] and epithelioid sarcoma,[7] which can infiltrate microscopically. Lesions that are smaller than 5 cm in diameter should be processed in their entirety. It is generally recommended that one block be taken per cm of the longest dimension of the tumor, up to a maximum of 12, though cases previously diagnosed on biopsy as of high-grade malignancy need fewer blocks. Areas that appear visibly different require appropriate extra sampling. In large liposarcomas, especially those from the retroperitoneum, any firmer or differently colored areas should be sampled to detect dedifferentiation.

DIAGNOSIS

Clinical Features

Before interpreting the biopsy, attention should be given to

(a) the patient's age and sex; (b) the size and duration of the tumor (e.g., a sarcoma is generally larger with a longer history, whereas nodular fasciitis is smaller and of very recent onset); and (c) its location, including anatomical plane (i.e., cutaneous, subcutaneous, fascial, or deep). Most pseudosarcomas and benign tumors, and less frequently sarcomas (e.g., myxofibrosarcoma, leiomyosarcoma, myxoinflammatory fibroblastic sarcoma, and epithelioid sarcoma) occur in the superficial soft tissues. Conversely, a mass located deep to the deep fascia is more likely to be a sarcoma. The plane in which the tumor is situated can also be determined by imaging (CT or magnetic resonance imaging), which can additionally suggest the composition of the lesion.

Diagnostic Techniques

Light microscopy is usually the only useful technique for distinguishing reactive lesions or benign tumors from malignant neoplasms. In the Royal Marsden series of 424 treated adult patients with soft tissue masses, 20% were benign.[8] In children, however, the majority of soft tissue masses are benign and the diagnostic spectrum of malignancies is different. Criteria of malignancy differ with lineage but commonly include nuclear pleomorphism, excessive or abnormal mitotic activity, necrosis, vascular invasion, and the fact of metastasis. However, benign lesions which are cellular, pleomorphic, or mitotically active can be mistaken for a similar-appearing sarcoma. Superficial benign lesions which simulate malignant tumors include cellular fibrous histiocytoma, the fasciitides, cellular myxoma, spindle cell and pleomorphic lipoma, chondroid lipoma, extraskeletal chondroma, solitary fibrous tumor, and pleomorphic hyalinizing angiectatic tumor. Examples in the deep soft tissues include cellular schwannoma and inflammatory myofibroblastic tumor, and fibromatoses can sometimes be difficult to distinguish from low-grade sarcomas. Conversely, some malignancies can be underdiagnosed, either because they have well-differentiated areas resembling their benign counterparts, such as atypical lipomatous tumor and well-differentiated leiomyosarcoma, or because they are deceptively bland, for example, epithelioid sarcoma, low-grade fibromyxoid sarcoma, and myxofibrosarcoma. Such problems can be resolved by careful assessment of often subtle features of architecture and cytomorphology, tumor-stromal interface and associated reaction; by immunohistochemical or genetic findings; and by awareness of the diagnostic possibilities and of the relevant criteria for malignancy.

Sarcomas with adipose or osteochondroid differentiation or vascular space formation can readily be diagnosed morphologically. Many others, however, are seen as spindle cell, epithelioid cell, clear cell, small round cell, or pleomorphic tumors which need to be characterized further with the aid of immunohistochemistry, ultrastructural examination, or genetic techniques.

Immunohistochemistry

Immunohistochemistry is an essential adjunct in soft tissue tumor diagnosis. In a few cases, specific antigens are expressed, but for most, a panel of antibodies is required, with a second panel according to the broad lineage indicated thereby, in conjunction with the morphology. Immunohistochemical markers useful in paraffin section are listed in detail for each tumor type, but some general comments are appropriate here. Antibodies are almost never 100% specific or sensitive, and overreliance on a single marker should be avoided. Familiarity with the pattern of reactivity for each antibody employed helps to avoid diagnostic error. Also, artifactually positive immunostaining can occur at the edges of small needle biopsy cores. A panel of antibodies should always be used; both positive and negative results are relevant and no finding should be taken out of the context of the morphologic findings and the clinical picture.

The initial panel will depend on the morphologic group into which the lesion falls and the clinical circumstances. However, for spindle cell and pleomorphic sarcomas, a first-line panel generally includes desmin, smooth muscle actin, S100 protein, a broad-spectrum cytokeratin, and CD34, perhaps with the addition of MDM2 and CDK4 for intra-abdominal pleomorphic sarcomas. For epithelioid and clear cell soft tissue tumors, an initial panel might include cytokeratin, EMA, CD34, CD31, CD30, desmin, and S100 protein, with addition of INI in selected cases. For small round cell tumors, a useful panel is CK, desmin, CD99, S100 protein, CD56, CD45, and TdT, with the addition of FLI-1, WT1, myogenin, TLE1, NB84a, synaptophysin, chromogranin, neurofilament, neuron-specific enolase, and other markers as indicated.

The results of these (e.g., Tables 1.1–1.3) will determine further investigations. Second-line panels apply more specific markers of epithelial, mesothelial, myoid, endothelial, neural, melanocytic, or other types of differentiation, or those useful for individual tumor types. Examples might include cytokeratin subtypes, calretinin, thrombomodulin, CEA, BerEp4, TLE1, GFAP; CD56, chromogranin, synaptophysin; myogenin, SMM, h-caldesmon, calponin, beta-catenin, TFE3; bcl-2; HMB45, melan A, inhibin; CD31, FLI-1, HHV8, CD117; CD45, CD30, CD21, CD23, CD35.

TABLE 1.1 Immunohistochemistry of Some CD34-Positive Soft Tissue Tumors

	CK	SMA	S100pr	Desmin	Other Diagnostic Markers
Dermatofibrosarcoma	–	–	+ (Bednar)	–	Apo D
Ectopic hamartomatous thymoma	+	–	–	–	EMA
Epithelioid angiosarcoma	±	–	–	–	CD31, FLI1, FVIIIRAg
Epithelioid sarcoma	+	±	–	–	INI negative
Gastrointestinal stromal tumor	–	+	±	±	CD117, DOG1, h-caldesmon
Mammary type myofibroblastoma	–	±	–	+	
Schwannoma	±	–	+ diffuse	–	
Spindle cell lipoma	–	–	–	±	
Perineurioma	–	–	–	–	EMA, claudin-1
Peripheral nerve sheath tumor, malignant	±	–	+ focal	+ (Triton)	
Solitary fibrous tumor	–	–	–	–	Bcl-2, CD99

TABLE 1.2 Immunohistochemistry of Selected Tumors with Desmin Positivity

	SMA	H-caldesmon	Myogenin	Other Markers
Mammary-type myofibroblastoma	±	±	–	CD34
Smooth muscle tumors	+	+	–	Calponin
Rhabdomyosarcoma	–	–	+	MyoD1
Myofibrosarcoma, low grade[a]	+	–	–	Calponin
Angiomatoid fibrous histiocytoma	–	+	–	CD68
Mesothelioma[a]	–	–	–	CK5/6, EMA, calretinin, thrombomodulin
Desmoplastic small round cell tumor	–	–	–	CK, WT1, NSE, NF
Alveolar soft part sarcoma[a]	–	–	–	TFE3
Melanoma[a]	–	–	–	S100 protein, HMB45, melan-A, MiTF, tyrosinase

[a] some examples are desmin-positive.

TABLE 1.3 Immunohistochemistry of Selected Tumors with S100 Protein Positivity

	HMB45	Melan-A	GFAP	CK	SMA	CD1a	Other Markers
Melanoma, clear cell sarcoma of soft tissue type	+[a]	+[a]	–	–	–	–	MiTF, tyrosinase
Schwannoma	–	–	+	+[b]	–	–	
MPNST	–	–	–	–	–	–	
Synovial sarcoma	–	–	–	+	–	–	TLE1, bcl-2, CD56, CD99
Myoepithelioma	–	–	+	+			H-caldesmon, calponin, CD10
Langerhans cell histiocytosis	–	–	–	–	–	+	Langerin
Rosai Dorfman disease	–	–	–	–	–	–	CD68
Follicular dendritic cell sarcoma	–	–	–	–	–	–	CD21/35, CD23, fascin, D2-40
Interdigitating dendritic cell sarcoma	–	–	–	–	–	+[b]	CD45, CD68, fascin, clusterin

[a] rarely positive in spindle cell melanoma; [b] occasionally.

A suspected diagnosis of gastrointestinal stromal tumor can be confirmed with CD117 and/or DOG1.

For grade 2 or 3 sarcomas, the proliferation index might have prognostic value[9,10] so that a proliferation marker such as Ki-67 (MIB1) can be added if required by clinicians.

Electron Microscopy

Ultrastructural examination now has a limited role,[11] but its use should be borne in mind where specifically indicated so that a small portion of tissue can be appropriately fixed and saved for referral to a specialist unit if this is subsequently needed. This technique remains of value where immunohistochemistry is inconclusive and genetic data are not available: examples include low-grade myofibrosarcoma, adult fibrosarcoma, S100 protein-negative malignant peripheral nerve sheath tumor (MPNST), and some synovial sarcomas. It can also be contributory to diagnosis of sarcomas with distinctive ultrastructural features such as the crystalline structures of alveolar soft part sarcoma.

Molecular Pathology

Molecular cytogenetic analysis can be used to identify specific chromosomal abnormalities, especially translocations, many of which have been consistently reported for certain soft tissue tumors (Table 1.4). The current most practical technique for this purpose is fluorescence *in situ* hybridization (FISH) using break-apart probes. For many of these translocations, the chimeric gene fusions can also be identified using molecular genetic techniques, including variations of the polymerase chain reaction (PCR) and sequence analysis. In general, FISH is more sensitive and PCR more specific, so both techniques can be used for optimum results. It should be noted that there is promiscuity among translocations, in that the same genetic rearrangement can be found in different tumors, such as in angiomatoid fibrous histiocytoma and clear cell sarcoma (Table 1.4).[12] Therefore, genetic information must always be integrated with clinical, morphologic, and immunohistochemical data by the surgical pathologist.[13]

Gene expression profiling studies of large numbers of tumors are beginning to find application in separating diagnostic and prognostic subgroups of tumor types[14] and in identifying new immunohistochemical reagents for diagnosis such as DOG1 for gastrointestinal stromal tumors and TLE1 for synovial sarcoma.[15–17]

REPORTING

Several bodies have published guidelines for reporting soft tissue sarcomas. They include in the United States those of the Association of Directors of Anatomic and Surgical Pathology[18] and the College of American

TABLE 1.4 Genetic Abnormalities in Selected Soft Tissue Tumors

Histologic Type	Chromosomal Abnormality	Fusion Gene or Other Genetic Change
Alveolar soft part sarcoma	t(X;17)(p11;q25)	*ASPL-TFE3*
Angiomatoid fibrous histiocytoma	t(12;22)(q13;q12) t(12;16)(q13;p11) t(2;22)(q33;q12)	*EWSR1-ATF1* *FUS-ATF1* *EWSR1-CREB1*
Clear cell sarcoma (soft tissue)	t(12;22)(q13;q12)	*EWSR1-ATF1*
Clear cell sarcoma (GIT)	t(2;22)(q33;q12)	*EWSR1-CREB1*
Dermatofibrosarcoma protuberans and variants	t(17;22)(q21;q13)	*COL1A1-PDGFB*
Desmoplastic SRCT	t(11;22)(p13;q12)	*EWSR1-WT*
Endometrial stromal sarcoma	t(7;17)(p15:q21)	*JAZF1-JJAZ1*
	t(6;7)(p21;p22)	*JAZF1-PHF1*
	t(10:17)(q22;p13)	
Epithelioid sarcoma (all histologic types)	Abnormalities of 22q	*INI1* inactivation
Ewing sarcoma/PNET (all histologic types)	t(11;22)(q24;q12)	*EWSR1-FLI1*
	t(21;22)(q12;q12)	*EWSR1-ERG*
	t(2;22)(q33;q12)	*EWSR1-FEV*
	t(7;22)(p22;q12)	*EWSR1-ETV1*
	t(17;22)(q12;q12)	*EWSR1-E1AF*
	inv(22)(q12;q12)	*EWSR1-ZSG*
Extraskeletal myxoid chondrosarcoma	t(9;22)(q22;q12) t(9;17)(q22;q11) t(9;15)(q22;q21)	*EWSR1-NR4A3* *TAF1168-NR4A3* *TCF12-NR4A3*
Fibrosarcoma, infantile	t(12;15)(p13;q26)	*ETV6-NTRK3*
	Trisomies 8, 11, 17, and 20	
Gastrointestinal stromal tumor		*Kit, PDGFRA* mutations
Inflammatory myofibroblastic tumor	2p23 rearrangement	*ALK* fusions with several different partners

(Continued)

TABLE 1.4 Genetic Abnormalities in Selected Soft Tissue Tumors (Continued)

Histologic Type	Chromosomal Abnormality	Fusion Gene or Other Genetic Change
Liposarcoma:		
Well-differentiated	Ring form of chromosome 12	12q13-12q15 amplification
Dedifferentiated	Rings and complex changes	12q13-12q15 amplification
Myxoid/round cell	t(12;16)(q13;p11)	*FUS-DDIT3*
	t(12;22)(q13;q12)	*EWSR1-DDIT3*
Pleomorphic	Complex changes	
Low-grade fibromyxoid sarcoma	t(7;16)(q33;p11)	*FUS-CREB3L2*
		FUS-CREB3L1 (exceptionally)
Malignant rhabdoid tumor	Deletion of 22q	*INI1* inactivation
MPNST	Complex changes	Loss of *NF1* at 17q11, *INK4A* deletion
Myofibrosarcoma, low-grade	Multiple ring chromosomes	12p11 and12q13-q22 amplification
Myxofibrosarcoma, all grades	Ring forms	
	Complex changes	
Myxoinflammatory fibroblastic sarcoma	t(1;10)(p22;q24) t(2;6)(q31;p21.3)	
Rhabdomyosarcoma:		
Embryonal	Trisomies 2q, 8, and 20	LOH at 11p15
Alveolar	t(1;13)(p36;q14)	*PAX7-FOXO1*
	t(2;13)(q35;q14)	*PAX3-FOXO1*
Pleomorphic	Complex changes	
Synovial sarcoma	t(X;18)(p11;q11)	*SS18-SSX1*
	t(X;20)(p11;q13)	*SS18-SSX2*
		SS18-SSX4 (rare)
		SS18L1-SSX1
Tenosynovial giant cell tumor	t(1;2)(q13;q37)	*COL6A3-CSF1*

GIT, gastrointestinal tract; SRCT, small round cell tumor; PNET, primitive neuroectodermal tumor; MPNST, malignant peripheral nerve sheath tumor; LOH, loss of heterozygosity.

Pathologists,[19] and in the United Kingdom the dataset of the Royal College of Pathologists.[20] The following information is generally included in the final report.

CLINICAL

Site
Depth from surface (tissue plane)

PATHOLOGICAL

Macroscopic

Tumor dimensions
Status of margins–Distance to nearest margin, type of tissue present at margin (e.g., fat, skeletal muscle)
Color, consistency–presence of cysts, calcification, necrosis (assess percentage)

Microscopic

Histological type and subtype. Soft tissue tumors are designated and categorized as in the WHO consensus classification of 2002.[1] This includes benign and malignant neoplasms and those of intermediate biologic potential. The latter category comprises locally aggressive neoplasms, for example, fibromatosis, and those that rarely metastasize, such as plexiform fibrohistiocytic tumor and angiomatoid fibrous histiocytoma.

Grade. The grading system in common use in Europe and elsewhere[21] and recommended by the European Organization for Research and Treatment of Cancer (EORTC) and the WHO consensus group[1] is that of the French Federation of Cancer Centers (FNCLCC).[22] This is a 3-step scoring system based on summation of independent scores for differentiation, mitotic index per 10 high power fields, and amount of necrosis (Table 1.5). Mitoses should be counted in the most mitotically active areas in ten successive fields using a ×40 objective and a standard ×10 eyepiece.[19] For low-grade smooth muscle tumors where the mitotic index is critical for assessing malignancy or metastatic potential,[23-25] mitoses should be counted in 50 high-power fields. The percentage of necrosis should be assessed macroscopically except in small biopsies.

Invasion of blood vessels, nerves, or bone

Ancillary Investigations

Immunohistochemistry (including Ki-67 index of proliferation)
Cytogenetic and molecular genetic findings

TABLE 1.5 French Federation of Cancer Centers System of Grading

Tumor Differentiation*	
Score	1 Sarcoma histologically very similar to normal adult mesenchymal tissue
	2 Sarcoma of defined histological subtype (e.g., myxofibrosarcoma)
	3 Sarcoma of uncertain type, embryonal and undifferentiated sarcomas
Mitotic count	
Score	1 0–9/10 hpf
	2 10–19/10 hpf
	3 >20/10 hpf
Microscopic tumor necrosis	
Score	0 No necrosis
	1 <50% tumor necrosis
	2 >50% tumor necrosis
Histological grade	
Grade 1	Total score 2 or 3
Grade 2	Total score 4 or 5
Grade 3	Total score 6, 7, or 8
Tumor differentiation scores**	
Well-differentiated liposarcoma	1
Well-differentiated fibrosarcoma	1
Well-differentiated MPNST	1
Well-differentiated chondrosarcoma	1
Myxoid liposarcoma	2
Conventional fibrosarcoma	2
Conventional MPNST	2
Well-differentiated malignant haemangiopericytoma	2
Myxoid MFH (myxofibrosarcoma)	2
Typical storiform/pleomorphic MFH	2
Conventional leiomyosarcoma	2
Extraskeletal myxoid chondrosarcoma	2
Conventional angiosarcoma[a]	2

(Continued)

TABLE 1.5 French Federation of Cancer Centers System of Grading (Continued)

Round cell liposarcoma	3
Pleomorphic liposarcoma	3
Dedifferentiated liposarcoma	3
Poorly differentiated fibrosarcoma	3
Epithelioid malignant schwannoma	3
Poorly differentiated MPNST	3
Malignant Triton tumor	3
Conventional malignant hemangiopericytoma	3
Giant cell and inflammatory MFH	3
Poorly differentiated/epithelioid/ pleomorphic leiomyosarcoma	3
Synovial sarcoma	3
Rhabdomyosarcoma	3
Mesenchymal chondrosarcoma	3
Poorly differentiated/epithelioid angiosarcoma	3
Extraskeletal osteosarcoma	3
Extraskeletal Ewing sarcoma/ PNET	3
Alveolar soft part sarcoma	3
Malignant rhabdoid tumor	3
Clear cell sarcoma	3
Undifferentiated sarcoma	3

Note that grading of MPNST has no prognostic value, and grading of embryonal and alveolar rhabdomyosarcoma, angiosarcoma, extraskeletal myxoid chondrosarcoma, alveolar soft part sarcoma, clear cell sarcoma, and epithelioid sarcoma is not recommended. The following tumors are graded by definition:

1. Well-differentiated liposarcoma, dermatofibrosarcoma protuberans, infantile fibrosarcoma, and angiomatoid fibrous histiocytoma are Grade 1.
2. Ewing's sarcoma/PNET, extra-renal malignant rhabdoid tumor soft tissue osteosarcoma, mesenchymal chondrosarcoma, and desmoplastic small round cell tumor are Grade 3.
3. Alveolar soft part sarcoma, clear cell sarcoma, and epithelioid sarcoma are not graded but are usually considered as high grade for management purposes.

* Modified from Trojani et al. *Int J Cancer* 1984;33:37–42) with permission from John Wiley and Sons, Ltd.

** Modified from Guillou et al. Comparative study of the National Cancer Institute and French Federation of Cancer Centers Sarcoma Group grading systems in a population of 410 adult patients with soft tissue sarcoma. *J Clin Oncol* 1997;15;350–362. Reprinted with permission from American Society of Clinical Oncology. All rights reserved © 2008.

Stage

Soft tissue sarcomas are staged using the staging systems of the American Joint Committee and the UICC (Table 1.6).[26,27] This currently uses a two-grade (high or low) system of tumor differentiation, in which high-grade tumors are regarded as equivalent to both grades 2 and 3 in the FNCLCC system.

TABLE 1.6 Staging System for Soft Tissue Sarcomas (UICC)[1]

The following histological types are included, with ICD-O9 morphology codes:	
Alveolar soft part sarcoma	9581/3
Epithelioid sarcoma	8804/3
Extraskeletal chondrosarcoma	9220/3
Extraskeletal osteosarcoma	9180/3
Extraskeletal Ewing sarcoma	9260/3
PNET	9473/3
Fibrosarcoma	8810/3
Leiomyosarcoma	8890/3
Liposarcoma	8850/3
Malignant fibrous histiocytoma	8830/3
Malignant hemangiopericytoma	9150/3
Malignant mesenchymoma	8990/3
MPNST	9540/3
Rhabdomyosarcoma	8900/3
Synovial sarcoma	9040/3
Sarcoma, not otherwise specified	8800/3
Primary Tumor (T)	
TX	Primary tumor cannot be assessed
T0	No evidence of primary tumor
T1	Tumor 5 cm or less in greatest dimension
T1a	Superficial tumor
T1b	Deep tumor
T2	Tumor more than 5 cm in greatest dimension
T2a	Superficial tumor
T2b	Deep tumor[2]
Regional Lymph Nodes (N)	
NX	Regional lymph nodes cannot be assessed

(Continued)

TABLE 1.6 Staging System for Soft Tissue Sarcomas (UICC)[1] (Continued)

N0	No regional lymph node metastasis			
N1	Regional lymph node metastasis			
Distant Metastasis (M)				
M0	No distant metastasis			
M1	Distant metastasis			
Histopathologic Grade				
GX	Grade cannot be assessed			
G1	Low grade (= FNCLCC grade 1)			
G2	High grade (= FNCLCC grades 2 and 3) [3,4]			
Stage Grouping				
Stage IA	T1 a	N0	M0	Low grade
	T1 b	N0	M0	Low grade
Stage IB	T2 a	N0	M0	Low grade
	T2 b	N0	M0	Low grade
Stage IIA	T1 a	N0	M0	High grade
	T1 b	N0	M0	High grade
Stage IIB	T2 a	N0	M0	High grade
Stage III	T2 b	N0	M0	High grade
	Any T	N1	M0	Any grade
Stage IV	Any T	Any N	M1	Any grade

SUMMARY: Soft Tissue Sarcoma	
T1	≤ 5 cm
T1 a	Superficial
T1 b	Deep
T2	>5 cm
T2 a	Superficial
T2 b	Deep
N1	Regional
	Low grade
	High grade

Notes:

1. The staging system applies to all soft tissue sarcomas except Kaposi sarcoma, dermatofibrosarcoma protuberans, desmoid fibromatosis, infantile fibrosarcoma, and angiosarcoma. In addition, sarcomas arising within the confines of the dura mater, including the brain, and sarcomas arising in parenchymatous organs (except breast) and from hollow viscera are not staged by this system.
2. Depth is assessed as follows:
   Superficial tumor is located exclusively above the superficial fascia without invasion of the fascia

TABLE 1.6 Staging System for Soft Tissue Sarcomas (UICC)[1] (Continued)

Deep tumor is located either exclusively beneath the superficial fascia or superficial to the fascia with invasion of or through the fascia. Retroperitoneal, mediastinal, visceral, paratesticular, and pelvic sarcomas and noncutaneous head and neck sarcomas are classified as deep tumors. modifed from Sobin LH, Gospodarowicz MK, Wittekind Ch eds. UICC, International Union against Cancer. TNM classification of malignant tumours. Chichester, Wiley-Blackwell, 2010. with permission from John Wiley and Sons Ltd)

3. Extraskeletal Ewing sarcoma is classified as high grade.
4. Use low grade for GX, and N0 for NX. The TNM protocol recommends that if grade cannot be assessed, the tumor should be classified as low grade. However, all tumors should be graded rather than arbitrarily classified.

Modified from Sobin LH, Gospodarowicz MK, Wittekind Ch eds. *UICC, International Union against Cancer. TNM classification of malignant tumours*. Chichester: Wiley-Blackwell, 2010 with permission from John Wiley and Sons Ltd.

REFERENCES

1. Fletcher C, Unni K, Mertens F, eds. *World Health Organization Classification of Tumours. Pathology and Genetics of Tumours of Soft Tissue and Bone*. Lyon, France: IARC Press, 2002.
2. Hoeber I, Spillane AJ, Fisher C, et al. Accuracy of biopsy techniques for limb and limb girdle soft tissue tumors. *Ann Surg Oncol*. 2001;8:80–87.
3. Akerman M. The cytology of soft tissue tumours. *Acta Orthop Scand Suppl*. 1997;273:54–59.
4. Akerman M. Fine-needle aspiration cytology of soft tissue sarcoma: benefits and limitations. *Sarcoma*. 1998;2:155–161.
5. Domanski HA, Akerman M, Carlen B, et al. Core-needle biopsy performed by the cytopathologist: a technique to complement fine-needle aspiration of soft tissue and bone lesions. *Cancer*. 2005;105:229–239.
6. Fanburg-Smith JC, Spiro IJ, Katapuram SV, et al. Infiltrative subcutaneous malignant fibrous histiocytoma: a comparative study with deep malignant fibrous histiocytoma and an observation of biologic behavior. *Ann Diagn Pathol*. 1999;3:1–10.
7. Fisher C. Epithelioid sarcoma of Enzinger. *Adv Anat Pathol*. 2006;13:114–121.
8. Pitcher ME, Fish S, Thomas JM. Management of soft tissue sarcoma. *Br J Surg*. 1994;81:1136–1139.
9. Engellau J, Persson A, Bendahl PO, et al. Expression profiling using tissue microarray in 211 malignant fibrous histiocytomas confirms the prognostic value of Ki-67. *Virchows Arch*. 2004;445:224–230.
10. Meister P. Histological grading of soft tissue sarcomas: stratification of G2-sarcomas in low- or high-grade malignant tumors. *Pathologe*. 2005;26:146–148.
11. Fisher C. The comparative roles of electron microscopy and immunohistochemistry in the diagnosis of soft tissue tumours. *Histopathology*. 2006;48:32–41.
12. Ordonez JL, Osuna D, Herrero D, et al. Advances in Ewing's sarcoma research: where are we now and what lies ahead? *Cancer Res*. 2009;69:7140–7150.
13. Fisher C. Soft tissue sarcomas with non-EWS translocations: molecular genetic features and pathologic and clinical correlations. *Virchows Arch*. 2010;456:153–166.
14. De Pitta C, Tombolan L, Albiero G, et al. Gene expression profiling identifies potential relevant genes in alveolar rhabdomyosarcoma pathogenesis and discriminates PAX3-FKHR positive and negative tumors. *Int J Cancer*. 2006;118:2772–2781.

15. West RB, Corless CL, Chen X et al. The novel marker, DOG1, is expressed ubiquitously in gastrointestinal stromal tumors irrespective of KIT or PDGFRA mutation status. *Am J Pathol.* 2004;165:107–113.
16. Trojani M, Contesso G, Coindre JM, et al. Soft-tissue sarcomas of adults; study of pathological prognostic variables and definition of a histopathological grading system. *Int J Cancer.* 1984;33:37–42.
17. Terry J, Saito T, Subramanian S, et al. TLE1 as a diagnostic immunohistochemical marker for synovial sarcoma emerging from gene expression profiling studies. *Am J Surg Pathol.* 2007;31:240–246.
18. Recommendations for reporting soft tissue sarcomas. Association of Directors of Anatomic and Surgical Pathology. *Am J Clin Pathol.* 1999;111:594–598.
19. Rubin BP, Fletcher CD, Inwards C, et al. Protocol for the examination of specimens from patients with soft tissue tumors of intermediate malignant potential, malignant soft tissue tumors, and benign/locally aggressive and malignant bone tumors. *Arch Pathol Lab Med.* 2006;130:1616–1629.
20. Dataset for cancer histopathology reports on soft tissue sarcomas. Royal College of Pathologists 2009: http://www.rcpath.org/resources/pdf/g094datasetsofttissue.pdf.
21. Golouh R, Bracko M. What is current practice in soft tissue sarcoma grading? *Radiol Oncol.* 2001;35:47–52.
22. Guillou L, Coindre JM, Bonichon F, et al. Comparative study of the National Cancer Institute and French Federation of Cancer Centers Sarcoma Group grading systems in a population of 410 adult patients with soft tissue sarcoma. *J Clin Oncol.* 1997;15:350–362.
23. Billings SD, Folpe AL, Weiss SW. Do leiomyomas of deep soft tissue exist? An analysis of highly differentiated smooth muscle tumors of deep soft tissue supporting two distinct subtypes. *Am J Surg Pathol.* 2001;25:1134–1142.
24. Paal E, Miettinen M. Retroperitoneal leiomyomas: a clinicopathologic and immunohistochemical study of 56 cases with a comparison to retroperitoneal leiomyosarcomas. *Am J Surg Pathol.* 2001;25:1355–1363.
25. Weiss SW. Smooth muscle tumors of soft tissue. *Adv Anat Pathol.* 2002;9:351–359.
26. Edge SB, Byrd DR, Carducci MA, et al. eds. *American Joint Committee on Cancer (AJCC) Cancer Staging Manual.* New York, NY: Springer, 2009.
27. Sobin LH, Gospodarowicz MK, Wittekind Ch, eds. UICC, International Union against Cancer. TNM classification of malignant tumours. Chichester: Wiley-Blackwell, 2010.

2

BENIGN AND INTERMEDIATE FIBROSING LESIONS

INTRODUCTION

A group of benign fibrosing spindle cell lesions is composed of various proportions of myofibroblasts, fibroblasts (see Chapter 3, Table 3.1 for comparison), collagenous or elastic tissue, and inflammatory cells of all types. They occur in all locations, and in some, the component elements change over time. This chapter includes those in which fibrosis is a prominent feature. Immunohistochemistry is of limited value, and diagnosis depends on attention to subtle morphologic features, but some entities cannot be identified by microscopy alone and careful clinicopathologic correlation is required. Cellular fibroblastic-myofibroblastic lesions are considered in Chapter 3, and tumors composed predominantly of myofibroblasts in Chapter 7. The differential diagnosis is summarized in Table 2.1.

ELASTOFIBROMA

Clinical Features

Elastofibroma is typically located in subcutis and muscles of the back near or beneath the inferior border of the scapula (elastofibroma dorsi) in adults over 50, with a female predominance, and sometimes with a history of physical labor or other repetitive activity. The lesion is probably an exaggerated reaction to trauma or friction since lesser but similar changes are found in some elderly persons at autopsy. There is an increased incidence in parts of Japan, and a familial predisposition to elastofibroma has been reported. Some cases are bilateral and examples have been described in other locations including oral cavity, rectum, and omentum. It is usually a painless infiltrative mass in which lesional tissue can extend deeply into subcutis, between muscles, and adhere to periosteum of middle ribs.

Pathologic Features

Elastofibroma forms an ill-defined firm tumor up to 10 cm diameter with fibrous and fatty areas. Infiltration of skeletal muscle imparts a variegated red, white, and yellow appearance. Microscopically, the appearances are characteristic, with numerous randomly orientated thick focally branching

TABLE 2.1 Differential Diagnosis of Fibrosing Lesions

	Typical Clinical Features	Microscopic Features	Ancillary Investigations
Elastofibroma	F>M, lower scapular area, beneath bone, infiltrative in subcutis and muscle	Poorly defined, infiltrative. Thick, focally beaded elastic fibers randomly dispersed in collagen	Elastic stain positive
Amyloidoma (tumoral amyloidosis)	Older adults, extremities, especially lower, in skin or subcutis. Idiopathic, or associated with myeloma, plasmacytoid lymphoma, long-term dialysis, chronic inflammation	Islands of amorphous eosinophilic material, plasma cells, multinucleated giant cells, calcification, metaplastic bone. Vessel walls involved	PASD+, apple green birefringence with Congo Red that persists after pre-treatment with permanganate in AL amyloid
Nuchal-type and Gardner fibroma	M>F, neck, shoulder, back, Associated with diabetes and Gardner syndrome. Can later develop desmoid fibromatosis	Poorly defined infiltrative lesion, dense collagen, very sparse cells, increased entrapped nerves	CD34+, CD99+
Nuchal fibrocartilaginous pseudotumor	Back of neck. History of trauma to neck. At junction of nuchal ligament and deep fascia	Dense fibrous tissue containing nodules of metaplastic mature cartilage	S100 protein+ in chondrocytes

(Continued)

TABLE 2.1 Differential Diagnosis of Fibrosing Lesions (Continued)

	Typical Clinical Features	Microscopic Features	Ancillary Investigations
Fibroma of tendon sheath	M > F, hands, feet, circumscribed. Slowly growing	Circumscribed, multinodular tumor, comprising hyalinized nodules, spindle cells, slits, or fasciitis-like more cellular areas	SMA+, CD34–. t(2;11)(q31–32;q12)
Calcifying fibrous tumor	Children, young adults, M = F Subcutaneous, subfascial, or intracavitary	Circumscribed, unencapsulated lesion. Hypocellular collagen, aggregates of lymphocytes, rounded calcifications, scanty fibroblasts	Occasionally CD34+, or SMA+
Calcifying aponeurotic fibroma	Childhood, extremities, digits, palm	Cords and files of spindle or rounded cells in fibrous stroma with focal calcification and chondroid metaplasia. Less commonly, osteoclast-like giant cells and ossification	S100 protein+ in chondrocytes
Fibromatosis-superficial	Palm, sole, penis; infiltrative plaque	Variable cellular nodules in dense collagen. Cells are parallel aligned, lack atypia. Mast cells	SMA+, nuclear beta-catenin+ occasionally, CD34–
Fibromatosis-desmoid type	Deep in limbs, head and neck, body cavities	Parallel myofibroblasts evenly dispersed in collagen, slit-like and thick-walled small-caliber vessels, perivascular and interstitial mast cells. Normal mitoses allowed but no atypia or necrosis	SMA+, nuclear beta-catenin+, CD34–

Low-grade fibromyxoid sarcoma	Skin, deep soft tissue, limbs/girdles	Fibromatosis-like areas, swirling fibromyxoid transitions, cellular myxoid areas without pleomorphism. Some nuclei lozenge shaped, inconspicuous nucleoli. Giant collagenous rosettes	Occasionally SMA+, EMA+, claudin-1 in some Nuclear beta-catenin usually negative t(7;16)(q34;p11), *FUS-CREB3L2* or *FUS-CREB3L1* fusion
Perineurioma	Skin, subcutis, most locations. Subset in colon Sclerosing variant: M > F, affects fingers, thumb, palm	Long thin nuclei, very long slender terminal cytoplasmic processes. Fascicles or perivascular whorls. Fibrous or myxoid stroma Sclerosing variant has cords and whorls of rounded or epithelioid cells in dense stroma	EMA+, claudin-1+, CD34+ in some, beta-catenin–negative
Sclerosing epithelioid fibrosarcoma	Deep soft tissue, limbs/girdles, head and neck Can involve or arise in bone	Multinodular, focally calcified. Cellular islands in dense fibrosis, Nests of ovoid cells, clear cytoplasm or single files simulating carcinoma. Fibrosarcoma-like spindle cell areas in many cases	Occasional and variable expression of bcl-2, EMA, CK, S100 protein. No specific immunophenotype
Infantile digital (inclusion body) fibromatosis	Congenital or up to about 2 years, rarely older. F > M Digits except first. Rarely other sites. Can be multiple. 50% of digital lesions recur	Infiltrative, moderately cellular, bland cells. Rounded eosinophilic paranuclear inclusions	SMA +, occasionally nuclear beta-catenin + or CD34+

(Continued)

TABLE 2.1 **Differential Diagnosis of Fibrosing Lesions (Continued)**

	Typical Clinical Features	Microscopic Features	Ancillary Investigations
Fibromatosis colli	Infants in first months, M > F Mass lower third of sternomastoid or trapezius Associated with torticollis. Eventual regression	Infiltrative, at first cellular, later fibrous, between muscle bundles that show focal atrophy or swelling	Nil specific
Juvenile hyaline fibromatosis	Childhood. Skin of head and neck, limbs, bones	Dense homogeneous eosinophilic stroma with small islands of ovoid cells with clear cytoplasm	Stroma is positive with PASD and Alcian blue
Desmoplastic fibroblastoma (collagenous fibroma)	M > F, mostly subcutaneous, limbs and limb girdles	Mostly circumscribed, unencapsulated, sparse stellate or spindle cells in dense collagenous stroma, occasional myxoid change, hyalinized vessels	Focal SMA +, rare nuclear beta-catenin +, t(2;11)(q31;q12)

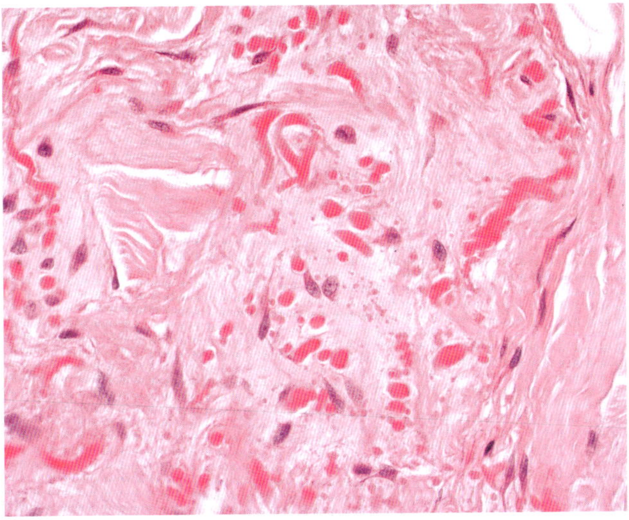

FIGURE 2.1 **Elastofibroma.** Wavy or fragmented eosinophilic elastic fibers are dispersed in sparsely cellular and focally hyalinized collagen.

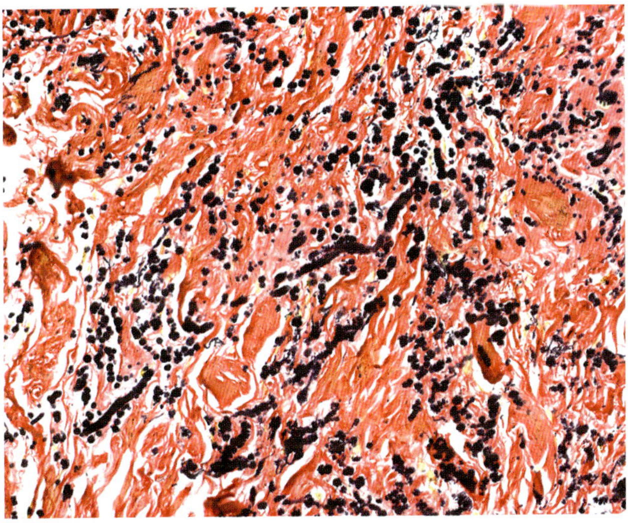

FIGURE 2.2. **Elastofibroma.** Elastic van Giesen stain highlights numerous globules of elastic fibers scattered throughout the lesion.

elastic fibers, in places fragmented into small bead-like spheroids or "globules," within collagen containing a few bland fibroblasts or myofibroblasts, admixed with mature adipocytes (Fig. 2.1, e-Figs. 2.1–2.3).

Ancillary Investigations

Histochemical stains such as Weigert's elastic, and immunohistochemistry with antielastin, highlight the elastic fibers, which also fluoresce with

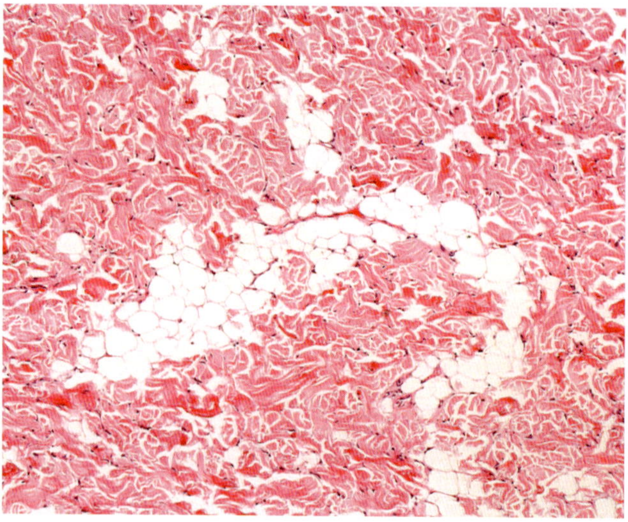

FIGURE 2.3 **Nuchal Fibroma.** Subcutaneous fat is irregularly infiltrated by confluent short bands of dense collagen with sparse fibroblastic spindle cells

ultraviolet illumination (Fig. 2.2, e-Fig. 2.4). This can be differentiated from amyloid deposits (e-Fig. 2.5), which shows apple-green birefringence after staining with Congo Red. Electron microscopy of elastofibroma shows irregular rounded mass of electron-dense pre-elastin surrounding less dense elastin, which is produced within rough endoplasmic reticulum of adjacent fibroblasts. Abnormalities in chromosome 1p and Xq[1] have been identified.

NUCHAL FIBROMA AND NUCHAL-TYPE FIBROMA

Clinical Features

Nuchal fibroma was originally described as predominantly occurring in the skin and subcutis of the back of the neck. Subsequently, it has been reported in other locations, including upper and lower back, buttock, shoulder, and face, indicating the term nuchal-type fibroma.[2] Over 80% arise in males, with a mean age of 40 years, and nearly half are associated with diabetes mellitus. Histologically identical lesions are associated with Gardner syndrome (see below). These are benign conditions which can recur if incompletely excised.

Pathologic Features

This is a poorly circumscribed firm mass usually <8 cm in maximum dimension, with similar histological appearances in all locations. The lesion infiltrates dermis (around adnexa), fat, and, sometimes, skeletal muscle and comprises very sparse fibroblasts dispersed in thick irregularly orientated collagen bundles with scattered fine elastic fibers, and, at most, a scanty lymphocytic infiltrate (Fig. 2.3, e-Figs. 2.6–2.8). Nerve bundles entrapped within the fibrous tissue (e-Fig. 2.9) can appear increased in number.

Ancillary Investigations

Immunohistochemistry is positive in the spindle cells for CD34 and CD99.

GARDNER (GARDNER-ASSOCIATED) FIBROMA

Clinical Features

Gardner syndrome is an autosomal dominant condition with variable penetrance associated with mutations in the adenomatous polyposis coli (*APC*) gene at 5q21.[3] The syndrome includes colonic and rectal polyps and multiple osteomas, as well as fibromatosis (in about 10% of patients) of mesentery or abdominal wall,[4] fibromas, leiomyomas, lipomas, and skin manifestations such as dermoid cysts, many of which have pilomatricoma-like features. Gardner-associated fibroma arises mostly in children and can be an antecedent marker for familial adenomatous polyposis (FAP)[5] or for Gardner syndrome, in which the osteomas appear later followed by the polyps. Some examples of Gardner fibroma eventuate in fibromatosis, especially after surgery to the lesion. Clinically, there is an infiltrative, subcutaneous plaque-like lesion in back, paraspinal region, chest wall, head and neck, and extremities. A similar desmoid-precursor lesion has been described in the mesentery.[6]

Pathologic Features

The microscopic features in Gardner fibroma are identical to those of nuchal-type fibroma with sparse fibroblastic spindle cells, randomly arranged thick collagen bundles showing focal cracking artifact, and occasional mast cells. Rarely there is mild atypia or multinucleation.

Ancillary Investigations

The spindle cells are immunoreactive for CD34 and CD99, and some cases show nuclear immunoreactivity for beta-catenin.[9] However, the cellularity is usually less and the collagen more coarse than in fibromatosis.

NUCHAL FIBROCARTILAGINOUS PSEUDOTUMOR

Clinical Features

This rare lesion, which is associated with prior soft tissue injury, is situated within the nuchal ligament in young adults, of either sex, and presents as a tender nodule up to 3 cm in diameter at the lower part of the back of the neck, where the nuchal ligament meets deep fascia.[7] It probably represents fibrocartilaginous metaplasia of the lower portion of the nuchal ligament, as a result of trauma.

Pathologic Features

This is a poorly circumscribed lesion composed of dense fibrous tissue with ill-defined foci of chondroid metaplasia containing mature chondrocytes (e-Figs. 2.10 and 2.11). Atypia, mitoses, inflammation, and calcification are absent.

Ancillary Investigations

The cartilage cells are immunoreactive for S100 protein. Ultrastructural examination shows fibroblastic and chondroid differentiation without features of myofibroblastic differentiation.

FIBROMA OF TENDON SHEATH

Clinical Features

Most commonly seen in males between 20 and 50 years, this is a small (<2 cm diameter) slowly growing lesion which forms a circumscribed lobulated firm mass attached to tendons in hands or, less commonly, feet. The thumb, first finger, dorsum and palm of hand, and wrist are the most frequently affected sites. Fibromas occasionally arise in other locations including the knee region, foot and ankle, and within a joint. Some cases have antecedent trauma. The lesions are benign but up to a quarter recur, usually within weeks.

Pathologic Features

Fibroma of tendon sheath is circumscribed but nonencapsulated. Histologically, the lobular architecture is emphasized by cleft-like spaces, at least some of which represent thin-walled blood vessels. (Fig. 2.4, e-Figs. 2.12 and 2.13) The lesions are mostly of low cellularity; scattered bland fibroblast-like spindle or stellate cells are dispersed in a densely collagenized stroma, with rare foci of myxoid change or occasionally osteochondroid

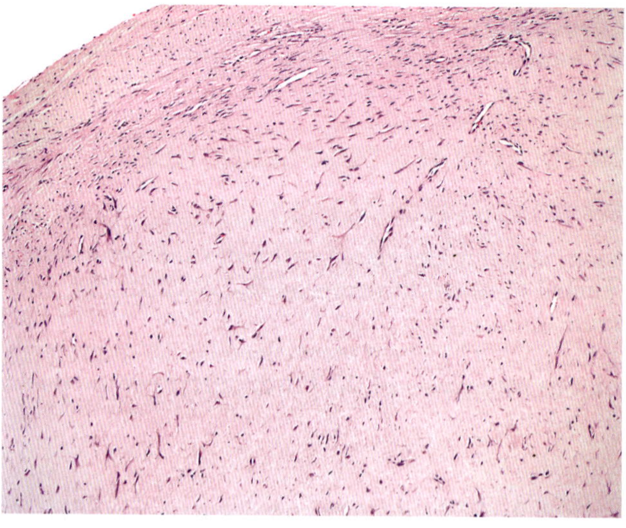

FIGURE 2.4 **Fibroma of Tendon Sheath.** Note circumscribed margin, sparse cellularity, hyalinized collagen, and thin-walled blood vessels.

metaplasia, and slit-like blood vessels. Some cases, however, display increased cellularity with nodular fasciitis-like areas (e-Fig. 2.14). These are presumed to represent an early stage of the lesion since transition to hyalinized areas is seen, and it has been suggested that fibroma of tendon sheath represents the tenosynovial counterpart of nodular fasciitis. More recent genetic findings, however, argue against this.[8] Multinucleated cells can be seen, but the range of appearances seen in giant cell tumor of tendon sheath is lacking and these are probably two separate entities. Some examples have diffuse nuclear atypia without mitotic activity; such lesions, termed pleomorphic fibroma of tendon sheath, behave in the same way as the usual fibroma of tendon sheath.

Ancillary Investigations

Some cells show positivity for smooth muscle actin (SMA), indicating focal myofibroblastic differentiation. Electron microscopy shows fibroblasts and myofibroblasts, with the latter being more prominent in the fasciitis-like areas. A chromosomal rearrangement t(2;11)(q31–32;q12) has been described in one case,[8] suggesting a possible relationship with desmoplastic fibroblastoma (collagenous fibroma) in which similar genetic findings have been reported.

CALCIFYING FIBROUS TUMOR

Clinical Features

This entity was described in 1988 as childhood fibrous tumor with psammoma bodies[9] and then in 1993 as calcifying fibrous pseudotumor.[10] It was designated calcifying fibrous tumor in the 2002 WHO consensus classification. Calcifying fibrous tumor favors children and young adults of either sex and arises in subcutaneous and subfascial locations, including in body cavities, as a mass up to 15 cm in diameter, with symptoms related to location. In the abdomen, where the lesions are occasionally multiple, it is included within the differential diagnosis of spindle cell lesions. It has been suggested that calcifying fibrous tumor might represent the end stage of inflammatory myofibroblastic tumor,[11] but subsequent studies have failed to support a relationship between the two entities. This is a benign lesion that occasionally recurs locally. A subset in the stomach occur in older patients, are usually solitary, and tend not to recur.[12]

Pathologic Features

Calcifying fibrous tumor is a generally circumscribed, unencapsulated lesion composed of hypocellular dense collagen with a scattered lymphoplasmacytic infiltrate, sometimes forming lymphoid follicles. There is a variable number of scattered psammomatous or amorphous dystrophic calcifications (Fig. 2.5, e-Figs. 2.15–2.17). The spindle cells are bland, sparse, and dispersed within the collagen.

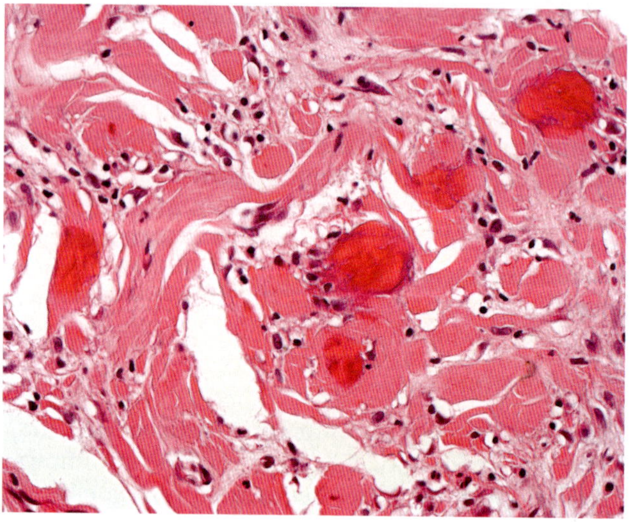

FIGURE 2.5 **Calcifying Fibrous Tumor.** The tumor is composed of dense collagen, with small foci of short spindle cells, and scattered rounded calcifications.

Ancillary Investigations

The lesional cells are occasionally C34-positive and rarely express SMA or desmin focally. ALK-1 is negative. The cells have ultrastructural features of fibroblasts, with electron-dense amorphous masses in the cytoplasm that are interpreted as the initial event in calcification.[13]

CALCIFYING (JUVENILE) APONEUROTIC FIBROMA

Clinical Features

This is a childhood tumor occurring more often in males and mostly in the first decade of life although cases are seen into adolescence and in adults. The occurrence of multiple lesions has been described. It is a slowly growing subcutaneous tumor, not exceeding 4 cm in diameter. The majority of cases involve the hands and feet, especially the palm of the hand and flexor aspects of digits, where the tumor can be adherent to a tendon sheath or aponeurosis. Rare examples affect other locations, including arm, thigh, knee, neck, and back.[14] The lesion is benign but prone to recur, sometimes after a long interval, and fibrosarcomatous transformation with metastasis[15] has been recorded.

Pathologic Features

Calcifying aponeurotic fibroma forms a firm or rubbery white poorly defined tumor sometimes with discernible flecks of calcification. Older lesions tend to become more circumscribed. Microscopically, variably cellular fibrous tissue infiltrates adjacent structures including skeletal muscle.

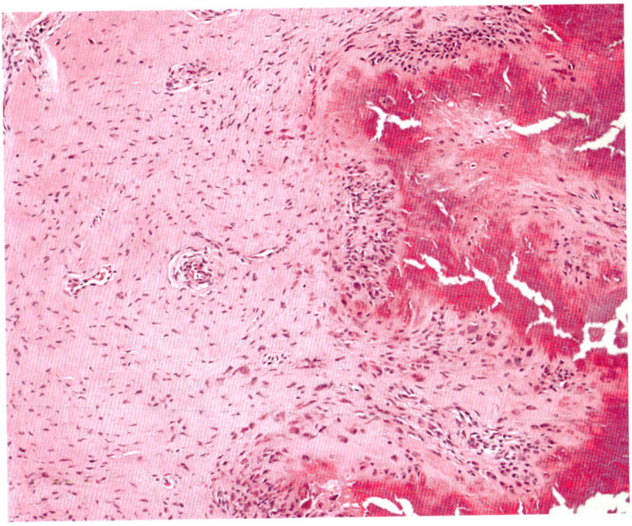

FIGURE 2.6 **Calcifying Aponeurotic Fibroma.** This lesion in the cellular phase demonstrates curved fascicles of bland spindle cells with vague storiform pattern, resembling nodular fasciitis.

The lesional cells are spindled but can be rounded or epithelioid and sometimes form radiating cords or palisades.(Fig. 2.6, e-Figs. 2.18–2.20) The distinctive feature is the presence of irregular deposits of amorphous calcification of varying size, with focal chondroid differentiation, that are more marked in older subjects and can be absent in younger ones. They tend to be centrally located within the lesion and often have an adjacent concentration of more rounded cells. Osteoclast-like giant cells can also be seen but are not a prominent feature (e-Fig. 2.20), and rarely there is also ossification.

Ancillary Investigations

Lesional cells can be immunoreactive for actins, CD99 and rarely epithelial membrane antigen (EMA) or CD34 but not for beta-catenin. The chondroid areas, and occasionally the spindle cells, express S100 protein.

INFANTILE DIGITAL FIBROMA (INCLUSION BODY FIBROMATOSIS)

Clinical Features

This lesion occurs usually in the first 2 years of life and can be present at birth.[16] There is a slight female predominance and occasional examples have been described in older subjects including adults. Typically there are one or more painless, flat-based, rounded dermal/subcutaneous nodules on the extensor or lateral surface of the fingers and, less often the toes. Most lesions involve the third to fifth digits; the thumb and the first toe

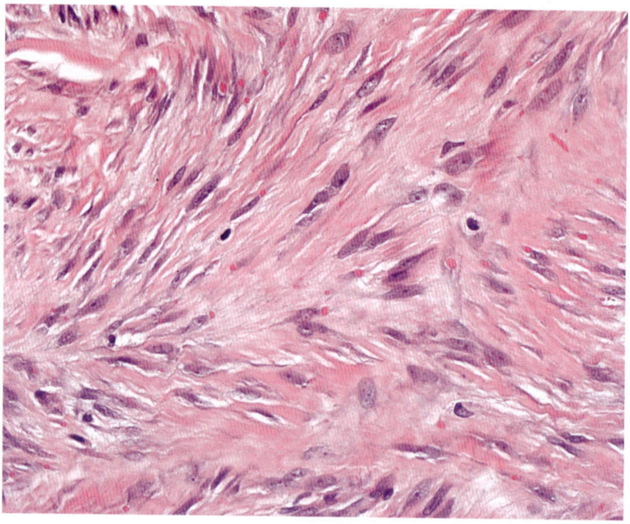

FIGURE 2.7 **Infantile Digital Fibromatosis (Inclusion Body Fibromatosis).** This is a moderately cellular lesion with fibroblastic spindle cells in fascicular orientation in collagen. Rounded eosinophilic paranuclear inclusions are seen, some of which are separated from the nucleus by a clear zone.

are very rare sites. In infants, over half of the lesions recur at the same site, but most eventually regress, although deformities or contractures can result. Rarely, the characteristic inclusion bodies are seen in extradigital lesions, especially in epithelial-stromal breast neoplasms,[17] prompting the term inclusion body fibromatosis.

Pathologic Features

Infantile digital fibroma is a firm white infiltrative dermal and subcutaneous lesion that is sparsely or moderately cellular, with bland spindle cells in a collagenous stroma (e-Figs. 2.21 and 22). The characteristic feature is the presence in variable number of cells of an intracytoplasmic rounded eosinophilic inclusion, in a paranuclear location with a narrow intervening clear zone. (Fig. 2.7, e-Figs. 2.23 and 2.24).

Ancillary Investigations

The lesional cells are myofibroblastic and are positive for SMA, desmin, and CD99 and occasionally for h-caldesmon, nuclear beta-catenin, and CD34.[16] The inclusions are apparently composed mostly of actin filaments and are PAS-negative but can be highlighted histochemically with a variety of stains (e.g., Masson trichrome which stains them red, e-Fig. 2.23) and, in some cases, by immunohistochemistry for SMA although this is inconsistent. Light h-caldesmon positivity has been reported in scattered inclusions in some cases.[16] Ultrastructurally, the cells show subplasmalemmal microfilament bundle with dense bodies. The inclusions comprise similar filaments and granular material, and contain scattered membrane-bound vesicles.

FIBROMATOSIS

Fibromatoses are locally infiltrative but nonmetastasizing myofibroblastic lesions which produce abundant extracellular collagen. In the WHO 2002 Classification, they are categorized as intermediate (locally aggressive) neoplasms. They are classified into superficial and deep (musculo-aponeurotic or desmoid) types, the latter being extra-abdominal or intra-abdominal.

Clinical Features

Superficial fibromatoses arise in the subcutis in palmar (Dupuytren disease, the most common), plantar (Ledderhose disease), and penile (Peyronie disease) locations, as well as knuckle pads. These four conditions can be associated in various combinations. For example, some patients with palmar fibromatosis also have metachronous plantar or, less often, penile lesions. Knuckle pads, which are nodules overlying extensor surfaces of proximal interphalangeal or metacarpophalangeal joints in the hand, are almost always associated with palmar or plantar fibromatosis. Pachydermodactyly is a variant of knuckle pads that occurs mostly in adolescent males over the proximal interphalangeal joints of the fingers[18] and is occasionally associated with plantar lesions. All four superficial fibromatoses predominantly affect adult males, although palmar and (more commonly) plantar fibromatoses can occur in childhood and adolescence.[19] Most patients are Caucasians, and the lesions are rare in black Africans. The relationship between manual work and Dupuytren disease remains debatable.[20] There is an increased incidence of superficial fibromatoses in patients with diabetes mellitus (types 1 and 2), related to duration of the disease, and in epilepsy, perhaps due to drug therapy. Palmar and plantar fibromatoses are also more frequently seen in patients with alcoholic liver disease.[21]

Dupuytren disease begins in the palmar fascia as a nodule that grows slowly, becomes cord-like, and can result in fixed contractures, especially of the fourth and fifth fingers. Both hands can eventually be affected. Plantar fibromatosis, which can also be bilateral, appears as a nodule beneath the skin in the medial plantar arch but rarely causes contracture. Peyronie disease presents with one or more plaques on the dorsal or lateral penile shaft associated with curvature on erection, especially in older patients.

Subfascial or deep fibromatoses can arise in any location including abdominal wall (especially during or shortly after pregnancy) and within the abdomen (mesentery or retroperitoneum), thorax or head and neck region. Most extra-abdominal tumors arise in young adults and more frequently in females, in the proximal limb girdle (especially the shoulder region and buttock), chest wall, neck and large thigh muscles. They are rare in infancy and childhood. Some cases follow irradiation, especially for Hodgkin disease. The lesions are usually solitary, but multiple tumors occur in up to 5% of patients. The recurrence rate averages up to 50%, with head and neck tumors having the highest incidence. Tumor size and incompleteness of excision are predictive factors[22] so that adequate local excision is indicated at the outset.

Fibromatoses of anterior abdominal wall arise in rectus sheath, rectus abdominis, or internal oblique muscles, almost always in women who are pregnant or recently (within 1 year) postpartum. Rare examples occur in males and in childhood. These lesions can recur, including in relation to subsequent pregnancies, and wide local excision is indicated.

Intra-abdominal fibromatosis arises in the pelvis, mesentery, peritoneal ligaments, or retroperitoneum, and since tumors in this location can attain a large size before coming to notice they present as a painless mass or via mass effects. Mesenteric tumors are more common in males, with a mean age of 41, and more frequent in patients with FAP or Gardner syndrome, up to 15% of whom develop intra-abdominal fibromatosis.[6] Such predisposed patients were found in one series to have a 65% chance of developing mesenteric fibromatosis after abdominal surgery.[23] Fibromatosis can also appear in a laparotomy scar.

Deep fibromatosis presents as a plaque-like or discrete hard mass which is usually slowly growing but which can reach a large size. Although fibromatosis does not metastasize, it can recur repeatedly (up to 23% of mesenteric lesions[24]). FAP-associated mesenteric tumors are more likely to recur. In the head and neck or abdomen, lesional tissue can infiltrate adjacent structures, causing difficulty in surgical excision and sometimes resulting in death.

Pathologic Features

Superficial fibromatoses have poorly demarcated, variably cellular nodules of myofibroblastic spindle cells within fibrous tissue. (Fig. 2.8, e-Fig. 2.25). Small giant cells have been described, especially in plantar fibromatosis (e-Fig. 2.26).[25] In penile fibromatosis, there are increased fibroblasts with focal chronic inflammation, followed by increased collagen and loss of elastic fibers with eventual hyalinization (e-Fig. 2.27 and 2.28), and sometimes calcification and osteochondroid metaplasia (e-Fig. 2.29). Knuckle pads are fibroblastic lesions which develop dense fibrosis.

Deep fibromatosis can be circumscribed but more frequently infiltrates surrounding tissues including skeletal muscle (e-Figs. 2.30 and 3.31) or intestinal wall. The lesion is composed of sweeping fascicles of parallel-aligned myofibroblasts evenly spaced in mature collagen. (Fig. 2.9) Myofibroblastic nuclei are ovoid and pale, with one or two small, punctate nucleoli, scanty or moderate amounts of amphophilic cytoplasm, and indistinct cell membranes. Pleomorphism and necrosis are absent but mitotic activity up to about 5 per 10 hpf can sometimes be found. Blood vessels are slit-like or small and thick walled, and occasionally in mesenteric fibromatoses, there are dilated or hemangiopericytoma-like vessels (e-Fig. 2.32). The stroma contains mast cells which often lie in perivascular spaces, and peripheral lymphoid aggregates. Focal myxoid change or edema associated with a loose storiform pattern can be seen in rapidly growing lesions, and especially in mesenteric fibromatoses (e-Fig. 2.33). Sometimes, especially in intra-abdominal tumors, there are thick, parallel, keloid-like collagen fibers (e-Fig. 2.34), and osseous metaplasia. When fibromatosis infiltrates skeletal muscle, damaged muscle fibers with hyperchromatic nuclei can be seen at the infiltrating margin of

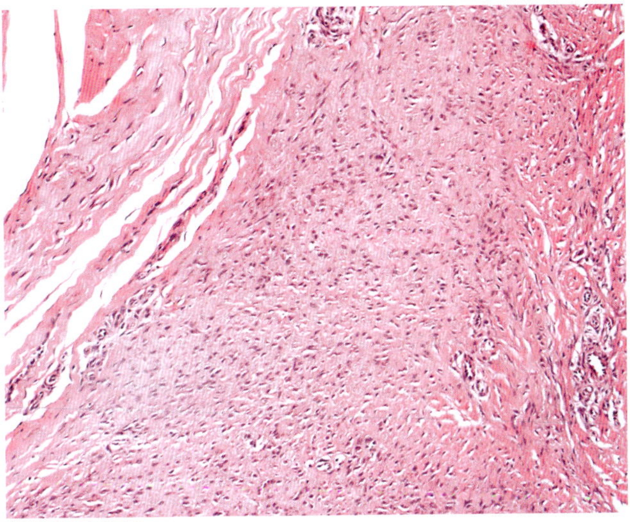

FIGURE 2.8 **Superficial (Palmar) Fibromatosis.** A moderately cellular nodule is well demarcated from the adjacent deep fascia.

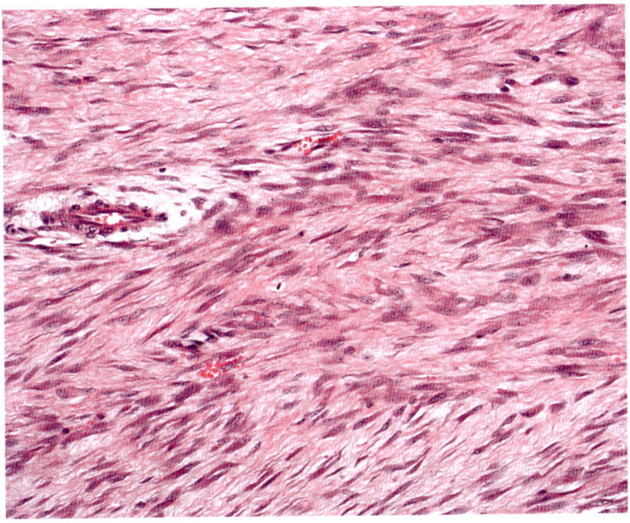

FIGURE 2.9 **Deep Fibromatosis.** Myofibroblastic cells are evenly dispersed in collagen with scattered mast cells. Note the small punctate nucleoli, and the perivascular space containing mast cells.

the tumor (e-Fig. 2.35 and 2.36); these are desmin-positive (e-Fig. 2.37) and should not be mistaken for rhabdomyoblasts or other malignant cells.

Low-grade fibromyxoid sarcoma (see Chapters 10 and 21) can resemble fibromatosis but lacks myofibroblastic nuclear features and has whorled fibromyxoid areas and cellular myxoid foci. In addition, it has diagnostic genetic abnormalities.

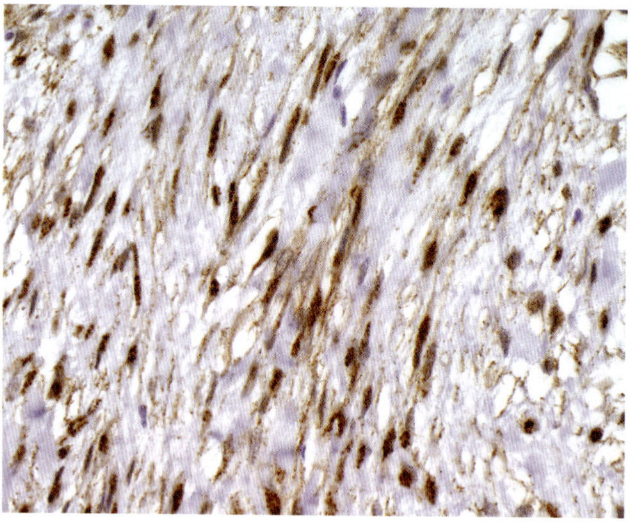

FIGURE 2.10 **Fibromatosis.** Nuclear immunoreactivity for beta catenin. The staining is finely granular. Careful observation is required as some cells have similar paranuclear positivity.

Ancillary Investigations

The lesional cells express SMA and occasionally (and very focally) desmin but lack h-caldesmon, CD34, and (usually) S100 protein. Many cases display estrogen receptor positivity, which might be relevant when antiestrogen therapy is under consideration. About 80% of deep fibromatoses, and a lesser proportion of superficial ones, show nuclear immunoreactivity for beta-catenin in a variable number of cells (Fig. 2.10).[26] There is a granular pattern of staining. Care must be taken in interpretation since the cytoplasm can stain similarly in a paranuclear distribution somewhat resembling a nucleus in shape (e-Fig. 2.38); this is not diagnostic. In deep fibromatosis, beta-catenin positivity relates to somatic mutations in codons 41 or 45 of exon 3 of the beta-catenin gene (*CTNNB1*), whereas fibromatosis in patients with FAP has inactivating germ-line mutations in the desmoid region of the *APC* gene.[27] Mutations in the APC and beta catenin genes are not detected in superficial fibromatoses.[28] These genes are part of the Wnt signaling pathway, and mutations in either result in stabilization of the beta-catenin protein and binding of beta-catenin to the TCF/Lef family of transcription factors.[29] Cytogenetic changes in fibromatosis include trisomy 8, trisomy 20, and loss of Y chromosome. Electron microscopy shows fibroblasts and myofibroblasts, often with abundant dilated rough endoplasmic reticulum.

GINGIVAL FIBROMATOSIS (HEREDITARY GINGIVAL HYPERPLASIA)

Clinical Features

This is a sporadic (two thirds of cases) or familial lesion which arises in children of either sex. Familial cases present at a younger age and can

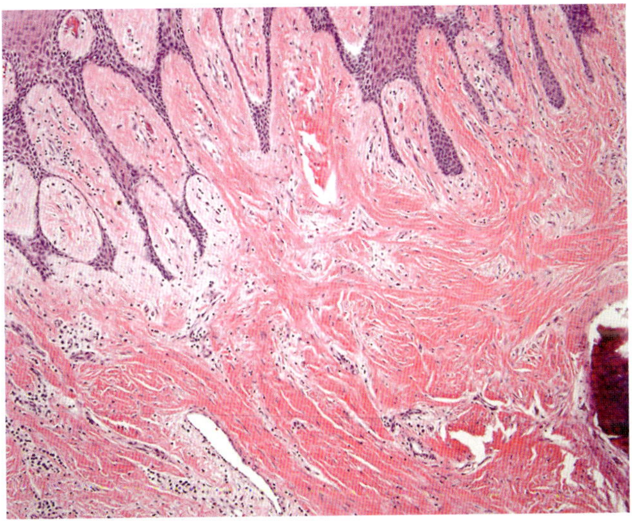

FIGURE 2.11 **Gingival Fibromatosis.** This is a subepithelial lesion. Note the epidermal hyperplasia, interlacing bundles of collagen, and focus of calcification.

be congenital. Mutations have been described at more than one genetic locus, including 2p21–22 and 5q13–q22[30]; most hereditary cases demonstrate autosomal dominant inheritance, but some are autosomally recessive. Some examples have been associated with hypertrichosis and developmental retardation, and others with various hereditary syndromes.[31] The disease can be localized, as a poorly circumscribed mass, or more often generalized, with widespread involvement of gums and adjacent structures. Lesional tissue gradually grows over the teeth and hard palate and can recur after excision although extraction of teeth can result in cure. Histologically the appearances are similar to those of gingival hyperplasia seen in pregnancy, in epilepsy especially following phenytoin use, or in association with use of some other drugs.

Pathologic Features

This is a paucicellular fibroblastic lesion with marked collagenization, mild focal inflammation, and occasional microcalcification. (Fig. 2.11) There is usually overlying epidermal hyperplasia (e-Fig. 2.39–2.41).

FIBROMATOSIS COLLI

Clinical Features

This usually appears in infants in the first month of life as a solitary mass in the lower third of sternomastoid muscle, and rarely also in trapezius, which can cause facial asymmetry. Fibromatosis colli accounts for a variable proportion of cases of muscular torticollis, which can be synchronous with the tumor or delayed. There is a slight male predominance, and the lesion is occasionally familial [32] and rarely bilateral. Obstetric trauma, including

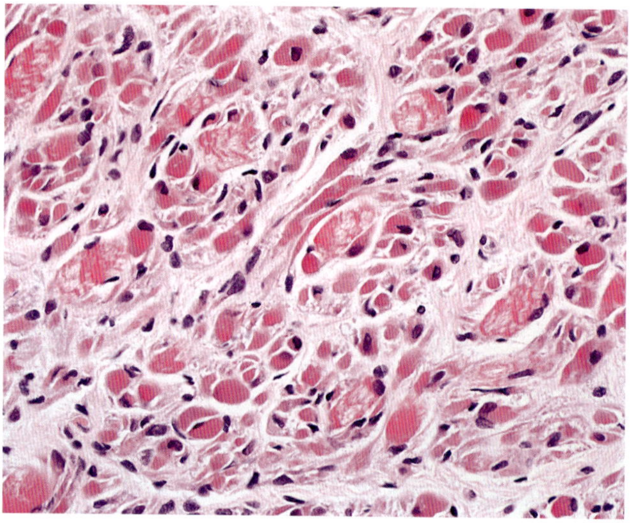

FIGURE 2.12 **Fibromatosis Colli.** This relatively advanced lesion shows skeletal muscle bundles separated by loose fibrous tissue.

breech and forceps deliveries, has been proposed as an associated factor.[33] The mass enlarges rapidly at first, then stops growing and persists. The majority of cases, however, eventually regress over many months, so that no intervention is required except surgery for lesions that are present for more than a year.

Pathologic Features

This is an infiltrative firm white lesion with an average size of 2 to 3 cm. Microscopically, there is a variably cellular fibroblastic proliferation that infiltrates between skeletal muscle bundles, which show focal atrophy or swelling (e-Fig. 2.42). Atypia, necrosis, mitoses, and an inflammatory component are absent. There is increased fibrosis in later stages, giving a characteristic fine "checkerboard" pattern (Fig. 2.12, e-Figs. 2.42 and 2.43).

Ancillary Investigations

The infiltrating fibroblasts were negative for beta-catenin in the one case so examined.[34]

JUVENILE HYALINE FIBROMATOSIS

Juvenile hyaline fibromatosis is a rare, hereditary (autosomal recessive) disease in which there is deposition in various organs of hyaline material containing type VI and some type I collagen, and the glycosaminoglycans dermatan sulfate, hyaluronic acid, and chondroitin sulfates. The disease is thought to be due to defects in collagen production and synthesis of glycosaminoglycans related to mutations in the *CMG2* (capillary morphogenesis protein)

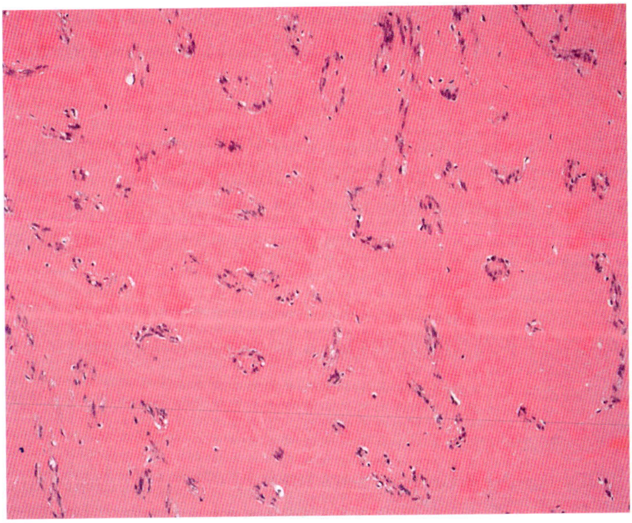

FIGURE 2.13 **Juvenile Hyaline Fibromatosis.** Clusters of short spindle cells with clear cytoplasm are dispersed in the characteristic homogeneous, acellular, eosinophilic stroma.

gene on chromosome 4q21. This is also found in infantile systemic hyalinosis[35], and the two conditions appear to overlap. Unique examples have been associated with bullous pemphigoid[36] and oral squamous cell carcinoma.[37]

Clinical Features

Though not strictly a neoplasm, this can present as multiple superficial and deep tumor-like masses which continue to grow. The disease has approximately equal sex incidence and usually presents in early childhood or congenitally, with rare examples first appearing in adult life. Cutaneous involvement is manifest as raised nodules in head and neck (especially periauricular) regions, and other locations including perianal skin. Other sites of involvement include gingivae scalp, trunk and limbs, especially fingers and periarticular soft tissues. The latter can result in contractures especially when involving elbow and knee joint regions. Bony manifestations include lytic lesions, present in over half of the cases, and generalized osteoporosis can occur. The lesions can progress and can recur after excision.

Pathologic Features

The nodules are firm with a pale, chondroid-like cut surface. They are composed of homogeneous, dense, eosinophilic material containing evenly dispersed, small groups of uniform, bland ovoid fibroblast-like cells with small amounts of clear cytoplasm (Fig. 2.13, e-Figs. 2.44 and 2.45). There are sometimes admixed macrophages. The cellularity decreases with duration of the lesion as stroma formation increases. Focal calcification and multinucleated giant cells are occasional but rare findings.

Ancillary Investigations

The stromal material is Alcian blue– and PAS-positive (diastase resistant). Apart from vimentin, the cells are nonimmunoreactive, and SMA and beta-catenin[38] are negative. Electron microscopy shows fibroblastic cells with abundant dilated rough endoplasmic reticulum containing precursor stromal material.

DESMOPLASTIC FIBROBLASTOMA (COLLAGENOUS FIBROMA)

Clinical Features

This is a solitary lesion which occurs mainly (75%) in males aged between 40 and 70 years, in the subcutis and sometime subfascial soft tissue of the arm, shoulder and back, and occasionally in lower limb and head and neck region.[39,40] The tumor is a painless mass that rarely exceeds 5 cm but examples up to 20 cm have been described.[40] No reported case has recurred or metastasized.

Pathologic Features

The typical desmoplastic fibroblastoma is a firm white tumor which is mainly sharply circumscribed but can be focally infiltrative (into fat or muscle) (Fig. 2.14, e-Fig. 2.46). Histologically, the lesion is composed of bland

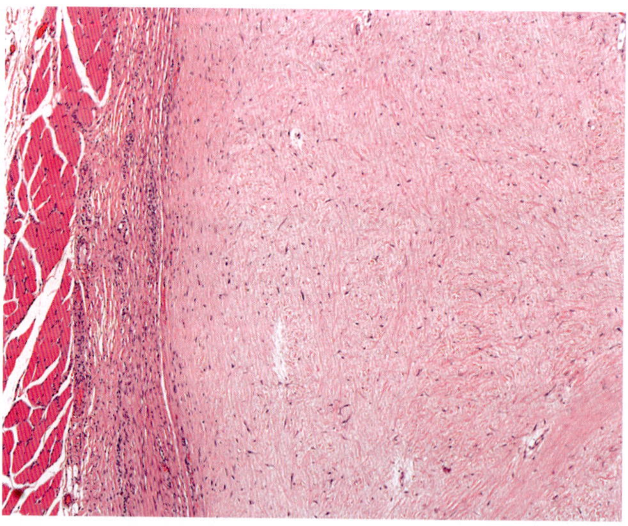

FIGURE 2.14 **Desmoplastic Fibroblastoma.** This intramuscular lesion shows characteristic sharp circumscription, and sparse spindle and stellate cells in collagenous stroma.

stellate or spindly myofibroblasts widely dispersed in a uniform densely fibrous stroma, rarely with focal myxoid change (e-Figs. 2.47–2.50), and with a paucity of blood vessels, some of which can be hyalinized. Mitoses are very rare and necrosis is absent.

Ancillary Investigations

Immunohistochemistry shows focal positivity for SMA and absence of CD34 and S100 protein. A very occasional case has demonstrated nuclear immunoreactivity for beta-catenin.[34] The cells have ultrastructural features of fibroblasts and myofibroblasts. A specific chromosomal rearrangement t(2;11)(q31;q12) has been identified in a number of cases[41] suggesting a genetic link with fibroma of tendon sheath in which a similar rearrangement with 11q12 abnormalities has also been found.

REFERENCES

1. Nishio JN, Iwasaki H, Ohjimi Y, et al. Gain of Xq detected by comparative genomic hybridization in elastofibroma. *Int J Mol Med.* 2002;10:277–280.
2. Michal M, Fetsch JF, Hes O, et al. Nuchal-type fibroma: a clinicopathologic study of 52 cases. *Cancer.* 1999;85:156–163.
3. Gardner EJ. Follow-up study of a family group exhibiting dominant inheritance for a syndrome including intestinal polyps, osteomas, fibromas and epidermal cysts. *Am J Hum Genet.* 1962;14:376–390.
4. Clark SK, Neale KF, Landgrebe JC, et al. Desmoid tumours complicating familial adenomatous polyposis. *Br J Surg.* 1999;86:1185–1189.
5. Coffin CM, Hornick JL, Zhou H, et al. Gardner fibroma: a clinicopathologic and immunohistochemical analysis of 45 patients with 57 fibromas. *Am J Surg Pathol.* 2007;31:410–416.
6. Clark SK, Smith TG, Katz DE, et al. Identification and progression of a desmoid precursor lesion in patients with familial adenomatous polyposis. *Br J Surg.* 1998;85:970–973.
7. Laskin WB, Fetsch JF, Miettinen M. Nuchal fibrocartilaginous pseudotumor: a clinicopathologic study of five cases and review of the literature. *Mod Pathol.* 1999;12:663–668.
8. Dal Cin P, Sciot R, De Smet L, et al. Translocation 2;11 in a fibroma of tendon sheath. *Histopathology.* 1998;32:433–435.
9. Rosenthal NS, Abdul-Karim FW. Childhood fibrous tumor with psammoma bodies. Clinicopathologic features in two cases. *Arch Pathol Lab Med.* 1988;112:798–800.
10. Fetsch JF, Montgomery EA, Meis JM. Calcifying fibrous pseudotumor. *Am J Surg Pathol.* 1993;17:502–508.
11. Van Dorpe J, Ectors N, Geboes K, et al. Is calcifying fibrous pseudotumor a late sclerosing stage of inflammatory myofibroblastic tumor? *Am J Surg Pathol.* 1999;23:329–335.
12. Agaimy A, Bihl MP, Tornillo L, et al. Calcifying fibrous tumor of the stomach: clinicopathologic and molecular study of seven cases with literature review and reappraisal of histogenesis. *Am J Surg Pathol.* 2010;34:271–278.
13. Maeda T, Hirose T, Furuya K, et al. Calcifying fibrous pseudotumor: an ultrastructural study. *Ultrastruct Pathol.* 1999;23:189–192.
14. Fetsch JF, Miettinen M. Calcifying aponeurotic fibroma: a clinicopathologic study of 22 cases arising in uncommon sites. *Hum Pathol.* 1998;29:1504–1510.

15. Lafferty KA, Nelson EL, Demuth RJ, et al. Juvenile aponeurotic fibroma with disseminated fibrosarcoma. *J Hand Surg [Am]*. 1986;11:737–740.
16. Laskin WB, Miettinen M, Fetsch JF. Infantile digital fibroma/fibromatosis: a clinicopathologic and immunohistochemical study of 69 tumors from 57 patients with long-term follow-up. *Am J Surg Pathol.* 2009;33:1–13.
17. Shin SJ, Rosen PP. Bilateral presentation of fibroadenoma with digital fibroma-like inclusions in the male breast. *Arch Pathol Lab Med.* 2007;131:1126–1129.
18. Sandobal C, Kuznietz A, Varizat A, et al. Pachydermodactyly: four additional cases. *Clin Rheumatol.* 2007;26:962–964.
19. Fetsch JF, Laskin WB, Miettinen M. Palmar-plantar fibromatosis in children and preadolescents: a clinicopathologic study of 56 cases with newly recognized demographics and extended follow-up information. *Am J Surg Pathol.* 2005;29:1095–1105.
20. Lucas G, Brichet A, Roquelaure Y, et al. Dupuytren's disease: personal factors and occupational exposure. *Am J Ind Med.* 2008;51:9–15.
21. Geoghegan JM, Forbes J, Clark DI, et al. Dupuytren's disease risk factors. *J Hand Surg [Br]*. 2004;29:423–426.
22. Pritchard DJ, Nascimento AG, Petersen IA. Local control of extra-abdominal desmoid tumors. *J Bone Joint Surg Am.* 1996;78:848–854.
23. Speake D, Evans DG, Lalloo F, et al. Desmoid tumours in patients with familial adenomatous polyposis and desmoid region adenomatous polyposis coli mutations. *Br J Surg.* 2007;94:1009–1013.
24. Burke AP, Sobin LH, Shekitka KM. Mesenteric fibromatosis. A follow-up study. *Arch Pathol Lab Med.* 1990;114:832–835.
25. Evans HL. Multinucleated giant cells in plantar fibromatosis. *Am J Surg Pathol.* 2002;26:244–248.
26. Ng TL, Gown AM, Barry TS, et al. Nuclear beta-catenin in mesenchymal tumors. *Mod Pathol.* 2005;18:68–74.
27. Tejpar S, Michils G, Denys H, et al. Analysis of Wnt/Beta catenin signalling in desmoid tumors. *Acta Gastroenterol Belg.* 2005;68:5–9.
28. Montgomery E, Lee JH, Abraham SC, et al. Superficial fibromatoses are genetically distinct from deep fibromatoses. *Mod Pathol.* 2001;14:695–701.
29. Kotiligam D, Lazar AJ, Pollock RE, et al. Desmoid tumor: a disease opportune for molecular insights. *Histol Histopathol.* 2008;23:117–126.
30. Ye X, Shi L, Cheng Y, et al. A novel locus for autosomal dominant hereditary gingival fibromatosis, GINGF3, maps to chromosome 2p22.3-p23.3. *Clin Genet.* 2005;68:239–244.
31. Chodirker BN, Chudley AE, Toffler MA, et al. Zimmerman-Laband syndrome and profound mental retardation. *Am J Med Genet.* 1986;25:543–547.
32. Tavill MA, Wetmore RF. A case of familial sternocleidomastoid tumor of infancy. *Int J Pediatr Otorhinolaryngol.* 1996;38:163–168.
33. Cheng JC, Tang SP, Chen TM, et al. The clinical presentation and outcome of treatment of congenital muscular torticollis in infants–a study of 1,086 cases. *J Pediatr Surg.* 2000;35:1091–1096.
34. Carlson JW, Fletcher CD. Immunohistochemistry for beta-catenin in the differential diagnosis of spindle cell lesions: analysis of a series and review of the literature. *Histopathology.* 2007;51:509–514.
35. Dowling O, Difeo A, Ramirez MC, et al. Mutations in capillary morphogenesis gene-2 result in the allelic disorders juvenile hyaline fibromatosis and infantile systemic hyalinosis. *Am J Hum Genet.* 2003;73:957–966.
36. Shimizu K, Ogawa F, Hamasaki Y, et al. A case of bullous pemphigoid arising in juvenile hyaline fibromatosis with oral squamous cell carcinoma. *J Dermatol.* 2005;32:650–653.

37. Kawasaki G, Yanamoto S, Mizuno A, et al. Juvenile hyaline fibromatosis complicated with oral squamous cell carcinoma: a case report. *Oral Surg Oral Med Oral Pathol Oral Radiol Endod.* 2001;91:200–204.

38. Thway K, Gibson S, Ramsay A, et al. Beta-catenin expression in pediatric fibroblastic and myofibroblastic lesions: s study of 100 cases. *Pediatr Dev Pathol.* 2009;12:292–296.

39. Evans HL. Desmoplastic fibroblastoma. A report of seven cases. *Am J Surg Pathol.* 1995;19:1077–1081.

40. Miettinen M, Fetsch JF. Collagenous fibroma (desmoplastic fibroblastoma): a clinicopathologic analysis of 63 cases of a distinctive soft tissue lesion with stellate-shaped fibroblasts. *Hum Pathol.* 1998;29:676–682.

41. Sakamoto A, Yamamoto H, Yoshida T, et al. Desmoplastic fibroblastoma (collagenous fibroma) with a specific breakpoint of 11q12. *Histopathology.* 2007;51:859–860.

3

CELLULAR BENIGN AND INTERMEDIATE LESIONS OF FIBROBLASTS AND MYOFIBROBLASTS

INTRODUCTION

Some soft tissue tumors are composed of a mixture of fibroblasts and myofibroblasts. Benign tumors in which myofibroblasts predominate are considered in Chapter 7, and myofibrosarcomas in Chapters 10 and 13. Fibroblasts are tapered cells with elongated slender, sometimes slightly wavy nuclei and scanty or indiscernible cytoplasm. Myofibroblasts are also tapered but tend to be plumper, with ovoid nuclei, small punctate nucleoli, variable amounts of eosinophilic or basophilic cytoplasm, and indistinct cell margins.[1] The differences between fibroblasts and myofibroblasts are summarized in Table 3.1. Many fibroblastic and myofibroblastic lesions are moderately or highly cellular and can show mitotic activity so that they can be mistaken for sarcomas. It is important to be aware of the clinical features, including history (reactive conditions can grow alarmingly rapidly but tend to stop and do not reach a large size), and location (reactive conditions are mostly subcutaneous). Some can also have nuclear pleomorphism, but they usually lack prominent nucleoli, abnormal mitotic figures, and necrosis. Conversely, it should also be noted the pseudocapsule adjacent to some sarcomas is composed of cellular fibrous tissue. Nonrepresentative sampling of this can lead to underdiagnosis of malignancy. Correlation with imaging is often helpful, and repeat biopsy might be indicated if the pathological findings are discordant. The differential diagnosis is summarized in Table 3.2.

NODULAR FASCIITIS

Clinical Features

Nodular fasciitis is a reactive condition which is frequently misdiagnosed clinically and microscopically as malignant. It occurs mostly in adults of either sex aged 20 to 40 years and can occur in almost any anatomical site, but favored locations include the upper limb, trunk, and head and neck.[2]

TABLE 3.1 **Features of Fibroblasts, Myofibroblasts, and Smooth Muscle Cells**

	Morphology	Immunohistochemistry	Electron Microscopy
Fibroblast	Tapered spindle cell with slender tapered or wavy nucleus, scanty, or indiscernible cytoplasm. Can assume epithelioid form (e.g., sclerosing epithelioid fibrosarcoma)	Vimentin+. Some subsets are CD34+. Focal SMA positivity suggests incipient myofibroblastic differentiation. Other markers negative	Variable, often abundant rough endoplasmic reticulum. No junctions, external lamina, or pinocytotic vesicles
Myofibroblast	Tapered or ovoid, oval nucleus with single punctate nucleolus, variable amounts of amphophilic cytoplasm. Indistinct cell membrane	SMA+ (subplasmalemmal "tram-track" distribution), desmin±, h-caldesmon−, SMM− Rarely CK+ (mostly in intra-abdominal lesions). CD34−, S100 protein–negative	Moderate amounts of rough endoplasmic reticulum, subplasmalemmal stress fiber continuous with fibronexus fibril No external lamina, junctions, or pinocytotic vesicles
Smooth muscle cell	Nontapered (parallel sided), abundant slightly fibrillary eosinophilic cytoplasm (also seen alongside nucleus). Nucleus has rounded or blunt ends, paranuclear vacuole. Can assume clear cell or epithelioid form	SMA+, desmin+, h-caldesmon+, calponin+ Some express CK (dot), EMA or S100 protein	Myofilaments with dense bodies throughout cytoplasm External lamina and pinocytosis often prominent

TABLE 3.2 Differential Diagnosis of Cellular Fibroblastic-Myofibroblastic Lesions

	Typical Clinical Features	Microscopic Features	Ancillary Investigations
Nodular fasciitis	Young adults, extremities, head, and neck. Short history–weeks; rarely up to a year. Rapid growth then stops <5 cm. Mostly subcutaneous or occasionally intramuscular. Similar lesions in bladder, spermatic cord, nerve	Circumscribed or minimally infiltrative. Variably myxoid, cellular, and collagenous areas. Normal mitoses acceptable but not atypia or necrosis Intravascular variant	SMA+, desmin±, h-caldesmon–
Myofibroma	Mostly in children, occasionally in adults, in head and neck, extremities, bone. Dermis or subcutis. Deep, visceral multicentric tumors can be fatal	Circumscribed, occasional central necrosis. Nodules of myofibroblasts, central smaller cells with pericytomatous pattern. Giant cells, ossification, intravascular spread	SMA+, desmin-negative, h-caldesmon–negative, S100 protein–negative, CK–
Low grade myofibrosarcoma	Head and neck sites (including bone), extremities, retroperitoneum. Infiltrative mass, Recurs and occasionally metastasizes	Infiltration of fat and muscle by cellular fascicles of tapered cells with mostly uniform nuclei but focal nuclear atypia. Occasional necrosis. Occasional myxoid change focally	SMA+, desmin±, h-caldesmon–
Leiomyosarcoma	Slowly growing. Tumors confined to dermis can recur but rarely metastasize. Those in subcutis have increased metastatic potential. NB leiomyoma occurs in skin but is very rare in deeper tissue especially in males	Fascicles intersect at right angles. Nontapered cells with eosinophilic cytoplasm and blunt-ended nuclei. Nuclear atypia, mitotic activity, and focal necrosis. Inflammatory variant has lymphocytic infiltrate, foamy macrophages, psammoma bodies	SMA+, desmin+, h-caldesmon+

Low-grade myxofibrosarcoma	Limbs, older adults, subcutaneous, fascial, or deeper Recurs, often with grade progression	Multinodular, myxoid, spindle cells with hyperchromatic nuclei and variable nuclear atypia, pleomorphic cellular areas	CD34± Lacks myoid antigens except in pleomorphic areas
Inflammatory myofibroblastic tumor	Mesenteric, retroperitoneal, other sites	Fascicular, myxoid, and sclerosing patterns. Mostly bland myofibroblasts, occasional atypical polygonal "ganglion-like" cells Marked inflammation, notably with plasma cells often in aggregates	SMA+, ALK1 55%
Proliferative fasciitis	Middle-aged adults, extremities, trunk. Rapid growth of firm subcutaneous nodule	Polygonal cells with prominent nucleoli in fasciitis-like background. No atypia, no acute inflammation	SMA+ in spindle cells, polygonal cells negative for CD34, S100 protein, desmin, CK, EMA
Myxoinflammatory fibroblastic sarcoma	Mostly extremities, adults. Cutaneous or subcutaneous, can involve tendons	Multinodular myxoid foci with vacuolated fibroblasts, cellular areas with Reed-Sternberg–like and atypical mononuclear cells. Eosinophils, plasma cells, hemosiderin	CD34+ in some. Rare cases with t(1;10)(p22;q24)

(Continued)

TABLE 3.2 **Differential Diagnosis of Cellular Fibroblastic-Myofibroblastic Lesions (Continued)**

	Typical Clinical Features	Microscopic Features	Ancillary Investigations
Solitary fibrous tumor	Subcutaneous or deep, circumscribed tumor. Can occur in any location, body cavity, or organ	Circumscribed, not usually encapsulated. Distinct cellular and fibrous areas, focal myxoid stroma, patternless short spindle cells. Hemangiopericytomatous pattern focally. Malignant variant has hypercellularity, mitoses >4 per 10 hpf, necrosis	CD34+, bcl-2+, CD99 +
Fibromatosis–superficial	Palm, sole, penis; infiltrative plaque	Variably cellular nodules, cells spindled or ovoid, evenly dispersed in dense collagen, mast cells. Normal mitoses acceptable but not atypia or necrosis	SMA+, nuclear beta-catenin+ occasionally, CD34–
Fibromatosis–desmoid type	Deep, limbs, head and neck, body cavities	Parallel-aligned myofibroblasts evenly dispersed in collagen, slit-like and thick-walled vessels, mast cells. Normal mitoses acceptable but not atypia or necrosis	SMA+, nuclear beta-catenin+, CD34–

Fibrous hamartoma of infancy	M>F, most appear in first 2 y of life. Axilla, trunk, inguinogenital region	Infiltrative tumor with variable mixture of (1) cellular fibrous bands containing small stellate or ovoid cells, (2) neurofibroma-like spindle cell component, (3) mature fat. Lipofibromatosis has morphologic similarities	SMA+ focally, rarely desmin+ or CD34+. S100 protein−
Cellular fibrous histiocytoma	Dermal nodule of varying size, extremities, trunk. Young adults, M>F	Fascicles of tapered spindle cells in dermis, radial extensions into subcutis. Mitoses variable. Peripheral collagen bundles, rare foamy, and giant cells. Central necrosis in some. Atypical variant has scattered enlarged hyperchromatic nuclei or multinucleation in background of typical cells	SMA+, desmin rarely+, h-caldesmon rarely+
Deep benign fibrous histiocytoma	Young adults, M>F, extremities, head and neck. Subcutaneous mass can reach large size. Can recur if incompletely excised, very rarely metastasizes	Circumscribed, often with fibrous capsule. Fascicles and storiform whorls of short spindle cells with variable mitotic activity. Lymphocyte sprinkling, multinucleated and foamy cells, hemosiderin, focal fibrosis, focal hemangiopericytomatous pattern. Rarely atypia or necrosis	CD34± (40%), SMA± (38%), desmin+ occasionally, S100 protein−

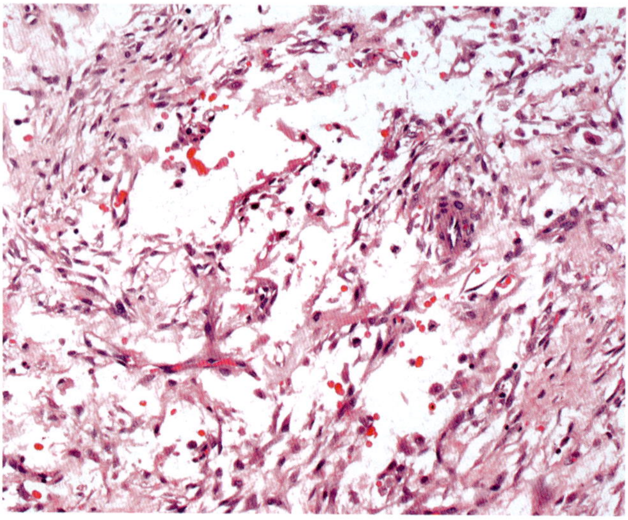

FIGURE 3.1. **Nodular Fasciitis.** This early stage lesion shows fascicles and files of myofibroblasts in myxoid stroma. There are lymphocytes and red blood cells in the stroma.

Rare examples arise within joints, especially the knee.[3] There is sometimes a history of local trauma. Clinical subsets include cranial fasciitis and proliferative funiculitis,[4] and the principal morphologic variants are intravascular, ossifying, and proliferative fasciitis. The typical lesion of nodular fasciitis grows rapidly over a period of weeks and then remains stable, rarely exceeding 5 cm in diameter. Most examples arise in subcutis but the process can extend from the deep aspect of the deep fascia to involve skeletal muscle (intramuscular fasciitis) or, rarely, be sited wholly within the dermis. Nodular fasciitis is benign and, except for occasional examples of intravascular fasciitis, very rarely recurs even when incompletely excised.[5] Those that do so should be carefully reviewed in case they are spindle cell sarcomas.[2]

Pathologic Features

Nodular fasciitis is usually a circumscribed lesion but can appear infiltrative. It is variously firm or soft according to the degree of fibrosis. Microscopically, the lesion can be based on deep fascia (on either aspect) or lie within the fat of the superficial fascia, extending along interlobular septa. Nodular fasciitis is composed of irregular fascicles of uniform myofibroblasts. These have ovoid pale nucleoli, single small nucleoli, and variable amounts of eosinophilic or amphophilic cytoplasm, sometimes with a paranuclear pale zone (Figs. 3.1 and 3.2). The cells are spindle shaped or (especially in early stages) stellate. Normal mitoses are frequent, but nuclear pleomorphism and atypical mitoses are absent. The presence of any nuclear atypia should raise concern for sarcoma, notably low-grade myofibrosarcoma. The stroma is at first myxoid (Fig. 3.1, e-Fig. 3.1). Later, there is increased cellularity with a vague storiform pattern (e-Fig. 3.2). Focally

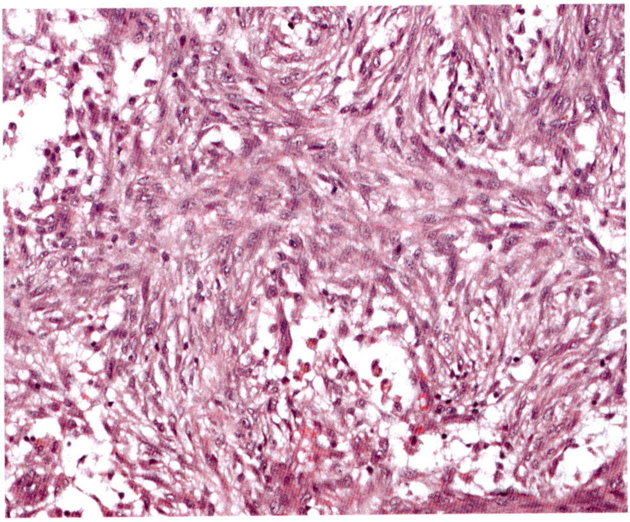

FIGURE 3.2. **Nodular Fasciitis.** Cellular phase displays sheets of bland cells with ill-defined storiform pattern. The cells have ovoid nuclei and small nucleoli, with scattered mitoses. Note the focal stromal microcysts.

there remain small microcysts containing a few extravasated red blood cells and lymphocytes, around which the spindle cells are curved (crescent sign) (e-Figs. 3.3 and 3.4). Small multinucleated cells can also be a feature (e-Fig. 3.5).[6] This is followed by fibrosis with distinct collagen bundles and fewer cells which are more slender with wavy nuclei (e-Figs. 3.6 and 3.7). Since the different stages usually coexist in the same lesion, there is a characteristic heterogeneity or "zoning" phenomenon which is helpful for diagnosis. Occasionally there is a central cyst containing fibrin, surrounded by radial leashes of elongated capillaries.

Ancillary Investigations

Nodular fasciitis, as a myofibroblastic lesion, expresses smooth muscle actin (SMA), calponin, and rarely desmin, but not h-caldesmon,[7] smooth muscle myosin (SMM), CD34, S100 protein, or beta catenin.[7] Electron microscopy shows cells with dilated rough endoplasmic reticulum and subplasmalemmal stress fibers with associated fibronexus fibrils.[8] Gene expression profiling of nodular fasciitis reveals a distinctive pattern unlike that in fibromatosis.[9] Many of the differentially expressed genes encode proteins that are associated with inflammation and tissue remodeling.

VARIANTS

Lesions with metaplastic bone formation are termed **ossifying fasciitis** (Fig. 3.3, e-Figs. 3.8 and 3.9). This starts centrally with maturation toward the periphery, but the ossification is more random than in myositis

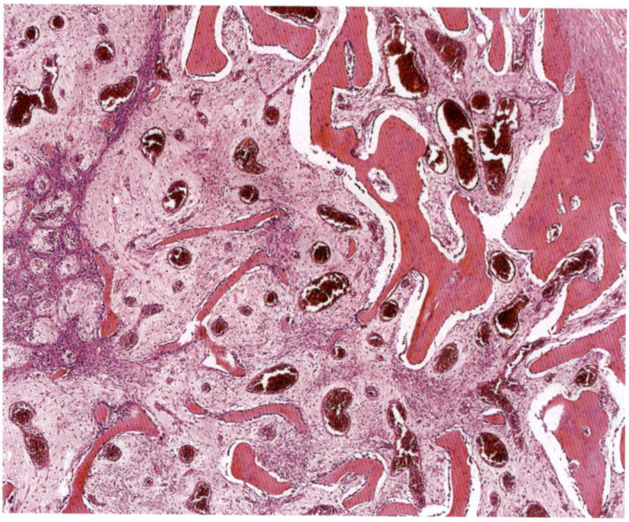

FIGURE 3.3. **Ossifying Fasciitis.** Within a cellular background of nodular fasciitis, there is bone formation with maturation and enlargement of trabeculae from left to right imparting a zoning appearance.

ossificans, and cartilage formation is usually lacking. However, the two processes occasionally appear contiguous across the deep fascia. A histologically similar phenomenon has been described in the abdomen in adult males following abdominal trauma or surgery as **heterotopic mesenteric ossification**.[9] This usually presents clinically as intestinal obstruction. **Intravascular fasciitis** (e-Figs. 3.10–3.13) arises mostly in the head and neck or arm (including hand) and affects small veins or occasionally arteries as an intraluminal or transmural mass with or without an extravascular component.[10] Conversely, usual-type nodular fasciitis can extend into adjacent vessels; in such cases, the intravascular component is minor. **Cranial fasciitis** (e-Figs. 3.14 and 3.15) occurs mostly in infancy and rarely in childhood or later life in the scalp with involvement of underlying bone, sometimes eroding through the skull to involve meninges.[11]

PROLIFERATIVE FASCIITIS

Clinical Features

This arises in adult males and females with a peak in the sixth decade and is by definition subcutaneous (similar subfascial lesions are mostly classified as proliferative myositis).[12] The most frequent locations are the upper limb, especially the forearm, and the trunk. The lesion is rapidly growing and forms a firm, sometimes painful, mobile subcutaneous nodule that rarely exceeds 5 cm in diameter and is usually smaller.

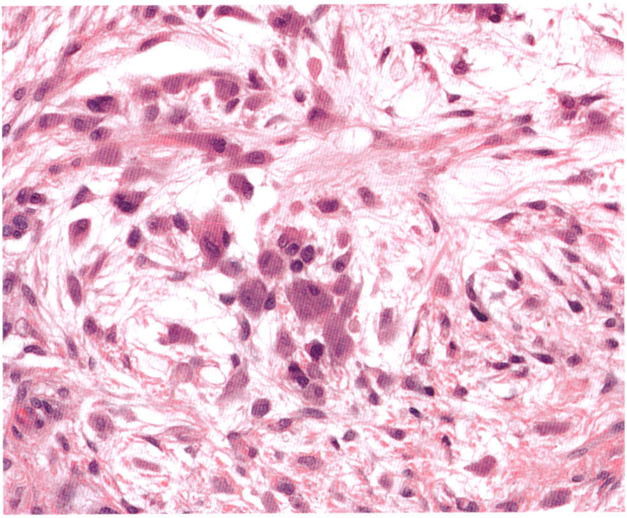

FIGURE 3.4. **Proliferative Fasciitis.** This shows typical clusters of rounded ganglion-like cells of varying size, with abundant darkly staining cytoplasm. There are also more spindled and stellate cells, which merge with the nodular fasciitis-like background.

Pathologic Features

Proliferative fasciitis is an infiltrative lesion which extends from the main mass along interlobular septa. In a background of a nodular fasciitis-like spindle cell proliferation, there are clusters of polygonal cells with one or two rounded nuclei containing prominent nucleoli, and amphophilic or basophilic cytoplasm (Fig. 3.4, e-Figs. 3.16 and 3.17). These are said to resemble ganglion cells. Necrosis and acute inflammation are absent except in pediatric cases,[13] and older lesions can become hyalinized but can also regress.

Ancillary Investigations

The spindled cells are SMA-positive. The ganglion-like cells have ultrastructural features of fibroblasts, with dilated rough endoplasmic reticulum and intracytoplasmic collagen fibrils.[14] With immunohistochemistry, they are reactive only for vimentin with very occasional focal positivity for actins and have a lower proliferation index than the adjacent spindle cells.[15] Importantly for diagnosis, they are nonimmunoreactive for desmin, S100 protein, and epithelial antigens. A clonal cytogenetic abnormality, trisomy 2, has been described in one case.[16]

PROLIFERATIVE MYOSITIS

Clinical Features

This resembles proliferative fasciitis in being a rapidly growing lesion but arises in older patients (median 50 years) and involves skeletal muscle of

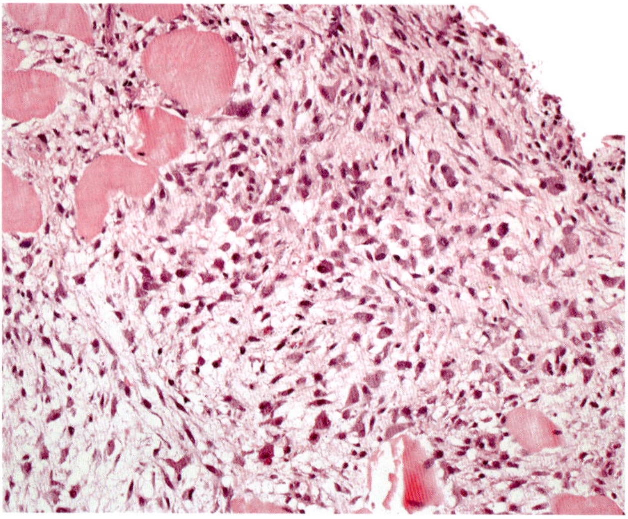

FIGURE 3.5. **Proliferative Myositis.** Skeletal muscle fibers are infiltrated and separated by a cellular infiltrate including proliferative fasciitis-like polygonal cells and fibroblastic spindle cells.

shoulder girdle or back, and thigh.[17] A painless mass up to 6 cm diameter appears in a matter of weeks.

Pathologic Features

Proliferative myositis begins beneath the deep fascia and extends along fibrous septa within the muscle. Bundles of skeletal muscle fibers are separated in a "checkerboard" pattern by spindle and polygonal "ganglion-like" cells in loosely cellular fibrous tissue (Fig 3.5, e-Figs. 3.18 and 3.19), with a microscopic picture identical to that seen in proliferative fasciitis.

Ancillary Investigations

The findings are similar to those in proliferative fasciitis. Reported examples have been diploid,[18] and one case with t(6;14)(q23;q32) has been described.[19]

ISCHEMIC FASCIITIS (ATYPICAL DECUBITAL FIBROPLASIA)

Clinical Features

This is a lesion characterized by necrosis in deep subcutis which occurs typically over bony prominences of hip or back in immobilized or debilitated, mostly elderly patients.[20] Examples are, however, increasingly becoming recognized in patients without the above predisposing features.[21] One example has been reported in association with bizarre parosteal osteochondromatous proliferation, a pseudosarcomatous proliferation of bone.[22]

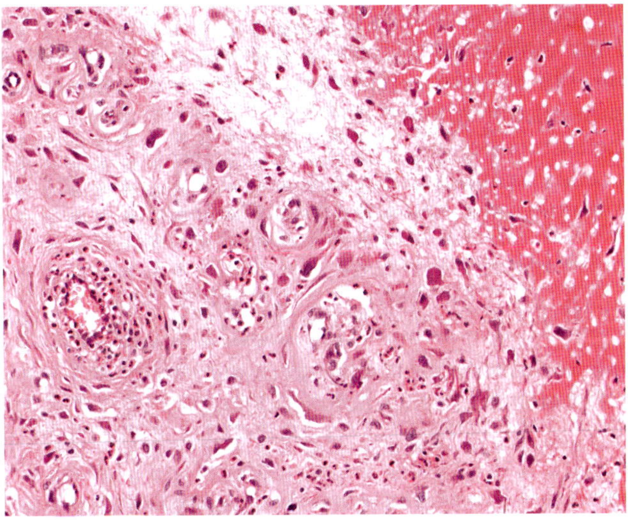

FIGURE 3.6. **Ischemic Fasciitis.** A zone of fibrinoid necrosis in subcutaneous fat (upper right) abuts a myxoid and cellular zone with clusters of hyaline-walled blood vessels and scattered spindle cells with irregularly enlarged hyperchromatic nuclei.

Pathologic Features

Ischemic fasciitis forms an ill-defined soft lesion usually 3 to 4 cm in diameter but occasionally up to 10 cm. It is centered in the subcutis but can extend into skeletal muscle. Microscopically, there is coagulative or liquefactive necrosis of fat with fibrinoid change, as well as an adjacent zone of granulation tissue-like proliferating blood vessels, with focal myxoid change, muciphages, and, rarely, hyalinization and calcification (Fig. 3.6, e-Figs. 3.20–3.24).[23] The additional distinctive feature is the presence of spindle and stellate fibroblasts, a variable number of which have enlarged hyperchromatic nuclei with nucleoli, somewhat similar to the cells of proliferative fasciitis (e-Figs. 3.23 and 3.24). Mitotic figures (though not abnormal ones) can also be seen. These features, and the presence of necrosis, can lead to a mistaken diagnosis of malignancy. However, the lesion is benign and rarely recurs.

Ancillary Investigations

The spindle cells stain focally for CD34 in some cases and occasionally for actin.

FIBROUS HAMARTOMA OF INFANCY

Clinical Features

This is a benign tumor that appears mostly during the first 2 years of life, with a male predominance.[24] Fibrous hamartoma can grow fairly rapidly until the child is about 5 years old, and thereafter more slowly without regressing. It presents as a mass averaging around 4 cm in diameter in the subcutis of the axillary folds, trunk, proximal limbs, or inguinal region, and as a subset in the genital region (scrotum or labium majus). Examples up to 15 cm in maximum dimension have been described. Similar lesions involving the extremities are usually now interpreted as lipofibromatosis.[25] There is no convincing evidence for a traumatic etiology. Up to 16% of cases recur, usually once, but none has metastasized.

Pathologic Features

Fibrous hamartoma is an infiltrative lesion with fibrous and fatty areas. Microscopically, it comprises three types of tissue. Branching cellular fibrous bands extend through lesional mature adipose tissue, with clusters of ovoid or stellate more primitive-looking cells which are sometimes perivascular (Fig. 3.7, e-Figs. 3.25–3.27).[25] The spindle component can be neurofibroma-like with increased cellularity, sinuous nuclei, and wavy collagen (e-Fig. 3.26). The proportions of the components vary; some cases have a predominance of adipose tissue, and not all components are present in every biopsy.

Ancillary Investigations

The spindle cells are focally positive for SMA and rarely for desmin or CD34, but nonimmunoreactive for S100 protein. They show ultrastructural evidence of fibroblastic or myofibroblastic differentiation, and features suggestive of smooth muscle differentiation have also been described.[26] The immature cellular component expresses vimentin only. Two translocations, t(2;3)

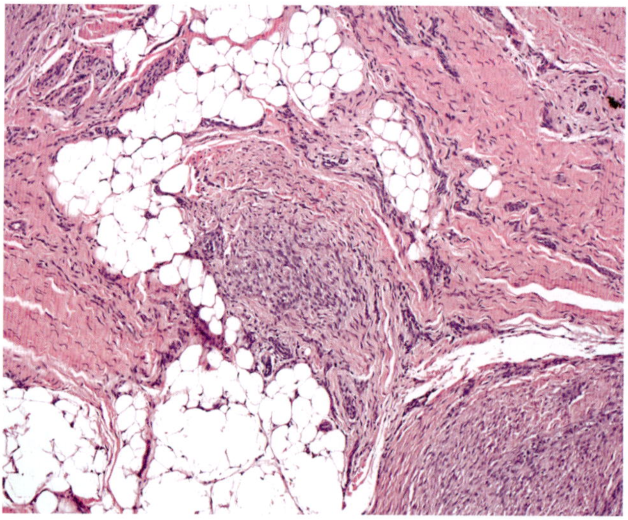

FIGURE 3.7. **Fibrous Hamartoma of Infancy.** Subcutaneous fat is infiltrated by broad bundles of fibroblastic spindle cells. The darker-staining central area represents the undifferentiated component.

(q31;q21)[27] and a complex t(6;12;8)(q25;q24.3;q13),[28] have been reported in examples of fibrous hamartoma of infancy, favoring a neoplastic nature.

LIPOFIBROMATOSIS

Clinical Features

This typically occurs in childhood with age range from 11 days to 12 years (median 1 year), as an ill-defined firm lesion principally in the hands and feet, including digits.[29] Examples have also been described in distal and proximal limbs, and trunk.

Pathologic Features

The excised specimen shows fat interspersed with firm white fibrous areas. On microscopy, bands of moderately cellular fibrous tissue infiltrate adipose tissue, and skeletal muscle or dermis, surrounding adnexa and nerves (Fig. 3.8, e-Figs. 3.28 and 3.29). The spindle cells lack atypia and mitoses are rare. The adipose tissue is histologically normal, but small univacuolated "microfat" cells can be seen at the interface with the fibrous bands; these should not be mistaken for lipoblasts. Lipofibromatosis lacks the 'primitive' round cell component of fibrous hamartoma of infancy which it otherwise resembles.

Ancillary Investigations

Lipofibromatosis is variably and focally immunoreactive for CD34, CD99, SMA, and EMA.[25]

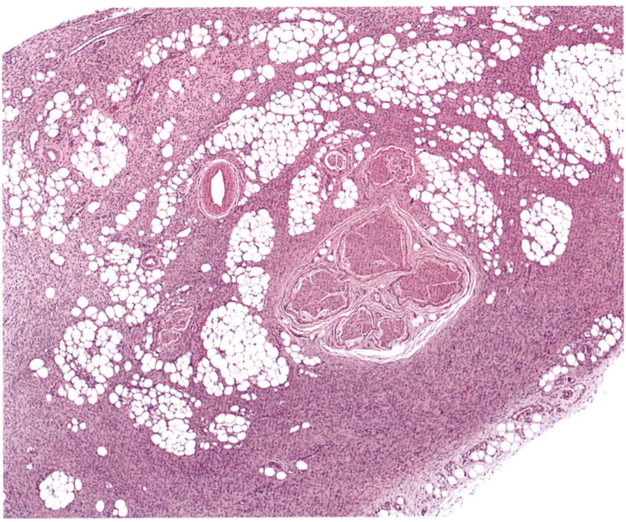

FIGURE 3.8. **Lipofibromatosis.** Cellular bands and trabeculae of fibroblastic spindle cells infiltrate adipose tissue in a complex anastomosing pattern, and surround nerves.

NASOPHARYNGEAL ANGIOFIBROMA

Clinical Features

Also termed juvenile nasopharyngeal angiofibroma, this lesion occurs mostly in pubertal or adolescent males aged 10 to 20 years (median age15[30]) with occasional cases in older males or in females. This arises in nasopharynx or paranasal sinuses, causing obstruction or epistaxis, and can extend into cheek or orbit producing related symptoms including facial swelling. Very rare extrapharyngeal examples have involved paranasal sinuses or nasal turbinate, and some cases have been associated with familial adenomatous polyposis.[31]

Pathologic Features

This appears as a smooth-surfaced highly vascular polypoid mass covered by mucosa and is spongy on section. Microscopy shows dilated endothelial-lined vessels that have no or only a focal smooth muscle layer and lack elastic (except in larger peripheral vessels) and lie within a moderately or sparsely cellular densely fibrous stroma.(Fig. 3.9, e-Figs. 3.30 and 3.31) The stromal cells are ovoid or spindle-shaped fibroblasts which sometimes show small nucleoli and mild nuclear pleomorphism.

Ancillary Investigations

The stromal cells are focally immunoreactive for SMA, and in all cases show diffuse nuclear positivity for beta-catenin (e-Fig. 3.32),[32] assisting diagnosis from sinonasal hemangiopericytoma. Immunoreactivity for

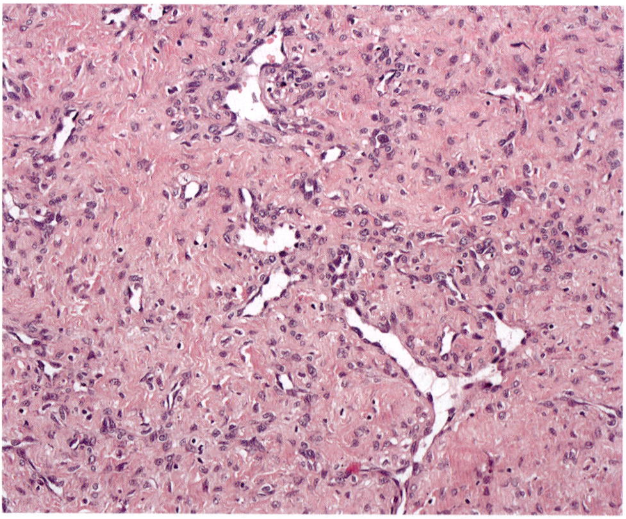

FIGURE 3.9. **Juvenile Angiofibroma.** This comprises branching, dilated thin-walled vessels within fibrous stroma containing dispersed ovoid or short spindle cells. Note the prominent endothelial cells.

androgen receptors is found in both endothelial and stromal cells.[33] In keeping with the overexpression of beta-catenin, mutations in the beta-catenin oncogene have been found.[32]

SOLITARY FIBROUS TUMOR

Clinical Features

The term solitary fibrous tumor (SFT) now subsumes most lesions that were previously termed hemangiopericytoma[34] based on the irregularly branching, dilated staghorn pattern of their vasculature, and absence of specific differentiation. Among specific subtypes, once SFTs have been separated out, infantile hemangiopericytoma is now categorized as part of the myofibroma spectrum,[35] sinonasal hemangiopericytoma is considered to show myopericytic or glomus-like differentiation,[36] and meningeal hemangiopericytoma is regarded as a SFT-like neoplasm distinct from meningioma.[37]

SFT arises mostly in adults of either sex and is found in any site[38] but mainly in deep soft tissue (with a subset in subcutis), pelvis, abdomen (including mesentery, retroperitoneum, and paratesticular region), and thorax (pleura, mediastinum, pericardium and lung), nasal cavity, orbit and meninges. Examples have also been described in viscera including thyroid, kidney, lower urinary tract, and salivary gland. SFT can present as a painless mass or by mass effects, and some intra-abdominal tumors cause symptomatic hypoglycemia because they secrete insulin-like growth factors (IGF), especially IGF-2, with activation of the insulin receptor pathway.[39] This tumor is categorized as intermediate (rarely metastasizing) in the WHO 2002 Classification.

Pathologic Features

SFT is a circumscribed, unencapsulated firm tumor usually up to 10 cm in diameter, although larger examples have been described. Rarely there is cyst formation. Pleural lesions can be pedunculated. Microscopically, the lesions display variable cellularity, including hypocellular fibrous areas and focal myxoid change (Fig. 3.10, e-Figs. 3.33–3.35). In the more cellular parts, the cells are typically arranged in a random ("patternless") fashion (Fig. 3.11, e-Figs. 3.36 and 3.37), although storiform areas can also be seen. The tumor cells are generally uniform but can vary in shape from spindled to ovoid, with darkly staining slender or paler, more ovoid nuclei, and scanty cytoplasm with indistinct cell boundaries (Fig. 3.12). Pleomorphism is unusual, but occasional larger mononuclear cells as well as small multinucleated cells can be encountered. The fibrous areas can vary from thick collagen bundles (e-Fig. 3.38), sometimes organized as amianthoid fibers (e-Figs. 3.39 and 3.40) to hyalinized sheets, and can be very sparsely cellular. As in many sclerosing tumors, the collagen contains artifactual linear cracks. Focal myxoid change is common, and rarely it is predominant (e-Figs.

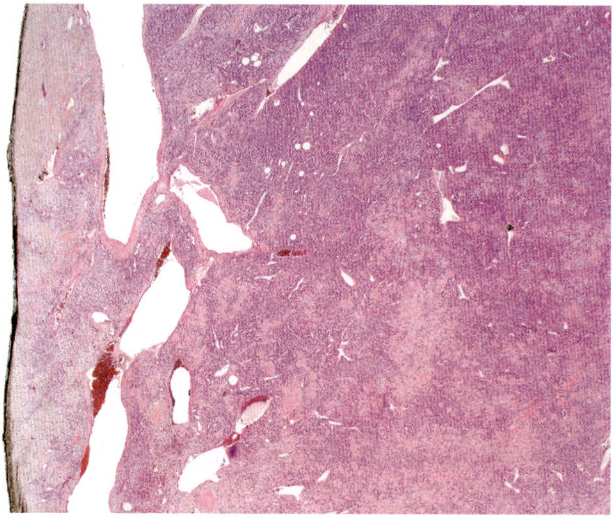

FIGURE 3.10. **Solitary Fibrous Tumor.** Low magnification shows a circumscribed tumor with peripheral hemangiopericytic vascular spaces, and central fibrous and cellular areas.

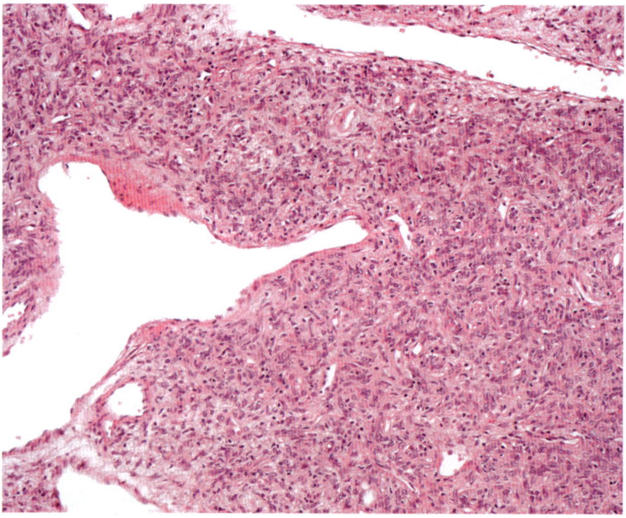

FIGURE 3.11. **Solitary Fibrous Tumor.** Cellular example showing patternless sheets of short spindle cells and dilated hemangiopericytomatous vascular spaces.

3.41 and 3.42).[40] The blood vessels have a focally pericytomatous pattern, often accentuated near the periphery of the lesion (Fig. 3.10, e-Fig. 3.34), and mast cells are prominent. Elsewhere there are numerous medium-sized and smaller vessels, many of which have perivascular hyalinization. Similar lesions that contain variable amounts of mature adipose tissue

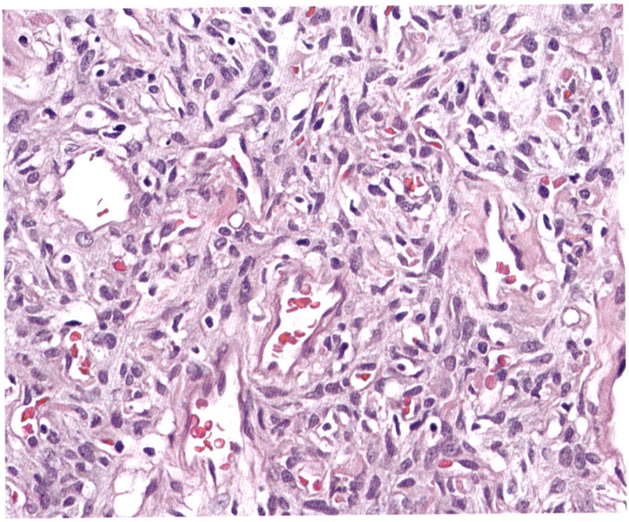

FIGURE 3.12. **Solitary fibrous tumor.** This typical pattern shows randomly orientated short spindle cells, in a fibrous stroma with inflammation and dilated thin-walled vessels.

(Fig. 3.12, e-Figs. 3.43–3.45) have been described as lipomatous hemangiopericytoma[41] and those with small giant cells as giant cell angiofibroma (e-Figs. 3.46 and 3.47).[42] Rationally, however, they might be designated as SFTs with an adipose tissue or giant cell component, respectively.[34]

Ancillary Investigations

The immunophenotype is summarized in Fig. 3.13. The lesional spindle and giant cells express CD34, either focally or diffusely (e-Figs. 3.48 and 3.49), and bcl-2 and CD99 are usually positive also. Some examples express beta-catenin and podoplanin.[43] Rarely, there is CD117 positivity; this is usually cytoplasmic and focal, but care should be taken with intra-abdominal tumors not to misdiagnose gastrointestinal stromal tumor. Electron microscopy reveals fibroblastic differentiation with rare cases containing some myofibroblasts. Chromosomal abnormalities have been described including trisomy 21, rearrangements at 4q13, and various translocations in tumors described as SFT[44] or hemangiopericytoma.[45] The findings are not consistent, though most rearrangements involve 12q, or less commonly 4q.

Criteria of Malignancy

Nuclear crowding or pleomorphism, more than 4 mitoses per 10 hpf (e-Fig. 3.50), and necrosis are indicators of malignant potential, although examples without these features have recurred or metastasized. Some SFT have a frankly sarcomatous component, with pleomorphism, high mitotic index, and necrosis, and this can sometimes appear in the course of recurrent

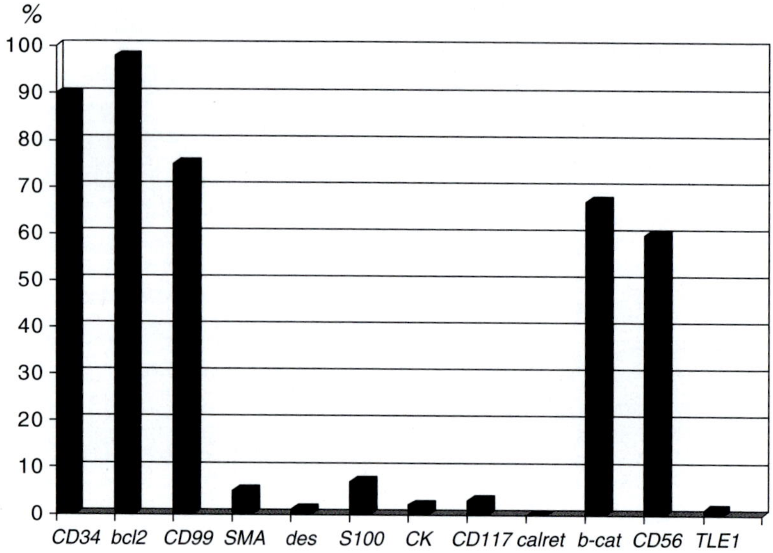

FIGURE 3.13. **Immunophenotype of SFT.**

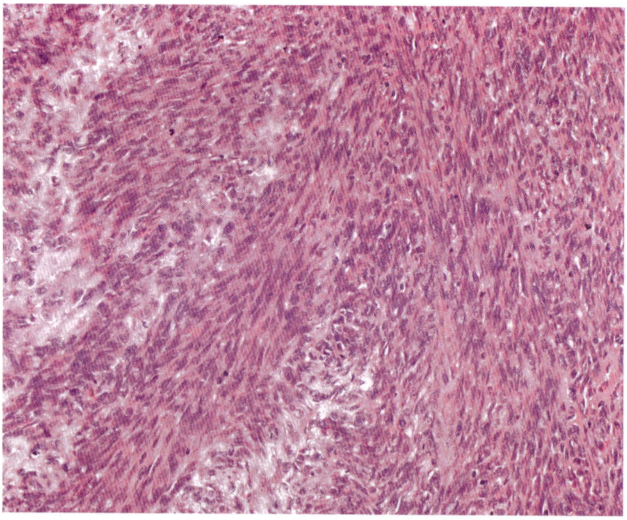

FIGURE 3.14. **Malignant SFT.** This is composed of highly cellular fibrosarcoma-like fascicles of short spindle cells with mitotic activity. This patient had typical SFT at this site some years earlier.

disease or as a presumed metastasis. Frankly malignant SFT resembles adult fibrosarcoma (Fig 3.14, e-Fig. 3.51) and can be CD34-positive (e-Fig. 3.52) or CD34-negative. In either event, diagnosis of sarcoma arising in SFT requires the presence of an adjacent typical component, or occurrence at

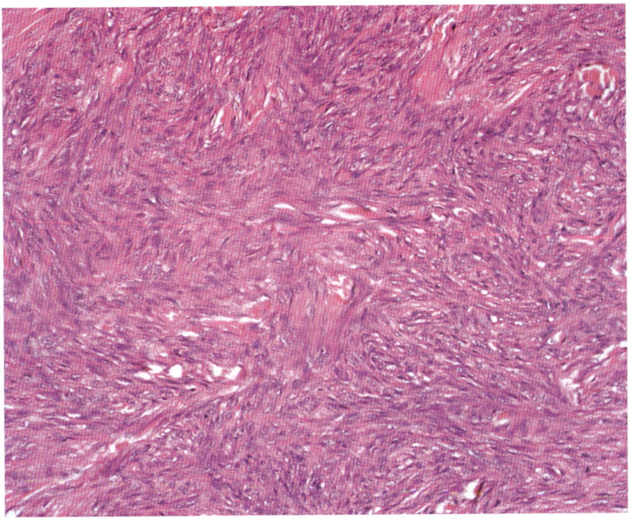

FIGURE 3.15. **Deep Benign Fibrous Histiocytoma.** Intersecting bundles of fibroblastic cells without significant atypia.

the site of a previously documented SFT.[46] Regular SFT with abrupt transition to a pleomorphic undifferentiated component can be referred to as dedifferentiation, but since both components have the same (fibroblastic) lineage, this is not an appropriate term.

DEEP BENIGN FIBROUS HISTIOCYTOMA

Clinical Features

This is a lesion that arises at any age but mostly in adults (mean 37 years) and more frequently in males.[47] Most examples arise in subcutaneous tissue of extremities or head and neck region but occasionally in retroperitoneum, mediastinum, or pelvis. The tumor presents as a discrete mass and is mostly small (mean 3 cm) but can reach 25 cm in diameter. Of 37 cases with follow-up, 22% recurred in relation to incomplete excision, and two metastasized including one with necrosis but no other distinguishing features.

Pathologic Features

Deep BFH is circumscribed (e-Fig. 3.53) and sometimes well encapsulated, and is composed of short spindle cells with storiform or focally fascicular architecture (Fig. 3.15, e-Fig. 3.54). There are scattered intralesional lymphocytes and variable features include multinucleated or osteoclast-like giant cells (e-Fig. 3.55), foamy macrophages, a hemangiopericytic vascular pattern, and stromal hyalinization or ossification. Mitotic activity can sometimes exceed 10 per 10 hpf, and rarely there is necrosis.

Ancillary Investigations

In a large series,[47] 40% of cases displayed focal positivity for CD34, and 38% for SMA, with 8% positive for desmin. Deep benign fibrous histiocytoma with CD34 expression can be misdiagnosed as dermatofibrosarcoma but differs in being circumscribed, and in displaying epiphenomena such as giant cells and foamy macrophages, as well as a pericytomatous pattern.

REFERENCES

1. Eyden B, Banerjee SS, Shenjere P, et al. The myofibroblast and its tumours. *J Clin Pathol.* 2009;62:236–249.
2. Bernstein KE, Lattes R. Nodular (pseudosarcomatous) fasciitis, a nonrecurrent lesion: clinicopathologic study of 134 cases. *Cancer.* 1982;49:1668–1678.
3. Hornick JL, Fletcher CD. Intraarticular nodular fasciitis–a rare lesion: clinicopathologic analysis of a series. *Am J Surg Pathol.* 2006;30:237–241.
4. Hollowood K, Fletcher CD. Pseudosarcomatous myofibroblastic proliferations of the spermatic cord ("proliferative funiculitis"). Histologic and immunohistochemical analysis of a distinctive entity. *Am J Surg Pathol.* 1992;16:448–454.
5. Thompson LD, Fanburg-Smith JC, Wenig BM. Nodular fasciitis of the external ear region: a clinicopathologic study of 50 cases. *Ann Diagn Pathol.* 2001;5:191–198.
6. Montgomery EA, Meis JM. Nodular fasciitis. Its morphologic spectrum and immunohistochemical profile. *Am J Surg Pathol.* 1991;15:942–948.
7. Ceballos KM, Nielsen GP, Selig MK, O'Connell JX. Is anti-h-caldesmon useful for distinguishing smooth muscle and myofibroblastic tumors? An immunohistochemical study. *Am J Clin Pathol.* 2000;114:746–753.
8. Eyden B. The fibronexus in reactive and tumoral myofibroblasts: further characterisation by electron microscopy. *Histol Histopathol.* 2001;16:57–70.
9. Patel RM, Weiss SW, Folpe AL. Heterotopic mesenteric ossification: a distinctive pseudosarcoma commonly associated with intestinal obstruction. *Am J Surg Pathol.* 2006;30:119–122.
10. Patchefsky AS, Enzinger FM. Intravascular fasciitis: a report of 17 cases. *Am J Surg Pathol.* 1981;5:29–36.
11. Sarangarajan R, Dehner LP. Cranial and extracranial fasciitis of childhood: a clinicopathologic and immunohistochemical study. *Hum Pathol.* 1999;30:87–92.
12. Chung EB, Enzinger FM. Proliferative fasciitis. *Cancer.* 1975;36:1450–1458.
13. Meis JM, Enzinger FM. Proliferative fasciitis and myositis of childhood. *Am J Surg Pathol.* 1992;16:364–372.
14. Ghadially FN, Thomas MJ, Jabi M, et al. Intracisternal collagen fibrils in proliferative fasciitis and myositis of childhood. *Ultrastruct Pathol.* 1993;17:161–168.
15. Sasano H, Yamaki H, Ohashi Y, et al. Proliferative fasciitis of the forearm: case report with immunohistochemical, ultrastructural and DNA ploidy studies and a review of the literature. *Pathol Int.* 1998;48:486–490.
16. Dembinski A, Bridge JA, Neff JR, et al. Trisomy 2 in proliferative fasciitis. *Cancer Genet Cytogenet.* 1992;60:27–30.
17. Enzinger FM, Dulcey F. Proliferative myositis. Report of thirty-three cases. *Cancer.* 1967;20:2213–2223.
18. el-Jabbour JN, Wilson GD, Bennett MH, et al. Flow cytometric study of nodular fasciitis, proliferative fasciitis, and proliferative myositis. *Hum Pathol.* 1991;22:1146–1149.

19. McComb EN, Neff JR, Johansson SL, et al. Chromosomal anomalies in a case of proliferative myositis. *Cancer Genet Cytogenet.* 1997;98:142–144.
20. Montgomery EA, Meis JM, Mitchell MS, et al. Atypical decubital fibroplasia. A distinctive fibroblastic pseudotumor occurring in debilitated patients. *Am J Surg Pathol.* 1992;16:708–715.
21. Liegl B, Fletcher CD. Ischemic fasciitis: analysis of 44 cases indicating an inconsistent association with immobility or debilitation. *Am J Surg Pathol.* 2008;32:1546–1552.
22. Boudova L, Michal M. Atypical decubital fibroplasia associated with bizarre parosteal osteochondromatous proliferation (Nora's reaction). *Pathol Res Pract.* 1999;195:99–103; discussion 104.
23. Fukunaga M. Atypical decubital fibroplasia with unusual histology. *Apmis.* 2001;109:631–635.
24. Dickey GE, Sotelo-Avila C. Fibrous hamartoma of infancy: current review. *Pediatr Dev Pathol.* 1999;2:236–243.
25. Fletcher CD, Powell G, van Noorden S, et al. Fibrous hamartoma of infancy: a histochemical and immunohistochemical study. *Histopathology.* 1988;12:65–74.
26. Groisman G, Lichtig C. Fibrous hamartoma of infancy: an immunohistochemical and ultrastructural study. *Hum Pathol.* 1991;22:914–918.
27. Lakshminarayanan R, Konia T, Welborn J. Fibrous hamartoma of infancy: a case report with associated cytogenetic findings. *Arch Pathol Lab Med.* 2005;129:520–522.
28. Rougemont AL, Fetni R, Murthy S, et al. A complex translocation (6;12;8)(q25;q24.3;q13) in a fibrous hamartoma of infancy. *Cancer Genet Cytogenet.* 2006;171:115–118.
29. Fetsch JF, Miettinen M, Laskin WB, et al. A clinicopathologic study of 45 pediatric soft tissue tumors with an admixture of adipose tissue and fibroblastic elements, and a proposal for classification as lipofibromatosis. *Am J Surg Pathol.* 2000;24:1491–1500.
30. Glad H, Vainer B, Buchwald C, et al. Juvenile nasopharyngeal angiofibromas in Denmark 1981–2003: diagnosis, incidence, and treatment. *Acta Otolaryngol.* 2007;127:292–299.
31. Giardiello FM, Hamilton SR, Krush AJ, et al. Nasopharyngeal angiofibroma in patients with familial adenomatous polyposis. *Gastroenterology.* 1993;105:1550–1552.
32. Abraham SC, Montgomery EA, Giardiello FM, et al. Frequent beta-catenin mutations in juvenile nasopharyngeal angiofibromas. *Am J Pathol.* 2001;158:1073–1078.
33. Hwang HC, Mills SE, Patterson K, et al. Expression of androgen receptors in nasopharyngeal angiofibroma: an immunohistochemical study of 24 cases. *Mod Pathol.* 1998;11:1122–1126.
34. Gengler C, Guillou L. Solitary fibrous tumour and haemangiopericytoma: evolution of a concept. *Histopathology.* 2006;48:63–74.
35. Mentzel T, Calonje E, Nascimento AG, et al. Infantile hemangiopericytoma versus infantile myofibromatosis. Study of a series suggesting a continuous spectrum of infantile myofibroblastic lesions. *Am J Surg Pathol.* 1994;18:922–930.
36. Thompson LD, Miettinen M, Wenig BM. Sinonasal-type hemangiopericytoma: a clinicopathologic and immunophenotypic analysis of 104 cases showing perivascular myoid differentiation. *Am J Surg Pathol.* 2003;27:737–749.
37. Tihan T, Viglione M, Rosenblum MK, et al. Solitary fibrous tumors in the central nervous system. A clinicopathologic review of 18 cases and comparison to meningeal hemangiopericytomas. *Arch Pathol Lab Med.* 2003;127:432–439.
38. Chan JK. Solitary fibrous tumour–everywhere, and a diagnosis in vogue. *Histopathology.* 1997;31:568–576.
39. Li Y, Chang Q, Rubin BP, et al. Insulin receptor activation in solitary fibrous tumours. *J Pathol.* 2007;211:550–554.
40. de Saint Aubain Somerhausen N, Rubin BP, Fletcher CD. Myxoid solitary fibrous tumor: a study of seven cases with emphasis on differential diagnosis. *Mod Pathol.* 1999;12:463–471.

41. Guillou L, Gebhard S, Coindre JM. Lipomatous hemangiopericytoma: a fat-containing variant of solitary fibrous tumor? Clinicopathologic, immunohistochemical, and ultrastructural analysis of a series in favor of a unifying concept. *Hum Pathol.* 2000;31:1108–1115.

42. Guillou L, Gebhard S, Coindre JM. Orbital and extraorbital giant cell angiofibroma: a giant cell-rich variant of solitary fibrous tumor? Clinicopathologic and immunohistochemical analysis of a series in favor of a unifying concept. *Am J Surg Pathol.* 2000;24:971–979.

43. Naito Y, Ishii G, Kawai O, et al. D2-40-positive solitary fibrous tumors of the pleura: diagnostic pitfall of biopsy specimen. *Pathol Int.* 2007;57:618–621.

44. Horton ES, Dobin SM, Donner LR. A clonal t(8;12)(p11.2;q24.3) as the sole abnormality in a solitary fibrous tumor of the pleura. *Cancer Genet Cytogenet.* 2007;172:77–79.

45. Henn W, Wullich B, Thonnes M, et al. Recurrent t(12;19)(q13;q13.3) in intracranial and extracranial hemangiopericytoma. *Cancer Genet Cytogenet.* 1993;71:151–154.

46. Vallat-Decouvelaere AV, Dry SM, Fletcher CD. Atypical and malignant solitary fibrous tumors in extrathoracic locations: evidence of their comparability to intra-thoracic tumors. *Am J Surg Pathol.* 1998;22:1501–1511.

47. Gleason BC, Fletcher CD. Deep “benign” fibrous histiocytoma: clinicopathologic analysis of 69 cases of a rare tumor indicating occasional metastatic potential. *Am J Surg Pathol.* 2008;32:354–362.

4

CUTANEOUS SPINDLE CELL LESIONS

INTRODUCTION

This chapter considers diagnosis of common spindle cell lesions predominantly occurring in dermis and superficial subcutis. They include reactive lesions and benign and malignant neoplasms, which can be cellular or accumulate variable amounts of myxoid or collagenous stroma. Many are fibroblastic or myofibroblastic but some melanocytic lesions also enter the differential diagnosis, as well as tumors with smooth muscle differentiation (Chapter 6) or nerve sheath differentiation (Chapters 9 and 10). Vascular tumors are discussed in Chapter 17, and predominantly myxoid lesions are discussed in Chapter 20. The differential diagnosis is summarized in Table 4.1.

KELOID

Clinical Features

This is an aberrant reaction to injury, especially surgical incision, or infection, often some time before the development of the lesion. It is most common in young adults, and more often seen in the upper part of the body, including anterior chest wall, head and neck, and upper limb and limb girdle. There is a familial component in some cases, an increased incidence in individuals with pigmented skin, and an association with scleroderma and other connective tissue diseases.[1] Mechanical factors such as stretching of the skin may also play a role in genesis of the lesions, which can enlarge during pregnancy. Keloid presents as a raised rounded or linear skin nodule, which is at first red and later paler. The lesions continue to grow, albeit slowly, and do not regress, but are prone to local recurrence following excision. Other available treatments include radiation therapy, and intralesional and topical application of various agents, including corticosteroids, interferon, 5-fluorouracil, and imiquimod.[2] However, most therapeutic applications for keloid (and hypertrophic scar) offer little improvement.[3]

TABLE 4.1 Differential Diagnosis of Cutaneous Spindle Cell Neoplasms

Tumor Type	Pattern	Morphology	Ancillary Investigations
Keloid	Randomly oriented thick collagen fibers in dermis, can extend beyond site of wound. Low cellularity	Eosinophilic thick collagen bundles, sparse bland fibroblastic spindle cells	Nil specific
Cellular (hypertrophic) scar	Variously oriented fibroblasts More cellular than keloid and restricted to site of wound	Bland tapered spindle cells, no nuclear atypia	SMA+, low MIB proliferation index
Cellular fibrous histiocytoma	Epidermal hyperplasia. Cellular fascicles in dermis, extensions into fat, short and pointed, radial to surface. Peripheral collagen bundles	Uniform tapered cells with ovoid nuclei and scanty cytoplasm, Touton giant cells, Hemorrhage and siderophages if aneurysmal component. Focal cellular pleomorphism in atypical variant	SMA+, FXIIIa+
Dermatofibrosarcoma	Diffusely storiform, infiltrates parallel to skin surface with extensive honeycombing of fat. Pattern changes to fascicular in fibrosarcomatous transformation.	Long cells, scanty cytoplasm, uniform tapered, slightly wavy nuclei. Focal or diffuse myxoid change Mitotic activity increases in fibrosarcomatous variant	CD34+, bcl2+. S100 protein+ in pigmented cells of Bednar variant. t(17;22)(q22;q13) with fusion gene *COL1A1-PDGFRB* Fibrosarcomatous variant similar but can be CD34-positive or CD34-negative

Giant cell fibroblastoma	Poorly circumscribed in skin and subcutis, variably cellular without distinct pattern except where coexistent dermatofibrosarcoma. Irregular pseudovascular spaces lined by lesional cells	Spindle and apparently multinucleated cells (in reality, each has a single highly convoluted nucleus) in fibrous and myxoid stroma.	CD34+, bcl2+, t(17;22)(q22;q13) with fusion gene *COL1A1-PDGFRB*
Dermal nerve sheath myxoma	Circumscribed multilobulated myxoid lesion, low cellularity	Spindle cells can show focal pleomorphism	S100 protein+ in myxoid areas, EMA+ at periphery of nodules
Superficial angiomyxoma	Non-circumscribed, multinodular, infiltrative in dermis and subcutis. Random pattern, not storiform or fascicular	Bland short to medium-length spindle or stellate fibroblasts in myxoid stroma, variable vascularity, scattered neutrophils	CD34+ (focally), S100 protein–
Neurofibroma, typical	Non-encapsulated, ill-defined fascicles, but not widely infiltrative except diffuse type.	Mixture of wavy cells, axons, collagen fibers, mast cells	S100 protein+ (not all cells), EMA+ very rarely focally, CD34+ focally. NF+ in axons
Neurofibroma, diffuse	Subcutaneous infiltrative plaque. Some associated with plexiform neurofibroma–extends outside nerve bundles into soft tissue	Sheets of short spindle cells in loose fibrous stroma, infiltrating between normal structures Wagner-Meissner bodies in various stages	S100 protein+ diffusely in nuclei

(Continued)

TABLE 4.1 **Differential Diagnosis of Cutaneous Spindle Cell Neoplasms (Continued)**

Tumor Type	Pattern	Morphology	Ancillary Investigations
Atypical fibroxanthoma	Dome-shaped with overlying epidermal thinning or ulceration. Dermal infiltrate is storiform, fascicular, or patternless	Pleomorphic spindle and polygonal cells throughout, abnormal mitoses. Clear cell, spindle cell and giant cell variants	SMA+ focally, CD10+
Kaposi sarcoma	Cellular, curved fascicles, sieve-like areas in cross-section, hemorrhage	Mildly pleomorphic cells, mitoses, hyaline globules, red cell extravasation	HHV8+, CD31+, CD34+, podoplanin (D2-40)+. S100 protein–
Angiosarcoma	Variable vascular channel formation and cellular areas, with hemorrhage	Spaces lined by atypical endothelial cells. Solid areas can have spindled or epithelioid cells.	CD34+, CD31+, FVIIIRAg+, FLI-1+, CK±, S100 protein–negative, desmin–
Leiomyoma	Nodular or diffuse, fascicles intersecting at right angles	Spindle cells with eosinophilic cytoplasm, non-tapering nuclei. No pleomorphism, mitotic activity, or necrosis	SMA+, desmin+, h-caldesmon+ S100 protein–
Leiomyosarcoma	Fascicles of varying size, intersecting at right angles	Spindle cells with eosinophilic cytoplasm, nontapering nuclei. Variable pleomorphism, mitotic activity, or necrosis according to grade	SMA+, desmin+, h-caldesmon+ S100 protein–
Spindle cell carcinoma	Sheets, nests, and storiform whorls. Areas of epithelial morphology. Overlying epithelial dysplasia or carcinoma	Pleomorphic spindle or epithelioid tumor cells. Sheet-like epithelial areas, transitions to sarcomatous morphology. Nested reticulin pattern.	CK+, EMA+, INI1+, CD34 negative, SMA+, P63+ in some, desmin-negative, h-caldesmon– S100 protein–

Myofibroma	Bundles or whorls of myofibroblastic spindle cells with foci of smaller darker cells, focal pericytomatous pattern. Can be focally necrotic or calcified	Spindle cells have ovoid nuclei, small nucleoli, tapering eosinophilic cytoplasm. Mitoses in some, but no atypia	SMA+, calponin+, desmin−, h-caldesmon−.
Dermatomyofibroma	Cellular fascicles run parallel (tangential) to skin surface. Mild adjacent epidermal hyperplasia.	Bland myofibroblastic spindle cells, ovoid nucleoli, small nucleoli, tapering cytoplasm.	SMA+, calponin+, desmin−, h-caldesmon−.
Nodular fasciitis	Variably myxoid, cellular, and collagenous areas. Mitoses but no nuclear atypia or necrosis	Spindle cells have ovoid nuclei, small nucleoli, tapering cytoplasm. Mitoses in some, but no atypia	SMA+, desmin±, h-caldesmon−
Spindle cell lipoma	Circumscribed, fatty component, collagen fibrils, mast cells. Myxoid variant	Short spindle cells, very occasional lipoblasts acceptable	CD34+, rarely S100 protein+, MDM2 & CDK4 usually−
Perineurioma	Circumscribed, variably cellular fascicles, with myxoid or fibrous stroma	Elongated bipolar or tripolar cells with very long terminal processes	EMA+, claudin-1+, GLUT-1+, CD34+,
Low grade fibromyxoid sarcoma	Ill-defined. Fibrous and myxoid areas with swirling pattern collagen cracking. Occasional hyaline rosettes	Bland cells with uniformly staining nuclei, sometimes rectangular, indiscernible cytoplasm	Occasional EMA+, claudin-1+. Rarely SMA+ or CD34+. t(7;16)(q34;p11) with fusion gene *FUS-CREB3L2* or *CREB3L1*

(Continued)

TABLE 4.1 Differential Diagnosis of Cutaneous Spindle Cell Neoplasms (Continued)

Tumor Type	Pattern	Morphology	Ancillary Investigations
Malignant melanoma, desmoplastic	Junctional activity present or absent. Spindle cells singly or in separated bundles infiltrating dermis and subcutis. Neurotropism	Spindle or focally epithelioid cells with nuclear pleomorphism, scanty cytoplasm, mitoses	S100 protein+ diffusely, HMB45 or melan-A+ rarely
Malignant Peripheral nerve sheatch tumor	No junctional activity. Bundles and sheaves of spindle cells. Occasional neurotropism	Elongated spindle cells, wavy or buckled nuclei. Epithelioid areas.	S100 protein+ focally
Clear cell sarcoma	Extremities especially lower limb, young adults.	Round or spindled cells in nests, round nuclei with central nucleolus, clear or granular cytoplasm, multinucleated cells, melanin pigment	S100 protein+, HMB45+ and melan A+ (other markers negative, t(12;22)(q13;q12), *EWSR1-ATF1* in soft tissue cases
PEComa	Can rarely arise in skin	Nests of ovoid or spindled cells with abundant clear or rarely granular cytoplasm, delicate fibrous septa	SMA+, HMB45+, melan-A+, desmin+ in some CD117+ in some, S100 protein+ rarely
Anaplastic large cell lymphoma	Cutaneous involvement can occur with or without nodal disease.	Sheets of cells with prominent nucleoli, multinucleated forms. Can be spindled.	CD30+, ALK+, CD43+, CD45+, CD3+, TIA1+, t(2;5)(p23;q35), *TMP3-ALK* fusion
Mycobacterial spindle cell pseudotumor	Sheets of spindle cells with storiform pattern and plump epithelioid macrophages	Cells have abundant eosinophilic cytoplasm. Foamy and multinucleated cells sometime seen	Ziehl-Neelsen stain for acid-fast bacilli is positive, revealing numerous organisms

Pathologic Features

The characteristic feature is the presence of thick, eosinophilic collagen fibers arranged randomly in the dermis (Fig. 4.1, e-Figs. 4.1–4.3). There are scattered bland spindle cells, and in older, more hyalinized lesions, there can be calcification or ossification. The overlying epidermis is thinned, and adnexa are separated by lesional tissue at the deep aspect. The lack of cellularity helps to exclude the rare dermatofibroma with focal keloidal change.[4]

Ancillary Investigations

Ultrastructurally, the lesional spindle cells are mostly fibroblastic and lack lineage markers including smooth muscle actin (SMA), which can help in diagnosis from other dermal myofibroblastic proliferations. Ki67 demonstrates proliferative activity, notwithstanding the sparse cellularity. Gene profiling has shown altered expression in multiple fibrosis-related pathways and differences in expression of caspase genes between normal skin of keloid-prone individuals and normal skin of keloid-resistant patients, which might contribute to susceptibility to develop keloids.[5]

Cellular scars are intradermal fibroblastic myofibroblastic lesions characterized by nodules of spindle cells orientated in various directions, without nuclear atypia or pleomorphism (e-Figs. 4.2 and 4.3). There is usually a recent history of trauma or surgery, and there is a predilection for flexor surfaces near joints, and the abdominal wall. They can be distinguished from keloid by their lack of infiltration beyond the original wound site, prominent blood vessels, absence of thick collagen fibers, SMA

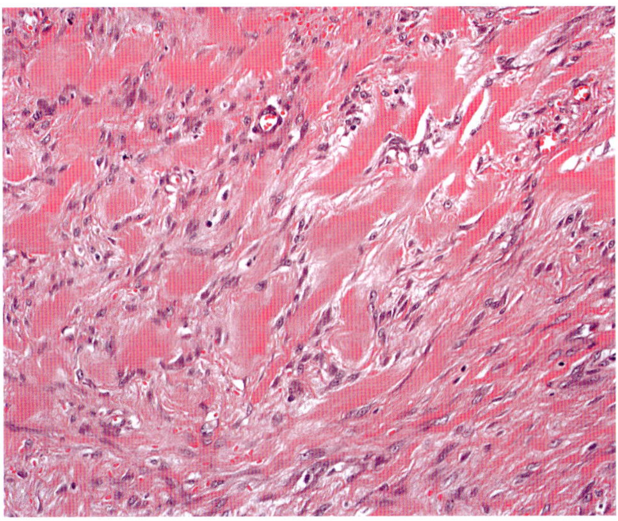

FIGURE 4.1. **Keloid.** Thick eosinophilic collagen fibers are disposed in a cellular fibroblastic stroma.

positivity, lower proliferation index with Ki67, and tendency to regress; from dermatomyofibroma by the lack of tangential orientation; and from fibromatosis by the hypocellularity, lack of alignment, and regular spacing of the lesional cells (e-Figs. 4.4 and 4.5).

SCLEROTIC FIBROMA (CIRCUMSCRIBED STORIFORM COLLAGENOMA)

Clinical Features

This is a solitary dermal nodule arising mainly on face, limbs, and trunk and presenting as a small pale well-demarcated papule. It is histologically identical to the multiple skin nodules that arise in Cowden syndrome.[6] The lesion is benign but an occasional example has recurred.

Pathologic Features

The lesions are rounded, sharply demarcated dermal nodules characterized by a whorled or laminated, thickened, collagen bundles containing scanty bland spindle cells and separated by clefts containing stromal mucin (Fig. 4.2, e-Figs. 4.6–4.9). The overlying epidermis is thinned. A pleomorphic variant, with a component resembling pleomorphic fibroma, has been described.[7] Similar features can be seen focally in the rare sclerotic fibroma-like dermatofibroma[8] and in a variety of other neoplastic and inflammatory skin lesions.

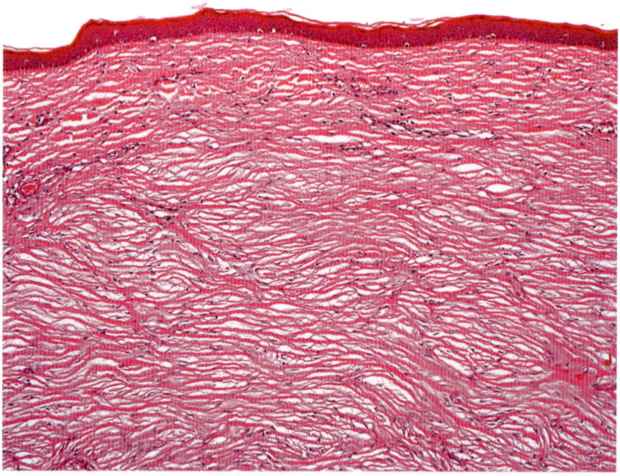

FIGURE 4.2. **Sclerotic Fibroma.** Interwoven laminae formed by collagen fibers form the lesion within the dermis. Bland fibroblasts are seen between the laminae. Note that the overlying epidermis is thinned.

Ancillary Investigations

Some sclerotic fibromas display immunoreactivity for CD34 and CD99. SMA positivity and the presence of FXIIIa-positive dermal dendrocytic cells have also been described.[9]

PLEOMORPHIC FIBROMA

Clinical Features

Pleomorphic fibroma is a rare dome-shaped or polypoid skin lesion occurring in adults of either sex, on extremities, trunk, or face. Reported cases have been benign, with occurrence only of an incompletely excised example. A relationship with sclerotic fibroma has been postulated.[10]

Pathologic Features

This is a circumscribed lesion with sparse spindle cells in a collagenous stroma with scattered cells with enlarged irregularly shaped degenerate-looking nuclei, or multinucleated cells, and rarely mitoses (Fig. 4.3, e-Figs. 4.10 and 4.11). The stroma contains mast cells and occasionally foamy macrophages, and a myxoid variant has been described.[11]

Ancillary Investigations

The lesional cells in some cases are positive for CD34 and CD99.

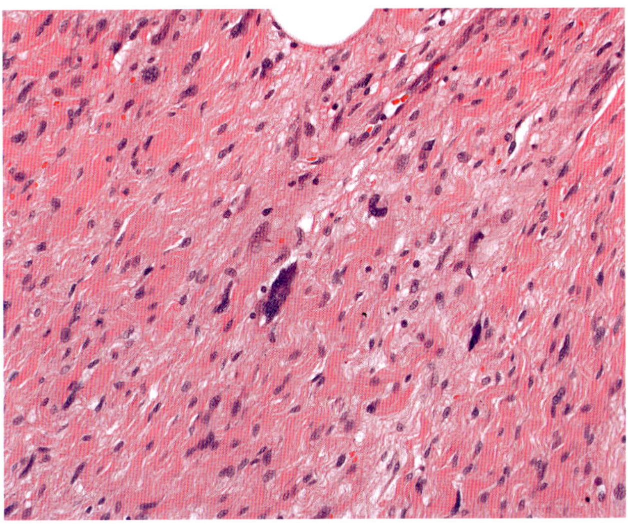

FIGURE 4.3. **Pleomorphic Fibroma.** Spindle cells with hyperchromatic enlarged nuclei are scattered between coarse collagen fibers. Occasional cells are multinucleated.

DERMATOMYOFIBROMA

Clinical Features

This is a dermal lesion that occurs mostly in young adult females and is mostly seen in the shoulder and axilla, with occasional lesions on the neck or trunk.[12] It forms a slowly growing ovoid erythematous plaque that can reach several centimeters in diameter or length. Multiple lesions have been described. The lesion is benign and does not usually recur after surgical excision.

Pathologic Features

Beneath mildly hyperplastic epidermis, the reticular dermis contains a noncircumscribed infiltrate comprising fascicles of bland myofibroblasts arranged tangentially or parallel to the skins surface (Fig. 4.4, e-Figs. 4.12–4.14). Rarely, lesional tissue extends into superficial subcutis. The stroma is collagenous with slightly increased and fragmented elastic fibers. A hemorrhagic variant has been described in male patients.[13]

Ancillary Investigations

The lesional cells are myofibroblasts and are positive for SMA, though not in all cases. Beta-catenin, desmin, h-caldesmon, and CD34 are negative.

CUTANEOUS FIBROUS HISTIOCYTOMA

Clinical Features

Dermatofibroma, or cutaneous fibrous histiocytoma, is a common lesion of young adults that forms a small, dome-shaped elevation that is sometimes

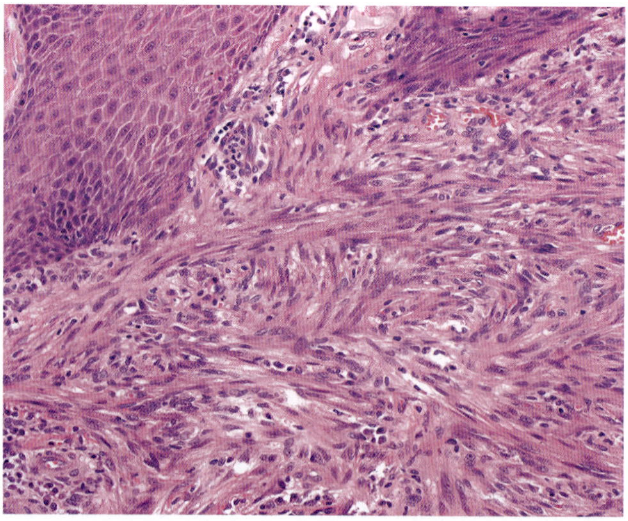

FIGURE 4.4. **Dermatomyofibroma.** Bundles of myofibroblasts are present in the dermis, mostly oriented parallel to the surface. The epidermis is mildly hyperplastic.

pigmented, and rarely multiple. This is usually a benign lesion though a small proportion recur and very rare examples have been reported to metastasize to lymph node and lung.[14]

Pathologic Features

The typical cutaneous fibrous histiocytoma is associated with hyperplasia of overlying epidermis, often with increased basal layers mimicking early basal cell carcinoma. The lesion is located in the dermis with ill-defined lateral margins and is composed of short spindle and ovoid cells with slightly irregularly shaped nuclei in a storiform or loose fascicular pattern (Figs. 4.5 and 4.6). Mitoses are usually few, but occasional enlarged or pleomorphic nuclei can be seen. Significant atypia and mitotic activity indicate categorization as atypical fibrous histiocytoma.[15] There is a variable admixture of lymphocytes, foamy macrophages, Touton giant cells, and siderophages (e-Fig. 4.15). At the lateral aspect, there are increased collagen bundles, which the lesional cells infiltrate (e-Fig. 4.16). The deep margin, when reaching subcutis, shows short radial extensions into the fat (e-Fig. 4.17), or occasionally is circumscribed. This differs from dermatofibrosarcoma, which shows honeycomb infiltration of subcutis with tangential (parallel to surface) spread along interlobular septa within fat. Cytological variants include those with granular (e-Fig. 4.18) or epithelioid (e-Figs. 4.19 and 4.20) cells. The latter can be distinguished from other epithelioid neoplasms by the absence of specific immunohistochemical markers (see Chapter 11). In aneurysmal fibrous histiocytoma (see Chapter 17), hemorrhage results in cyst formation and marked hemosiderin deposition (e-Figs. 4.21 and 4.22). This should not be confused with angiomatoid fibrous histiocytoma (see Chapter 17), which is more deeply located, has a fibrous and lymphoid cuff, expresses desmin, and has characteristic chromosomal translocations.

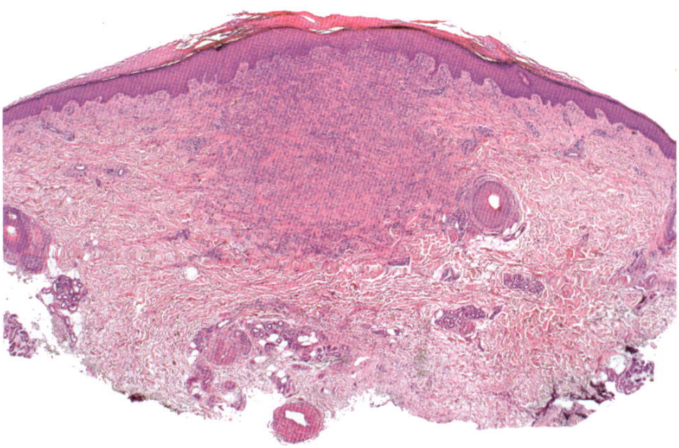

FIGURE 4.5. **Cutaneous Fibrous Histiocytoma.** This scanning view shows epidermal thickening with hyperkeratosis overlying an ill-defined cellular dermal lesion. Note the accentuated collagen bundles at the lateral and deep aspects of the lesion.

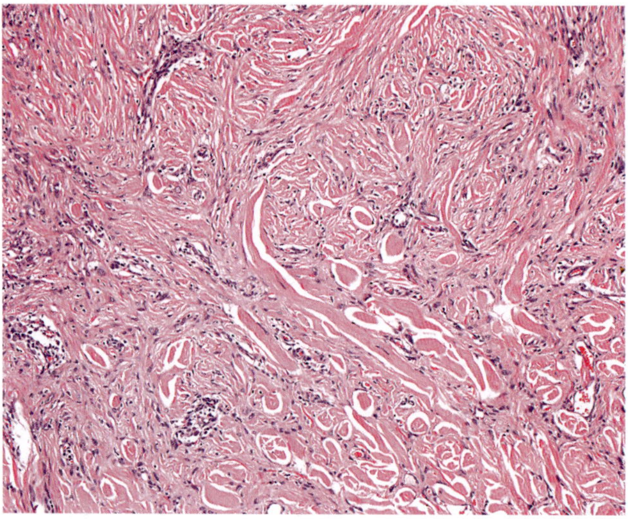

FIGURE 4.6. **Cutaneous Fibrous Histiocytoma.** At the lateral borders of the lesion, spindle cells infiltrate between coarse collagen bundles. This appearance is characteristic of cutaneous fibrous histiocytoma and assists diagnosis from dermatofibrosarcoma.

Ancillary Investigations

Cutaneous fibrous histiocytomas are focally immunoreactive for SMA and FXIIIa, and desmin, CD34, S100 protein, and CK are usually negative. Electron microscopy shows a mixture of fibroblastic, myofibroblastic, and histiocytic features.

VARIANTS

There are numerous cytomorphologic variants of cutaneous fibrous histiocytoma, and many cases show overlapping features of more than one subtype. Relevant here are the cellular variant, which can be confused with malignant spindle cell lesions involving the cutis and subcutis, and the atypical variant, which can be mistaken for pleomorphic sarcoma.

Cellular cutaneous fibrous histiocytoma is seen more frequently in males.[16] It is characterized by a predominantly fascicular spindle cell proliferation with increased mitotic activity and extension into subcutis (Fig. 4.7, e-Figs. 4.23–4.26). Up to 25% of these lesions recur, possibly in relation to incomplete excision, and metastasis to lung has been documented.[17] The cells are elongated with tapered nuclei and scanty cytoplasm, and pleomorphism is not a feature but occasionally there is central necrosis or surface ulceration. Epiphenomena of lymphocytic infiltration, foamy cells, and giant cells can be seen, although to a lesser extent than in usual cutaneous fibrous histiocytomas. Cellular fibrous histiocytoma is often

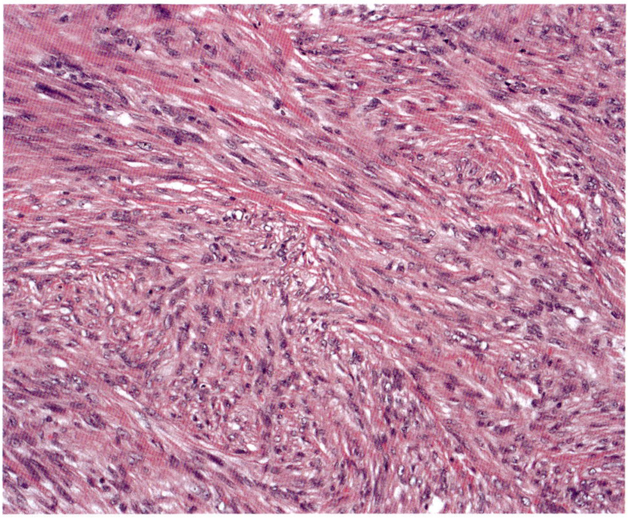

FIGURE 4.7. **Cellular Cutaneous Fibrous histiocytoma.** Fascicles of uniform slender spindle cells stream between collagen fibers. In places, there is a poorly defined whorled pattern.

misdiagnosed as leiomyosarcoma, but the latter lacks epidermal hyperplasia, lateral fibrosis, and epiphenomena, and in leiomyosarcoma, the cells have blunt-ended, parallel-sided nuclei, more eosinophilic cytoplasm, and express desmin and h-caldesmon as well as SMA.

Atypical cutaneous fibrous histiocytoma displays significant pleomorphism and mitotic activity, occasional necrosis, and extension into subcutis.[15] The pleomorphic cells vary in number and have large, hyperchromatic irregularly shaped nuclei and atypical multinucleated forms, with atypical mitoses (Fig. 4.8, e-Figs. 4.27–4.30). Of 21 cases with follow-up information, three recurred but two metastasized.[15] This lesion can be distinguished from atypical fibroxanthoma (see Chapter 13) or superficial pleomorphic sarcoma by the younger age incidence, the extremity location, the epidermal hyperplasia and the background of typical fibrous histiocytoma: in atypical fibroxanthoma, there is epidermal thinning or ulceration and the lesional cells are pleomorphic throughout.

DERMATOFIBROSARCOMA PROTUBERANS

Clinical Features

Dermatofibrosarcoma is a relatively common lesion, which is more frequent in males, with a peak age incidence of 25 to 45 years; some also occur in childhood and congenitally.[18] Most lesions occur on the trunk and upper limbs as well as, to a lesser extent, other locations, including a subset in the vulva.[19] The tumor begins as a dermal plaque or nodule and grows slowly, sometimes becoming multinodular. Dermatofibrosarcoma

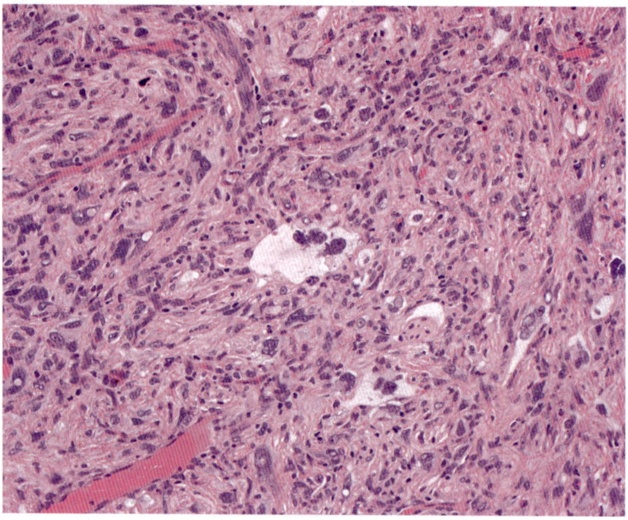

FIGURE 4.8. **Atypical Cutaneous Fibrous Histiocytoma.** There are scattered cells with irregularly shaped enlarged hyperchromatic nuclei, some with abundant foamy cytoplasm.

recurs, especially if incompletely excised; metastasis occurs in fewer than 5% of cases and follows multiple recurrences; exceptionally, there is fibrosarcomatous or pleomorphic sarcomatous transformation, which can be regarded as a form of dedifferentiation and is associated with a more aggressive course. Platelet-derived growth factor (PDGFR) is a receptor tyrosine kinase, which has suggested the use of the tyrosine kinase inhibitors imatinib and, more recently, sunitinib or sorafenib in locally advanced or metastatic disease. However, tumors without the translocation do not respond[20] so that genetic analysis is indicated before targeted therapy.

Pathologic Features

Macroscopically, the skin has one or more raised nodules with pale thickening of dermis and subcutis. Microscopically, the overlying epidermis is thinned and separated by a grenz zone from the lesion that is infiltrative, forming a nodule or ill-defined dermal plaque that extends into subcutaneous fat with a characteristic honeycomb pattern. This includes infiltration in layers parallel to the skin surface (Fig. 4.9, e-Figs. 4.31 and 4.32). The tumor is composed of uniformly elongated thin spindle cells with minimal cytoplasm and indistinct margins, arranged in a striking and monotonous storiform pattern (Fig. 4.10, e-Figs. 4.33 and 4.34). At the periphery, the lesion is often less cellular, and more subtly infiltrative, so that it can be missed in a core biopsy. However, the tumor cells can be highlighted by immunostaining for CD34. Rarely, foci of "myoid" (or more likely myofibroblastic) differentiation are seen as paler nodules of cells with eosinophilic cytoplasm, centered on a small blood vessel. This might represent a

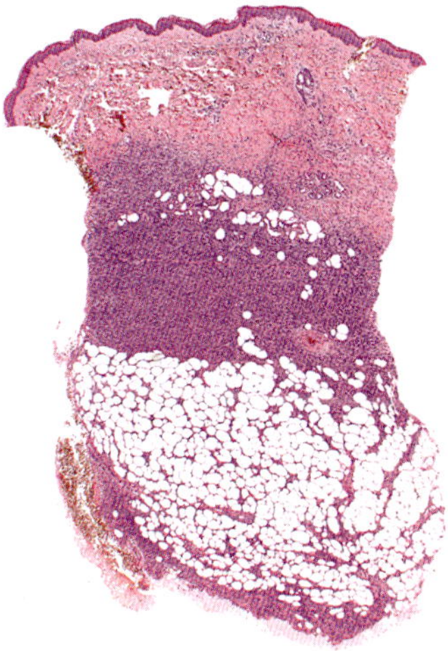

FIGURE 4.9. **Dermatofibrosarcoma.** This punch biopsy shows a deep dermal tumor extending into subcutis. Note the irregular 'honeycombing' extensions of tumor into fat, and the horizontal spread of lesional tissue just above deep fascia (at lower margin of biopsy).

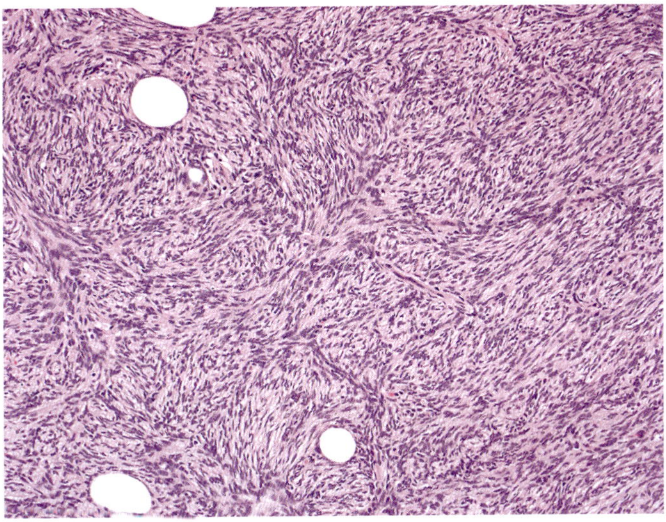

FIGURE 4.10. **Dermatofibrosarcoma.** Spindle cells are disposed in a uniform whorled or storiform pattern, infiltrating fat.

change in the stromal rather than the lesional cells.[21] Scattered cells with melanin pigment are also seen in some cases (Bednar tumor), a finding of no prognostic significance. Some cases have a component of giant cell fibroblastoma. Rarer atrophic,[22] palisading,[23] and granular cell[24] variants of dermatofibrosarcoma are also recognized.

Ancillary Investigations

Dermatofibrosarcoma characteristically has strong, diffuse CD34 expression (e-Figs. 4.35 and 4.36). There is occasional focal reactivity for SMA but usually no significant staining for S100 protein. Apolipoprotein D has also been advocated as a diagnostic immunohistochemical marker.[25] Some cases show focal epithelial membrane antigen (EMA) positivity, and occasional cases are CD117-positive. Factor XIIIa (which is expressed in a subset of dermal "dendrocytes") is generally not detectable in the principal lesional cells of dermatofibrosarcoma. Ultrastructurally, the cells mostly display features of fibroblasts (notably rough endoplasmic reticulum) and are similar to dermal dendrocytes.[26] The foci of "myoid" differentiation are immunoreactive for SMA but not for desmin or CD34, and electron microscopy has shown myofibroblastic differentiation.

Genetically, dermatofibrosarcoma has a reciprocal translocation, t(17;22)(q22;q13) (with a supernumerary ring chromosome in adult cases) resulting in fusion of the genes *COL1A* (collagen type 1 alpha 1) on 17q21–22, and *PDGFB1* (platelet-derived growth factor beta chain) at 22q13.[27] The same abnormalities have also been shown in fibrosarcoma arising in dermatofibrosarcoma.[28] Other rearrangements, including t(2;17) and t(9;22), are found rarely.[29] Gene expression profiling has shown high expression of a group of genes, which included *PDGFB* and osteonectin.[30]

VARIANTS

Myxoid Dermatofibrosarcoma Many dermatofibrosarcomas have small myxoid areas, but extensive myxoid change is rare.[31] This variant is clinically, pathologically, and behaviorally similar to regular dermatofibrosarcoma, foci of which are usually found somewhere in the lesion. Myxoid dermatofibrosarcoma has evenly spaced, elongated, uniform spindle cells and, in common with other myxoid lesions, a vasculature of thin-walled vessels. (Fig. 4.11, e-Figs. 4.37–4.39) The cellularity, and the absence of atypia, lipoblasts and S100 protein, respectively allow distinction from myxoma, myxofibrosarcoma, myxoid liposarcoma, and nerve sheath tumors.

Pigmented dermatofibrosarcoma (Bednar tumor) has melanin-containing cells singly or in small clusters (Fig. 4.12, e-Figs. 4.40–4.42). The cells are immunoreactive for S100 protein (e-Fig. 4.38) and HMB-45. This variant, which is incidentally more common in individuals with pigmented skin, is cytogenetically identical to regular dermatofibrosarcoma[32] and can undergo fibrosarcomatous change with pigmentation also present in metastases.

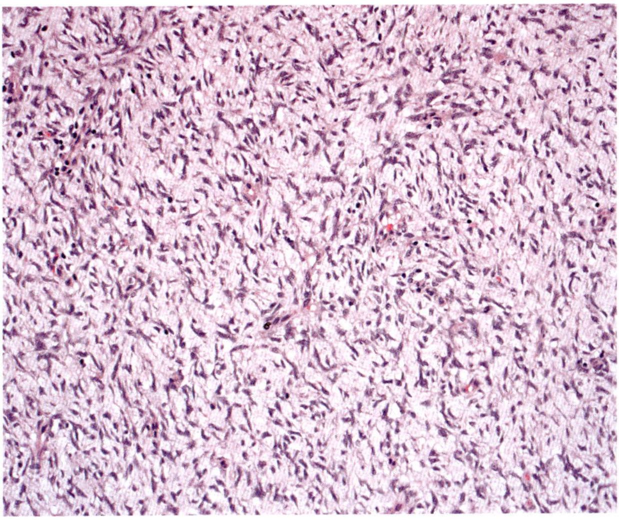

FIGURE 4.11. **Myxoid Dermatofibrosarcoma.** Slender elongated spindle cells in a myxoid stroma, focally with a delicate vasculature. A residual storiform pattern can be seen.

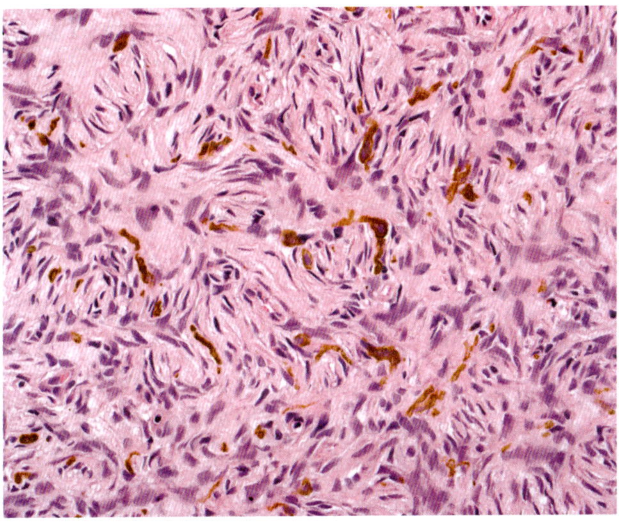

FIGURE 4.12. **Pigmented Dermatofibrosarcoma.** Dendritic cells containing melanin pigment are present within dermatofibrosarcoma displaying typical storiform pattern.

Fibrosarcoma in dermatofibrosarcoma usually arises either de novo but sometimes in the course of recurrence of dermatofibrosarcoma. The fibrosarcomatous component is characterized by greater cellularity, increased mitotic activity (>5 per 10 hpf), and fascicular rather than storiform architecture (Fig. 4.13, e-Figs. 4.43–4.45). "Myoid" foci (e-Figs. 4.46–4.49) and melanin-containing cells can also be seen. Immunoreactivity for CD34 is variously retained (e-Fig. 4.44), reduced or lost in the fibrosarcomatous area, and proliferative index (MIB1) (e-Fig. 4.45) and p53 expression are increased.[33] The genetic changes are identical to those in regular dermatofibrosarcoma and have also been found in superficial adult fibrosarcomas without evidence of antecedent dermatofibrosarcoma.[34] Fibrosarcoma in dermatofibrosarcoma behaves relatively aggressively, with local recurrence in over 50% and metastasis in 10% to 15% of cases.[33] However, adequate local control, with clear surgical margins, can reduce both local recurrence and the incidence of metastasis.[35]

Giant cell fibroblastoma occurs in childhood and occasionally in adults predominantly arising, like dermatofibrosarcoma, in proximal lower limb and trunk.[36] It is a poorly circumscribed tumor that infiltrates skin and subcutis and is composed of spindle and bland multinucleate cells in a fibrous and myxoid stroma (Fig. 4.14, e-Figs. 4.48–4.52). Cystic spaces lined by tumor (not endothelial) cells (e-Fig. 4.51) are a characteristic feature. Both hypercellular and hypocellular (fibrous) areas occur. The multinucleate cells ultrastructurally have a single, markedly indented, and convoluted nucleus. Dermatofibrosarcoma can contain areas of giant cell fibroblastoma, which when pure can recur partially or completely as dermatofibrosarcoma, of either classical or

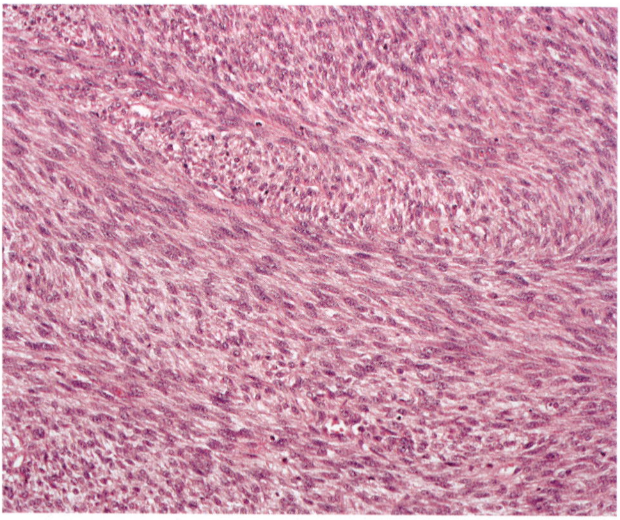

FIGURE 4.13. **Fibrosarcoma in Dermatofibrosarcoma.** In contrast to regular dermatofibrosarcoma, fibrosarcomatous change is indicated by arrangement of lesional cells in a fascicular, herring-bone architecture, and increased mitotic activity.

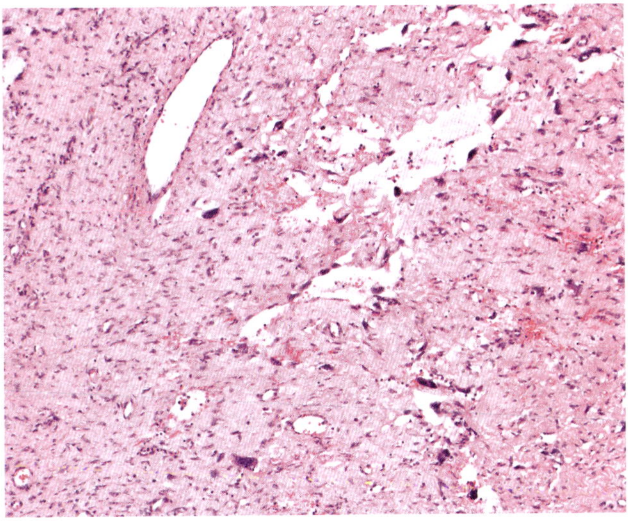

FIGURE 4.14. **Giant Cell Fibroblastoma.** Spindle cells are dispersed unevenly in myxoid stroma, with scattered multinucleated giant cells. The latter also line irregular "pseudovascular" spaces (compare with blood vessel at upper left of field).

pigmented types. The lesional cells are CD34-positive. Giant cell fibroblastoma and dermatofibrosarcoma are genetically identical,[37] and giant cell fibroblastoma is therefore regarded as a (juvenile) variant of dermatofibrosarcoma.

DESMOPLASTIC MELANOMA

Clinical Features

This is a rare variant of melanoma characterized by spindling of cells and stromal fibrosis. It occurs mostly in older patients (mean age 71[38]) with slight male predominance[39] and favors the head and neck region, presenting as a slowly growing nodule or broader plaque. This lesion has a tendency to infiltrate small nerves (neurotropism) and is prone to local recurrence, although the figures vary between 4%[38] and 40%.[39] Significant predictors of recurrence after excision are positive margin status, presence of neurotropism, and stage, and predictors of overall survival are patient age, mitotic rate, and stage.[39] Notwithstanding their generally greater depth at presentation (over half of the cases have a Breslow thickness exceeding 4 mm), pure desmoplastic melanomas spread to lymph nodes less frequently than mixed desmoplastic melanomas or conventional melanomas of similar stage, with a 5-year survival of about 70%. About 10% metastasize to lung, liver, and bone.[38,39]

Pathologic Features

Most but not all cases have a junctional component, resembling lentigo maligna or superficial spreading melanoma. Desmoplastic melanomas in which the invasive component exceeds 90% are designated "pure" and the others as "mixed"[40] or "combined."[38] The dermal lesion is noncircumscribed; nests or files of spindle cells infiltrate the dermis in an irregular fashion (Fig. 4.15, e-Figs. 4.53–4.60). The cells have scanty cytoplasm and hyperchromatic elongated nuclei, which can look bland and tapered and resemble fibroblasts, or be wavy-like cells of a neurofibroma and, and are often arranged radially, at right angles to the surface. Mitoses are often scanty. The majority of cases are amelanotic. The lesional cells lie in a fibrous stroma, often with inflammation, and can be overlooked when dispersed singly, especially as they can infiltrate deeply around adnexa, and closely around and within nerves. Cases with pure histology or lacking an in situ component can be difficult to distinguish from cutaneous malignant peripheral nerve sheath tumor (MPNST).

Ancillary Investigations

Desmoplastic melanoma is diffusely positive for S100 protein (e-Fig. 4.56) but very rarely expresses markers of melanocytic differentiation (HMB45, melan-A). Microphthalmia transcription factor is positive in up to 40% of desmoplastic melanomas but is not specific. Immunoreactivity for clusterin can also be useful as it is rarely expressed in conventional melanomas but

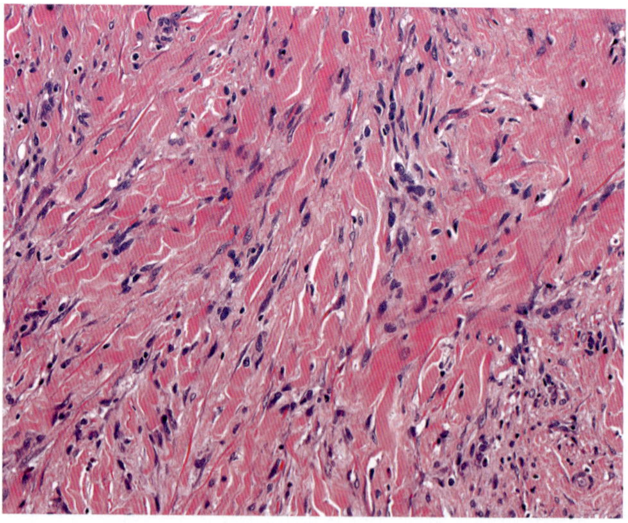

FIGURE 4.15. **Desmoplastic Melanoma.** Atypical spindle cells with scanty cytoplasm infiltrate between thickened collagen bundles in deep dermis.

is also found in only 30% of desmoplastic melanoma and is not specific.[41] Ultrastructurally, there is either fibroblast-like or, often, focal schwannian differentiation without melanosomes so that the distinction from MPNST can be very difficult in cases without an overlying in situ melanomatous component. Immunohistochemistry for collagen IV is occasionally useful in such cases as it is disposed around groups of cells in melanoma and around single cells in MPNST. Clinically, however, the distinction between desmoplastic melanoma and superficial MPNST might not be immediately clinically significant.

SPINDLE CELL CARCINOMA

Clinical Features

In the skin, sarcomatoid carcinoma can occur in association with a previous or synchronous in situ or invasive squamous cell carcinoma, or appear de novo. It is seen most frequently in the head and neck region including scalp and oral mucosa and can also arise in extremities including in the nail bed.

Pathologic Features

Spindle cell carcinoma forms sheets and fascicles of pleomorphic spindle and epithelioid cells with mitotic activity and sometimes necrosis (e-Figs. 4.61 and 4.62). Morphologic clues to its nature include foci of (squamous) epithelial differentiation, dysplasia or in situ carcinoma in the overlying or (if ulcerated) the adjacent epithelium, and a nested reticulin pattern.

Ancillary Investigations

Immunostains usually show focal positivity for epithelial markers (cytokeratins, EMA) (e-Fig. 4.63) and often for p63, with none for CD34 or S100 protein.

KAPOSI SARCOMA

This is considered in Chapters 10 and 17. In the plaque stage, it is recognized by fascicles of long spindle cells with mitoses and interstitial hemorrhage and by its specific nuclear immunoreactivity for HHV8.

ANGIOSARCOMA

This is considered in Chapter 18. Patients with cutaneous angiosarcoma usually have a history of ultraviolet or therapeutic irradiation. Histologically, there is often vascular channel formation with spindled or epithelioid tumor cells which display immunoreactivity for endothelial antigens and in some cases cytokeratins also.

REFERENCES

1. Barzilai A, Lyakhovitsky A, Horowitz A, et al. Keloid-like scleroderma. *Am J Dermatopathol.* 2003;25:327–330.
2. Kelly AP. Medical and surgical therapies for keloids. *Dermatol Ther.* 2004;17:212–218.
3. Leventhal D, Furr M, Reiter D. Treatment of keloids and hypertrophic scars: a meta-analysis and review of the literature. *Arch Facial Plast Surg.* 2006;8:362–368.
4. Kuo T-t, Hu S, Chan H-L. Keloidal dermatofibroma. Report of 10 cases of a new variant. *Am J Surg Pathol.* 1998;22:564–568.
5. Nassiri M, Woolery-Lloyd H, Ramos S, et al. Gene expression profiling reveals alteration of caspase 6 and 14 transcripts in normal skin of keloid-prone patients. *Arch Dermatol Res.* 2009;301:183–188.
6. Al-Daraji WI, Ramsay HM, Ali RB. Storiform collagenoma as a clue for Cowden disease or PTEN hamartoma tumour syndrome. *J Clin Pathol.* 2007;60:840–842.
7. Chen TM, Purohit SK, Wang AR. Pleomorphic sclerotic fibroma: a case report and literature review. *Am J Dermatopathol.* 2002;24:54–58.
8. Gonzalez-Vela MC, Val-Bernal JF, Martino M, et al. Sclerotic fibroma-like dermatofibroma: an uncommon distinctive variant of dermatofibroma. *Histol Histopathol.* 2005;20:801–806.
9. Wilk M, Kaiser HW, Steen KH, et al. Sclerotic fibroma. *Hautarzt.* 1995;46:413–416.
10. Garcia-Doval I, Casas L, Toribio J. Pleomorphic fibroma of the skin, a form of sclerotic fibroma: an immunohistochemical study. *Clin Exp Dermatol.* 1998;23:22–24.
11. Miliauskas JR. Myxoid cutaneous pleomorphic fibroma. *Histopathology.* 1994;24:179–181.
12. Kamino H RV, Gero M, Alba Greco M. Dermatomyofibroma. A benig cutaneous, plaque-like proliferation of fibroblasts and myofibroblasts in young adults. *J Cutan Pathol.* 1992;19:85–93.
13. Mentzel T, Kutzner H. Haemorrhagic dermatomyofibroma (plaque-like dermal fibromatosis): clinicopathological and immunohistochemical analysis of three cases resembling plaque-stage Kaposi's sarcoma. *Histopathology.* 2003;42:594–598.
14. Guillou L, Gebhard S, Salmeron M, et al. Metastasizing fibrous histiocytoma of the skin: a clinicopathologic and immunohistochemical analysis of three cases. *Mod Pathol.* 2000;13:654–660.
15. Kaddu S, McMenamin ME, Fletcher CD. Atypical fibrous histiocytoma of the skin: clinicopathologic analysis of 59 cases with evidence of infrequent metastasis. *Am J Surg Pathol.* 2002;26:35–46.
16. Calonje E, Mentzel T, Fletcher CD. Cellular benign fibrous histiocytoma. Clinicopathologic analysis of 74 cases of a distinctive variant of cutaneous fibrous histiocytoma with frequent recurrence. *Am J Surg Pathol.* 1994;18:668–676.
17. De Hertogh G, Bergmans G, Molderez C, et al. Cutaneous cellular fibrous histiocytoma metastasizing to the lungs. *Histopathology.* 2002;41:85–86.
18. Maire G, Fraitag S, Galmiche L, et al. A clinical, histologic, and molecular study of 9 cases of congenital dermatofibrosarcoma protuberans. *Arch Dermatol.* 2007;143:203–210.
19. Edelweiss M, Malpica A. Dermatofibrosarcoma protuberans of the vulva: a clinicopathologic and immunohistochemical study of 13 cases. *Am J Surg Pathol.* 2010;34:393–400.
20. McArthur GA. Molecular targeting of dermatofibrosarcoma protuberans: a new approach to a surgical disease. *J Natl Compr Canc Netw.* 2007;5:557–562.
21. Sanz-Trelles A. Myoid cells in the fibrosarcomatous variant of dermatofibrosarcoma protuberans. Are they neoplastic? *Histopathology.* 1999;34:179–180.

22. Zelger BW, Ofner D, Zelger BG. Atrophic variants of dermatofibroma and dermatofibrosarcoma protuberans. *Histopathology.* 1995;26:519–527.

23. Llatjos R, Fernandez-Figueras MT, Diaz-Cascajo C, et al. Palisading and verocay body-prominent dermatofibrosarcoma protuberans: a report of three cases. *Histopathology.* 2000;37:452–455.

24. Maire G, Pedeutour F, Coindre JM. COL1A1-PDGFB gene fusion demonstrates a common histogenetic origin for dermatofibrosarcoma protuberans and its granular cell variant. *Am J Surg Pathol.* 2002;26:932–937.

25. Lisovsky M, Hoang MP, Dresser KA, et al. Apolipoprotein D in CD34-positive and CD34-negative cutaneous neoplasms: a useful marker in differentiating superficial acral fibromyxoma from dermatofibrosarcoma protuberans. *Mod Pathol.* 2008;21:31–38.

26. Dominguez-Malagon H, Valdez-Carrillo Mdel C, Cano-Valdez AM. Dermatofibroma and dermatofibrosarcoma protuberans: a comparative ultrastructural study. *Ultrastruct Pathol.* 2006;30:283–291.

27. Sirvent N, Maire G, Pedeutour F. Genetics of dermatofibrosarcoma protuberans family of tumors: from ring chromosomes to tyrosine kinase inhibitor treatment. *Genes Chromosomes Cancer.* 2003;37:1–19.

28. Patel KU, Szabo SS, Hernandez VS, et al. Dermatofibrosarcoma protuberans COL1A1-PDGFB fusion is identified in virtually all dermatofibrosarcoma protuberans cases when investigated by newly developed multiplex reverse transcription polymerase chain reaction and fluorescence in situ hybridization assays. *Hum Pathol.* 2008;39:184–193.

29. Sonobe H, Furihata M, Iwata J, et al. Dermatofibrosarcoma protuberans harboring t(9;22)(q32;q12.2). *Cancer Genet Cytogenet.* 1999;110:14–18.

30. Sandberg AA, Bridge JA. Updates on the cytogenetics and molecular genetics of bone and soft tissue tumors. Dermatofibrosarcoma protuberans and giant cell fibroblastoma. *Cancer Genet Cytogenet.* 2003;140:1–12.

31. Mentzel T, Scharer L, Kazakov DV, et al. Myxoid dermatofibrosarcoma protuberans: clinicopathologic, immunohistochemical, and molecular analysis of eight cases. *Am J Dermatopathol.* 2007;29:443–448.

32. Nishio J, Iwasaki H, Ishiguro M, et al. Supernumerary ring chromosome in a Bednar tumor (pigmented dermatofibrosarcoma protuberans) is composed of interspersed sequences from chromosomes 17 and 22: a fluorescence in situ hybridization and comparative genomic hybridization analysis. *Genes Chromosomes Cancer.* 2001;30:305–309.

33. Abbott JJ, Oliveira AM, Nascimento AG. The prognostic significance of fibrosarcomatous transformation in dermatofibrosarcoma protuberans. *Am J Surg Pathol.* 2006;30:436–443.

34. Sheng WQ, Hashimoto H, Okamoto S, et al. Expression of COL1A1-PDGFB fusion transcripts in superficial adult fibrosarcoma suggests a close relationship to dermatofibrosarcoma protuberans. *J Pathol.* 2001;194:88–94.

35. Goldblum JR, Reith JD, Weiss SW. Sarcomas arising in dermatofibrosarcoma protuberans: a reappraisal of biologic behavior in eighteen cases treated by wide local excision with extended clinical follow up. *Am J Surg Pathol.* 2000;24:1125–1130.

36. Terrier-Lacombe MJ, Guillou L, Maire G, et al. Dermatofibrosarcoma protuberans, giant cell fibroblastoma, and hybrid lesions in children: clinicopathologic comparative analysis of 28 cases with molecular data–a study from the French Federation of Cancer Centers Sarcoma Group. *Am J Surg Pathol.* 2003;27:27–39.

37. Maire G, Martin L, Michalak-Provost S, et al. Fusion of COL1A1 exon 29 with PDGFB exon 2 in a der(22)t(17;22) in a pediatric giant cell fibroblastoma with a pigmented Bednar tumor component. Evidence for age-related chromosomal pattern in dermatofibrosarcoma protuberans and related tumors. *Cancer Genet Cytogenet.* 2002;134:156–161.

38. de Almeida LS, Requena L, Rutten A, et al. Desmoplastic malignant melanoma: a clinicopathologic analysis of 113 cases. *Am J Dermatopathol.* 2008;30:207–215.

39. Posther KE, Selim MA, Mosca PJ, et al. Histopathologic characteristics, recurrence patterns, and survival of 129 patients with desmoplastic melanoma. *Ann Surg Oncol.* 2006;13:728–739.

40. George E, McClain SE, Slingluff CL, et al. Subclassification of desmoplastic melanoma: pure and mixed variants have significantly different capacities for lymph node metastasis. *J Cutan Pathol.* 2009;36:425–432.

41. Busam KJ, Kucukgol D, Eastlake-Wade S, et al. Clusterin expression in primary and metastatic melanoma. *J Cutan Pathol.* 2006;33:619–623.

5

INTRA-ABDOMINAL SPINDLE CELL LESIONS

INTRODUCTION

Although most soft tissue tumors can occur in intra-abdominal locations, including retroperitoneum, there are several benign and malignant lesions that are peculiar to this anatomical region, and others that can appear in a variety of sites but which form distinct and clinically important subsets within the abdomen, and often present a diagnostic challenge, especially in core biopsies. They are mostly spindle cell lesions that can be predominantly fibrous or mainly cellular, but some epithelioid and pleomorphic tumors also enter the diagnosis. These are considered in Chapters 11 and 13, respectively. Smooth muscle tumors are considered in Chapter 6. The differential diagnosis is summarized in Table 5.1.

REACTIVE NODULAR FIBROUS PSEUDOTUMOR

Clinical Features

First described in 2003,[1] reactive nodular fibrous pseudotumor is a lesion that predominantly affects males, with a mean age of 45 years. The usual presentation is with abdominal pain or a mass, and some patients have a history of abdominal surgery. The lesions can be solitary or multiple and involve mesentery, surface of small or large intestine or peripancreatic tissue. They vary between 3 and 10 cm. Reported examples have not recurred after excision.

Pathologic Features

This is a circumscribed firm lesion that is microscopically infiltrative at the margin. Reported lesions are of low or moderate cellularity and composed of stellate or spindled fibroblastic cells arranged in intersecting fascicles in a focally hyalinized or keloidal collagenous stroma with scattered lymphocytes forming aggregates peripherally (Fig. 5.1, e-Figs. 5.1 and 5.2). *Heterotopic mesenteric ossification* can also occur after abdominal surgery but differs in having a nodular fasciitis-like background and foci of metaplastic ossification (e-Fig. 5.3).[2]

TABLE 5.1 **Differential Diagnosis of Intra-abdominal Spindle Cell Tumors**

	Typical Clinical Features	Microscopic Features	Ancillary Investigations
Calcifying fibrous tumor	Children, young adults, M = F Abdomen up to 15 cm. Can be multiple. Also in subcutaneous and deep soft tissue	Circumscribed, unencapsulated tumor with hypocellular collagen containing scanty fibroblasts, inflammatory aggregates, and rounded calcifications	Occasionally CD34+ or SMA+
Reactive nodular fibrous pseudotumor	M > F, solitary or multiple, mesentery and surface of small or large bowel, circumscribed. History of abdominal surgery in some	Nodules of mildly to moderately cellular stellate and spindle cells in fascicles in collagen, lymphoid aggregates	SMA+, desmin±, CK ±
Heterotopic mesenteric ossification	Follows abdominal surgery or trauma, can present with intestinal obstruction	Resembles ossifying fasciitis with nodular fasciitis-like background and foci of metaplastic bone formation	SMA+, desmin−, h-caldesmon−
Retroperitoneal fibrosis	M > F, plaque at aortic bifurcation, ureters retract	Collagen bands, mixed inflammation, vasculitis, few spindle cells	SMA+, IgG4+ in plasma cells
Sclerosing mesenteritis	M > F, ill-defined mesenteric mass. Can be associated with other sclerosing fibroinflammatory diseases	Fibrosis, inflammation, fat necrosis, foamy cells, sparse spindle cells	SMA+, IgG4+ in plasma cells
Fibromatosis - desmoid type	Any age, deep, limbs, head and neck, body cavities. Association with familial adenomatous polyposis	Parallel myofibroblasts evenly dispersed in collagen, slit-like and muscular-walled small vessels, and mast cells. Focally myxoid or with keloidal fibers	SMA+, beta-catenin+ (nuclear)
Sclerosing well-differentiated liposarcoma	Older adults. Often multicentric	Variable admixture of paucicellular sclerosis and adipose tissue, with scattered enlarged hyperchromatic nuclei mostly in fibrous areas. Rare lipoblasts	CDK4+, MDM2+, P16 +, CD34+, FISH shows amplification of CDK4, MDM2

Solitary fibrous tumor	Mass in pelvis, abdomen or retroperitoneum	Circumscribed, not usually encapsulated, distinct cellular and fibrous areas, focal myxoid stroma, patternless short spindle cells. Hemangiopericytomatous pattern focally. Malignant variant has hypercellularity, mitoses >4 per 10 hpf, necrosis	CD34+, bcl-2+, CD99+
Inflammatory myofibroblastic tumor	Childhood or adult. Single mass or multicentric. Mesenteric, retroperitoneal, other sites	Spindle cells in fascicles or myxoid fasciitis-like patterns. Occasional larger polygonal cells. Focal sclerosis without spindle cells. Marked inflammation, plasma cells prominent especially in areas of sclerosis	SMA+, ALK+ (about 55%, especially childhood visceral tumors) ALK gene rearrangements
Leiomyosarcoma	F>M. Retroperitoneum, bowel wall or wall of vessel including IVC, renal vein	Fascicles at right angles. Cells elongated with eosinophilic cytoplasm and nontapered nuclei. Paranuclear vacuoles. Myxoid change, fibrosis. Inflammatory variant has bland spindle cells, marked lymphocytic infiltrate, foamy macrophages, psammoma bodies	SMA+, desmin+, h-caldesmon+, CD117−
Gastrointestinal stromal tumor	Related to wall of any part of alimentary tract (most commonly stomach, small intestine), Also, in retroperitoneum, omentum. Metastatic potential varies with site, size, and mitotic index per 50 hpf	Fascicles of long spindle cells, nuclei with blunt or tapered ends, paranuclear vacuoles. Organoid pattern, palisading. Focal or widespread epithelioid morphology common. Occasional clear cell, plasmacytoid, or rhabdoid change	CD117+, DOG1+, CD34+, h-caldesmon+. SMA variable, desmin+ rarely, S100 protein+ rarely. CK sometimes+ after therapy. *KIT* or *PDGFRA* mutations

(Continued)

TABLE 5.1 **Differential Diagnosis of Intra-abdominal Spindle Cell Tumors (Continued)**

	Typical Clinical Features	Microscopic Features	Ancillary Investigations
Inflammatory fibroid polyp	Submucosa and mucosa of esophagus, stomach or intestine	Bland spindle and stellate cells in inflamed stroma including eosinophils. Perivascular whorls.	CD34+, CD117-negative, h-caldesmon–negative. *PDGFRA* mutations
Clear cell sarcoma of GI tract	Occurs in stomach or small intestine	Nested pattern, round nuclei with central nucleolus, clear or granular cytoplasm, sometimes spindling, osteoclast-like giant cells	S100 protein+, HMB45+ and melan A usually negative, other markers negative. t (2;22)(q33;q12), *EWSR1-CREB1*, rarely t(12;22)(q13;q12), *EWSR1-ATF1*
PEComa	Falciform ligament, mesentery, retroperitoneum, uterus	Nests of ovoid or spindled cells with clear or granular cytoplasm, delicate fibrous septa. Malignant variants often epithelioid	SMA+, HMB45+, melan-A+, desmin+ in some CD117+ in some, S100 protein+ rarely
Cellular schwannoma	F>M, Middle age. Paravertebral in retroperitoneum or pelvis, can erode bone. Also submucosal in stomach or intestine	Thick capsule, subcapsular lymphoid aggregates. Fascicles of cells with eosinophilic cytoplasm, focal pleomorphism, occasional mitoses. Lacks Antoni A and B areas. Lymphocytes, clusters of foamy cells, thick-walled vessels, hemosiderin.	S100 protein diffusely+, CD117–. Some cases express CK
Dedifferentiated liposarcoma	Older adults, large retroperitoneal tumor, recurrences frequent	Low-grade dedifferentiation: cellular fascicles with mild pleomorphism	CDK4+, MDM2+, variable desmin, SMA, CD34 positivity

		High-grade dedifferentiation: pleomorphic undifferentiated sarcoma, or myofibrosarcoma-like, Heterologous osteochondroid or rhabdomyosarcomatous elements	FISH shows amplification of *CDK4, MDM2*
Sarcomatoid mesothelioma	Sheet-like mass involving peritoneal surface or omentum. History of asbestos exposure	Fascicles of pleomorphic spindle cells, tapered nuclei, scanty cytoplasm, mitoses, necrosis. Desmoplastic or hyalinized stroma. Epithelioid component in some	CK focal+, calretinin+, CD34- and bcl2–
Follicular dendritic cell sarcoma	Omentum, GI tract, liver, spleen, soft tissue	Sheets, whorls, and fascicles of ovoid cells. Prominent nuclear membranes, speckled chromatin. Intimate admixture of lymphocytes. Rarely giant cells, pleomorphism, necrosis	CD21/35+, CD23+, S100 protein+, EMA+, D2-40+, fascin+, clusterin+, desmoplakin+. CD45–
Synovial sarcoma, monophasic	Very rare in abdomen. Mass in retroperitoneum or pelvis	Sheets of uniform short spindle cells with minimal cytoplasm, focal pericytomatous pattern. Poorly differentiated synovial sarcoma is a small round cell tumor	CK, EMA, CD99, S100pr focally+, bcl2+, TLE1+ CD34– and CD117–, t(X;18)(p11;q11), *SSX-SS18* fusion gene
Endometrial stromal sarcoma	F. Can arise in a focus of endometriosis or present as metastasis in abdomen or elsewhere	Short closely packed spindle cells, variable focal myoid differentiation. Thick-walled vessels	CD10+, SMA+, occasional des+, CK+ Nuclear beta catenin+ in 50% ER, PgR+ *JAZF1-JJAZ1, JAZF1-PHF1*, and *EPC1-PHF1* fusion genes
Sclerosing lymphoma	Adults, associated lymphadenopathy	Cords and nests of atypical lymphoid cells with fibrous stroma Absence of prominent spindle cell component	Lymphoid markers, often large B-cell lymphoma

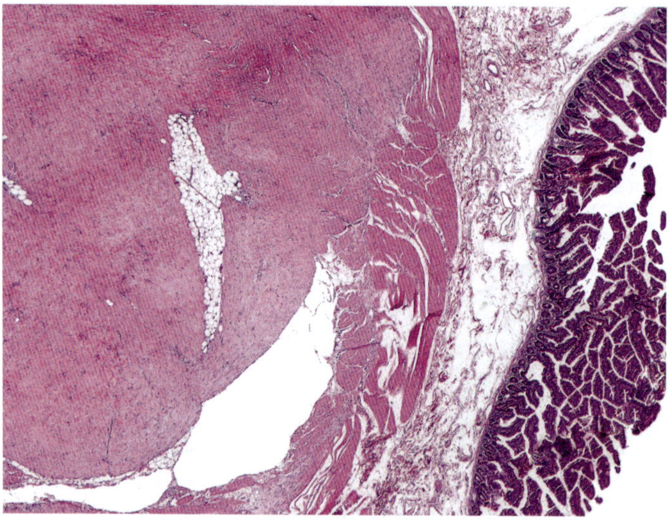

FIGURE 5.1. **Reactive Nodular Fibrous Pseudotumor.** (Courtesy of Dr. GP Nielsen). This is a moderately cellular spindle cell lesion in fibrous stroma. The lesion is adherent to muscularis propria of small intestine.

Ancillary Investigations

Immunohistochemistry is diffusely positive for vimentin and focally positive for smooth muscle actin (SMA), and desmin, and for cytokeratins AE1/AE3, and CAM5.2 in some cases. CD34, S-100 protein, and anaplastic lymphoma kinase (ALK) are negative. The initial report of immunoreactivity for CD117[1] was not confirmed in a subsequent study in which, additionally, no abnormalities were found in exons 11 or 9 of the *KIT* gene,[3] unlike in gastrointestinal stromal tumor (GIST). The tumor cells have ultrastructural features of myofibroblasts, with the cytokeratin positivity suggesting origin from submesothelial cells.

RETROPERITONEAL FIBROSIS, IDIOPATHIC

Clinical Features

Retroperitoneal fibrosis has a distinct clinico-radiologic profile, presenting most commonly in males aged 40 to 60 years with abdominal pain and sometimes generalized systemic symptoms with associated biochemical or hematologic abnormalities. Retroperitoneal fibrosis can arise secondary to other local conditions including aortic aneurysm and neoplasms and, historically, in patients treated with methysergide for migraine. At least some idiopathic cases appear to arise in aortitis[4] or secondary to atheroma. There is an association with immune-mediated diseases such as systemic lupus erythematosus, renal glomerular disease, and autoimmune pancreatitis[5] and also with histologically similar lesions in other anatomic locations

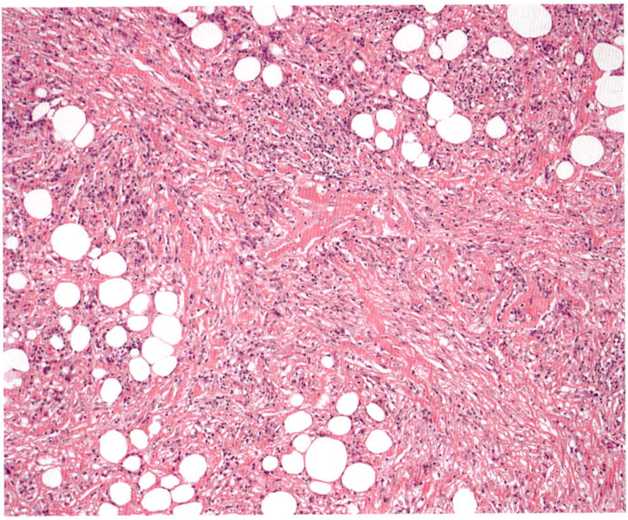

FIGURE 5.2. **Retroperitoneal Fibrosis.** In the early stages, the lesion has a mixed inflammatory infiltrate with coarse collagen bundles infiltrating fat.

collectively termed idiopathic fibrosclerotic (or sclerosing fibroinflammatory) diseases.[6] These include mediastinal fibrosis, sclerosing cholangitis, Riedel thyroiditis, and orbital fibrous pseudotumor. Many examples of these have an infiltrate of IgG4-secreting plasma cells in increased numbers, and they have been grouped together as IgG4-related sclerosing disorders, or hyper-IgG4 disease (since there is an increased serum level of IgG4 during the acute phase).[7] Retroperitoneal fibrosis forms a plaque-like lesion based at the bifurcation of the aorta which infiltrates adjacent tissues. In most cases, this includes the ureters, involvement of the middle portions of which can result in their displacement medially and also cause urinary obstruction.

Pathologic Features

The biopsy or excision specimen is generally received in several pieces. Microscopic examination (Figs. 5.2 and 5.3, e-Figs. 5.4–5.7) shows collagenous bands with hyalinization and a variable diffuse and perivascular infiltrate of mixed inflammatory cells including eosinophils (but rarely neutrophils) and sometimes lymphoid follicles with germinal centers. Older lesions have less inflammation. Small vessel vasculitis is occasionally seen (e-Fig. 5.5). A paucicellular, bland fibro-myofibroblastic spindle cell component is sometimes present but less than that seen in inflammatory myofibroblastic tumor.

Ancillary Investigations

The lymphoid infiltrate comprises a mixture of B and T cells, aiding in the distinction from sclerosing lymphomas that can enter the differential

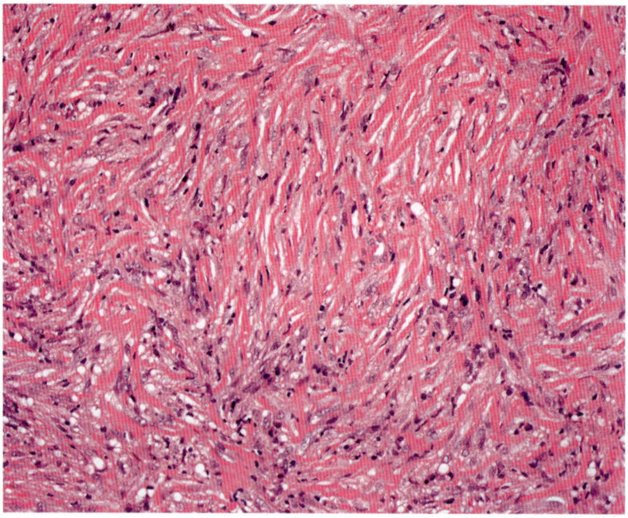

FIGURE 5.3. **Retroperitoneal Fibrosis.** At a later stage, there is dense fibrosis (as discrete bands rather than confluent hyalinization) and sparse inflammation.

diagnosis of retroperitoneal fibrosis in its early, cellular phase. Many of the plasma cells are IgG4-positive (e-Fig. 5.7), especially in cases associated with autoimmune pancreatitis.[8] The myofibroblastic spindle cells are SMA-positive but nonimmunoreactive for ALK or for beta-catenin in nuclei.

SCLEROSING MESENTERITIS

Clinical Features

Sclerosing mesenteritis is the preferred term for lesions also reported as retractile mesenteritis, mesenteric panniculitis, or mesenteric lipodystrophy.[9] It is a chronic fibrosing lesion that presents in adults (70% in males, mean age 60 to 65 years) with abdominal pain sometimes due to intestinal obstruction, a mass, diarrhea, or weight loss.[10] The lesions can be discrete or poorly defined, forming one or more firm irregularly shaped masses within the mesentery of small (or occasionally large) intestine, or more diffuse mesenteric thickening, with resultant retraction and adhesion of bowel loops. The pancreas can be involved, mimicking carcinoma.[11] Diagnostic imaging features have been described.[12] Although histologically benign, this can have a long course with a sometimes fatal outcome due to complications of the disease or its management. Examples have been associated with other sclerosing or immune-related diseases such as retroperitoneal fibrosis and giant cell temporal arteritis.[13]

Pathologic Features

This comprises sparse myofibroblasts without atypia in chronically inflamed fibrous tissue that infiltrates fat, and also shows fat necrosis at

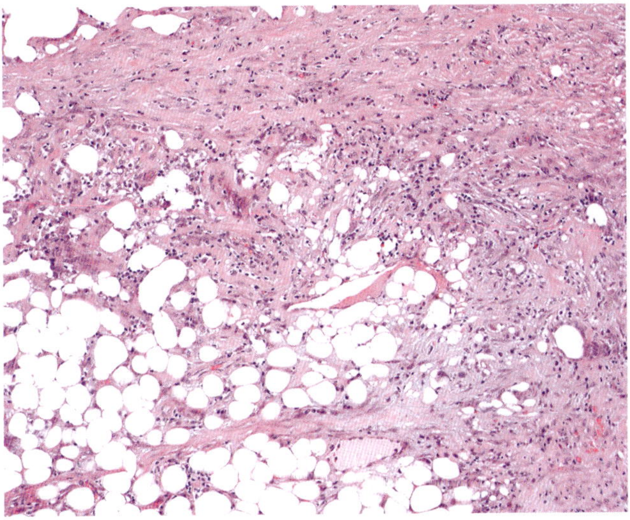

FIGURE 5.4. **Sclerosing Mesenteritis.** There is irregular infiltration of mesenteric fat by fibrous tissue with focal chronic inflammation including plasma cells.

various stages, with associated foamy macrophages. (Fig. 5.4, e-Fig. 5.8) Lymphocytes and plasma cells are present but the latter are not as prominent as in the sclerosing areas of inflammatory myofibroblastic tumor. Care should be taken not to overlook metastatic carcinoma with marked stromal fibrosis.

Ancillary Investigations

The lesional fibroblasts are focally immunoreactive for SMA and negative for CD117 and nuclear beta-catenin,[14] the latter observations aiding the distinction from fibromatosis. In about a third of cases, the plasma cells express IgG4.[10]

INFLAMMATORY MYOFIBROBLASTIC TUMOR (INFLAMMATORY FIBROSARCOMA)

Clinical Features

Inflammatory myofibroblastic tumor[15] most commonly arises in the abdomen, especially retroperitoneum or mesentery, and rarely in other soft tissue sites.[16,17] Similar tumors have been described in the lung under a variety of terms, and a distinct subset arise in the urinary tract,[17,18] especially in the bladder.[18,19] Other pelvic sites can be involved in both sexes.[20,21] The peak incidence is in the first decade of life, followed by adolescence, although examples occur in older adults. Patients present with symptoms relating to the mass lesion or with systemic symptoms including fever, anemia, and leukocytosis. Bladder tumors occur more frequently in males with a

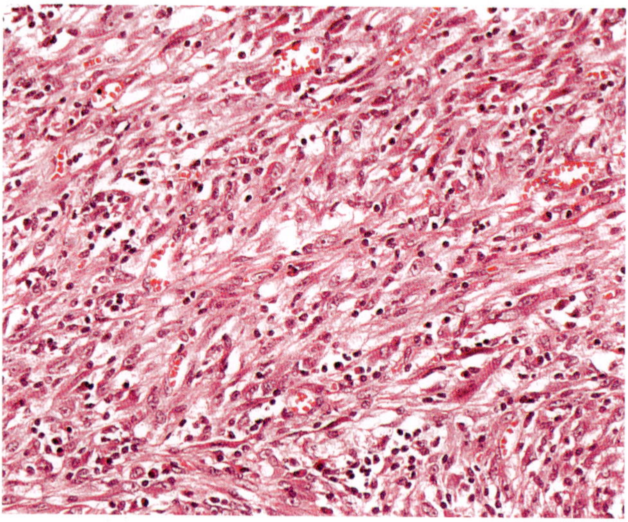

FIGURE 5.5. **Inflammatory Myofibroblastic Tumor.** One of the typical patterns is a loose fasciitis-like proliferation of bland spindle cells with interspersed inflammatory cells including a predominance of plasma cells.

peak in the fifth decade, and about a quarter of the cases are associated with prior instrumentation. Inflammatory myofibroblastic tumor can be solitary or multicentric, and around a third of cases recur after excision. Inflammatory myofibroblastic tumor is categorized as intermediate (rarely metastasizing) in the WHO 2002 Classification. A small number of cases undergo frank sarcomatous transformation,[22] but there are no histologic features predictive of this, or of recurrent potential. However, absence of immunoreactivity for ALK is associated with a worse outcome.[23] This tumor should not be confused with inflammatory fibroid polyps of the bowel which are benign lesions of CD34-positive focally whorled spindle and stellate cells in an inflamed fibromyxoid stroma (including eosinophils) in the submucosa and mucosa of the stomach, small bowel, colon, and rarely esophagus. The presence of *PDGFRA* mutations in these lesions has been reported. [24]

Pathologic Features

The typical intra-abdominal lesion is a firm white irregular mass extending into the mesentery and often adherent to wall of bowel, which can be infiltrated. Bladder tumors form a polypoid mass up to 12 cm in diameter which can infiltrate the muscularis propria. Histologically, inflammatory myofibroblastic tumor is composed of fibroblasts and myofibroblasts,[15,25] with characteristic spindle or stellate shape, pale nuclei, and single small nucleoli (Figs. 5.5 and 5.6, e-Figs. 5.9–5.14). The cytoplasm is amphophilic and cell boundaries are indistinct. Pleomorphism is rare, although rare atypical cells, often with epithelioid morphology, can sometimes be found.

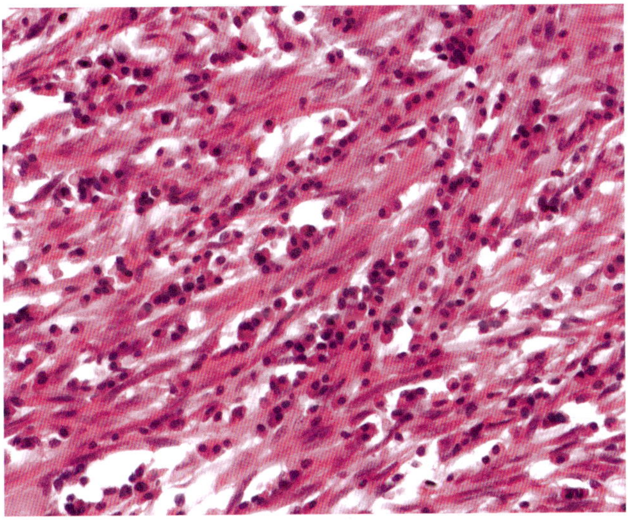

FIGURE 5.6. **Inflammatory Myofibroblastic Tumor.** A fascicular pattern is also commonly seen, with a marked plasmacytic infiltrate as here.

The cellularity varies; cellular areas can have loose, fasciitis-like (e-Fig. 5.9) or more compact fascicular patterns (e-Fig. 5.10), and paucicellular zones, with sclerosis (e-Fig. 5.13) and calcification, are commonly seen. In all patterns, there is an inflammatory infiltrate composed predominantly of plasma cells, with lymphocytes and sometimes eosinophils and neutrophils in the fasciitis-like areas. Necrosis is uncommon except in the bladder where it is a feature in up to 50% of cases.

Ancillary Investigations

The spindle cells are immunoreactive for SMA, and, in fewer cases, for desmin. Cytokeratin positivity is occasionally seen, especially in intra-abdominal tumors. Bladder tumors are positive for cytokeratins in about 75% of cases, SMA and desmin in about 75%, and h-caldesmon in over half the cases examined.[19] Just over half of inflammatory myofibroblastic tumors express ALK (e-Fig. 5.14), mostly in intra-abdominal, visceral, or pulmonary tumors, and especially in those occurring in childhood.[17,22] ALK-positive cases appear to have a better outcome than those which are negative.[23] The ALK positivity is related to clonal abnormalities involving the *ALK* gene, located on 2p23, which encodes a tyrosine kinase receptor. In inflammatory myofibroblastic tumor, this is rearranged with one of several other genes, including tropomyosin 3 at 1p13 (resulting in *TPM3-ALK*), tropomyosin 4 at 19–13, *CLTC* (clathrin heavy chain gene, localized to 17q23), *ATIC* at 2q35, *SEC31L1* at 4q21, *CARS* at 11p15 and *RANBP2* at 2q13. The pattern and distribution of ALK staining relate to the fusion gene; it is diffuse and cytoplasmic except for the fusions with *CLTC* (granular) and *RANBP2* (nuclear membrane).[26] It should be noted that immunoreactivity for ALK has also been reported in a few examples of malignant peripheral nerve sheath tumor (MPNST), rhabdomyosarcoma, and leiomyosarcoma.[27] Lesions arising following instrumentation to the bladder (postoperative spindle cell nodule) are more fasciitis-like and might represent pseudosarcomatous fasciitis-like myofibroblastic lesions rather than inflammatory myofibroblastic tumors. However, some are reportedly ALK-positive[20] and they also have a wider immunophenotype, with expression of cytokeratins, desmin, and h-caldesmon, than is usually seen in fasciitis-like proliferations.[26]

GASTROINTESTINAL STROMAL TUMOR

Clinical Features

GISTs have an incidence in the population of 10 to 15 per million and occur in either sex and at any age but are most common over the age of 50. Familial cases show autosomal dominant inheritance, and there is an increased incidence in neurofibromatosis type 1, in Carney triad,[27] and in Carney-Stratakis syndrome.[29] Fifty percent of GISTs occur in the stomach and a quarter in the small intestine, with smaller numbers in esophagus and large intestine (mostly rectum).[28] Evidence has recently accrued of single or multiple microscopic or small (<6 mm) precursor lesions, mainly in the stomach, which bear the typical kit mutations. These were found in 35% of gastrectomies for carcinoma,[29] and in 22.5% of consecutive autopsy specimens,[30] some with calcification. The findings suggest that this is a common event and that most such lesions do not progress to clinical significance. In about 10% of cases, the tumor arises outside the gastrointestinal tract (extra-GIST) in retroperitoneum, omentum, or mesentery.

Bowel lesions present with a mass, hemorrhage, pain, or intestinal obstruction depending on the location, but the presenting symptoms sometimes relate to metastatic disease in liver or peritoneum. Small lesions (<1 cm) can be found incidentally during unrelated procedures. Over the years, numerous pathologic features have been proposed to identify malignant GISTs and predict their behavior. However, the current practice is to consider all GISTs as potentially malignant with variable risk, which can be assessed by a combination of three parameters—tumor size, mitotic index, and location (Table 5.2).[30,31] A staging system for GIST has been included in the 7th edition of the UICC TNM classification[32] (Table 5.3), and a protocol for the examination of specimens has been published.[33]

Pathologic Features

GISTs are circumscribed or multinodular firm white masses which can show cyst formation, hemorrhage and necrosis. They can reach 35 cm in diameter but most are between 5 and 10 cm. Most arise in the muscular

TABLE 5.2 Risk of Progression* in GISTs (%)

Mitotic Index per 50 hpf	Tumor Size cm	Risk	Stomach	Duodenum	Jejunum/Ileum	Rectum
<5	<2	None	0	0	0	0
<5	2–5	Very low or low	1.9	8.3	4.3	8.5
<5	>5–10	Low or moderate	3.6	–	24	–
<5	>10	Moderate or high	10	34	52	57
>5	<2	None or high	None	–	–	54
>5	2–5	Moderate	16	50	73	52
>5	>5–10	High	55	–	85	–
>5	>10	High	86	86	90	71

* = metastasis or tumor-related death.
– = insufficient data
Modified from Miettinen M, Lasota J. Gastrointestinal stromal tumors: pathology and prognosis at different sites. *Semin Diagn Pathol.* 2006;23:70–83, by permission of Elsevier.

TABLE 5.3 Staging System for Gastrointestinal Stromal Tumors

T–Primary Tumor				
TX–Primary tumor cannot be assessed				
T0–No evidence for primary tumor				
T1–Tumor 2 cm or less				
T2–Tumor more than 2 cm but not more than 5 cm				
T3–Tumor more than 5 cm but not more than 10 cm				
T4–Tumor more than 10 cm in greatest dimension				
N–Regional lymph nodes				
NX–Regional lymph nodes cannot be assessed[a]				
N0–No regional lymph node metastasis				
N1–Regional lymph node metastasis				
M–Distant metastasis				
M0–No distant metastasis				
M1–Distant metastasis				
Histopathological grading				
Grading for GIST is dependent on mitotic rate.[b]				
Low mitotic rate: 5 or fewer per 50 hpf				
High mitotic rate: over 5 per 50 hpf				
STAGE GROUPING				
Gastric GIST				
				Mitotic rate
Stage IA	T1, T2	N0	M0	Low
Stage IB	T3	N0	M0	Low
Stage II	T1, T2	N0	M0	High
	T4	N0	M0	Low
Stage IIIA	T3	N0	M0	High
Stage IIIB	T4	N0	M0	High
Stage IV	Any T	N1	M0	Any rate

(Continued)

TABLE 5.3 Staging System for Gastrointestinal Stromal Tumors (Continued)

	Any T	Any N	M1	Any rate
Small Intestinal GIST[c]				
				Mitotic rate
Stage I	T1, T2	N0	M0	Low
Stage II	T3	N0	M0	Low
Stage IIIA	T1	N0	M0	High
	T4	N0	M0	Low
Stage IIIB	T2, T3, T4	N0	M0	High
Stage IV	Any T	N1	M0	Any rate
	Any T	Any N	M1	Any rate
SUMMARY Gastrointestinal Stromal Tumour				
T1	≤ 2 cm			
T2	> 2–5 cm			
T3	> 5–10 cm			
T4	> 10 cm			

[a] NX: Regional lymph node involvement is rare for GISTs so that cases in which the nodal status is not assessed clinically or pathologically could be considered N0 instead of NX or Pnx.

[b] The mitotic rate of GIST is best expressed as the number of mitoses per 50 high-power fields (hpf) using the 40× objective (total area 5 mm^2 in 50 fields).

[c] Staging criteria for gastric tumors can be applied in primary, solitary omental GISTs. Staging criteria for intestinal tumours can be applied to GISTs in less common sites such as esophagus, colon, rectum, and mesentery.

Sobin LH, Gospodarowicz MK, Wittekind Ch, eds. *UICC, International Union Against Cancer. TNM Classification of Malignant Tumours*. Chichester: Wiley-Blackwell, 2010. With permission from John Wiley and Sons Ltd

wall of the bowel (e-Fig. 5.15) though some are serosal or centered on muscularis mucosae. Microscopically, they comprise spindled or epithelioid cells, or a mixture.[31] The spindle cells are elongated, with nuclei displaying pointed or blunt ends (Figs. 5.7 and 5.8, e-Fig. 5.15), paranuclear vacuoles (which can be a prominent feature, e-Fig. 5.16), and moderate amounts of eosinophilic cytoplasm. The cells are arranged in fascicles, sometimes with nuclear palisading. Epithelioid cells can also show prominent vacuolation or a clear cell appearance, and be arranged in organoid nests (e-Figs. 5.17–5.20). Variations include plasmacytoid and rhabdoid change (e-Fig. 5.19), and degenerative nuclear change is sometimes seen (e-Fig. 5.21) but true pleomorphism is uncommon. However, dedifferentiated GIST, with

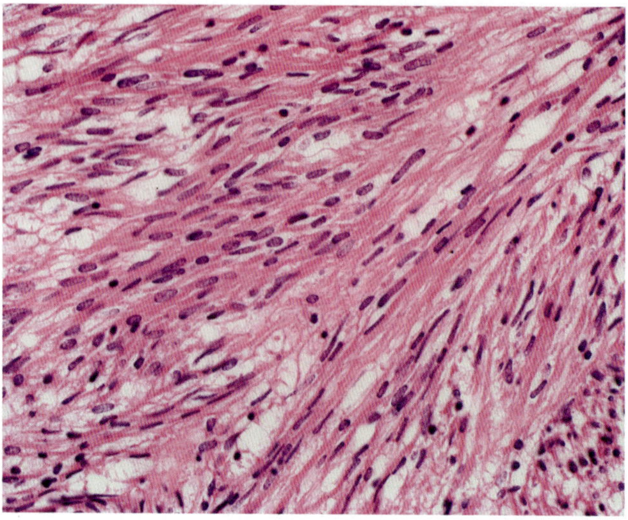

FIGURE 5.7. **Gastrointestinal Stromal Tumor.** The spindle cells have long slender nuclei with rounded ends and are arranged in fascicles. Note the focal myxoid stromal change.

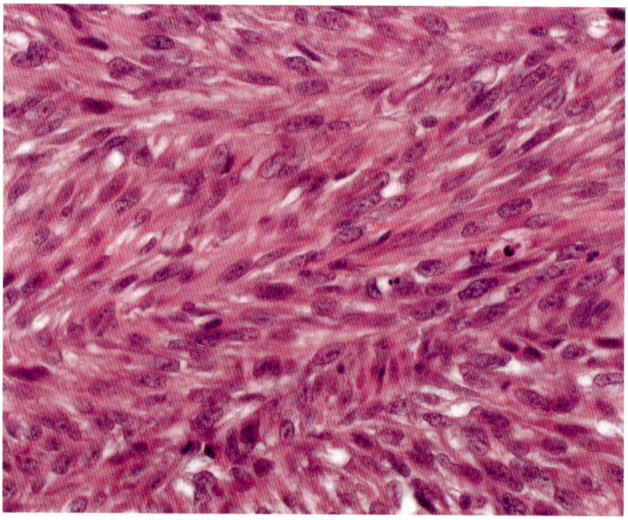

FIGURE 5.8. **Gastrointestinal Stromal Tumor.** The cells are closely packed and uniform and here resemble peripheral nerve sheath tumor.

a component of high-grade sarcoma, has recently been recognized. The stroma can be myxoid or hyalinized and can contain giant cells (e-Fig. 5.22); eosinophilic cytoplasmic bodies (skeinoid fibers) are sometimes seen, especially in GIST in the small intestine (e-Fig. 5.23). These contain tangled collagen fibers and are PASD-positive (e-Fig. 5.24).

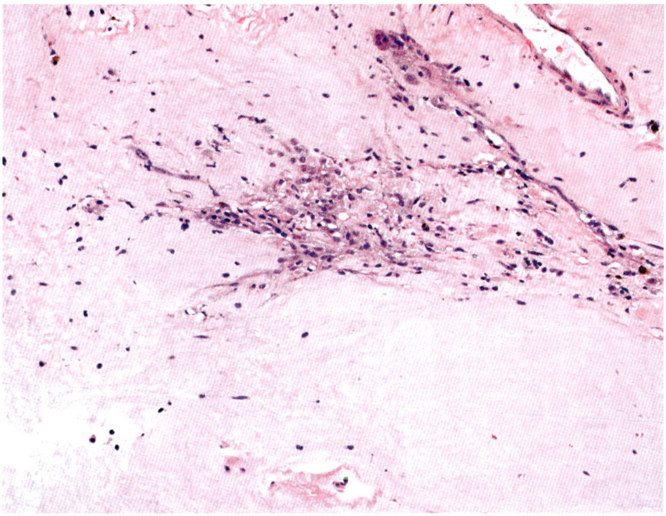

FIGURE 5.9. **Gastrointestinal Stromal Tumor.** Biopsy appearances following therapy with imatinib. There is loss of tumor cells with scattered foamy macrophages in a fibromyxoid stroma.

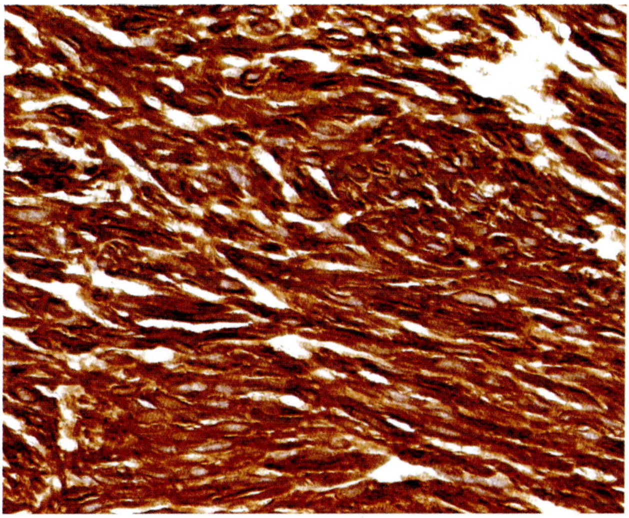

FIGURE 5.10. **Gastrointestinal Stromal Tumor.** Diffuse membranous immunoreactivity for CD117 is characteristic of this tumor. Immunoperoxidase

Biopsies and excision specimens taken after targeted therapy with imatinib or sunitinib show hypocellularity, necrosis, myxoid change, and clusters of foamy cells with variable amounts of residual tumor (Fig. 5.9, e-Fig. 5.25). Identification (but not yet quantification) of the latter is sometimes requested by clinicians although the need for this in determining management is unclear.

Ancillary Investigations

GISTs are considered to show differentiation toward the interstitial cell of Cajal. Almost all GISTs show diffuse membranous (Fig. 5.10) and cytoplasmic immunoreactivity for CD117 (KIT), sometimes with a paranuclear dot pattern. Depending on location, 60% to 70% are immunoreactive for CD34, 30% to 40% for SMA, 5% for S100 protein, and 1% to 2% for cytokeratin.[28] Desmin is positive in only about 1% of cases, but h-caldesmon is often positive in GIST, which can cause misdiagnosis as leiomyosarcoma; smooth muscle tumors, however, are negative for CD117. About 5% of GIST are KIT-negative and DOG1, an immunohistochemical marker derived from gene expression profiling studies with high specificity and sensitivity for GIST, is useful for diagnosis of KIT-negative GIST.[37] Over 75% of these also show diffuse positivity for protein kinase C theta.[36]

On genetic examination, mutations in one or other (but not both) of the genes for the receptor tyrosine kinases *KIT* or platelet-derived growth factor A (*PDGFRA*), which lead to constitutional (ligand-independent) activation of the receptors, are found in over 90% of GISTs. *KIT* mutations mostly involve exon 11 (juxtamembranous domain) and less commonly exons 9, 8 (extracellular domain), 13, and 17 (kinase I and II domains). *PDGFRA* mutations are identifiable in up to 8% of tumors, in exons 12 (juxtamembranous), 14, or 18 (kinase II domain), and are usually found in epithelioid gastric tumors that tend to be less aggressive, but GISTs with the most common one, an Asp842Val substitution in exon 18, are resistant to imatinib.[35] GISTs associated with NF-1, and a subset of those in pediatric age groups, lack mutations of both *KIT* and *PDGFRA*. Similar germline mutations are found in patients with familial GISTs, with 100% penetrance.[36] Mutational analysis is increasingly used for assessing management and outcome. For example, the best responses to imatinib (about 65% of cases) are seen in tumors with exon 11 mutations, whereas those with *KIT* exon 9 Ala502_Tyr503dup mutants occur predominantly in GISTs in small intestine and right colon are more aggressive and less responsive to imatinib (34% to 40%).[37] Additional mutations can arise in the course of therapy and impart secondary resistance to imatinib.[38] Sunitinib, another kinase inhibitor, is currently advocated as second-line therapy in this situation.

DEDIFFERENTIATED LIPOSARCOMA (SEE ALSO CHAPTER 16)

Clinical Features

Dedifferentiated liposarcoma arises de novo or in the course of recurrence of atypical lipomatous tumor/well-differentiated liposarcoma (WDL).[39] The risk of dedifferentiation varies with location; subcutaneous tumors rarely dedifferentiate, subfascial tumors in extremities have a 6% risk, and intra-abdominal tumors have the highest risk with dedifferentiation in

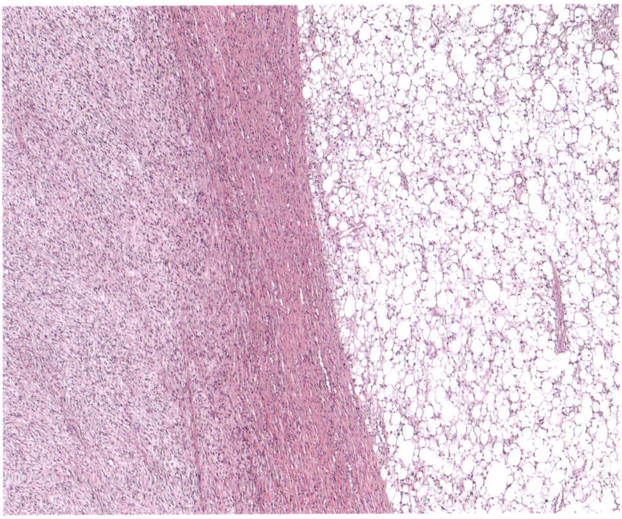

FIGURE 5.11. **Dedifferentiated Liposarcoma.** This spindle cell sarcoma (left) is clearly demarcated from the adjacent WDL (right).

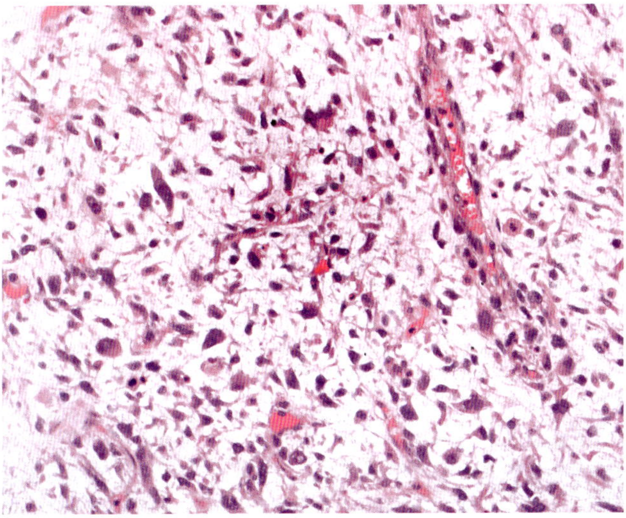

FIGURE 5.12. **Dedifferentiated Liposarcoma.** Myxofibrosarcoma-like component, with pleomorphic polygonal and spindle cells in myxoid stroma.

about 25% of cases. Most pleomorphic sarcomas and myxofibrosarcomas in the abdomen[40] and rhabdomyosarcomas in the internal trunk[41] are now considered to represent dedifferentiated liposarcoma so that the incidence has increased. Clinically, dedifferentiation in liposarcoma manifests an increased rate of growth compared with WDL.

Pathologic Features

The dedifferentiated areas can be of high or low grade. The former resemble either pleomorphic undifferentiated sarcoma, with pleomorphic spindle, polygonal and multinucleated cells (Fig. 5.11, e-Fig. 5.26), or with marked inflammation (inflammatory malignant fibrous histiocytoma, Figs. 13.6, e-Figs. 13.22–13.24), or myxofibrosarcoma (Fig. 5.12, e-Fig. 5.27). An unusual feature is the presence of whorls of spindle cells around a small blood vessel, often near to a focus of metaplastic bone (e-Figs. 5.28 and 5.31), and divergent differentiation, notably to osteosarcoma, chondrosarcoma (e-Fig. 5.29), or rhabdomyosarcoma, can be seen in occasional cases. Low-grade dedifferentiation, which is less common, resembles low-grade fibrosarcoma, with cellular fascicles of focally atypical spindle cells (Fig 5.13, e-Fig. 5.30). This differs from sclerosing well-differentiated liposarcoma in being much more cellular, and in lacking lipoblasts; typically, no lipogenic component is seen in several contiguous low-power microscopic fields. The well-differentiated (lipogenic) component in dedifferentiated liposarcoma is mostly discrete, but the two components can be intermingled in a mosaic pattern.

Ancillary Investigations

Immunohistochemistry is positive for CDK4 and MDM2 in nuclei of tumor cells in both the well-differentiated and the dedifferentiated component (e-Figs. 5.32 and 5.33). Amplification of these genes can be detected by molecular genetic techniques. Results of gene expression profiling have suggested the therapeutic use of mdm2 antagonists.[42] The spindle component can also show variable positivity for SMA, desmin, and CD34, but beta-catenin and CD117 are negative.

SARCOMATOID MESOTHELIOMA

Identification of mesothelioma is important for clinical and medico-legal reasons. This neoplasm can assume biphasic, epithelioid, spindle cell or, exceptionally, pleomorphic cytomorphology both in the thorax when the lung or chest wall can be involved and in the abdomen where there can be visceral involvement. Sarcomatoid (spindle cell) mesothelioma is an uncommon but aggressive mesothelioma variant which needs to be distinguished from sarcomatoid carcinoma, synovial sarcoma, MPNST, leiomyosarcoma, fibrosarcoma, and solitary fibrous tumor. Notwithstanding the use of an extensive panel of antibodies, the diagnosis can require careful synthesis of clinical, radiological, and pathological findings. This is especially so in small samples such as core biopsies.

Clinical Features

Mesothelioma can arise in pleural or pericardial cavities and in the abdominal cavity including the paratesticular region. The best known predisposing factor is occupational or other exposure to asbestos, especially of the

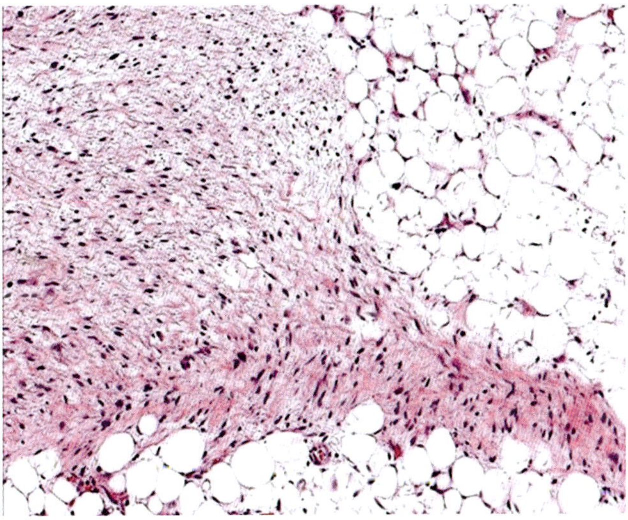

FIGURE 5.13. **Dedifferentiated Liposarcoma with Low-Grade Dedifferentiation.** This resembles low-grade fibrosarcoma, here seen infiltrating into the well-differentiated liposarcomatous component.

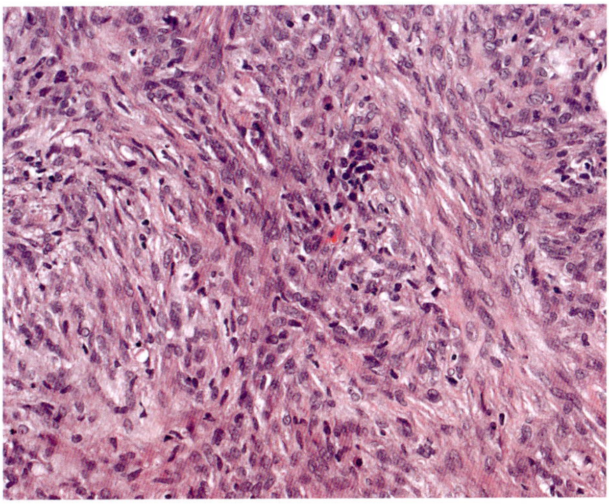

FIGURE 5.14. **Sarcomatoid Mesothelioma.** This tumor comprises fascicles of uniform spindle cells with a focal storiform pattern, infiltrating fibrous stroma.

amphibole type (of which crocidolite and amosite have the highest risk). There is usually a long latent period of at least 15 years before the development of mesothelioma. Some examples have been associated with prior irradiation or fibrosing chronic inflammation. Mesothelioma affects mainly adults in fifth to eighth decades and is more common in males. Diffuse

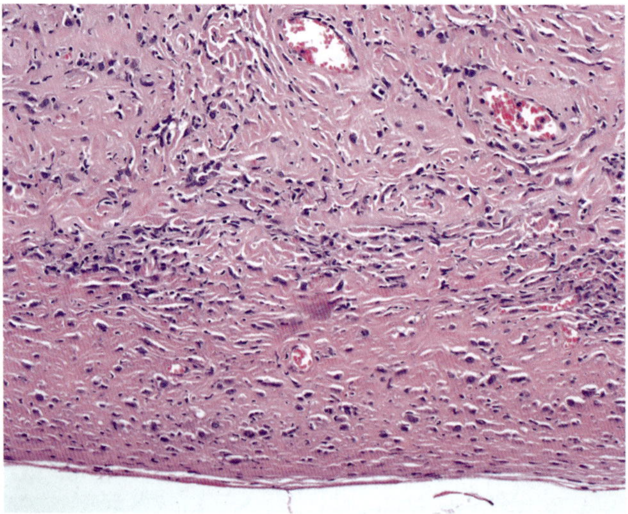

FIGURE 5.15. **Desmoplastic Sarcomatoid Mesothelioma.** Pleomorphic spindle cells with hyperchromatic nuclei are dispersed in dense fibrous tissue. This variant is often hypocellular so that the neoplastic cells can be overlooked.

mesothelioma forms an ill-defined sheet-like mass that can infiltrate underlying structures. It can manifest in the abdomen as an omental tumor.

Pathologic Features

In sarcomatoid mesothelioma, the cells are elongated with variably pleomorphic tapered nuclei and scanty cytoplasm. They are arranged in parallel fascicles and can show mitotic activity and necrosis (Fig. 5.14, e-Figs. 5.34–5.36). Rarely there are foci resembling undifferentiated pleomorphic sarcoma (malignant fibrous histiocytoma). Stromal desmoplasia (with relatively bland scattered cells) (Fig. 5.15, e-Figs. 5.35 and 5.36) or hyalinization, multinucleated giant cells, and a hemangiopericytomatous pattern can be seen. Rarely, there are vacuolated cells or histiocyte-like cells with marked mixed inflammation (e-Fig. 5.37). Asbestos bodies (e-Fig. 5.38) can sometimes be identified in the lung tissue adjacent to intrathoracic tumors. Desmoplastic mesothelioma differs from a pleural plaque by increased cellularity, mitotic activity, pleomorphism and necrosis, as well as infiltration of adjacent structures. Immunohistochemistry is unhelpful in this situation.

Ancillary Investigations

Epithelioid mesothelioma can express cytokeratins (especially CAM5.2 and CK5/6), EMA, calretinin, thrombomodulin, WT1, HBME-1, mesothelin, podoplanin (D2-40)[43] and SMA, and lack CD34, bcl2, S100 protein, TTF1, CEA, and BerEP4. However, in the spindle cells of biphasic mesothelioma and in the sarcomatoid variant, expression of many of these antigens is variable. For example, CK5/6, D2-40, and mesothelin are rarely expressed.[43] However, the combination of a broad-spectrum cytokeratin with calretinin can be diagnostically specific and sensitive for sarcomatoid mesothelioma. Those cases that express only cytokeratins can be difficult to distinguish from monophasic synovial sarcoma and spindle cell carcinoma. The former lacks pleomorphism and usually has very focal expression of epithelial antigens, as well as diffuse immunoreactivity for bcl-2. The diagnosis can be confirmed by genetic demonstration of the specific (X;18) and fusion gene products, which are absent from mesothelioma. Sarcomatoid carcinoma also has widespread positivity for cytokeratins but is usually more pleomorphic and reticulin staining can reveal a pattern of small nests. Electron microscopy can be diagnostic by revealing elongated microvilli but these are less frequent in the spindle cells of mesothelioma which generally show features of fibroblasts or occasionally myofibroblasts.

FOLLICULAR DENDRITIC CELL SARCOMA

The follicular dendritic (dendritic reticulum) cell is considered to be a mesenchymal-derived cell in the lymphoid follicle which is involved in "antigen processing." It has pale nuclei with distinct nuclear membrane, long cell processes, and a characteristic CD21/CD35-positive immunophenotype. Its rare malignant counterpart, follicular dendritic cell sarcoma (FDCS), was initially described chiefly in lymphoid tissue. However, over a third of published cases have involved extranodal locations, including oral cavity (tonsil, palate) pharynx, neck, axilla, GI tract (stomach, colon), spleen, mediastinum, lung, mesentery, mesocolon, and breast. A proportion of cases of hyaline-vascular type of Castlemans disease is associated with or eventuates in FDCS, accounting for 10% to 15% of reported examples, often with antecedent FDC hyperplasia and dysplasia (e-Figs. 5.39–5.42).[44]

Clinical Features

FDCS is a tumor of young and middle-aged adults which presents as localized lymphadenopathy or with symptoms related to a mass (up to 20 cm in maximum dimension in reported cases). Although many are indolent, a proportion are aggressive with a 3-year mortality of up to 20%.[45] In an analysis of 46 extranodal cases with a median follow-up of 18 months, 43% of the cases recurred and 7% died of disease, with a 5-year recurrence-free survival of only 27.4%.[46]

Pathologic Features

FDC sarcomas are composed of sheets or vaguely storiform whorls of ovoid cells with pale cytoplasm and indistinct cell boundaries giving a focally syncytial appearance (Figs. 5.16 and 5.17, e-Figs. 5.43–5.45). Their nuclei have distinctive speckled chromatin and prominent nuclear membranes, and there is a characteristic infiltrate of small lymphocytes which adhere

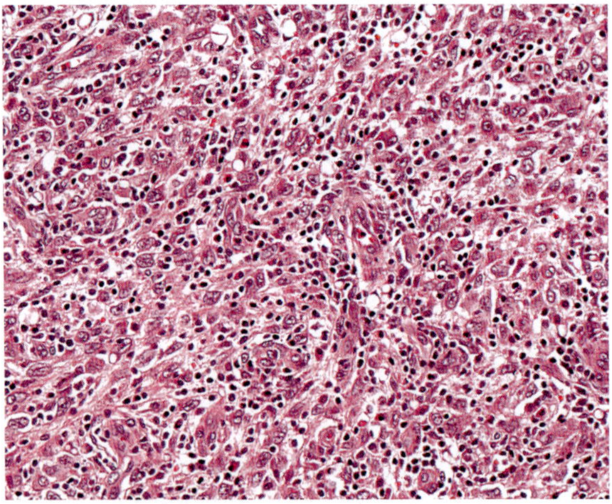

FIGURE 5.16. **Follicular Dendritic Cell Sarcoma.** Ovoid cells with vesicular nuclei are typically arranged in loosely cohesive sheets. Note the moderate to marked lymphocytic infiltrate closely associated with the tumor cells.

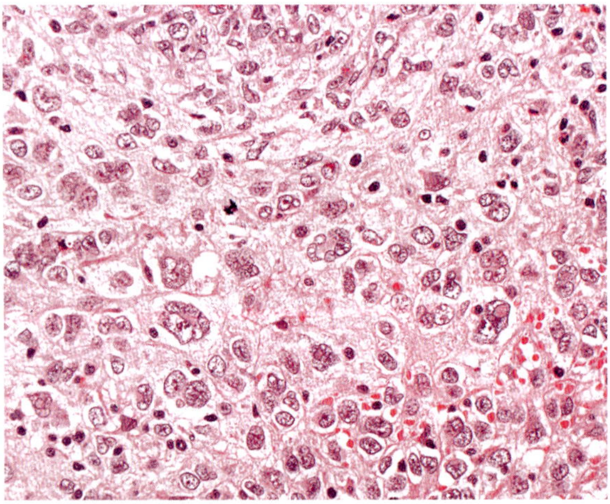

FIGURE 5.17. **Follicular Dendritic Cell Sarcoma.** This tumor has a less prominent lymphocytic component. The nuclei have distinct nuclear membranes, small nucleoli, and occasional intranuclear inclusions.

to the bodies and processes of the tumor cells, and also form perivascular cuffs. Other occasional features include giant cells, pleomorphism, and necrosis.

Ancillary Investigations

These tumors are readily diagnosed by their expression of FDC antigens, notably CD21, CD35 (most sensitive when their antibodies are used together as a cocktail[47]) (e-Fig. 5.46) and CD23. Because of the specificity of these markers, FDCS is readily identified once the diagnosis has come to mind. Other antigens expressed include S100 protein, EMA, desmoplakin, D2-40, fascin, clusterin, and epidermal growth factor receptor. Epstein Barr virus-encoded RNA (EBER) can be demonstrated, by immunohistochemistry or in situ hybridization, in the inflammatory variant. The lesional cells lack CD45 and other lymphocytic markers, and the infiltrating lymphocytes are a mixture of T and (fewer) B cells. Electron microscopy shows interdigitating cytoplasmic processes with poorly formed desmosomes but no external lamina and no Birbeck granules.

VARIANTS

Inflammatory pseudotumor-like FDC sarcoma occurs mainly in females, in liver, spleen or peripancreatic retroperitoneum and is an EBV-associated neoplasm which can cause systemic symptoms.[48] The lesional cells are inconspicuous and dispersed within a dense mixed inflammatory infiltrate including lymphocytes, plasma cells, and giant cells (e-Fig. 5.47).

Myxoid FDC sarcoma has so far been described only in the breast.[49] There is a focally prominent myxoid stroma that separates the tumor cells and their adherent lymphocytes (e-Figs. 5.48 and 5.49).

ENDOMETRIAL STROMAL SARCOMA

This can arise in the abdomen from a focus of endometriosis, or be metastatic there and in other locations. There may be a remote history of hysterectomy with or without a diagnosis of stromal sarcoma. Endometrial stromal sarcoma is composed of closely packed short spindle cells which resemble those of synovial sarcoma (e-Figs. 5.50–5.52). There can be variable smooth muscle differentiation, and immunohistochemically, there is immunoreactivity for CD10 and focally for SMA, desmin, and occasionally cytokeratins. Endometrial stromal sarcomas also display nuclear staining for ER and PgR, and 40% have nuclear positivity for beta-catenin.[50] Specific chromosomal rearrangements t(7;17)(p15;q21), t(6p;7p), and t(6p;10q;10p) have been described in some endometrial stromal sarcomas, resulting respectively in *JAZF1-JJAZ1*, *JAZF1-PHF1*, and *EPC1-PHF1* fusion genes.

Sometimes the stroma represents part of a deposit of endometriosis in which the glands are not represented. Cutting into the block can reveal the glandular component Endometriosis can be found almost anywhere within the abdomen and pelvis and occasionally in extra-abdominal locations (e-Figs. 5.53 and 5.54).

REFERENCES

1. Yantiss RK, Nielsen GP, Lauwers GY, et al. Reactive nodular fibrous pseudotumor of the gastrointestinal tract and mesentery: a clinicopathologic study of five cases. *Am J Surg Pathol*. 2003;27:532–540.

2. Patel RM, Weiss SW, Folpe AL. Heterotopic mesenteric ossification: a distinctive pseudosarcoma commonly associated with intestinal obstruction. *Am J Surg Pathol* 2006;30:119–122.
3. Daum O, Vanecek T, Sima R, et al. Reactive nodular fibrous pseudotumors of the gastrointestinal tract: report of 8 cases. *Int J Surg Pathol.* 2004;12:365–374.
4. Baker LR. Auto-allergic periaortitis (idiopathic retroperitoneal fibrosis). *BJU Int* 2003;92:663–665.
5. Kuwatani M, Kawakami H, Makiyama H, et al. Autoimmune pancreatitis with retroperitoneal fibrosis which responded to steroid therapy but was complicated with refractory renal dysfunction. *Intern Med.* 2007;46:1557–1564.
6. Dehner LP, Coffin CM. Idiopathic fibrosclerotic disorders and other inflammatory pseudotumors. Semin Diagn Pathol 1998;15:161–173.
7. Kamisawa T, Nakajima H, Egawa N, et al. IgG4-related sclerosing disease incorporating sclerosing pancreatitis, cholangitis, sialadenitis and retroperitoneal fibrosis with lymphadenopathy. *Pancreatology*. 2006;6:132–137.
8. Miyajima N, Koike H, Kawaguchi M, et al. Idiopathic retroperitoneal fibrosis associated with IgG4-positive-plasmacyte infiltrations and idiopathic chronic pancreatitis. *Int J Urol* 2006;13:1442–1444.
9. Emory TS, Monihan JM, Carr NJ, et al. Sclerosing mesenteritis, mesenteric panniculitis and mesenteric lipodystrophy: A single entity? *Am J Surg Pathol.* 1997;21:392–398.
10. Akram S, Pardi DS, Schaffner JA, et al. Sclerosing mesenteritis: clinical features, treatment, and outcome in ninety-two patients. *Clin Gastroenterol Hepatol.* 2007;5:589–596; quiz 523–584.
11. Scudiere JR, Shi C, Hruban RH, et al. Sclerosing mesenteritis involving the pancreas: a mimicker of pancreatic cancer. *Am J Surg Pathol.* 2010;34:447–453.
12. Sabate JM, Torrubia S, Maideu J, et al. Sclerosing mesenteritis: imaging findings in 17 patients. AJR Am J Roentgenol 1999;172:625–629.
13. Howaizi M, Kanate A. Sclerosing mesenteritis associated with giant-cell temporal arteritis. *Eur J Intern Med.* 2006;17:511–513.
14. Montgomery E, Torbenson MS, Kaushal M, et al. Beta-catenin immunohistochemistry separates mesenteric fibromatosis from gastrointestinal stromal tumor and sclerosing mesenteritis. *Am J Surg Pathol.* 2002;26:1296–1301.
15. Meis JM, Enzinger FM. Inflammatory fibrosarcoma of the mesentery and retroperitoneum. A tumor closely simulating inflammatory pseudotumor. *Am J Surg Pathol.* 1991;15:1146–1156.
16. Coden DJ, Hornblass A. Orbital hemangiopericytoma. *JAMA*. 1990;264:1861.
17. Coffin CM, Humphrey PA, Dehner LP. Extrapulmonary inflammatory myofibroblastic tumor: a clinical and pathological survey. *Semin Diagn Pathol.* 1998;15:85–101.
18. Harik LR, Merino C, Coindre JM, et al. Pseudosarcomatous myofibroblastic proliferations of the bladder: a clinicopathologic study of 42 cases. *Am J Surg Pathol.* 2006;30:787–794.
19. Sukov WR, Cheville JC, Carlson AW, et al. Utility of ALK-1 protein expression and ALK rearrangements in distinguishing inflammatory myofibroblastic tumor from malignant spindle cell lesions of the urinary bladder. *Mod Pathol.* 2007;20:592–603.
20. Montgomery EA, Shuster DD, Burkart AL, et al. Inflammatory myofibroblastic tumors of the urinary tract: a clinicopathologic study of 46 cases, including a malignant example inflammatory fibrosarcoma and a subset associated with high-grade urothelial carcinoma. *Am J Surg Pathol.* 2006;30:1502–1512.
21. Hirsch MS, Dal Cin P, Fletcher CD. ALK expression in pseudosarcomatous myofibroblastic proliferations of the genitourinary tract. *Histopathology.* 2006;48:569–578.
22. Hussong JW, Brown M, Perkins SL, et al. Comparison of DNA ploidy, histologic, and immunohistochemical findings with clinical outcome in inflammatory myofibroblastic tumors. *Mod Pathol.* 1999;12:279–286.

23. Coffin CM, Hornick JL, Fletcher CD. Inflammatory myofibroblastic tumor: comparison of clinicopathologic, histologic, and immunohistochemical features including ALK expression in atypical and aggressive cases. *Am J Surg Pathol.* 2007;31:509–520.
24. Schildhaus HU, Cavlar T, Binot E, et al. Inflammatory fibroid polyps harbour mutations in the platelet-derived growth factor receptor alpha (PDGFRA) gene. *J Pathol.* 2008;216:176–182.
25. Meis-Kindblom JM, Kjellstrom C, Kindblom LG. Inflammatory fibrosarcoma: update, reappraisal, and perspective on its place in the spectrum of inflammatory myofibroblastic tumors. *Semin Diagn Pathol.* 1998;15:133–143.
26. Eyden B, Banerjee SS, Shenjere P, et al. The myofibroblast and its tumours. *J Clin Pathol.* 2009;62:236–249.
27. Matyakhina L, Bei TA, McWhinney SR, et al. Genetics of carney triad: recurrent losses at chromosome 1 but lack of germline mutations in genes associated with paragangliomas and gastrointestinal stromal tumors. *J Clin Endocrinol Metab.* 2007;92:2938–2943.
28. Rubin BP, Heinrich MC, Corless CL. Gastrointestinal stromal tumour. *Lancet.* 2007;369:1731–1741.
29. Kawanowa K, Sakuma Y, Sakurai S, et al. High incidence of microscopic gastrointestinal stromal tumors in the stomach. *Hum Pathol.* 2006;37:1527–1535.
30. Demetri GD, Benjamin RS, Blanke CD, et al. NCCN Task Force report: management of patients with gastrointestinal stromal tumor (GIST)–update of the NCCN clinical practice guidelines. *J Natl Compr Canc Netw.* 2007;5(suppl 2):S1–S29; quiz S30.
31. Miettinen M, Lasota J. Gastrointestinal stromal tumors: pathology and prognosis at different sites. *Semin Diagn Pathol.* 2006;23:70–83.
32. Sobin LH, Gospodarowicz MK, Wittekind Ch, eds. *UICC, International Union Against Cancer. TNM Classification of Malignant Tumours.* Chichester: Wiley-Blackwell, 2010.
33. Rubin BP, Blanke CD, Demetri GD, et al. Protocol for the examination of specimens from patients with gastrointestinal stromal tumor. *Arch Pathol Lab Med.* 2010;134:165–170.
34. Miettinen M, Lasota J. Gastrointestinal stromal tumors: review on morphology, molecular pathology, prognosis, and differential diagnosis. *Arch Pathol Lab Med.* 2006;130:1466–1478.
35. Lasota J, Corless CL, Heinrich MC, et al. Clinicopathologic profile of gastrointestinal stromal tumors (GISTs) with primary KIT exon 13 or exon 17 mutations: a multicenter study on 54 cases. *Mod Pathol.* 2008;21:476–484.
36. McWhinney SR, Pasini B, Stratakis CA. Familial gastrointestinal stromal tumors and germ-line mutations. *N Engl J Med.* 2007;357:1054–1056.
37. Heinrich MC, Corless CL, Demetri GD, et al. Kinase mutations and imatinib response in patients with metastatic gastrointestinal stromal tumor. *J Clin Oncol.* 2003;21:4342–4349.
38. Heinrich MC, Corless CL, Blanke CD, et al. Molecular correlates of imatinib resistance in gastrointestinal stromal tumors. *J Clin Oncol.* 2006;24:4764–4774.
39. Evans HL. Atypical lipomatous tumor, its variants, and its combined forms: a study of 61 cases, with a minimum follow-up of 10 years. *Am J Surg Pathol.* 2007;31:1–14.
40. Coindre JM, Mariani O, Chibon F, et al. Most malignant fibrous histiocytomas developed in the retroperitoneum are dedifferentiated liposarcomas: a review of 25 cases initially diagnosed as malignant fibrous histiocytoma. *Mod Pathol.* 2003;16:256–262.
41. Binh MB, Guillou L, Hostein I, et al. Dedifferentiated liposarcomas with divergent myosarcomatous differentiation developed in the internal trunk: a study of 27 cases and comparison to conventional dedifferentiated liposarcomas and leiomyosarcomas. *Am J Surg Pathol.* 2007;31:1557–1566.
42. Singer S, Socci ND, Ambrosini G, et al. Gene expression profiling of liposarcoma identifies distinct biological types/subtypes and potential therapeutic targets in well-differentiated and dedifferentiated liposarcoma. *Cancer Res.* 2007;67:6626–6636.

43. Ordonez NG. D2-40 and podoplanin are highly specific and sensitive immunohistochemical markers of epithelioid malignant mesothelioma. *Hum Pathol.* 2005;36:372–380.
44. Chan AC, Chan KW, Chan JK, et al. Development of follicular dendritic cell sarcoma in hyaline-vascular Castleman's disease of the nasopharynx: tracing its evolution by sequential biopsies. *Histopathology.* 2001;38:510–518.
45. Kairouz S, Hashash J, Kabbara W, et al. Dendritic cell neoplasms: an overview. *Am J Hematol.* 2007;82:924–928.
46. Shia J, Chen W, Tang LH, et al. Extranodal follicular dendritic cell sarcoma: clinical, pathologic, and histogenetic characteristics of an underrecognized disease entity. *Virchows Arch.* 2006;449:148–158.
47. Chan JKC. Proliferative lesions of follicular dendritic cells: an overview, including a detailed account of follicular dendritic cell sarcoma, a neoplasm with many faces and uncommon etiologic associations. *Adv Anat Pathol.* 1997;6:387–411.
48. Cheuk W, Chan JK, Shek TW, et al. Inflammatory pseudotumor-like follicular dendritic cell tumor: a distinctive low-grade malignant intra-abdominal neoplasm with consistent Epstein-Barr virus association. *Am J Surg Pathol.* 2001;25:721–731.
49. Fisher C, Magnusson B, Hardarson S, et al. Myxoid variant of follicular dendritic cell sarcoma arising in the breast. *Ann Diagn Pathol.* 1999;3:92–98.
50. Ng TL, Gown AM, Barry TS, et al. Nuclear beta-catenin in mesenchymal tumors. *Mod Pathol.* 2005;18:68–74.

6

SMOOTH MUSCLE TUMORS

INTRODUCTION

Tumors with smooth muscle differentiation occur in skin, subcutis, and deep soft tissue, as well as pelvis, retroperitoneum (including paratesticular structures), male and female genital tracts, and other viscera. Many of these form distinct clinicopathologic subsets since behavior and criteria of malignancy relate primarily to location. However, the constituent cells have common morphologic and immunohistochemical properties. Some tumors termed myofibroblastoma have characteristics more suggestive of smooth muscle differentiation, but for reasons of terminology and differential diagnosis, they are discussed in Chapter 7.

GENERAL FEATURES OF SMOOTH MUSCLE TUMORS

Pathologic Features

Microscopically, smooth muscle tumors are characterized by elongated cells which are parallel sided with eosinophilic, finely fibrillary cytoplasm and nuclei which are blunt ended and sometimes have paranuclear vacuoles. The latter are more prominent in sections where the spindle cells are cut transversely. The cells are typically arranged in fascicles disposed at right angles to each other, and nuclear palisading can be seen, imparting a resemblance to schwannoma. Stromal features include separation of the cells by myxoid change or fibrosis (the latter sometimes with calcification) and presence of osteoclast-like giant cells. "Degenerative" nuclear change, characterized by enlargement, irregular shape, and uniform hyperchromasia, is a relatively common feature of smooth muscle tumors. This can be seen without mitotic activity (symplastic leiomyoma) or with a prominence disproportionate to the low level of mitotic activity in low-grade leiomyosarcomas. In higher grades of leiomyosarcoma, there is more marked nuclear pleomorphism including prominent nucleoli and more frequent and abnormal mitoses, as well as necrosis.

Ancillary Investigations

Smooth muscle tumors are usually diffusely positive for smooth muscle and muscle-specific actins and calponin and at least focally so for desmin and h-caldesmon. Some smooth muscle tumors additionally express epithelial markers (cytokeratins–often in a dot-like pattern–and epithelial membrane antigen) and S100 protein, but usually in such cases, there is coexistent immunoreactivity for smooth muscle antigens. Occasional leiomyosarcomas, including intra-abdominal tumors, are also CD34 positive but lack CD117 and DOG1, facilitating the distinction from gastrointestinal stromal tumors. Many smooth muscle tumors, especially in females, display positivity for estrogen (ER) and progesterone (PgR) receptors. A subset in the female genital tract, including those with epithelioid morphology, expresses HMB45.[1] Ultrastructurally, smooth muscle cells have longitudinal thin filaments (myofilaments) with dense bodies, present throughout the cytoplasm, pinocytosis, intercellular junctions, and continuous external lamina. There are no consistent molecular genetic abnormalities that are diagnostically useful.

SMOOTH MUSCLE TUMORS OF SKIN AND SUPERFICIAL SUBCUTIS

Clinical Features

Cutaneous leiomyoma can be solitary or multiple (leiomyomatosis), and a familial form is associated with an autosomal dominant inheritance of mutations in the *MCUL-1* gene at 1q42.3–q43, a tumor suppressor gene encoding fumarate hydratase. This genetic abnormality is also implicated in the syndrome of hereditary leiomyomatosis and renal cell cancer.[2] The cutaneous lesions occur mostly in young adults on extensor surfaces of limbs as well as trunk and face. They form small pink to brown papules or nodules in a dermatome distribution and can be painful or tender especially in the cold.

Subcutaneous leiomyoma is rare (see below). Vascular leiomyoma (angioleiomyoma, angiomyoma) is a painful, tender, and cold-sensitive tumor in subcutaneous tissue of head and neck or extremities favoring middle-aged females. A similar lesion has recently been described in the myometrium as a leiomyoma variant.[3]

Cutaneous and superficial subcutaneous leiomyosarcomas also occur on extensor surfaces of limbs and in the head and neck region but more frequently in older adults and predominantly in males. They present as a firm nodule with or without skin discoloration, depending on the tissue plane involved, and can be painful, ulcerated, or bleeding. In one large series of cutaneous leiomyosarcomas, 27% recurred locally and 7% (four cases) metastasized.[4] The latter included one case of dermal leiomyosarcoma with minimal extension into subcutis.

Pathologic Features

Cutaneous (pilar) leiomyomas are noncircumscribed lesions composed of intersecting fascicles of highly differentiated, closely packed smooth muscle cells which infiltrate dermal collagen (Figs. 6.1 and 6.2, e-Figs. 6.1

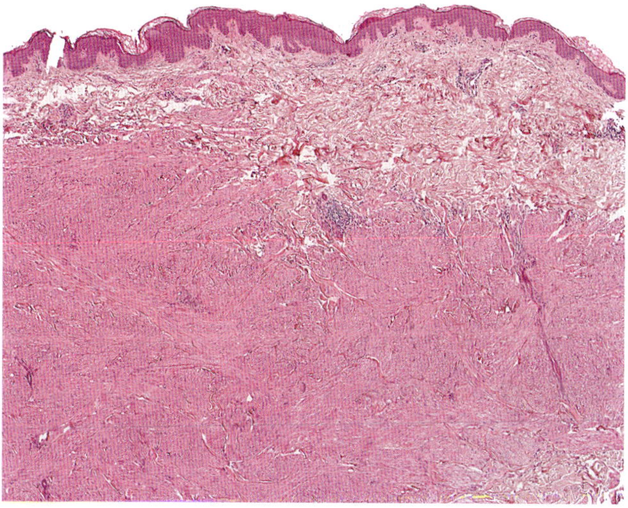

FIGURE 6.1 **Cutaneous Leiomyoma.** This is a dermal tumor composed of tight fascicles of uniform epidermal spindle cells. The lesion is relatively circumscribed but non-encapsulated and does not extend to dermal-epidermal junction.

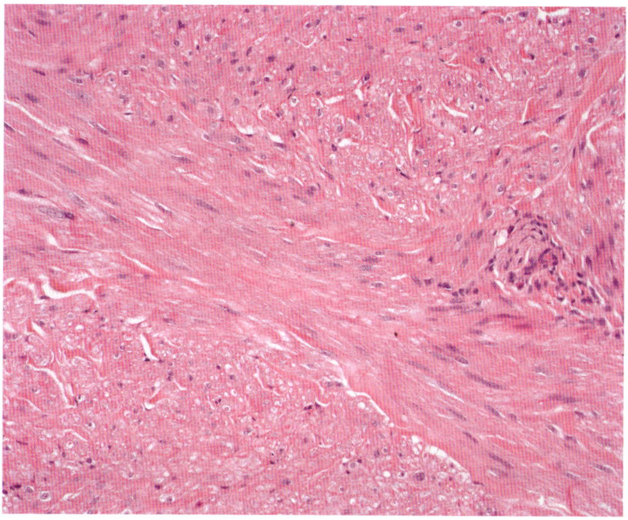

FIGURE 6.2 **Cutaneous Leiomyoma.** The tumor comprises bundles of smooth muscle cells without nuclear atypia, mitotic activity, or necrosis.

and 6.2). The tumor is separated from the epidermis by a grenz zone but sometimes extends into subcutaneous fat.

Vascular leiomyoma is circumscribed, usually <1 cm in diameter, and microscopically composed of smooth muscle bundles in layers, which blend with muscle walls of blood vessels (Fig. 6.3, e-Figs. 6.3–6.7). Three histologic subtypes have been described–solid (with sheets of smooth muscle

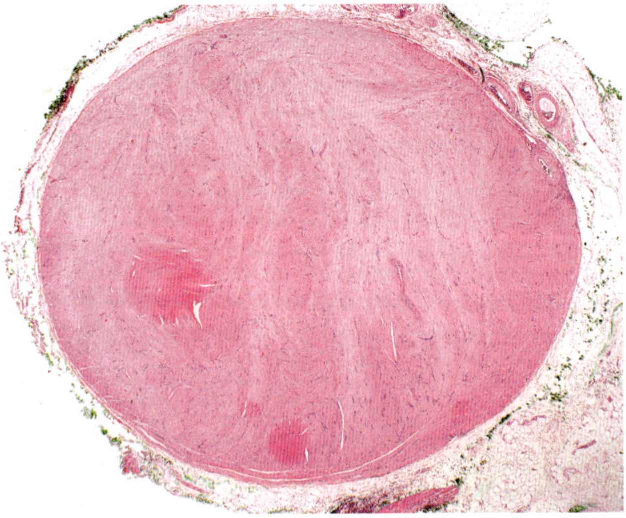

FIGURE 6.3 **Angiomyoma.** A sharply circumscribed subcutaneous lesion comprising whorls of smooth muscle cells with dispersed slit-like vascular spaces.

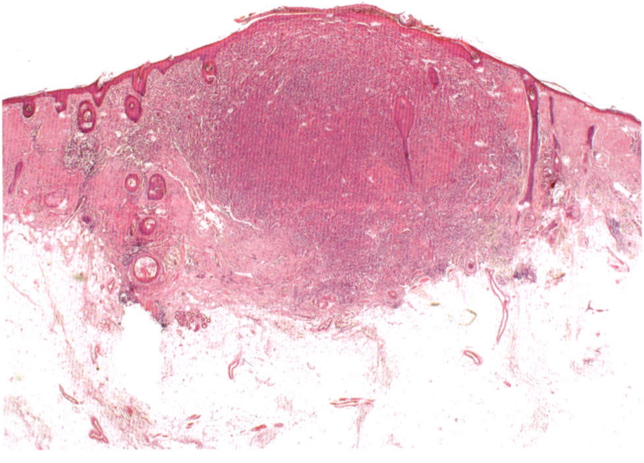

FIGURE 6.4 **Cutaneous Leiomyosarcoma.** The tumor is cellular, infiltrates the dermis, and has irregular margins. Note overlying epidermal hyperplasia with hyperkeratosis and absence of grenz zone.

cells and slit-like vessels), venous (in which smooth bundles blend with the muscular venous wall), and cavernous (which has minimal extravascular smooth muscle). The morphologic features overlap to some extent with those of myopericytoma, and the two entities are probably related.[5]

Cutaneous leiomyosarcomas can have a diffuse or nodular growth pattern (Figs. 6.4 and 6.5, e-Figs. 6.8–6.11). The former, of presumed arrector

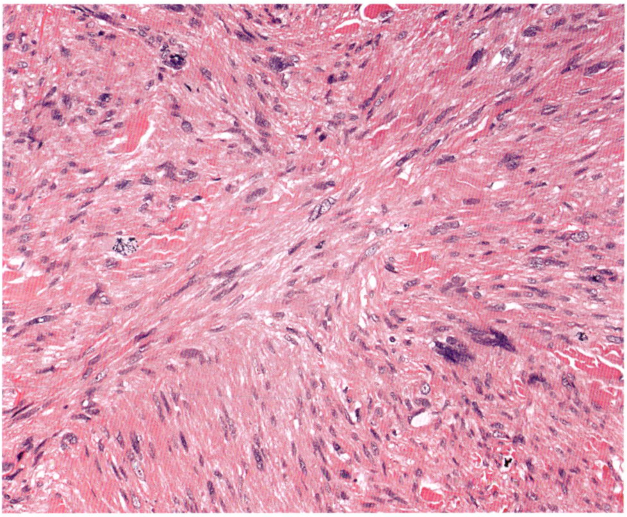

FIGURE 6.5 **Cutaneous Leiomyosarcoma.** Fascicles of elongated spindle cells arranged at right angles. The cells show focal nuclear pleomorphism.

pili origin, are usually better differentiated and confined to dermis. The latter, considered to be tumors of vascular origin, are circumscribed but often more pleomorphic and mitotically active, with deeper extension.

Criteria of Malignancy

In cutaneous leiomyomas, the discovery of a single mitotic figure in a section is not conclusive of malignancy, but such lesions should be completely excised with observation in case of recurrence. For cutaneous and superficial subcutaneous lesions, an index of more than 1 mitosis per 10 hpf, the presence of necrosis, or any significant pleomorphism with or without mitoses indicates a diagnosis of leiomyosarcoma. Knowledge of the precise location of the lesion is essential: leiomyosarcomas confined to the dermis or very superficial subcutis have high (25% to 50%) recurrent but very low metastatic potential,[4] whereas those involving subcutis have recurrence rates of over 50% and metastatic rates of over 30%. The aim should be to obtain clear excision margins although there is no precise recommendation for the minimum width of the clearance. Grade is also a prognostic factor, although tumor size and mitotic index alone have less predictive value.

Ancillary Investigations

Cutaneous differentiated smooth muscle neoplasms usually express desmin, smooth muscle actin (SMA), and h-caldesmon but lack ER and PgR.[6] In vascular leiomyoma, desmin expression is variable, with the solid type mostly being positive and the perivascular myoid whorls negative.[5]

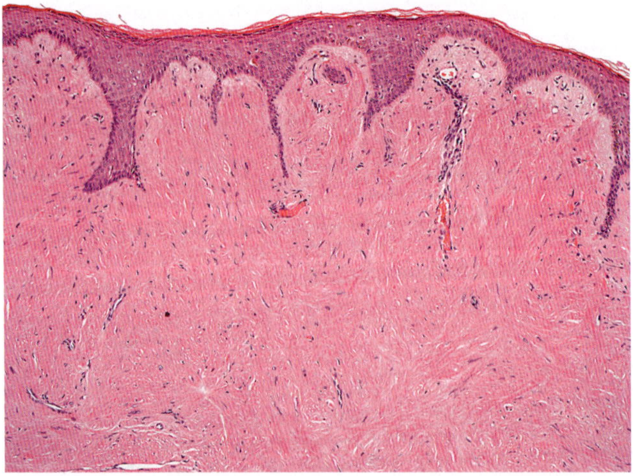

FIGURE 6.6 **Leiomyoma of Nipple.** A homogeneous hypocellular smooth muscle lesion fills the dermis. The cells lack atypia and mitotic activity.

Genital Leiomyoma

A subset of benign smooth muscle tumors arise in the vulva, scrotum, or nipple. Their features differ slightly according to the site.

Clinical features. Nipple lesions present in young adults of either sex as a painful nodule involving the areola.7 Scrotal tumors arise in middle age in the dartos muscle and can form a large painless mass. Vulval leiomyoma occurs in young or middle-aged females as a painless mass, usually in the labium majus, which clinically resembles a Bartholin gland cyst.[8]

Pathologic features and criteria of malignancy. Leiomyoma of nipple resembles other cutaneous leiomyomas, with infiltrative fascicles of bland smooth muscle cells in mid or upper dermis (Fig. 6.6, e-Figs. 6.12–6.14), sometimes with overlying epidermal hyperplasia. Scrotal leiomyomas show similar infiltration of dartos muscle fibers (distinguished from tumor cells by their better organization) but can additionally be hypercellular or show enlarged hyperchromatic nuclei with large nucleoli or multinucleated cells and lymphoid aggregates (Fig. 6.7, e-Figs. 6.15 and 6.16). These bizarre (symplastic) leiomyomas behave in a benign fashion, but the presence of any mitoses in an atypical or hypercellular leiomyoma indicates a diagnosis of leiomyosarcoma. Vulval tumors are often circumscribed rather than infiltrative and can have epithelioid cell morphology and stromal myxoid change or hyalinization. Size >5 cm in diameter, infiltrative margins, moderate to severe cytologic atypia, and a mitotic count of more than 5 mitoses per 10 hpf are features indicative of potential malignant behavior in vulval smooth muscle tumors; it has been suggested that the finding of three or more of these features indicates management as leiomyosarcoma, that is,

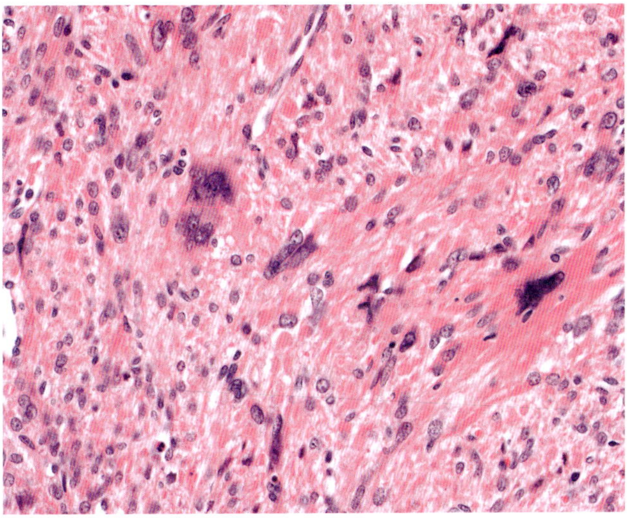

FIGURE 6.7 **Bizarre Leiomyoma of Scrotum.** Scattered cells have hyperchromatic irregularly shaped nuclei, without nucleoli or mitotic activity.

excision with wide negative margins.[8] Tumors with one feature are considered benign and those with two are termed atypical leiomyoma; both can be managed by conservative local excision.

Ancillary investigations. In addition to the usual muscle antigens, leiomyomas of both nipple and vulva are frequently positive for ER and PgR. A clonal translocation t(7;8)(p13;q11.2) has been identified in a leiomyoma of vulva.[9]

SMOOTH MUSCLE TUMORS OF DEEP SUBCUTANEOUS AND SUBFASCIAL SOFT TISSUE

Deeply located smooth muscle tumors present distinct clinical and pathological challenges and require detailed consideration of the separate entities.

DEEP LEIOMYOMA

Clinical Features

Leiomyomas of deep soft tissue are very rare and should be diagnosed only after careful exclusion of malignant features. They are slowly growing tumors which can reach a large size and form a circumscribed mass. Two types are recognized according to the site: tumors in deep subcutaneous or subfascial somatic soft tissue and those within the abdomen. Leiomyoma in deep somatic soft tissue arises in limbs, is rarely associated with blood vessel walls, and occurs equally in either sex. Pelvic and retroperitoneal leiomyomas, which resemble uterine leiomyoma, are more common and

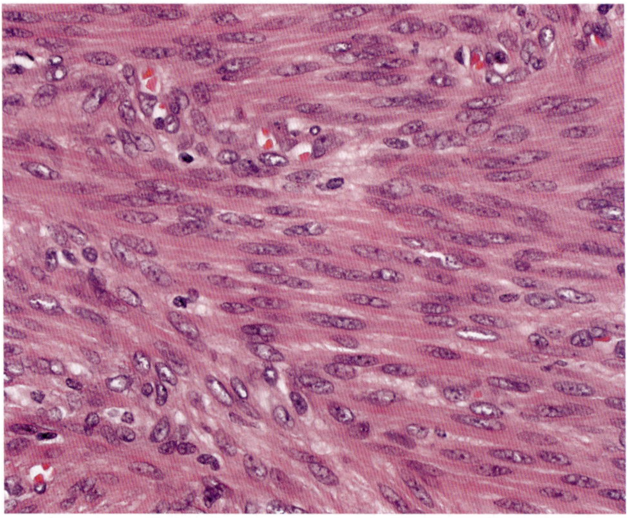

FIGURE 6.8 **Deep Leiomyoma of Thigh.** The lesion is cellular but mitoses, atypia, and necrosis are absent.

the large majority occurs in females.[10,11] Like other retroperitoneal tumors, these can grow to a large size before presentation. By definition, in deep soft tissue leiomyoma, there should be infrequent recurrence and no metastases. In two series, no deep somatic leiomyomas and only 3 of 64 (2%) retroperitoneal cases recurred and none metastasized.[10,11]

Pathologic Features

Microscopically, deep leiomyomas display the usual fascicles of well-differentiated smooth muscle cells and are considered to resemble vascular smooth muscle (Fig. 6.8, e-Figs. 6.17–6.25). In somatic deep leiomyoma, there can be clear cell areas and calcification is common. In retroperitoneal tumors, a range of changes similar to those of uterine leiomyoma can be found. These include hyalinization of blood vessels, focal calcification or ossification, old hemorrhage, and cyst formation. Degenerative nuclear atypia without mitoses (symplastic change) does not indicate malignancy.[12,13] In males, retroperitoneal leiomyomas are more cellular with solid and trabecular patterns, and occasional clear cell areas, but hyalinization, calcification, and ossification can also be seen.[11] Some smooth muscle tumors have a component of differentiated adipose tissue, without atypia. These can be considered as neoplasms with divergent differentiation and are known as lipoleiomyoma or myolipoma according to the dominant component. They occur in the uterus, pelvis, or groin area; in one series of nine myolipomas,[14] seven occurred in deep soft tissue including three in retroperitoneum.

Ancillary Investigations

In addition to the usual markers of smooth muscle differentiation (above), the majority of gynecologic-type deep leiomyomas show nuclear positivity for

ER and PgR.[10,11] Deep leiomyomas elsewhere lack these hormone receptors, but they can be expressed in a proportion of leiomyosarcomas in females and are not therefore a criterion of benignity. They are, however, more weakly and focally expressed in retroperitoneal leiomyosarcoma than in leiomyoma (or uterine leiomyosarcoma).[15] Also, some well-differentiated retroperitoneal leiomyosarcomas which are positive for ER and PgR have a low mitotic index and can be underdiagnosed.[11] Retroperitoneal leiomyomas in males lack ER but an occasional case shows focal positivity for PgR. An occasional retroperitoneal leiomyoma expresses CD34, but CD117 and DOG1 are always negative,[11] aiding in the distinction from gastrointestinal stromal tumor.

Criteria of Malignancy

Excision specimens should be thoroughly sampled. The diagnosis of malignancy in well-differentiated deep smooth muscle tumors is especially problematic in a small or core biopsy. The following recommendations are based on published findings and the authors' personal practice.

1. Lesions without atypia, pleomorphism, or mitoses can be reported (in an excision specimen) as leiomyoma or (in a core biopsy) as smooth muscle tumor without features of malignancy with the caveat that the biopsy might not be representative.
2. The presence of necrosis indicates leiomyosarcoma.[13,16,17]
3. The presence of atypia alone or with any mitoses can be taken as evidence of leiomyosarcoma.[11]
4. In deep leiomyoma of somatic soft tissue with mitoses but no nuclear atypia or necrosis, <1 mitosis per 50 hpf has been considered acceptable for the diagnosis, although one group reported no malignant behavior in tumors with up to 4 per 50 hpf with mean follow-up of 58 months.[10] However, recurrences have been reported by others with 1 mitosis per 50 hpf[13] so that tumors with 1 to 5 mitoses per 50 hpf should be regarded as of at least uncertain malignant potential.[17]
5. In the retroperitoneum, leiomyoma with <1 mitosis per 50 hpf (<3 mitoses per 50 hpf in one series[11]) can be considered as benign. Retroperitoneal leiomyosarcomas generally have >5 mitoses per 10 hpf,[11] but some have fewer (yet have behaved well), so there is overlap in the mitotic indices with a zone of uncertainty. In retroperitoneal uterine-type tumors with up to 5 mitoses per 10 hpf, a small number recurred but none metastasized with median follow-up period of 42[10] and 142[11] months. Such tumors in females with 5 to 10 mitoses per 50 hpf, and in males with 1 to 5 mitoses per 50 hpf, and no other worrisome features should, therefore, be regarded as of uncertain malignant potential.

DEEP LEIOMYOSARCOMA

Clinical Features

The vast majority of smooth muscle tumors of deep soft tissue are malignant. Leiomyosarcoma can occur at any age. The most common, in retroperitoneum, favor adult females between the ages of 40 and 70 years. A subset arises in association with a large vein, notably the inferior vena cava (most commonly in its suprarenal, infrahepatic portion and less frequently in the infrarenal or suprahepatic segments), other large intracavitary or lower extremity veins, and occasionally from a pulmonary or peripheral artery. Such tumors can be associated with obstruction or thrombosis of the vessel, producing a clinical picture related to the site, and can extend beyond the vessel to form a large circumscribed mass with hemorrhage and necrosis. Those within the abdomen usually attain a large size before becoming manifest and often invade adjacent organs. Pelvic smooth muscle tumors need to be distinguished from those of uterine origin since the criteria for malignancy differ. For example, the concept of mitotically active leiomyoma as seen in myometrium[18] is not recognized in deep soft tissue. Leiomyosarcoma of deep somatic soft tissue is less frequent and occurs mostly in the thigh and trunk, in both males and females. Smooth muscle tumors that arise in immunocompromised patients can be associated with **Epstein-Barr virus** (EBV) infection (see below).

The metastatic rate in deep leiomyosarcomas is 45% with a 5-year survival of 64%.[19] Retroperitoneal leiomyosarcoma has an especially poor outcome with survival rates between 10% and 50%.[20] Tumor grade is a general prognostic factor in smooth muscle tumors.[21,22] Age, large size, and vascular invasion are adverse predictive factors, and " disruption" due to prior biopsy or incomplete excision (while correlated with size and depth) has been identified as an additional risk factor for metastasis.[22] Small leiomyosarcomas and those with very low mitotic activity have metastasized.[23] Leiomyosarcomas with >50% of myxoid stromal change are mostly of low-grade malignancy; however, in one series, 5/13 cases recurred and 2/13 metastasized.[24]

Pathologic Features

Deep leiomyosarcoma forms a solid tumor mass which can be circumscribed or infiltrative (especially in retroperitoneum) and displays hemorrhage and necrosis, especially in retroperitoneal tumors. Most deep somatic leiomyosarcomas are of vascular origin and many can be seen to arise from a vessel wall (e-Figs. 6.26 and 6.27). Microscopically, the cells are arranged in fascicles at right angles to each other and are parallel sided with typically blunt-ended nuclei, sometimes with paranuclear vacuoles (Fig. 6.9). The cytoplasm is eosinophilic and occasionally clumped. In relation to grade, there is a range of histologic appearances from well-differentiated leiomyosarcomas that resemble leiomyoma, including nuclear palisading, through those with loss of orderly pattern and increasing pleomorphism and mitotic activity (e-Fig. 6.28), to frankly pleomorphic sarcomas. Epithelioid leiomyosarcoma (e-Figs. 6.29 and 6.30) is uncommon and mostly occurs in the female genital tract. Some tumors show marked myxoid change (e-Figs. 6.31 and 6.32), in which cells are dispersed singly or in clusters. These are mostly found in the uterus but examples occur in soft tissue sites. In the myxoid areas, the mitotic index can be misleadingly low,

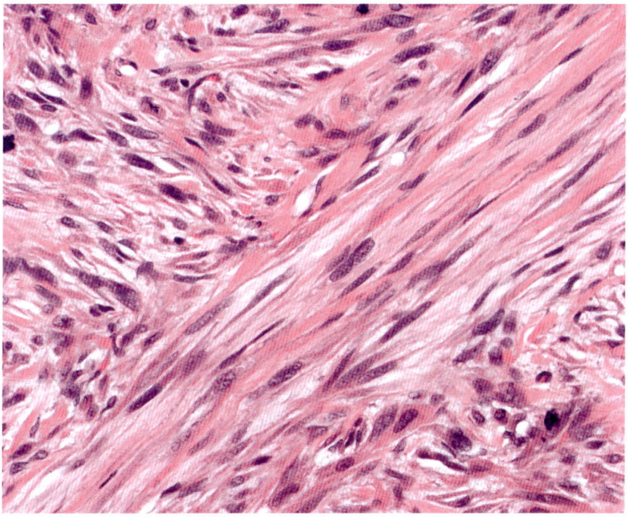

FIGURE 6.9 **Deep Leiomyosarcoma.** This tumor from retroperitoneum shows fascicular pattern with distinctive rectilinear architecture. The cells have parallel-sided, blunt-ended nuclei with tiny paranuclear vacuoles and eosinophilic cytoplasm. Mitoses are apparent.

but as mentioned myxoid leiomyosarcomas are mostly low-grade tumors.[24] Other changes include hyalinization and the presence of osteoclast-like cells which are sometimes a prominent feature.[25]

Ancillary Investigations

The expression of muscle antigens in leiomyosarcoma is variable. There is usually diffuse positivity for SMA and more focal staining for desmin and h-caldesmon. Antigen expression diminishes and becomes more focal with decreasing differentiation. Similarly, the ultrastructural features of smooth muscle cells can be incompletely developed in leiomyosarcomas, with loss of external lamina and pinocytosis. Various nonspecific genetic changes have been described.[26]

Variants

Inflammatory leiomyosarcoma occurs in deep soft tissue of trunk and proximal extremities and can cause systemic symptoms. It is a relatively bland spindle cell lesion that is heavily infiltrated by lymphocytes and can also have foci of xanthoma cells and psammomatous calcification (Fig. 6.10, e-Figs. 6.33 and 6.34).[27] It is further characterized by a distinctive immunophenotype with diffuse positivity for desmin but only focal reactivity for SMA and none for h-caldesmon.[28] A few cases have shown genetic abnormalities with a near-haploid karyotypes,[28] but no ultrastructural data are available for inflammatory leiomyosarcoma, and it is not certain that these tumors show smooth muscle differentiation. The striking desmin positivity raises the differential diagnosis of spindle cell

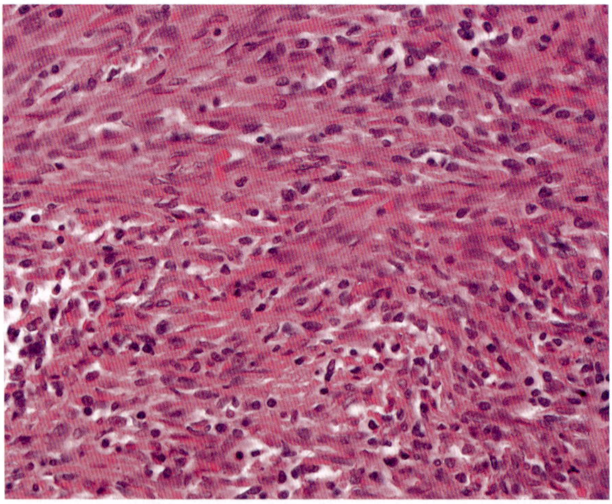

FIGURE 6.10 **Inflammatory Leiomyosarcoma.** Ill-formed fascicles of spindle cells interspersed with mixed inflammatory cells. This tumor displayed diffuse positivity for desmin but only focal immunoreactivity for smooth muscle actin.

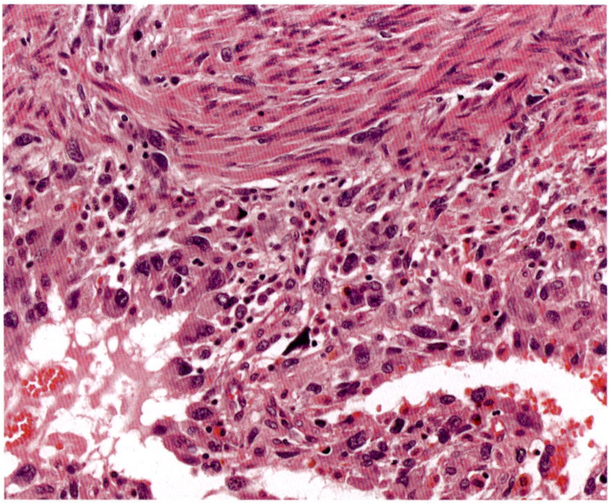

FIGURE 6.11 **Pleomorphic Leiomyosarcoma.** Typical leiomyosarcoma, at upper part of the field, is juxtaposed to a pleomorphic sarcomatous component. The latter component should comprise at least two thirds of the tumor for this diagnosis.

rhabdomyosarcoma, but relevant lineage markers (myogenin and MyoD1) are lacking. The immunophenotype also differs from that in inflammatory myofibroblastic tumor in which SMA positivity predominates, desmin is scanty, and ALK positivity can be found in over 50% of cases.

Pleomorphic leiomyosarcoma has been defined as a pleomorphic sarcoma with MFH-like areas in which less than one third of the tumor shows smooth muscle differentiation with fascicular architecture (Fig. 6.11,

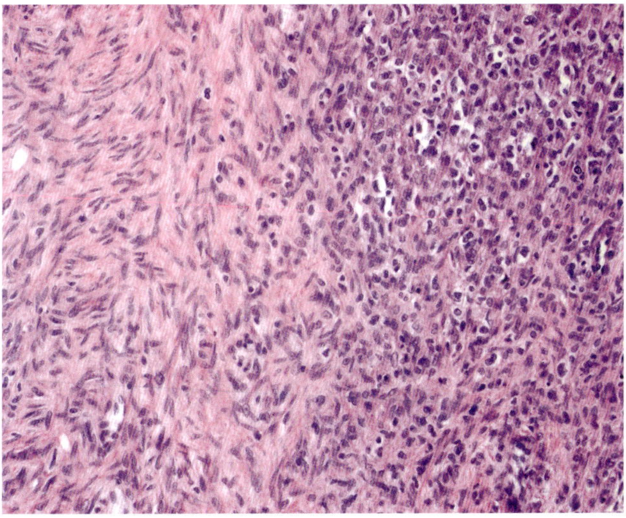

FIGURE 6.12 **EBV-associated Smooth Muscle Tumor.** This is composed of spindle cells in loosely arranged fascicles and areas of smaller rounded cells. Note the characteristic lymphocytic infiltrate (from a slide courtesy of Dr SW Weiss).

e-Fig. 6.35).[29] Many pleomorphic sarcomas have focal expression of smooth muscle antigens (SMA, desmin, and h-caldesmon), but this is insufficient for a diagnosis of leiomyosarcoma in the absence of the appropriate morphologic features. However, this affects prognosis and such tumors should be reported as pleomorphic sarcomas with immunohistochemical evidence of myoid differentiation.

EBV-associated smooth muscle tumors arise in patients who are immunocompromised for any reason[30] and occur in soft tissue, gastrointestinal tract, lung, liver, spleen, adrenal gland, and other sites. They can be multifocal due to clonally distinct tumors.[31] These are typically low-grade lesions with minimal atypia and mitotic activity. They have mostly spindle cell morphology but can also display primitive-looking round cell areas and prominent infiltration by T lymphocytes (Fig. 6.12, e-Figs. 6.36–6.38). Immunohistochemistry shows consistent actin positivity but desmin in only 14/26 cases.[31] In situ hybridization for EBV early RNAs (EBER) is positive in all cases.

Lipoleiomyoma and lipoleiomyosarcoma: Some smooth muscle tumors have a component of adipose tissue (Fig. 6.13, e-Figs. 6.39–6.42). These can be considered as neoplasms with divergent differentiation and both components can be benign or malignant. The former, known as lipoleiomyomas or myolipomas according to the dominant component, occur in uterus, pelvis, or groin area. Well-differentiated liposarcoma can have a leiomyosarcomatous component,[32] and dedifferentiated liposarcoma can show divergent myosarcomatous differentiation.[33]

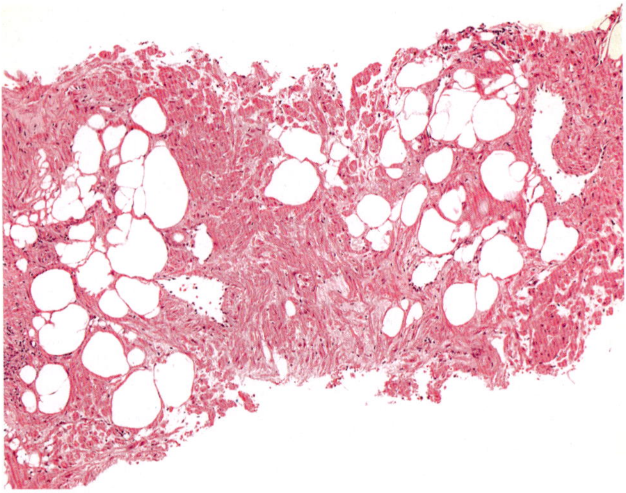

FIGURE 6.13 **Lipoleiomyoma (Myolipoma).** Needle core biopsy showing bland smooth muscle tumor with irregular islands of mature fat. Adipocytes vary in size but no nuclear atypia is seen.

OTHER SMOOTH MUSCLE TUMORS

A group of largely benign lesions arising from or associated with uterine smooth muscle proliferations or other gynecologic-type lesions is considered here.

LEIOMYOMATOSIS PERITONEALIS DISSEMINATA

Clinical Features

In this condition, multiple deposits of smooth muscle are found in the abdomen and pelvis on the peritoneum and surfaces of viscera, in females in the fertile period, and commonly associated with pregnancy, hormonal therapy, hormone-secreting ovarian tumors, and endometriosis.[34] This is usually an incidental finding. Familial clustering has been reported.[35] This condition probably originates from subserosal cells which undergo myofibroblastic or smooth muscle differentiation, possibly in relation to levels of estrogen and progesterone. The lesions regress after pregnancy or when the hormonal stimulus is removed.[34,36]

Pathologic Features

The nodules, which can number hundreds and appear to stud visceral and parietal surfaces, are subperitoneal and circumscribed or infiltrative. They are usually composed of mature smooth muscle cells in fascicles, without atypia or significant mitotic activity (Fig. 6.14, e-Figs. 6.43 and 6.44). A subset has more myofibroblast-like cells, and there can be

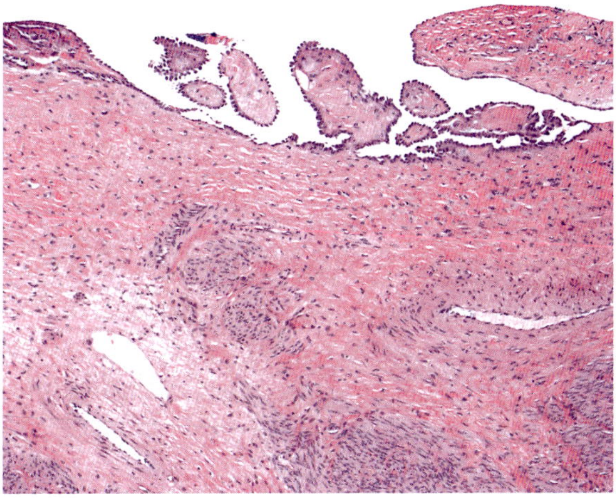

FIGURE 6.14 **Leiomyomatosis Peritonealis Disseminata.** An ill-defined focus of differentiated smooth muscle cells is present in subperitoneal connective tissue. The peritoneal surface shows mild papillation.

focal decidualization, with hyalinization in regressing lesions. Occasional examples of endometriosis within the smooth muscle lesions have been reported.[37]

Ancillary Investigations

Lesions with smooth muscle differentiation are immunoreactive for SMA, desmin, and h-caldesmon, whereas those that are myofibroblastic usually express actin only. ER and PgR can be positive in nuclei of the smooth muscle cells. Genetic investigation has shown clonality of multiple lesions.[38]

INTRAVENOUS LEIOMYOMATOSIS

Clinical Features

This is a smooth muscle proliferation that grows within veins in myometrium and sometimes extends into adjacent gynecologic organs and less often to inferior vena cava and pulmonary veins.[39] Secondary extravascular extension might be a source of extrauterine pelvic or retroperitoneal smooth muscle tumors, or of benign metastasizing leiomyoma. Intravenous leiomyomatosis occurs mostly in premenopausal or perimenopausal females with uterine fibroids and presumably represents intravascular spread from one or more thereof. Some examples are unassociated with fibroids, but origin from vessel walls is unlikely since most tumors so arising are frank leiomyosarcomas. In a majority of patients, the lesion is benign and cured by hysterectomy although (intrathoracic) spread can cause severe symptoms and be fatal in some cases.

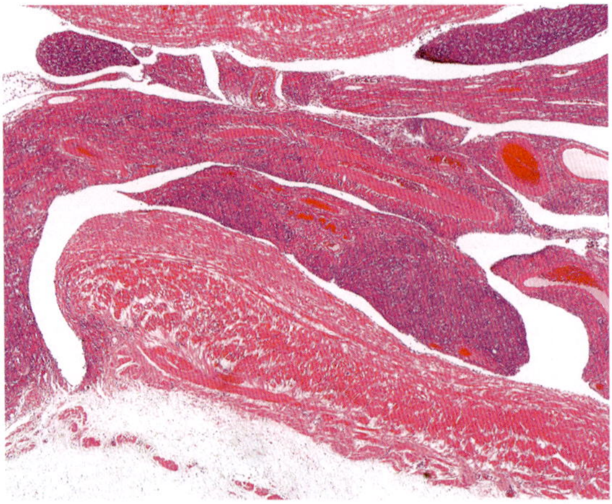

FIGURE 6.15 **Intravenous Leiomyomatosis.** Tongues of tumor are seen within dilated vascular channels adjacent to the uterus.

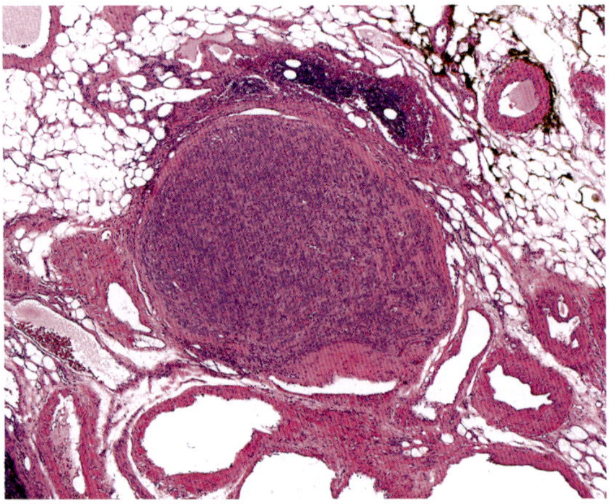

FIGURE 6.16 **Benign Metastasizing Leiomyoma.** Vein distended by plug of smooth muscle tumor in intra-abdominal soft tissue.

Pathologic Features

The veins contain nodules of differentiated smooth muscle surfaced by endothelium and containing thick-walled vessels (Fig. 6.15, e-Figs. 6.45 and 6.46). The lesions can show cytologic variations and secondary changes similar to those seen in uterine leiomyomata. Atypia is occasionally seen but mitotic activity is minimal.

Ancillary Investigations

In addition to the usual markers of smooth muscle, the cells of intravenous leiomyomatosis show variable nuclear immunoreactivity for ER and PgR.

A specific chromosomal abnormality, der(14)t(12;14)(q15;q24), has been described which has led to the suggestion that intravenous leiomyomatosis arises from a uterine leiomyoma with a t(12;14)(q15;q24).[40]

BENIGN METASTASIZING LEIOMYOMA

Clinical Features

Benign metastasizing leiomyoma occurs as one or more extrauterine nodules in a patient with a history (including prior hysterectomy) for uterine fibroids. It is most common in the lungs but can also be found in the abdomen, lymph nodes, peritoneal sites, and large veins. Some examples appear to arise from intravenous leiomyomatosis, and genetic evidence suggests possible clonal derivation from benign-appearing uterine leiomyomas.[41]

Pathologic Features

The nodules, located within pulmonary vessels or veins on other locations (Fig. 6.16, e-Figs. 6.47 and 6.48), are composed of well-differentiated smooth muscle cells without atypia and with no or very rare mitoses. Immunohistochemistry is positive for smooth muscle antigens and for ERs.[42]

REFERENCES

1. Vang R, Kempson RL. Perivascular epithelioid cell tumor ('PEComa') of the uterus: a subset of HMB-45-positive epithelioid mesenchymal neoplasms with an uncertain relationship to pure smooth muscle tumors. *Am J Surg Pathol.* 2002;26:1–13.
2. Lehtonen HJ, Kiuru M, Ylisaukko-Oja SK, et al. Increased risk of cancer in patients with fumarate hydratase germline mutation. *J Med Genet.* 2006;43:523–526.
3. McCluggage WG, Boyde A. Uterine angioleiomyomas: a report of 3 cases of a distinctive benign leiomyoma variant. *Int J Surg Pathol.* 2007;15:262–265.
4. Massi D, Franchi A, Alos L et al. Cutaneous leiomyosarcoma: clinico-pathologic analysis of 76 cases. *Lab Invest.* 2008;88:98A–98A.
5. Matsuyama A, Hisaoka M, Hashimoto H. Angioleiomyoma: a clinicopathologic and immunohistochemical reappraisal with special reference to the correlation with myopericytoma. *Hum Pathol.* 2007;38:645–651.
6. McGinley KM, Bryant S, Kattine AA, et al. Cutaneous leiomyomas lack estrogen and progesterone receptor immunoreactivity. *J Cutan Pathol.* 1997;24:241–245.
7. Nascimento AG, Karas M, Rosen PP, et al. Leiomyoma of the nipple. *Am J Surg Pathol.* 1979;3:151–154.
8. Nielsen GP, Rosenberg AE, Koerner FC, et al. Smooth-muscle tumors of the vulva. A clinicopathological study of 25 cases and review of the literature. *Am J Surg Pathol.* 1996;20:779–793.
9. Horton E, Dobin SM, Debiec-Rychter M, et al. A clonal translocation (7;8)(p13;q11.2) in a leiomyoma of the vulva. *Cancer Genet Cytogenet.* 2006;170:58–60.
10. Billings SD, Folpe AL, Weiss SW. Do leiomyomas of deep soft tissue exist? An analysis of highly differentiated smooth muscle tumors of deep soft tissue supporting two distinct subtypes. *Am J Surg Pathol.* 2001;25:1134–1142.

11. Paal E, Miettinen M. Retroperitoneal leiomyomas: a clinicopathologic and immunohistochemical study of 56 cases with a comparison to retroperitoneal leiomyosarcomas. *Am J Surg Pathol.* 2001;25:1355–1363.
12. Kilpatrick SE, Mentzel T, Fletcher CD. Leiomyoma of deep soft tissue. Clinicopathologic analysis of a series. *Am J Surg Pathol.* 1994;18:576–582.
13. Fletcher CD, Kilpatrick SE, Mentzel T. The difficulty in predicting behavior of smooth-muscle tumors in deep soft tissue. *Am J Surg Pathol.* 1995;19:116–117.
14. Meis JM, Enzinger FM. Myolipoma of soft tissue. *Am J Surg Pathol.* 1991;15:121–125.
15. Rao UN, Finkelstein SD, Jones MW. Comparative immunohistochemical and molecular analysis of uterine and extrauterine leiomyosarcomas. *Mod Pathol.* 1999;12:1001–1009.
16. Miettinen M, Fetsch JF. Evaluation of biological potential of smooth muscle tumours. *Histopathology.* 2006;48:97–105.
17. Weiss SW. Smooth muscle tumors of soft tissue. *Adv Anat Pathol.* 2002;9:351–359.
18. Bell SW, Kempson RL, Hendrickson MR. Problematic uterine smooth muscle neoplasms. A clinicopathologic study of 213 cases. *Am J Surg Pathol.* 1994;18:535–558.
19. Gustafson P, Willen H, Baldetorp B, et al. Soft tissue leiomyosarcoma. A population-based epidemiologic and prognostic study of 48 patients, including cellular DNA content. *Cancer.* 1992;70:114–119.
20. Stoeckle E, Coindre JM, Bonvalot S, et al. Prognostic factors in retroperitoneal sarcoma: a multivariate analysis of a series of 165 patients of the French Cancer Center Federation Sarcoma Group. *Cancer.* 2001;92:359–368.
21. Fisher C, Goldblum JR, Epstein JI, et al. Leiomyosarcoma of the paratesticular region: a clinicopathologic study. *Am J Surg Pathol.* 2001;25:1143–1149.
22. Farshid G, Pradhan M, Goldblum J, et al. Leiomyosarcoma of somatic soft tissues: a tumor of vascular origin with multivariate analysis of outcome in 42 cases. *Am J Surg Pathol.* 2002;26:14–24.
23. Berlin O SB, Kindblom L-G, Angervall L. Leiomyosarcomas of venous origin in the extremities. A correlated clinical, roentgenologic, and morphologic study with diagnostic and surgical implications. *Cancer.* 1984;54:2147–2159.
24. Rubin BP, Fletcher CD. Myxoid leiomyosarcoma of soft tissue, an underrecognized variant. *Am J Surg Pathol.* 2000;24:927–936.
25. Mentzel T, Calonje E, Fletcher CD. Leiomyosarcoma with prominent osteoclast-like giant cells. Analysis of eight cases closely mimicking the so-called giant cell variant of malignant fibrous histiocytoma. *Am J Surg Pathol.* 1994;18:258–265.
26. Wang R, Titley JC, Lu YJ, et al. Loss of 13q14–q21 and gain of 5p14-pter in the progression of leiomyosarcoma. *Mod Pathol.* 2003;16:778–785.
27. Merchant W, Calonje E, Fletcher CD. Inflammatory leiomyosarcoma: a morphological subgroup within the heterogeneous family of so-called inflammatory malignant fibrous histiocytoma. *Histopathology.* 1995;27:525–532.
28. Chang A, Schuetze SM, Conrad EU, III, et al. So-called "inflammatory leiomyosarcoma": a series of 3 cases providing additional insights into a rare entity. *Int J Surg Pathol.* 2005;13:185–195.
29. Oda Y, Miyajima K, Kawaguchi K, et al. Pleomorphic leiomyosarcoma: clinicopathologic and immunohistochemical study with special emphasis on its distinction from ordinary leiomyosarcoma and malignant fibrous histiocytoma. *Am J Surg Pathol.* 2001;25:1030–1038.
30. Lee ES, Locker J, Nalesnik M, et al. The association of Epstein-Barr virus with smooth-muscle tumors occurring after organ transplantation. *N Engl J Med.* 1995;332:19–25.
31. Deyrup AT, Lee VK, Hill CE, et al. Epstein-Barr virus-associated smooth muscle tumors are distinctive mesenchymal tumors reflecting multiple infection events: a

clinicopathologic and molecular analysis of 29 tumors from 19 patients. *Am J Surg Pathol.* 2006;30:75–82.

32. Folpe AL, Weiss SW. Lipoleiomyosarcoma (well-differentiated liposarcoma with leiomyosarcomatous differentiation): a clinicopathologic study of nine cases including one with dedifferentiation. *Am J Surg Pathol.* 2002;26:742–749.
33. Tallini G, Erlandson RA, Brennan MF, et al. Divergent myosarcomatous differentiation in retroperitoneal liposarcoma. *Am J Surg Pathol.* 1993;17:546–556.
34. Tavassoli FA, Norris HJ. Peritoneal leiomyomatosis (leiomyomatosis peritonealis disseminata): a clinicopathologic study of 20 cases with ultrastructural observations. Int J Gynecol Pathol 1982;1:59–74.
35. Halama N, Grauling-Halama SA, Daboul I. Familial clustering of Leiomyomatosis peritonealis disseminata: an unknown genetic syndrome? *BMC Gastroenterol.* 2005;5:33.
36. Crosland DB. Leiomyomatosis peritonealis disseminata: a case report. *Am J Obstet Gynecol.* 1973;117:179–181.
37. Kaplan C, Benirschke K, Johnson KC. Leiomyomatosis peritonealis disseminata with endometrium. *Obstet Gynecol.* 1980;55:119–122.
38. Quade BJ, McLachlin CM, Soto-Wright V, et al. Disseminated peritoneal leiomyomatosis. Clonality analysis by X chromosome inactivation and cytogenetics of a clinically benign smooth muscle proliferation. *Am J Pathol.* 1997;150:2153–2166.
39. Clement PB, Young RH, Scully RE. Intravenous leiomyomatosis of the uterus. A clinicopathological analysis of 16 cases with unusual histologic features. *Am J Surg Pathol.* 1988;12:932–945.
40. Dal Cin P, Quade BJ, Neskey DM, et al. Intravenous leiomyomatosis is characterized by a der(14)t(12;14)(q15;q24). *Genes Chromosomes Cancer.* 2003;36:205–206.
41. Patton KT, Cheng L, Papavero V, et al. Benign metastasizing leiomyoma: clonality, telomere length and clinicopathologic analysis. *Mod Pathol.* 2006;19:130–140.
42. Esteban JM, Allen WM, Schaerf RH. Benign metastasizing leiomyoma of the uterus: histologic and immunohistochemical characterization of primary and metastatic lesions. *Arch Pathol Lab Med.* 1999;123:960–962.

7

MYOFIBROMA, MYOPERICYTIC TUMORS, MYOEPITHELIOMA, AND MYOFIBROBLASTOMA

INTRODUCTION

This chapter concerns tumors that are usually benign and show predominant myofibroblastic or partial myoid differentiation. The former are distinguished from tumors composed of reactive or neoplastic myofibroblasts admixed with fibroblasts (see Chapter 3) and from low-grade and pleomorphic myofibrosarcoma (Chapters 10 and 13 respectively). Many tumors discussed in this chapter have similar or overlapping features and are terminologically similar, which can cause confusion. The features of the different cell types are summarized in Table 7.1.

Myofibroma is a tumor of myofibroblasts with morphologic features that overlap with those of pericytic neoplasms. The latter are derived from vascular pericytes that proliferate and manifest myoid or glomus cell differentiation, giving rise to hemangiopericytomatous tumors with a variety of patterns. Myoepithelioma shows, in varying degree, both myoid and epithelial differentiation. Apart from those in the genital tract (see Chapter 8), soft tissue neoplasms termed myofibroblastomas are probably composed of specialized or modified smooth muscle cells rather than myofibroblasts. The differential diagnosis is summarized in Table 7.2.

MYOFIBROMA

Clinical Features

Although predominantly a lesion of early life, including congenital incidence, myofibroma can also occur in adults.[1] It can be single or multicentric, and familial forms have been described with autosomal dominant inheritance. Solitary lesions usually arise in dermis or subcutis, and occasionally skeletal muscle especially in the head and neck region (with a subset within the oral cavity[2,3]), and in bone, trunk, and proximal extremities. They are benign and many cases regress spontaneously, apparently by apoptosis, although about 10% recur. Multicentric tumors are more common in females, involve bone and viscera (gastrointestinal tract, heart, lung), and can be fatal.[4]

TABLE 7.1 Features of Selected Spindle Cell Types

	Morphology	Immunohistochemistry	Electron Microscopy
Myofibroblast	Tapered or ovoid, oval nucleus with single punctate nucleolus, variable amounts of amphophilic cytoplasm. Indistinct cell membrane	SMA+ (subplasmalemmal "tram-track" distribution), desmin±, h-caldesmon−, SMM−. Rarely CK+ (mostly in intra-abdominal lesions)	Moderate amounts of rough endoplasmic reticulum, subplasma-lemmal stress fiber continuous with fibronexus fibril. No significant external lamina, junctions, or pinocytotic vesicles
Myopericyte	Short, tapered, elongated, or plump spindle cell with ovoid or tapered nucleus, moderate eosinophilic cytoplasm. Glomus cell interpreted as specialized rounded form	SMA+, h-caldesmon+, desmin+ occasionally, CD34+ rarely+	Resembles smooth muscle cell–abundant cytoplasmic filaments with dense bodies, continuous external lamina, micropinocytotic vesicles
Myoepithelial cell	Usually tapered spindle cell with moderate amounts of eosinophilic cytoplasm. Can assume polygonal, clear cell, plasmacytoid, or rhabdoid form	CK+, S100 protein+, calponin+, P63+, desmin−	Intercellular junctions (desmosomes), tonofilaments, bundles of myofilaments with dense bodies
Smooth muscle cell	Nontapered (parallel-sided), abundant slightly fibrillary eosinophilic cytoplasm (also seen alongside nuclei). Nucleus has rounded or blunt ends, paranuclear vacuole. Can assume clear cell or epithelioid form	SMA+, desmin+, h-caldesmon+, calponin+ some express CK (dot), EMA, S100 protein	Myofilaments with dense bodies throughout cytoplasm. Continuous or interrupted (fragmented) external lamina, micropinocytotic vesicles often prominent

TABLE 7.2 **Differential Diagnosis of Myofibroma, Myopericytoma, Myoepithelioma, and Myofibroblastoma**

	Typical Clinical Features	Microscopic Features	Ancillary Investigations
Myofibroma	Mostly in children, occasionally in adults Head and neck, extremities, bone. Dermis or subcutis. Occasionally visceral and multicentric. Mostly benign but deep multicentric forms can be fatal	Circumscribed, occasionally central necrosis. Nodules of myofibroblasts, central smaller cells with pericytomatous pattern. Giant cells, ossification, intravascular spread	SMA+, desmin–, h-caldesmon–, S100 protein–, CK–
Nodular fasciitis	Young adults, extremities, head and neck. Short history–weeks; rarely up to a year. Rapid growth then stops <5 cm	Circumscribed or mildly infiltrative myofibroblastic tumor. Variably myxoid, cellular and collagenous areas. Normal mitoses acceptable but not atypia or necrosis	SMA+, desmin±, h-caldesmon–
Myopericytoma	M > F, limbs, head and neck, trunk, in dermis, or subcutis. Single or multiple. Intravascular and malignant variants occur	Circumscribed, encapsulated. Prominent pericytomatous pattern. Myoid or glomus cells around vessels or in nodules, or slender spindle cells in perivascular whorls Malignant variants have infiltration, pleomorphism, mitoses, necrosis	SMA+, caldesmon+, desmin–, CD34–, S100 protein–, CK–
Myoepithelioma/ mixed tumor	Adults, limbs and girdles, rarely head and neck or trunk. Dermis, subcutis or deep soft tissue Malignant variants occur.	Resembles salivary tumor. Epithelial cords, nests, or sheets, plasmacytoid change, and rarely pure spindle cell pattern. Ductules in mixed tumor. Chondromyxoid stroma	Variable expression of S100 protein, CK, EMA, GFAP, SMA, h-caldesmon, calponin

Mammary-type myofibroblastoma	Breast M = F. Inguinal region M > F, buttock, abdominal wall Painless, slow-growing, rarely >6 cm diameter Benign	Circumscribed tumor comprising irregular fascicles of spindle cells, collagenous bands, variable adipose tissue, mast cells. Resembles spindle cell lipoma. Atypical and epithelioid variants occur	CD34+, desmin+ SMA± h-caldesmon–, S100 protein–, CK–
Intranodal myofibroblastoma	Inguinal lymph node, rarely submandibular node Very rarely recurs	Rim of lymph node. Solid, hemorrhagic cut surface. Cellular, fascicles of slender spindle cells with nuclear palisading. Extravasated erythrocytes, hemosiderin. Hyaline-walled vessels, amianthoid fibers	SMA+, other markers negative
Kaposi sarcoma, intranodal	Children or young adults in lymph node draining skin lesion, or rarely primary generalized lymphadenopathy	Curved fascicles of spindle cells, pleomorphism, and mitoses. Hemorrhage, hyaline globules	HHV8+, CD34+, CD31+, SMA–, S100 protein–, CK–
Cellular schwannoma	M > F. Deep soft tissue, retroperitoneum, pelvis, rare in lymph node. Firm mass up to 20 cm diameter Can recur but does not metastasize	Encapsulated (fragment of capsule often present in core biopsy), subcapsular lymphoid aggregates, sheets of elongated spindle cells with eosinophilic cytoplasm. Clusters of foamy macrophages, lymphocytes	S100 protein+ diffusely, GFAP+, CK+ rarely

(Continued)

TABLE 7.2 Differential Diagnosis of Myofibroma, Myopericytoma, Myoepithelioma, and Myofibroblastoma (continued)

	Typical Clinical Features	Microscopic Features	Ancillary Investigations
Fibromatosis–desmoid type	Deep soft tissue, limbs, head and neck, body cavities	Parallel-aligned myofibroblasts evenly dispersed in collagen, slit-like and thick-walled vessels, mast cells. No nuclear atypia or necrosis	SMA+, beta-catenin+ in nuclei. CD34–
Low-grade myofibrosarcoma	Head and neck, extremities, retroperitoneum, bone, infiltrative mass, recurs	Cellular fascicles infiltrate muscle. Myofibroblastic morphology, mostly uniform but focal nuclear atypia is diagnostic. Occasional necrosis	SMA+, desmin±, h-caldesmon–, S100 protein–, CD34–
Leiomyosarcoma	Dermis, subcutis or (mostly) deep soft tissue. Slowly growing. Some related to obvious blood vessel. Recurs	Well-defined fascicles at right angles. Nontapered cells, eosinophilic cytoplasm, nuclear atypia, abnormal mitoses	SMA+, desmin+, h-caldesmon+, CK in some (dot), CD34+ rarely

Pathologic Features

Myofibroma forms a circumscribed nodule up to 5 cm in diameter, and unlike in nodular fasciitis there can sometimes be central necrosis. Superficial lesions can involve dermis and subcutis (e-Fig. 7.1). Histologically, there is a biphasic pattern with whorled lobules of palely eosinophilic myofibroblastic cells around a central focus of smaller, more darkly staining cells, with ovoid nuclei, scanty cytoplasm and focal mild pleomorphism, associated with a hemangiopericytomatous pattern (Figs. 7.1 and 7.2, e-Figs. 7.2–7.6). Multinucleated cells (e-Figs. 7.5 and 7.6) are occasionally seen and intravascular extension (e-Fig. 7.7) is relatively common. Mitoses can be frequent, and the central necrosis is sometime extensive, leaving only a thin rim of viable lesional tissue. This can result in hyalinization, calcification, or ossification (e-Fig. 7.8). Some cases show morphologic overlap with myopericytoma.[5]

Ancillary Investigations

The spindle cells of myofibroma are positive for smooth muscle actin (SMA) (e-Fig. 7.9) and negative for desmin, h-caldesmon, CD34, and S100 protein.[6] Electron microscopy shows the spindle cells to be myofibroblasts rather than smooth muscle cells, with rough endoplasmic reticulum, stress fibers, and rare fibronexus structures.[6,7]

MYOPERICYTOMA

The concept of hemangiopericytoma as a distinct tumor type has been challenged in recent years, on the basis that a pericytomatous vascular pattern is seen in a wide variety of soft tissue tumor types, and that it is not therefore specific to any cell lineage.[8] Many tumors previously termed

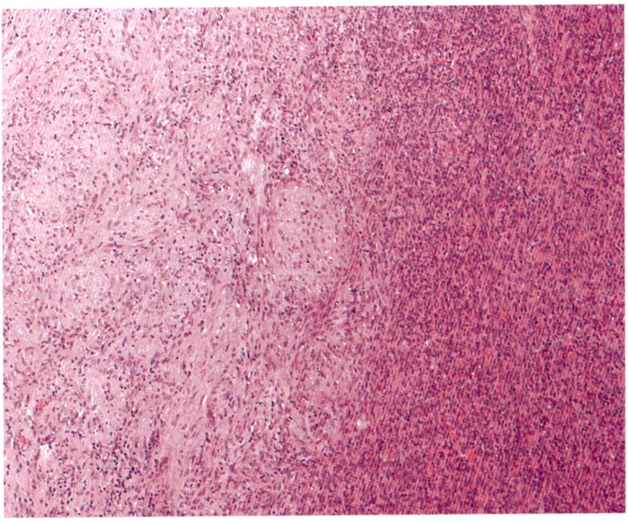

FIGURE 7.1 **Myofibroma.** A zone of closely packed cells merges with paler nodules with peripheral spindle cells. There is a poorly defined hemangiopericytic pattern.

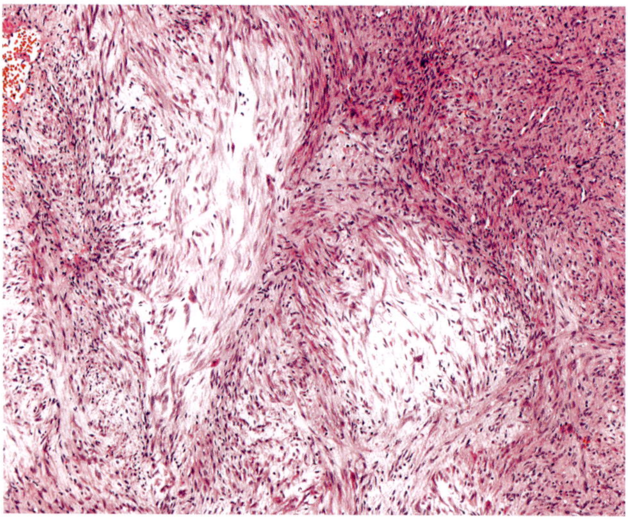

FIGURE 7.2 **Myofibroma.** Nodules of myofibroblasts with myxoid change and mild inflammation, more cellular at periphery. There is an adjacent more cellular zone with residual vascular pattern.

hemangiopericytoma have been recategorized as solitary fibrous tumor,[9] and infantile hemangiopericytoma is now regarded as a variant of myofibroma or, occasionally, myopericytoma. Meanwhile, tumors considered to show true pericytic differentiation have become defined.[5,10] The pericyte is a spindle-shaped or rounded cell which surrounds and is closely related to endothelium in capillary blood vessels and can exhibit variable smooth muscle ("myopericytic"[10]) or glomus-like differentiation. Tumors with pericytic differentiation can therefore resemble leiomyomas, myofibromas, or glomus tumors, often with the addition of a prominent hemangiopericytomatous pattern.[5] Since the latter, however, is now regarded as a nonspecific finding unrelated to differentiation, this is presumably adventitious. Myopericytomas can have various combinations of patterns. This has led to division into a number of morphologic subtypes, but these have no prognostic significance.

Clinical Features

Myopericytoma is more common in males, in adult life, and occurs principally in the upper and lower extremities, with occasional cases in the head and neck region and on the trunk. Most myopericytomas arise in dermis or subcutis or involve both, with occasional deeper examples. They present as slowly growing single or rarely multiple nodules. The behavior is generally benign, with only an occasional recurrence,[11] but rare malignant examples have been described with aggressive behavior.[12]

Pathologic Features

Myopericytoma is a circumscribed nonencapsulated lesion with variable hemangiopericytomatous vascular pattern, which displays a variety

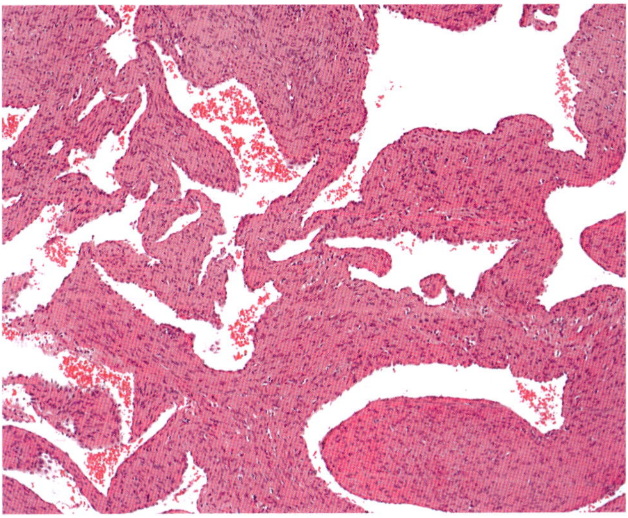

FIGURE 7.3 **Myofibroma-like Myopericytoma.** Branching dilated vascular channels are surrounded by small ovoid or spindle-shaped lesions cells with eosinophilic cytoplasm.

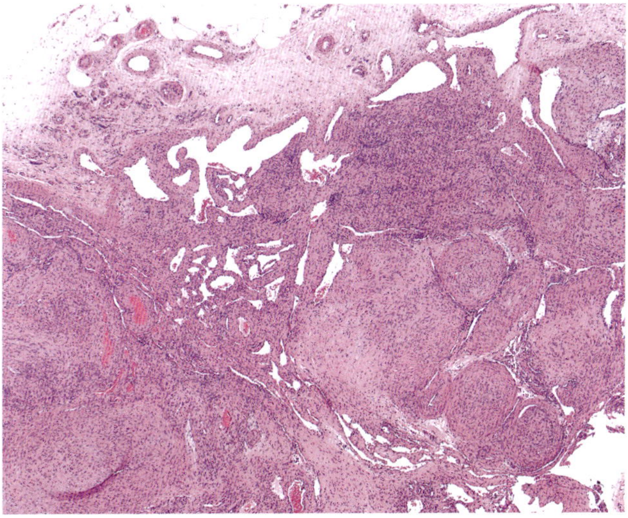

FIGURE 7.4 **Pericytomatous Myopericytoma.** Peripheral hemangiopericytomatous pattern and cellular areas containing perivascular whorls of cells.

of overlapping cytological features. In the myofibroma-like variant, the cells are spindle shaped with eosinophilic cytoplasm (Fig. 7.3, e-Figs. 7.10 and 7.11). In the pericytomatous subtype, the striking feature of spindle cells with elongated nuclei disposed in concentric layers in the walls of small vessels and spinning off into adjacent tissues, which often contain dilated thin walled vessels (Figs. 7.4 and 7.5, e-Figs. 7.12–7.18). The cells

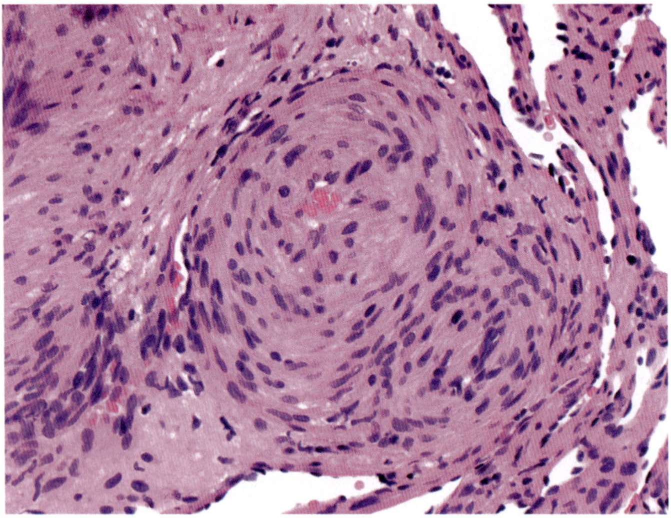

FIGURE 7.5 **Pericytomatous Myopericytoma.** Higher magnification shows concentric whorls of pericytes in an "onion-skin" pattern surrounding a vascular lumen.

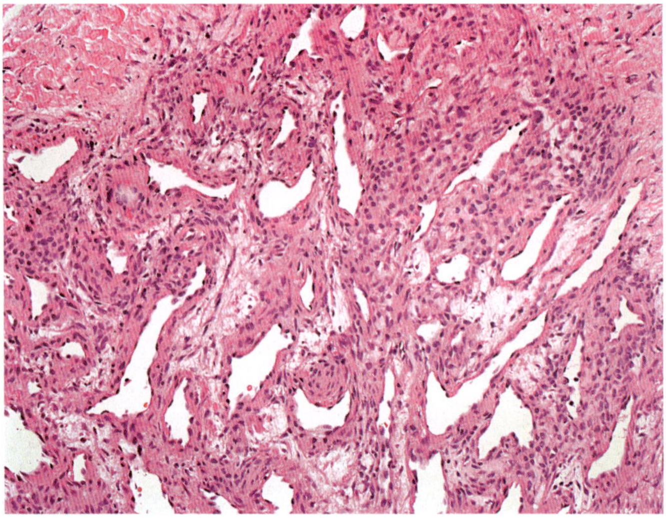

FIGURE 7.6 **Glomangiomatous Myopericytoma.** Rounded glomus cells form a layer surrounding vascular spaces.

have bland nuclei, indiscernible cell boundaries, and varying amounts of eosinophilic cytoplasm. Other examples display focal or widespread glomus cell differentiation, usually as a single perivascular layer displaying a glomangiomatous pattern (Fig. 7.6, e-Figs. 7.19 and 7.20). They differ from regular glomus tumor in the vascular architecture and usually in having only focal glomus cell differentiation. Enlarged or multinucleated cells can occasionally be seen. Mitoses usually do not exceed 2 per 10 hpf. Rare malignant examples have more mitoses, including atypical forms, nuclear pleomorphism, infiltration, and necrosis.[12] Some tumors are predominantly hemangiopericytomatous, and solid, angiomyoma-like, and hypocellular fibroma-like variants have been defined, but combinations of these patterns can be seen (e-Fig. 7.18).[11] The picture can be complicated by the presence of hemorrhage or infarction, hyalinizing fibrosis, edema, or inflammation. Intravascular myopericytoma, arising within a larger vessel, has also been described.[13]

Ancillary Investigations

The myopericytes are immunoreactive for SMA and h-caldesmon but rarely for desmin.[5,11] Myofibroblastic lesions (including myofibroma) differ in lacking h-caldesmon,[14] and angiomyoma typically expresses desmin also. Examples of myopericytoma have been described with a t(7;12)(p21–22;q13–15), resulting in *ACTB-GLI* fusion with activation of the *GLI* oncogene. This is step in the sonic hedgehog signaling pathway, which is involved in tissue-specific cell proliferation during embryogenesis.[15]

GLOMUS TUMOR

Glomus tumors show differentiation along the lines of glomus cells, which are probably modified smooth muscle cells derived from pericytes. The normal glomus body, usually situated in the distal extremities and in the precoccygeal tissues, regulates temperature. It is composed of an afferent arteriole leading into an endothelial-lined pocket (Sucquet-Hoyer canal) supported by round epithelioid glomus cells.

Clinical Features

Glomus tumors affect adults (20–40 years) without gender predominance overall. Their classic location is the subungual region of the fingers (in this site there is a female predominance) followed by the distal upper extremity and the distal lower extremity. They are also reported near the end of the spine in the area of the glomus coccygeum, although some lesions reported as such may simply be the glomus coccygeum, a normal structure. Glomus tumors have been reported in multiple anatomic sites including deep soft tissue, bone, and female genital tract. They are also rarely encountered in the gastrointestinal tract.[16] Occasional examples are associated with neurofibromatosis.[17] Most glomus tumors manifest as small bluish nodules or, when subungual, as discoloration of the nail bed. Classic skin lesions cause considerable pain that can be elicited by changes in temperature and pressure. Rare malignant examples are known.[18]

Pathologic Features

Glomus tumors are well-marginated lesions comprising sheets and nests of cells containing perfectly round nuclei, amphophilic cytoplasm, and prominent basement membrane (Fig. 7.7, e-Figs. 7.21–7.23). The latter imparts sharp demarcations between the individual rounded cells in a lace-like network. The tumor is richly vascularized with a variable hemangiopericytoma-like pattern (and can overlap with glomangiopericytoma as described above), and nests of tumor cells can often be seen within vessel walls. There is sometimes a more solid pattern, especially in deeper lesions. Occasional examples display oncocytic change or even symplastic change (e-Fig. 7.24) in which atypical cells are encountered, without mitotic activity. Criteria that have been suggested for malignancy in glomus tumor include deep location and a size of more than 2 cm, or atypical mitotic figures, or moderate to high nuclear grade and ≥5 mitotic figures per 50 hpf[18] (e-Fig. 7.25). Lesions regarded as "glomus tumors of uncertain malignant potential" have some but not all the features of malignancy.[18] However, occasional otherwise typical lesions have behaved aggressively.[16] Glomangiosarcoma is a very rare tumor in which foci of glomus tumor are associated with a spindle cell sarcoma, sometimes showing smooth muscle differentiation.

Ancillary Investigations

Glomus tumors are immunoreactive with antibodies to SMA (e-Fig. 7.26) and h-caldesmon (e-Fig. 7.27) but usually negative for desmin. CD34 is occasionally positive. The basement membrane can be highlighted by

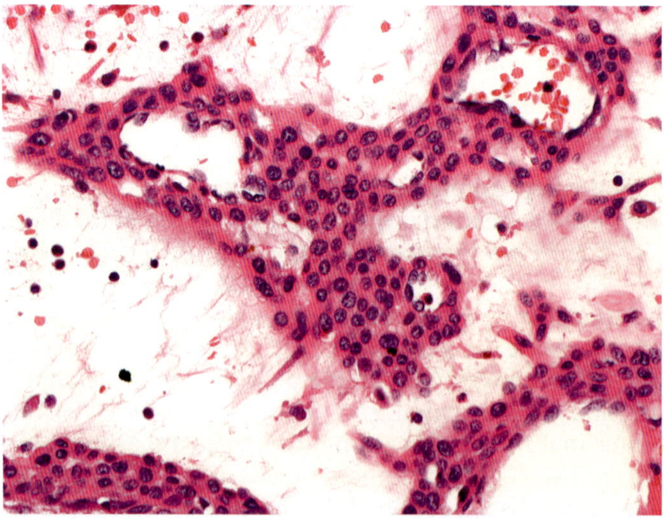

FIGURE 7.7 **Glomus Tumor.** Several layers of glomus cells are arranged around blood vessels. Note the myxohyaline stroma.

laminin and type IV collagen staining. Gastrointestinal tract examples have consistently lacked *KIT* mutations.[16]

SINONASAL-TYPE HEMANGIOPERICYTOMA

Clinical Features

This is now regarded as a myopericytic neoplasm with glomus-like differentiation. It arises predominantly in older adults as a polypoid tumor in the nasal cavity where it causes obstruction or bleeding, and can extend into paranasal sinuses. Most lesions are benign, although up to a third of cases recur, especially if incompletely excised.[19]

Pathologic Features

The tumor is nonencapsulated and extends beneath surface epithelium in cellular sheets or fascicles composed of ovoid cells with uniform (or sometimes mildly pleomorphic) nuclei and variable amounts of eosinophilic cytoplasm (e-Figs. 7.28 and 7.29). Occasional mitoses are seen. There is usually a prominent vascular pattern, including dilated hemangiopericytomatous thin-walled vessels. The stroma has mast cells, occasional eosinophils, and variable amounts of myxoid change, hemorrhage, and fibrosis. Rare examples have increased mitotic activity, pleomorphism, and necrosis and can be regarded as having malignant potential.

Ancillary Investigations

The lesional cells are positive for SMA, but not for desmin or CD34.

MYOEPITHELIOMA OF SOFT TISSUES

Neoplasms with myoepithelial differentiation, resembling those occurring in salivary glands, have recently been recognized in soft tissue locations. They can have a range of appearances, including spindle cell, plasmacytoid, epithelioid, or clear cell morphology, and a fascicular or sheet-like architecture with fibrous or myxoid stromal change. By analogy with salivary gland neoplasms, mixed tumors also have gland-like tubular (ductal) formations or chondroid change. Tumors previously designated as parachordoma have been subsumed into the category of myoepithelioma,[20] although there are subtle differences between the two entities.[21] Some examples of ectomesenchymal chondromyxoid tumor, a rarity occurring in the anterior tongue, have a myoepithelial immunophenotype,[22] and ectopic hamartomatous thymoma also has features suggestive of myoepithelial differentiation (see below).

Clinical Features

Soft tissue myoepithelioma occurs in either sex, at any age but mainly in adults. The tumor, which can reach 20 cm in diameter, presents as a painless or painful mass, in dermis,[23,24] subcutis or deep soft tissue,[25] and predominantly arises in limbs and limb girdles with smaller numbers originating in head and neck or trunk. Most are benign but up to 18% recur locally, and histologically malignant variants are described that recur more frequently and metastasize.[25]

Pathologic Features

Myoepithelioma forms a circumscribed (though often microscopically infiltrative), pseudoencapsulated mass with focal myxoid change or, rarely, necrosis. Microscopically, most often there are spindled or epithelioid cells in small nests or cords in a reticular or trabeculated pattern, within chondromyxoid, myxoid, or fibrous stroma resembling extraskeletal myxoid chondrosarcoma (Figs. 7.8–7.10, e-Figs. 7.30–7.35) and which can also show osteochondroid or adipocytic differentiation. As mentioned, tubule formation is seen in soft tissue mixed tumors and squamous change can occur. The purely spindle cell variant is uncommon; it is composed of sheets of cells of variable length with tapered nuclei and eosinophilic or granular cytoplasm (e-Figs. 7.36–7.39). Malignant myoepithelioma (myoepithelial carcinoma) has pleomorphic nuclei with prominent nucleoli, mitotic activity, and necrosis. Malignant mixed tumors additionally have a sarcomatous component (e-Fig. 7.40). About 40% of malignant myoepithelial neoplasms recur and 30% metastasize.[25]

Ancillary Investigations

Myoepithelial neoplasms express to a variable extent S100 protein, cytokeratins (especially with broad spectrum reagents, CAM 5.2 or antibodies to high molecular weight cytokeratins) (e-Fig. 7.41), epithelial membrane

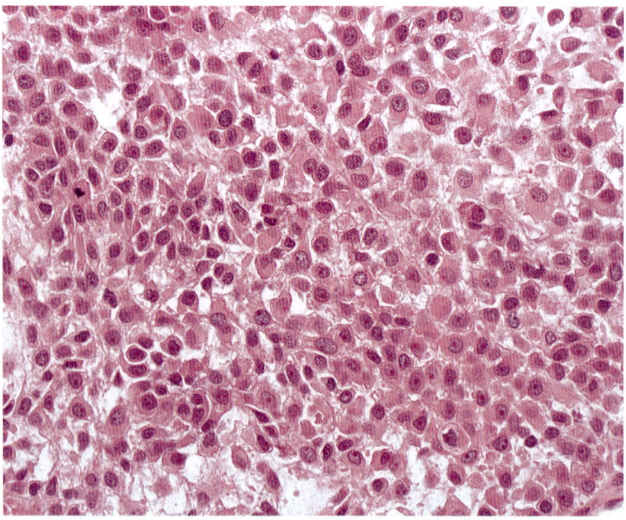

FIGURE 7.8 **Soft Tissue Myoepithelioma.** Sheets of ovoid and focally plasmacytoid cells are seen in this example.

antigen (EMA), glial fibrillary acidic protein (GFAP), calponin, h-caldesmon, and SMA. CK 14, desmin, CD10, and p63 are less frequently positive, and CD34 is negative.[23,25,26] Some cases lack nuclear immunoreactivity for INI1. The diagnosis of myoepithelioma should be considered in tumors

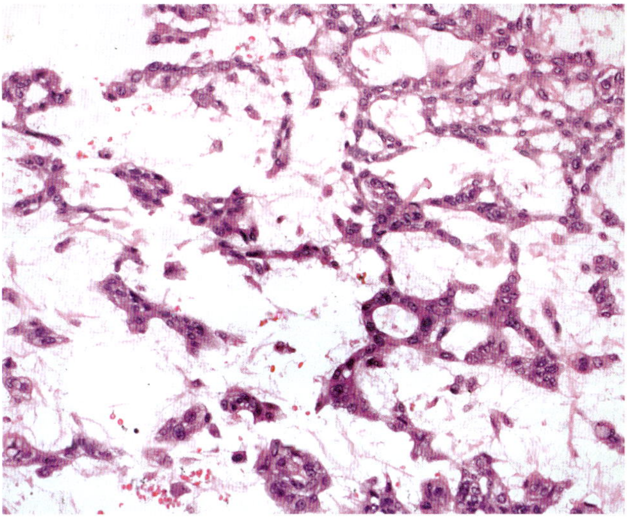

FIGURE 7.9 **Soft Tissue Myoepithelioma.** Strands and cords of cells in a myxoid stroma. This pattern is seen in tumors termed parachordoma and resembles extraskeletal myxoid chondrosarcoma.

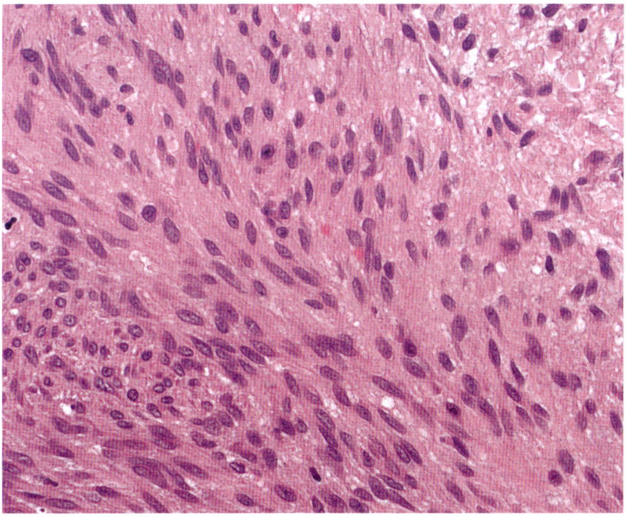

FIGURE 7.10 **Soft Tissue Myoepithelioma, Spindle Variant.** This tumor comprises plump spindle cells with eosinophilic cytoplasm, arranged in a fascicular pattern. Distinguishing this from smooth muscle and myofibroblastic tumors and from schwannoma requires the use of an immunohistochemical panel.

coexpressing S100 protein and cytokeratins/EMA, although the diagnosis can be made in the absence of one or more marker when the morphology is typical. Single cases have been reported of a myoepithelioma with t(1;22)(q23;q12) translocation resulting in *EWSR1-PBX*,[27] and a soft tissue myoepithelial carcinoma with t(19;22)(q13;q12) translocation leading to the novel fusion gene *EWSR1-ZNF444*.[28]

Electron microscopy shows variably differentiated desmosomes, tonofilaments, and mainly peripheral myofilaments.

ECTOPIC HAMARTOMATOUS THYMOMA

Clinical Features

These tumors are found in the inferior neck (supraclavicular, presternal) region almost exclusively in adult males. They are slowly growing and mostly small but can reach 19 cm in diameter. Reported cases have behaved in a benign fashion.

Pathologic Features

They are composed of plump or slender spindle cells arranged in fascicles and also have solid, cystic, glandular, or tubular epithelial elements and adipose tissue (e-Figs. 7.42 and 7.43). Mitoses can be seen but atypia and necrosis are lacking.

Ancillary Investigations

Immunohistochemistry shows expression of cytokeratins (AE1/3, CK5/6, CK14), EMA, CD10 CD34, and SMA[29] (e-Figs. 7.44 and 7.45), but not S100 protein. Based on these findings, it has been suggested that this tumor is not related to thymus but represents a branchial anlage mixed tumor.

MAMMARY AND MAMMARY-TYPE (EXTRA-MAMMARY) MYOFIBROBLASTOMA

This benign lesion was first reported in the breast, and histologically identical tumors were subsequently identified in other locations. In spite of the name, the ultrastructure and immunophenotype suggest modified smooth muscle rather than myofibroblastic differentiation.[30,31]

Clinical Features

Mammary myofibroblastoma was initially described more frequently in the male than the female breast where it clinically resembles (and can be associated with) gynecomastia, but subsequent experience indicates a more equal gender distribution, in older males and postmenopausal females.[32] Mammary-type (extra-mammary) myofibroblastoma is a rare subcutaneous tumor that arises mostly in the inguinal region, and occasionally in other locations, including buttock or abdominal wall, with a male predominance.[33] The lesion presents as a slowly growing, usually painless mass that rarely exceeds 4 cm in maximum dimension in the breast, and 6 cm in extramammary locations.

Pathologic Features

The tumor is circumscribed, firm, and rubbery with a pale cut surface, and resembles fibroadenoma. Microscopically, irregular fascicles of bland, elongated spindle cells infiltrate between bands of fibrous tissue with focal myxoid change (Figs. 7.11 and 7.12, e-Figs. 7.46–7.51). Most examples have a variably prominent component of normal adipose tissue, imparting a resemblance to spindle cell lipoma. Focally the cells can resemble smooth muscle. Mitotic activity, atypical and multinucleated cells can be seen, and rarely the tumor cells assume epithelioid morphology (e-Figs. 7.50 and 7.51). The stroma contains mast cells and can show chondroid differentiation, hyalinized blood vessels, and focally a hemangiopericytomatous pattern.

Ancillary Investigations

Typically, immunohistochemistry shows positivity for CD34 (e-Fig. 7.52) and desmin (e-Fig. 7.53) with a smaller proportion expressing SMA. H-caldesmon is usually negative. The myoid markers help to distinguish this from solitary fibrous tumor. Genetic studies have shown partial monosomy of 13q and 16q and loss at *RB*/13q14 and *FKHR*/13q14 loci.[34] Similar changes have been found in spindle cell lipoma (Chapter 15)[35] and in cellular angiofibroma (Chapter 8).[36]

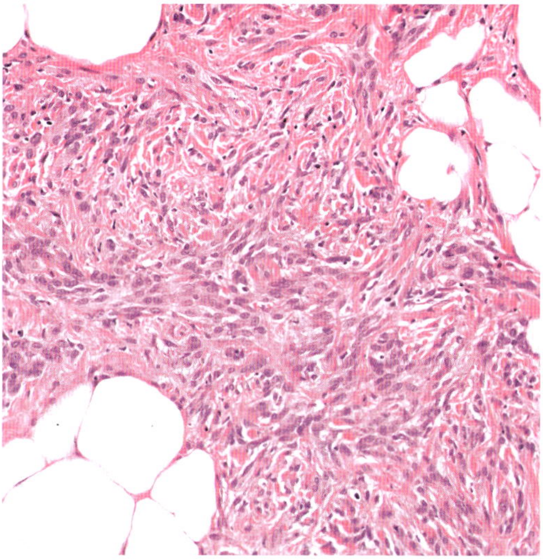

FIGURE 7.11 **Mammary-type Myofibroblastoma, Lesion in Male Breast.** Short spindle cells are interspersed with collagen fibers, with an adjacent fatty component.

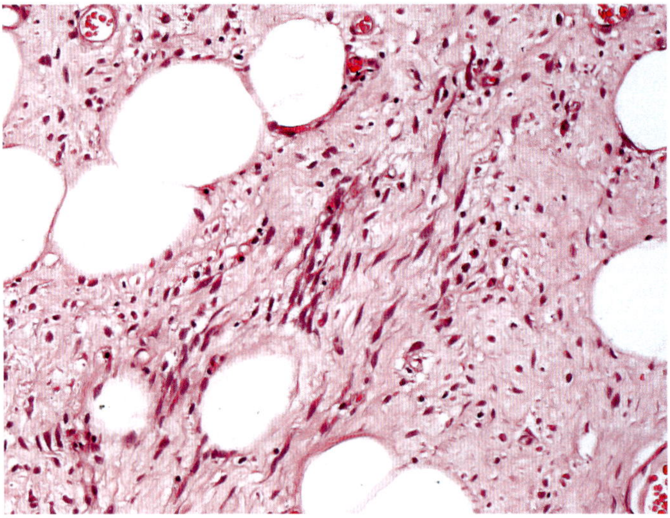

FIGURE 7.12 **Mammary-type Myofibroblastoma.** This example shows wavy spindle cells in small clusters in myxoid stroma, with scattered mast cells.

INTRANODAL (PALISADED) MYOFIBROBLASTOMA

This lesion was originally described in 1989 under three different terms: intranodal hemorrhagic spindle cell tumor with "amianthoid" fibers,[37] palisaded myofibroblastoma,[38] and solitary spindle cell tumor with myoid differentiation of the lymph node.[39] It occurs within lymph nodes but in a biopsy is often misinterpreted as a primary or metastatic sarcoma.

Clinical Features

The lesion is more frequent in men in the fifth and sixth decades, and most cases involve inguinal lymph nodes. However, examples have been described in the submandibular region[40] and multicentrically.[41] Reported examples have behaved in a benign fashion although an occasional recurrence has been reported (including one with metaplastic bone formation[42]).

Pathologic Features

This is typically a circumscribed lesion up to 5 cm in diameter with a solid, often dark red or black cut surface with interspersed paler firm areas. Microscopically, a cellular spindle tumor replaces the majority of the node that can persist as a rim within the node capsule (Fig. 7.13, e-Figs. 7.54 and 7.55). The spindle cells are uniform with minimal mitotic activity, elongated round or slightly pointed-ended nuclei and pale eosinophilic cytoplasm. Rarely, epithelioid cell morphology is seen. The cells are arranged in fascicles with areas of vague palisading (e-Figs. 7.56 and 7.57) around variably sized hyalinized areas, some of which have centrally located blood vessels (e-Figs. 7.58 and 7.59). There is also an admixture of blood vessels

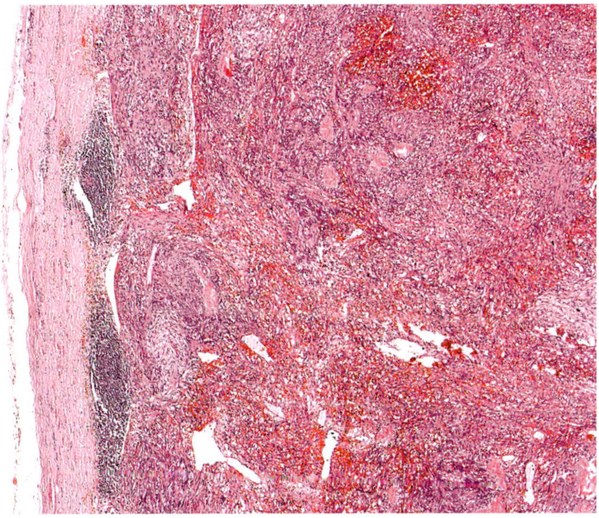

FIGURE 7.13 **Palisaded Myofibroblastoma, Lymph Node.** There is a rim of lymphoid tissue within a thickened fibrous capsule. The lesion has cellular areas with vague palisading, and foci of hemorrhage.

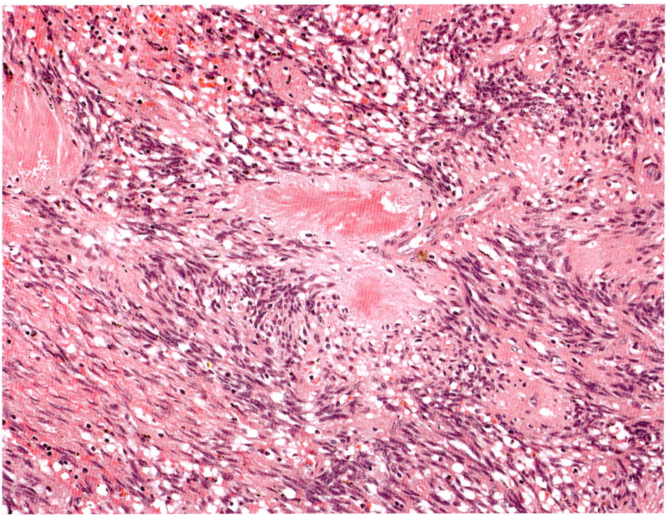

FIGURE 7.14 **Palisaded Myofibroblastoma.** Slender spindle cells are arranged in fascicles with focal nuclear palisading. At the center is a focus of amianthoid collagen and there are microhemorrhages (top) with intercellular spaces, imparting resemblance to Kaposi sarcoma.

and scattering of lymphocytes, and microhemorrhages and hemosiderin deposition can be prominent (e-Figs. 7.60 and 7.61). Occasionally, there are stellate areas with thick collagen fibers (so called amianthoid fibers), and irregularly sized clusters of small eosinophilic globules (Fig. 7.14, e-Fig. 7.62). Amianthoid fibers are abnormal collagen fibers with the same periodicity as collagen but much thicker (from 280 up to 1,000 nm, compared with the normal fiber diameter of 80–150 nm). They are arranged in a radial fashion rather than in parallel, and appear to be focused on blood vessels. Occasionally they calcify in the center. These structures have also been described in some sarcomas (chondrosarcoma, synovial sarcoma, malignant peripheral nerve sheath tumor), in solitary fibrous tumor, and in a so-called benign amianthioma.[43]

Ancillary Investigations

The spindle cells show cytoplasmic positivity for SMA and calponin and focally for muscle specific actin (HHF35) but are negative for desmin, h-caldesmon, S100 protein, CD31, and CD34. Overexpression of cyclin D1 has been reported.[44] Electron microscopy shows moderate amounts of RER, peripheral bundles of myofilaments and fragments of external lamina, which are features of myofibroblasts. However, based on ultrastructural studies, it has also been suggested that the cells show incomplete smooth muscle differentiation.[45]

REFERENCES

1. Daimaru Y, Hashimoto H, Enjoji M. Myofibromatosis in adults (adult counterpart of infantile myofibromatosis). *Am J Surg Pathol.* 1989;13:859–865.
2. Montgomery E, Speight PM, Fisher C. Myofibromas presenting in the oral cavity: A series of 9 cases. *Oral Surg Oral Med Oral Pathol Oral Radiol Endod.* 2000;89:343–348.
3. Foss RD, Ellis GL. Myofibromas and myofibromatosis of the oral region: a clinicopathologic analysis of 79 cases. *Oral Surg Oral Med Oral Pathol Oral Radiol Endod.* 2000;89:57–65.
4. Wiswell TE, Davis J, Cunningham BE, et al. Infantile myofibromatosis: the most common fibrous tumor of infancy. *J Pediatr Surg.* 1988;23:315–318.
5. Granter SR, Badizadegan K, Fletcher CD. Myofibromatosis in adults, glomangiopericytoma, and myopericytoma: a spectrum of tumors showing perivascular myoid differentiation. *Am J Surg Pathol.* 1998;22:513–525.
6. Hicks J, Mierau G. The spectrum of pediatric fibroblastic and myofibroblastic tumors. *Ultrastruct Pathol.* 2004;28:265–281.
7. Eyden B. Electron microscopy in the study of myofibroblastic lesions. *Semin Diagn Pathol.* 2003;20:13–24.
8. Nappi O, Ritter JH, Pettinato G, et al. Hemangiopericytoma: histopathological pattern or clinicopathologic entity? *Semin Diagn Pathol.* 1995;12:221–232.
9. Gengler C, Guillou L. Solitary fibrous tumour and haemangiopericytoma: evolution of a concept. *Histopathology.* 2006;48:63–74.
10. Dictor M, Elner A, Andersson T, et al. Myofibromatosis-like hemangiopericytoma metastasizing as differentiated vascular smooth-muscle and myosarcoma. Myopericytes as a subset of "myofibroblasts." *Am J Surg Pathol.* 1992;16:1239–1247.
11. Mentzel T, Dei Tos AP, Sapi Z, et al. Myopericytoma of skin and soft tissues: clinicopathologic and immunohistochemical study of 54 cases. *Am J Surg Pathol.* 2006;30:104–113.
12. McMenamin ME, Fletcher CD. Malignant myopericytoma: expanding the spectrum of tumours with myopericytic differentiation. *Histopathology.* 2002;41:450–460.
13. McMenamin ME, Calonje E. Intravascular myopericytoma. *J Cutan Pathol.* 2002;29:557–561.

14. Fisher C. Myofibrosarcoma. *Virchows Arch.* 2004;445:215–223.
15. Dahlen A, Fletcher CD, Mertens F, et al. Activation of the GLI oncogene through fusion with the beta-actin gene (ACTB) in a group of distinctive pericytic neoplasms: pericytoma with t(7;12). *Am J Pathol.* 2004;164:1645–1653.
16. Miettinen M, Paal E, Lasota J, et al. Gastrointestinal glomus tumors: a clinicopathologic, immunohistochemical, and molecular genetic study of 32 cases. *Am J Surg Pathol.* 2002;26:301–311.
17. Sawada S, Honda M, Kamide R, et al. Three cases of subungual glomus tumors with von Recklinghausen neurofibromatosis. *J Am Acad Dermatol.* 1995;32:277–278.
18. Folpe AL, Fanburg-Smith JC, Miettinen M, et al. Atypical and malignant glomus tumors: analysis of 52 cases, with a proposal for the reclassification of glomus tumors. *Am J Surg Pathol.* 2001;25:1–12.
19. Thompson LD, Miettinen M, Wenig BM. Sinonasal-type hemangiopericytoma: a clinicopathologic and immunophenotypic analysis of 104 cases showing perivascular myoid differentiation. *Am J Surg Pathol.* 2003;27:737–749.
20. Kilpatrick SE, Limon J. Mixed tumour/myoepithelioma/parachordoma. In: Fletcher CD, Unni K, Mertens F, eds. *WHO Classification of Tumours. Pathology and Genetics. Tumours of Soft Tissue and Bone.* Lyon: IARC Press, 2002:198–199.
21. Fisher C. Parachordoma exists–but what is it? *Adv Anat Pathol.* 2000;7:141–148.
22. Allen CM. The ectomesenchymal chondromyxoid tumor: a review. *Oral Dis.* 2008;14:390–395.
23. Michal M, Miettinen M. Myoepitheliomas of the skin and soft tissues. Report of 12 cases. *Virchows Arch.* 1999;434:393–400.
24. Hornick JL, Fletcher CD. Cutaneous myoepithelioma: a clinicopathologic and immunohistochemical study of 14 cases. *Hum Pathol.* 2004;35:14–24.
25. Hornick JL, Fletcher CD. Myoepithelial tumors of soft tissue: a clinicopathologic and immunohistochemical study of 101 cases with evaluation of prognostic parameters. *Am J Surg Pathol.* 2003;27:1183–1196.
26. Mentzel T. Myoepithelial neoplasms of skin and soft tissues. *Pathologe.* 2005;26:322–330.
27. Brandal P, Panagopoulos I, Bjerkehagen B, et al. Detection of a t(1;22)(q23;q12) translocation leading to an EWSR1-PBX1 fusion gene in a myoepithelioma. *Genes Chromosomes Cancer.* 2008;47:558–564.
28. Brandal P, Panagopoulos I, Bjerkehagen B, et al. t(19;22)(q13;q12) translocation leading to the novel fusion gene EWSR1-ZNF444 in soft tissue myoepithelial carcinoma. *Genes Chromosomes Cancer.* 2009;48:1051–1056.
29. Fetsch JF, Laskin WB, Michal M, et al. Ectopic hamartomatous thymoma: a clinicopathologic and immunohistochemical analysis of 21 cases with data supporting reclassification as a branchial anlage mixed tumor. *Am J Surg Pathol.* 2004;28:1360–1370.
30. Eyden BP, Shanks JH, Ioachim E, et al. Myofibroblastoma of breast: evidence favoring smooth-muscle rather than myofibroblastic differentiation. *Ultrastruct Pathol.* 1999;23:249–257.
31. Magro G, Gurrera A, Bisceglia M. H-caldesmon expression in myofibroblastoma of the breast: evidence supporting the distinction from leiomyoma. *Histopathology.* 2003;42:233–238.
32. Wargotz ES, Weiss SW, Norris HJ. Myofibroblastoma of the breast. Sixteen cases of a distinctive benign mesenchymal tumor. *Am J Surg Pathol.* 1987;11:493–502.
33. McMenamin ME, Fletcher CD. Mammary-type myofibroblastoma of soft tissue: a tumor closely related to spindle cell lipoma. *Am J Surg Pathol.* 2001;25:1022–1029.
34. Maggiani F, Debiec-Rychter M, Verbeeck G, et al. Extramammary myofibroblastoma is genetically related to spindle cell lipoma. *Virchows Arch.* 2006;449:244–247.

35. Mandahl N, Mertens F, Willen H, et al. A new cytogenetic subgroup in lipomas: loss of chromosome 16 material in spindle cell and pleomorphic lipomas. *J Cancer Res Clin Oncol.* 1994;120:707–711.

36. Maggiani F, Debiec-Rychter M, Vanbockrijck M, et al. Cellular angiofibroma: another mesenchymal tumour with 13q14 involvement, suggesting a link with spindle cell lipoma and (extra)-mammary myofibroblastoma. *Histopathology.* 2007;51:410–412.

37. Suster S, Rosai J. Intranodal hemorrhagic spindle-cell tumor with "amianthoid" fibers. Report of six cases of a distinctive mesenchymal neoplasm of the inguinal region that simulates Kaposi's sarcoma. *Am J Surg Pathol.* 1989;13:347–357.

38. Weiss SW, Gnepp DR, Bratthauer GL. Palisaded myofibroblastoma. A benign mesenchymal tumor of lymph node. *Am J Surg Pathol.* 1989;13:341–346.

39. Lee JY, Abell E, Shevechik GJ. Solitary spindle cell tumor with myoid differentiation of the lymph node. *Arch Pathol Lab Med.* 1989;113:547–550.

40. Alguacil-Garcia A. Intranodal myofibroblastoma in a submandibular lymph node. A case report. *Am J Clin Pathol.* 1992;97:69–72.

41. Rahimi S, Onetti Muda A, Faraggiana T. Multicentric intranodal myofibroblastoma in an infant. *Histopathology.* 1995;27:477–478.

42. Creager AJ, Garwacki CP. Recurrent intranodal palisaded myofibroblastoma with metaplastic bone formation. *Arch Pathol Lab Med.* 1999;123:433–436.

43. Connolly CE. "Crystalline" collagen production by an unusual benign soft tissue tumour ("amianthioma"). *Histopathology.* 1981;5:11–20.

44. Kleist B, Poetsch M, Schmoll J. Intranodal palisaded myofibroblastoma with overexpression of cyclin D1. *Arch Pathol Lab Med.* 2003;127:1040–1043.

45. Eyden B, Chorneyko KA. Intranodal myofibroblastoma: study of a case suggesting smooth-muscle differentiation. *J Submicrosc Cytol Pathol.* 2001;33:157–163.

8

TUMORS OF SPECIALIZED LOWER GENITAL TRACT MESENCHYME

INTRODUCTION

A number of cellular and myxoid soft tissue lesions of the skin can be encountered in the vulva, including dermatofibrosarcoma protuberans (Chapter 4), vascular lesions (Chapters 16 and 17), and superficial myxoid tumors (see detailed discussion in Chapter 20). A host of sarcoma types has been described in the female genital tract, especially alveolar soft part sarcoma[1] (Chapter 12). However, a group of myxoid lesions is often considered somewhat site specific, the prototype of which is aggressive angiomyxoma (AAM). These myxoid lesions are also found in men but were first described in women.

In some respects, classification of the various angiomyxoid lesions of the genital region is much ado about very little. They are benign but, when infiltrative (AAM), they can be locally aggressive. They all tend to express hormone receptors with variable desmin, actin, and CD34 and may form a spectrum despite many publications delineating their distinguishing features. In reality, some cases are not clearly recognizable as either AAM, angiomyofibroblastoma (AMF), cellular angiofibroma, or pseudosarcomatous fibroepithelial stromal polyps of the lower genital tract. In such a situation, it is probably most important to simply assure that the lesion is not a rhabdomyosarcoma. Many of the lesions in this category express desmin, so use of a specific skeletal muscle marker (MyoD1 or myogenin) is recommended in evaluating such tumors. Of these genital region lesions, AAM is the most likely to be overtly myxoid, but any such case always has a differential diagnosis that includes the other lesions in this group of neoplasms (Table 8.1).

DEEP (AGGRESSIVE) ANGIOMYXOMA

AAM is a well-vascularized, myxedematous spindled cell tumor that presents in the deep soft tissues of the pelvic and perineal regions. It is prone to recurrences owing to its infiltrative growth pattern but does not metastasize. This distinctive tumor was first delineated by Steeper and Rosai in 1983.[2] Subsequent series of AAM have reported nearly identical histologic findings and have confirmed the tumor's proclivity for local recurrence in both female and male patients.[3–9]

TABLE 8.1 Differential Diagnosis of Selected Lesions Presenting in the Genital Region

Lesion	Gross Features	Morphologic Features
Aggressive angiomyxoma	Usually large (>5 cm), infiltrative	Infiltrative, myxoid, Medium- to large-sized vessels with clusters of smooth muscle cells "spinning off" from the main vessel wall
Angiomyofibroblastoma	Well marginated and small	Plump, epithelioid cells concentrated around vessels
Cellular angiofibroma	Well marginated and small	Uniform short spindle-shaped cells proliferating in edematous to fibrous stroma, wiry collagen akin to that in spindle cell lipomas
Fibroepithelial polyp	Under mucosal surfaces, small	Spindled and stellate with pale tapering cytoplasmic processes. Multinucleate cells common
Superficial myofibroblastoma of the lower female genital tract	Small subepithelial lesions	Bland ovoid, stellate, or spindled cells in a delicately collagenized stroma just under the epithelium
Mammary-type myofibroblastoma	Inguinal region, buttock, abdominal wall.	Circumscribed. Irregular fascicles of spindle cells, collagenous bands, adipose tissue, mast cells. Resembles spindle cell lipoma. Atypical and epithelioid variants occur
	Painless, slow-growing, rarely >6 cm diameter Benign	CD34+, desmin+ SMA±, h-caldesmon–

Clinical Features

AAM shows a striking female predominance with a female to male ratio of about 6:1.[2–7,9–11] The age of patients at presentation ranges from the teens to 70 years with a peak incidence in the fourth decade of life. In females, the vast majority of tumors present in the deep soft tissues of the vulvovaginal and pelviperineal regions. Less common sites include the

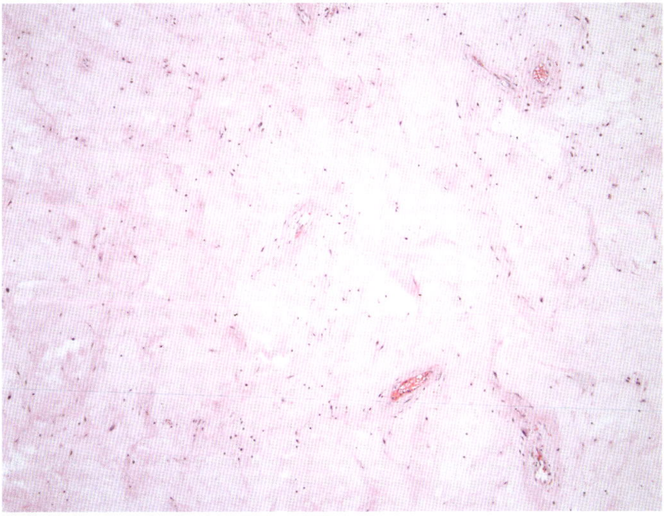

FIGURE 8.1 **Aggressive Angiomyxoma.** At low magnification, the lesion is hypocellular, myxoid, and features large vessels.

buttock, retroperitoneum, and inguinal region. The scrotum and spermatic cord, inguinal area (including presentation within hernia sacs), perianal area and pelviperineal region are primary sites for AAM in men.[6,12]

The most common presenting signs and symptoms are pain or pressure in the vulvovaginal or pelviperineal areas, dyspareunia, and increased frequency of urination. In males, AAM presents in a similar fashion to a hernia. AAM is benign, but may locally infiltrate adjacent soft tissue, including fascia and muscle. The reported recurrence rate of AAM ranges from 36% to 72%.[7] Late and multiple recurrences are not uncommon and presumably reflect inadequate initial resection. The ability of CT, ultrasound, and MRI to better assess invasion of AAM into adjacent organs and soft tissue makes these radiologic techniques important in the planning of a surgical approach. The recommended treatment of AAM is to surgically excise as much of the tumor as technically possible.

Pathologic Features

AAM range in size from 3 cm to as large as 60 cm with the majority of lesions measuring at least 5 cm in greatest dimension.[2,3] On gross examination, AAM is a large, lobulated mass that generally appears deceptively well circumscribed. The tumor is soft to rubbery in consistency. The cut surface has a glistening, gelatinous appearance and a gray-white to pink-tan color. Small cystic areas and foci of hemorrhage are occasionally observed.

Microscopically, AAM exhibits low to moderate cellularity and is composed of haphazardly arranged, short spindled, and stellate-shaped cells set a myxoid-appearing, edematous stroma containing fine strands of collagen and a prominent component of variably sized vessels (Fig. 8.1, e-Figs. 8.1–8.3). Multinucleated cells are infrequently observed. An increase in the

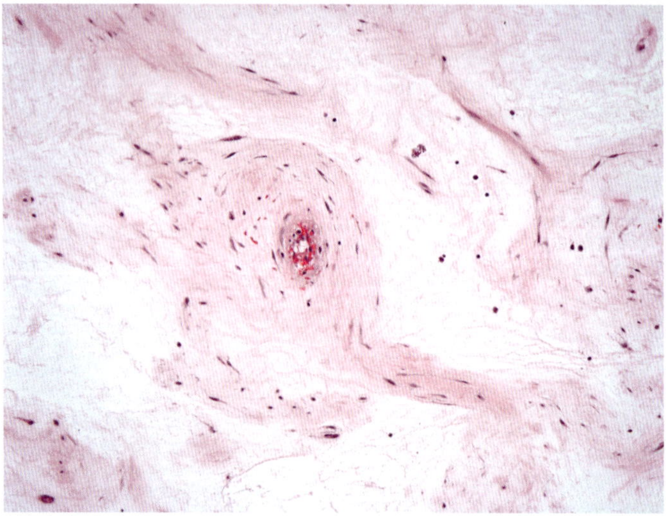

FIGURE 8.2 **Aggressive Angiomyxoma.** Note the appearance of strands of cells emanating from the vessel in the center of the field.

cellularity is occasionally observed around vessels or at the periphery of the lesion where microscopic evidence of infiltration into surrounding tissue with entrapment of fat, peripheral nerve, or muscle is common. Mitotic activity is negligible.

Medium- to large-sized vessels with clusters of smooth muscle cells "spinning off" from the main vessel wall are found (Fig. 8.2). Capillary-sized thin-walled vessels are found as scattered units or organized into tight collections. Extravasation of red blood cells is commonly noted around these fragile capillary structures.

The stroma consists of a loose meshwork of delicate, wavy collagen fibers set in a myxedematous matrix. Thin bundles or fascicles of mature smooth muscle can be identified within the stroma, generally running parallel to vessels or nerves. Microcysts occasionally form within the stroma.

Ancillary Investigations

Histochemical stains demonstrate that the noncollagenous stroma consists of a small quantity of acidic mucopolysaccharide, chiefly hyaluronic acid.[7]

The cells strongly express vimentin and variably express muscle-specific and alpha-smooth muscle actin, desmin and CD34 (e-Figs. 8.4 and 8.5). The tendency is toward expression of desmin and lack of CD34, but some cases do have this pattern. The nuclei show strong expression of estrogen and progesterone receptor proteins (e-Fig. 8.6).[7]

There are a few reports of cytogenetic alterations in these lesions, but none is sufficiently characteristic to be exploited for diagnosis.[9,11,13–15] The most promising is *HMGA2* gene rearrangements, which are detected in about a third of cases.[16]

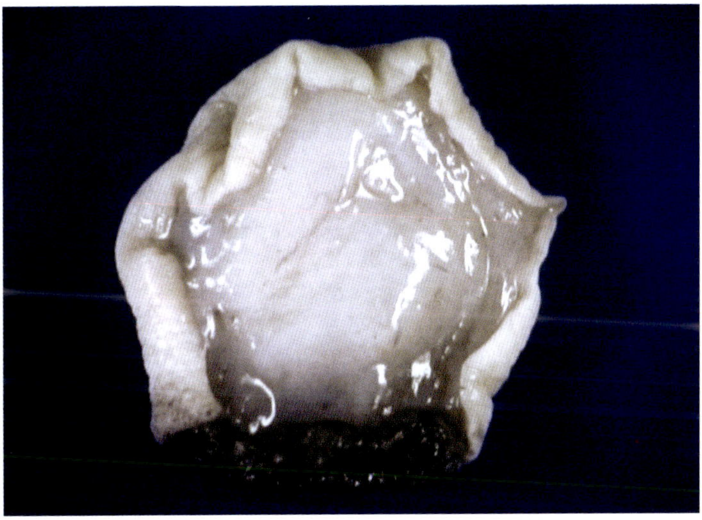

FIGURE 8.3 **Angiomyofibroblastoma.** This well-marginated lesion was resected from the vaginal wall. The mucosa has curled back on the edges of the excised sample, which is viewed here from its deep aspect.

ANGIOMYOFIBROBLASTOMA

Clinical Features

AMF arises principally within the vulvar region[8,17–24] but has also been reported in the male genital region[19] and has a peak incidence in the fifth decade of life. In contrast to AAM, AMF is typically small, well circumscribed, and subcutaneous in location.

Pathologic Features

Grossly these tumors are well marginated with a firm rather than gelatinous cut surface (Fig. 8.3). Microscopically, the cells comprising AMF differ from the short spindled and stellate-shaped cells of AAM by their plump, epithelioid appearance and their proclivity to concentrate around vessels in a nested and cord-like arrangement (Figs. 8.4 and 8.5). The vessels of AMF are more numerous and more evenly distributed throughout the process than the vessels of AAM. Vessels with muscular walls and entrapped nerves are commonly identified in AAM, but typically absent in AMF. Occasional cases display prominent fat that appears to be an integral part of the lesion (Fig. 8.6, e-Fig. 8.7).[17,24] Rare cases purportedly show malignant transformation.[22,25]

Ancillary Investigations

The immunohistochemical profile of these neoplasms is essentially the same as that of AAM, with variable actin, desmin, and CD34 labeling, and with a similar trend to desmin expression with absent CD34 labeling[8,17–21,23,24,26]

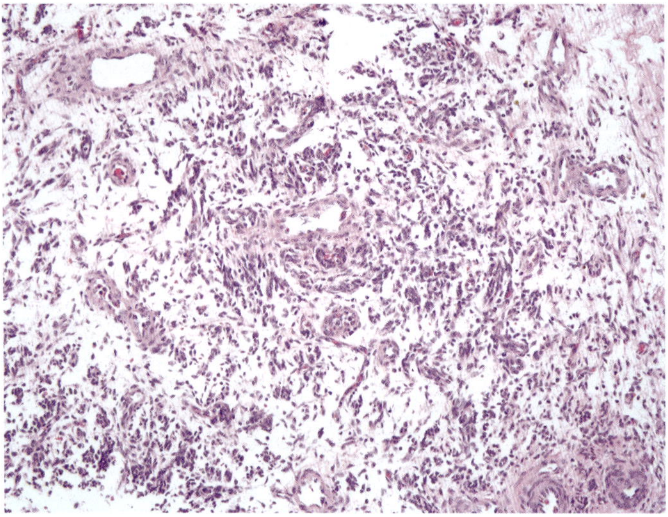

FIGURE 8.4 **Angiomyofibroblastoma.** Plump epithelioid cells are arranged around vessels.

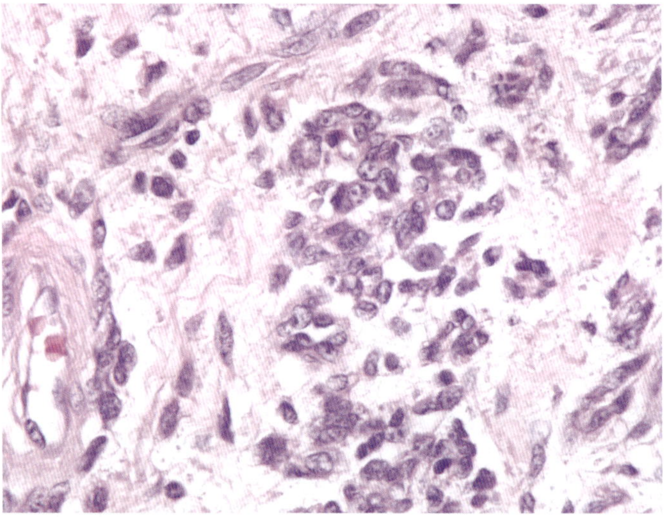

FIGURE 8.5 **Angiomyofibroblastoma.** At high magnification, the nuclei are bland, and smaller than the adjacent endothelial cell nuclei.

such that immunohistochemistry does not allow their separation. Both AAM and AMF can express hormone receptors.[17,24] There are few data concerning genetic alterations in such lesions but, in contrast to AAM, AMF lacks *HMGA2* gene rearrangements, which supports viewing it as a distinct entity. Flow cytometric results have been inconsistent.[26]

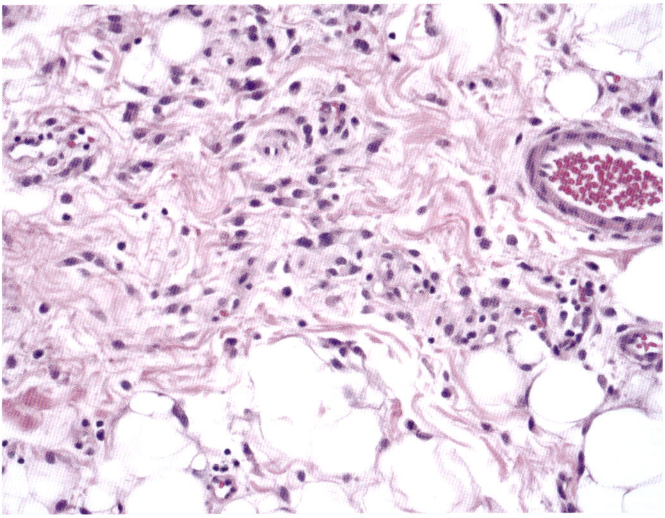

FIGURE 8.6 **Angiomyofibroblastoma.** This example featured areas in which fat was a part of the lesion.

CELLULAR ANGIOFIBROMA (ANGIOMYOFIBROBLASTOMA-LIKE TUMOR)

Clinical Features

Cellular angiofibroma[27,28] (also called AMF -like tumor of the male genital tract[29]) is found in both women and men with similar incidence in patients with a median age in the sixth decade. In women, the most common location is the vulva and in men, the inguinoscrotal region. Those lesions in men tend to attain a larger size (median, about 7 cm) than those of the vulva (median, about 3 cm) at the time of resection. These lesions are benign with minimal tendency for local recurrence.

Pathologic Features

Grossly these lesions are well marginated, with a multilobulated appearance in a subset of cases. Their cut surface is similar to that of AMF, that is, firm to rubbery rather than gelatinous. Microscopically the tumors consist of uniform short spindle-shaped cells proliferating in edematous to fibrous stroma punctuated by wiry collagen akin to that in spindle cell lipomas (Fig. 8.7, e-Fig. 8.8). In fact, a subset has an adipose tissue component as per AMF (e-Fig. 8.9). Some cases have zones of palisaded nuclei in a pattern reminiscent of that seen in schwannomas. The cells feature pale eosinophilic bipolar cytoplasm (e-Fig. 8.10). The vessels in these tumors are variable, but all lesions have foci with thick walled vessels with mural hyalinization (Fig. 8.8). In contrast to AMF or AAM, there is no proliferation of either lesional cells (AMF) or smooth muscle (AAM) around the vessels in cellular angiofibromas.

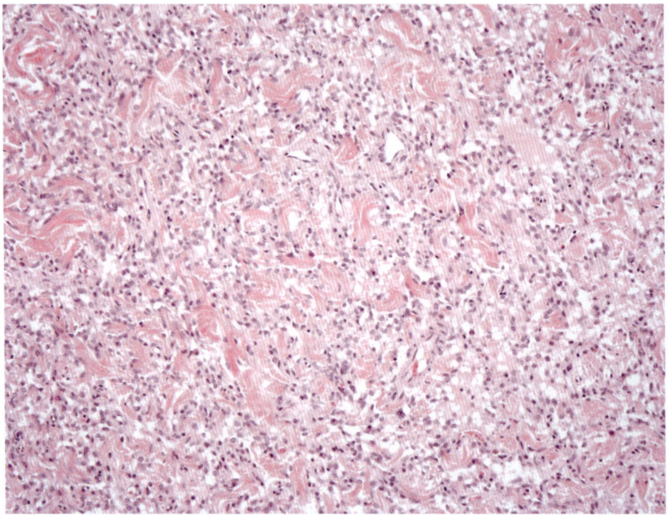

FIGURE 8.7 **Cellular Angiofibroma (Also Called "Angiomyofibroblastoma-like Tumor of the Male Genital Tract") has overlapping features with AMF.** At low magnification, this example is cellular with abundant wiry collagen.

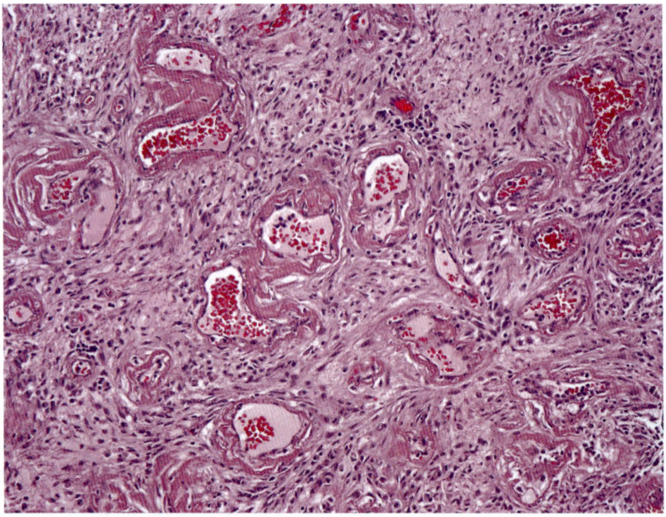

FIGURE 8.8 **Cellular Angiofibroma.** A characteristic feature of this tumor is thick-walled vessels with fibrinoid change.

Ancillary Investigations

Like AMF and AAM, cellular angiofibromas have variable actin, desmin (e-Fig. 8.11), and CD34 expression, but the trend is expression of CD34 and lack of desmin in cellular angiofibroma. There may be estrogen (e-Fig. 8.12) or progesterone receptor expression in lesions from either men or

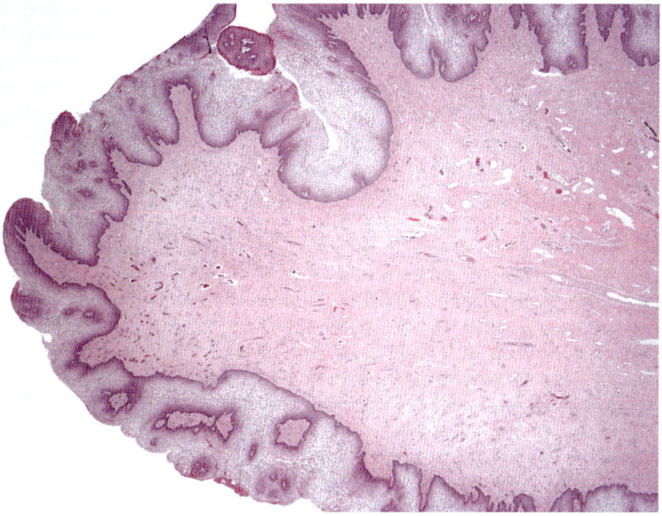

FIGURE 8.9 **Vaginal Stromal Polyp.** These are similar to fibroepithelial polyps of the skin, but they can sometimes have alarmingly cellular stroma.

women. These tumors, like the others in this family of lesions, lack keratins and S100 protein.

FIBROEPITHELIAL STROMAL POLYPS OF THE LOWER FEMALE GENITAL TRACT

These lesions can be myxoid but differ from the others by having an epithelial component and, of course, by being polypoid as the name indicates. They have been known for years [30] and are most common in the vagina followed by the vulva and cervix, and they are detected during pregnancy about 20% of the time.[31] The epithelial surface in these is often hyperplastic and beneath it a stromal lesion, which can feature markedly atypical cells, proliferates (Fig. 8.9, e-Figs. 8.13–8.15). The stroma is edematous with prominent often dilated vessels and only rarely myxoid. The proliferating cells are spindled and stellate with pale tapering cytoplasmic processes. Multinucleate cells are a frequent finding. Occasionally, the stromal cells can appear hyperchromatic and bizarre. In these polyps, many mitoses, including aberrant forms, can be encountered.[32] A percentage of these polyps express desmin or smooth muscle actin, but they lack keratins, S100 protein, and specific markers of skeletal muscle differentiation.

SUPERFICIAL MYOFIBROBLASTOMA OF THE LOWER FEMALE GENITAL TRACT

Although these lesions are not as overtly myxoid as the previously mentioned entities, they are part of the differential diagnosis of benign spindle

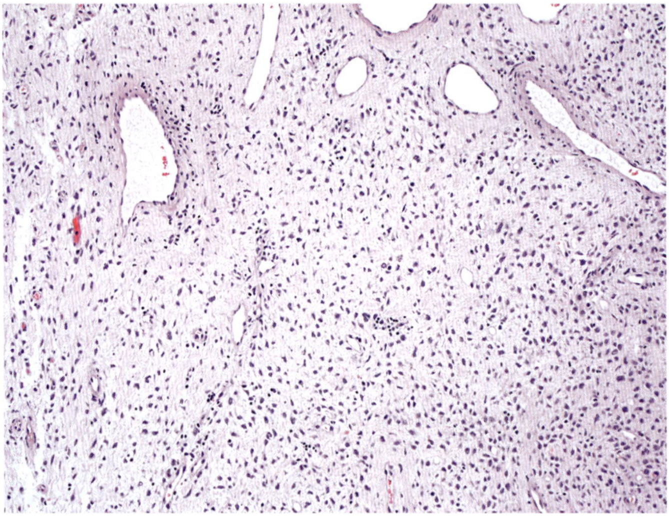

FIGURE 8.10 **Superficial Myofibroblastoma of the Lower Female Genital Tract.** These well-circumscribed tumors consist of ovoid to spindled cells in delicately collagenized stroma.

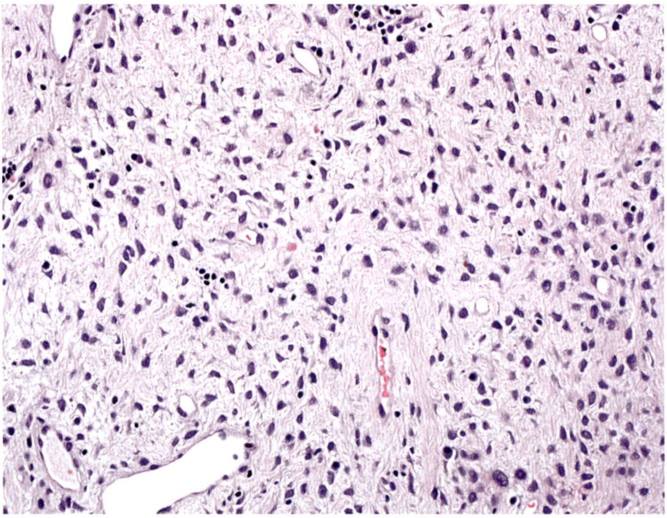

FIGURE 8.11 **Superficial Myofibroblastoma of the Lower Female Genital Tract.** At high magnification, the nuclei are bland and uniform appearing.

cell tumors of the genital region. They have been termed "superficial cervicovaginal myofibroblastoma" [33] and "superficial myofibroblastoma of the lower female genital tract."[34] The reported lesions have arisen in mostly adult patients ranging from 23 to 80 years (median about 60 years) and are small (up to 6 cm), well-marginated subepithelial lesions that involve the vagina, cervix, and vulva. There is a history of hormonal manipulation (tamoxifen use) in some of the patients. The lesions proliferate just under the epithelium with a spared Grenz zone and consist of bland ovoid, stellate, or spindled cells in a delicately collagenized stroma (Figs. 8.10 and 8.11). Mitoses are sparse. Most examples express desmin on immunohistochemistry and most express estrogen and progestogen receptors. A subset of cases label with CD34 and actin antibodies, but the lesions are negative for S100 protein and cytokeratins. In other words, these have the same immunoprofile as all of the other members of the family of gynecologic mesenchymal lesion.

REFERENCES

1. Nielsen GP, Oliva E, Young RH, et al. Alveolar soft-part sarcoma of the female genital tract: a report of nine cases and review of the literature. *Int J Gynecol Pathol.* 1995;14:283–292.
2. Steeper TA, Rosai J. Aggressive angiomyxoma of the female pelvis and perineum. Report of nine cases of a distinctive type of gynecologic soft-tissue neoplasm. *Am J Surg Pathol.* 1983;7:463–475.
3. Begin LR, Clement PB, Kirk ME, et al. Aggressive angiomyxoma of pelvic soft parts: a clinicopathologic study of nine cases. *Hum Pathol.* 1985;16:621–628.
4. Smith HO, Worrell RV, Smith AY, et al. Aggressive angiomyxoma of the female pelvis and perineum: review of the literature. *Gynecol Oncol.* 1991;42:79–85.
5. Tsang WY, Chan JK, Lee KC, et al. Aggressive angiomyxoma. A report of four cases occurring in men. *Am J Surg Pathol.* 1992;16:1059–1065.
6. Clatch RJ, Drake WK, Gonzalez JG. Aggressive angiomyxoma in men. A report of two cases associated with inguinal hernias. *Arch Pathol Lab Med.* 1993;117:911–913.
7. Fetsch JF, Laskin WB, Lefkowitz M, et al. Aggressive angiomyxoma: a clinicopathologic study of 29 female patients. *Cancer.* 1996;78:79–90.
8. Granter SR, Nucci MR, Fletcher CD. Aggressive angiomyxoma: reappraisal of its relationship to angiomyofibroblastoma in a series of 16 cases. *Histopathology.* 1997;30:3–10.
9. Nucci MR, Weremowicz S, Neskey DM, et al. Chromosomal translocation t(8;12) induces aberrant HMGIC expression in aggressive angiomyxoma of the vulva. *Genes Chromosomes Cancer.* 2001;32:172–176.
10. Amr SS, el-Mallah KO. Aggressive angiomyxoma of the vagina. *Int J Gynaecol Obstet.* 1995;48:207–210.
11. Kazmierczak B, Wanschura S, Meyer-Bolte K, et al. Cytogenic and molecular analysis of an aggressive angiomyxoma. *Am J Pathol.* 1995;147:580–585.
12. Iezzoni JC, Fechner RE, Wong LS, et al. Aggressive angiomyxoma in males. A report of four cases. *Am J Clin Pathol.* 1995;104:391–396.
13. Rabban JT, Dal Cin P, Oliva E. HMGA2 rearrangement in a case of vulvar aggressive angiomyxoma. *Int J Gynecol Pathol.* 2006;25:403–407.
14. Micci F, Panagopoulos I, Bjerkehagen B, et al. Deregulation of HMGA2 in an aggressive angiomyxoma with t(11;12)(q23;q15). *Virchows Arch.* 2006;448:838–842.
15. Kenny-Moynihan MB, Hagen J, Richman B, et al. Loss of an X chromosome in aggressive angiomyxoma of female soft parts: a case report. *Cancer Genet Cytogenet.* 1996;89:61–64.
16. Medeiros F, Erickson-Johnson MR, Keeney GL, et al. Frequency and characterization of HMGA2 and HMGA1 rearrangements in mesenchymal tumors of the lower genital tract. *Genes Chromosomes Cancer.* 2007;46:981–990.

17. Laskin WB, Fetsch JF, Tavassoli FA. Angiomyofibroblastoma of the female genital tract: analysis of 17 cases including a lipomatous variant. *Hum Pathol.* 1997;28:1046–1055.
18. Fletcher CD, Tsang WY, Fisher C, et al. Angiomyofibroblastoma of the vulva. A benign neoplasm distinct from aggressive angiomyxoma. *Am J Surg Pathol.* 1992;16:373–382.
19. Ockner DM, Sayadi H, Swanson PE, et al. Genital angiomyofibroblastoma. Comparison with aggressive angiomyxoma and other myxoid neoplasms of skin and soft tissue. *Am J Clin Pathol.* 1997;107:36–44.
20. Silverman JS, Albukerk J, Tamsen A. Comparison of angiomyofibroblastoma and aggressive angiomyxoma in both sexes: four cases composed of bimodal CD34 and factor XIIIa positive dendritic cell subsets. *Pathol Res Pract.* 1997;193:673–682.
21. Bigotti G, Coli A, Gasbarri A, et al. Angiomyofibroblastoma and aggressive angiomyxoma: two benign mesenchymal neoplasms of the female genital tract. An immunohistochemical study. *Pathol Res Pract.* 1999;195:39–44.
22. Nielsen GP, Young RH, Dickersin GR, et al. Angiomyofibroblastoma of the vulva with sarcomatous transformation ("angiomyofibrosarcoma"). *Am J Surg Pathol.* 1997;21:1104–1108.
23. Nielsen GP, Rosenberg AE, Young RH, et al. Angiomyofibroblastoma of the vulva and vagina. *Mod Pathol.* 1996;9:284–291.
24. Cao D, Srodon M, Montgomery EA, et al. Lipomatous variant of angiomyofibroblastoma: report of two cases and review of the literature. *Int J Gynecol Pathol.* 2005;24:196–200.
25. Satheshkumar T, Saklani AP, Banerjee D, et al. Angiomyofibrosarcoma: a rare ischiorectal fossa swelling. *Hosp Med.* 2003;64:244–245.
26. Fukunaga M, Nomura K, Matsumoto K, et al. Vulval angiomyofibroblastoma. Clinicopathologic analysis of six cases. *Am J Clin Pathol.* 1997;107:45–51.
27. Nucci MR, Granter SR, Fletcher CD. Cellular angiofibroma: a benign neoplasm distinct from angiomyofibroblastoma and spindle cell lipoma. *Am J Surg Pathol.* 1997;21:636–644.
28. Iwasa Y, Fletcher CD. Cellular angiofibroma: clinicopathologic and immunohistochemical analysis of 51 cases. *Am J Surg Pathol.* 2004;28:1426–1435.
29. Laskin WB, Fetsch JF, Mostofi FK. Angiomyofibroblastomalike tumor of the male genital tract: analysis of 11 cases with comparison to female angiomyofibroblastoma and spindle cell lipoma. *Am J Surg Pathol.* 1998;22:6–16.
30. Norris HJ, Taylor HB. Polyps of the vagina. A benign lesion resembling sarcoma. *Cancer.* 1966;19:227–232.
31. Tobon H, McIntyre-Seltman K, Rubino M. 'Polyposis vaginalis' of pregnancy. *Arch Pathol Lab Med.* 1989;113:1391–1393.
32. Nucci MR, Young RH, Fletcher CD. Cellular pseudosarcomatous fibroepithelial stromal polyps of the lower female genital tract: an underrecognized lesion often misdiagnosed as sarcoma. *Am J Surg Pathol.* 2000;24:231–240.
33. Laskin WB, Fetsch JF, Tavassoli FA. Superficial cervicovaginal myofibroblastoma: fourteen cases of a distinctive mesenchymal tumor arising from the specialized subepithelial stroma of the lower female genital tract. *Hum Pathol.* 2001;32:715–725.
34. Ganesan R, McCluggage WG, Hirschowitz L, et al. Superficial myofibroblastoma of the lower female genital tract: report of a series including tumours with a vulval location. *Histopathology.* 2005;46:137–143.

9

BENIGN PERIPHERAL NERVE SHEATH TUMORS

INTRODUCTION

The principal cells of the nerve sheath are the Schwann cell and the perineurial cell. Schwann cells form the inside layer of the endoneurium, surround the axon, and produce myelin, external lamina, and collagen. In myelinated nerves there is one Schwann cell per axon, and in nonmyelinated nerves there are several axon segments within a single Schwann cell, but with only very few layers of schwannian plasmalemma. Ultrastructurally, the Schwann cell has elongated processes with a continuous external lamina covering these and the cell body (e-Fig. 9.1). The Schwann cell is neural crest derived and is immunoreactive for S100 protein (e-Fig. 9.2), Leu7, laminin, and myelin basic protein, and usually negative for cytokeratin, epithelial membrane antigen (EMA), desmin, and muscle actins. However, schwannomas expressing cytokeratin have been described.[1] The external lamina of the Schwann cell stains mainly for laminin (and less so for collagen IV).

Perineurial cells form a few circumferential layers each within continuous external lamina outside the endoneurium (e-Fig. 9.3). The perineurial cell differs ultrastructurally from a fibroblast by the presence of external lamina (continuous or interrupted), pinocytosis, and intercellular junctions (e-Fig. 9.4).[2] Perineurial cells are continuous with and similar to cells of the arachnoid mater, and are immunoreactive for EMA (e-Fig. 9.3),[3] claudin-1,[4] and GLUT1,[5] but not usually for cytokeratin or S100 protein. The external lamina of the perineurial cell is immunoreactive for collagen IV and to a lesser extent laminin.

A third cell type identified within the endoneurium is a slender dendritic spindle cell that displays CD34 and appears to be distinct from Schwann, perineurial, or endothelial cells.[6] It might be analogous to the dermal dendritic fibroblast. CD34-positive cells are found in increased numbers in neurofibromas and in Antoni B (but not A) areas of schwannomas, but only in about 25% of malignant peripheral nerve sheath tumors (MPNST).

Benign nerve sheath tumors comprise one or more cell types, although usually a single one is predominant. Malignant nerve sheath tumors usually have one direction of differentiation although this is often incomplete. In biopsies of nerve sheath tumors, the difficulty is less often assessing the lineage than whether a tumor is likely to behave in a malignant fashion. The differential diagnosis is summarized in Table 9.1.

TABLE 9.1 **Differential Diagnosis of Nerve Sheath Tumors**

	Typical Clinical Features	Microscopic Features	Ancillary Investigations
Neuroma, traumatic	Painful nodule on or near nerve, following trauma	Nonencapsulated,multiple nerve bundles of varying size randomly dispersed in fibrous tissue	S100pr+ (Schwann cells), EMA+ (perineurial cells), NF+ (axons)
Neuroma, mucosal	Oral cavity, eyelids, GI tract. Associated with MEN type IIb	Nonencapsulated aggregate of uniformly sized nerve bundles	S100pr+ (Schwann cells), EMA+ (perineurial cells), NF+ (axons)
Neurofibroma, regular	Any location, associated NF-1. Nonencapsulated	Mixture of wavy spindle cells, collagen fibers ("shredded-carrot"), mast cells	S100 protein+ (not all cells), EMA+ very rarely focally, CD34+ focally. NF+ in axons
Neurofibroma, diffuse	Some associated with NF-1. Children and young adults. Head and neck, subcutaneous infiltrative plaque	Sheets of short spindle cells in loose fibrous stroma, infiltrating between normal structures	S100 protein+ diffusely in nuclei
	Associated with plexiform neurofibroma–extends outside nerve bundles into soft tissue	Wagner-Meissner bodies in various stages	
Neurofibroma, plexiform	Associated with NF-1. Can involve large nerves in deep locations or more superficial ones. Can undergo malignant change. Can extend extraneurally as diffuse neurofibroma	Transitions from normal nerve. Nerve expanded by variable myxoid stroma and increased cellularity. Atypical variant has nuclear crowding, pleomorphism. Diffuse extraneural component in some	S100 protein+ focally, EMA+ in peripheral perineurial cells. NF+ in axons

Perineurioma	Skin, subcutis, most locations. Subset in colon. Intraneural, sclerosing, reticular and plexiform variants	Spindle cells with long thin nuclei and very long slender terminal processes, in fascicles or perivascular whorls. Fibrous or myxoid stroma	EMA+, claudin-1+, CD34+ in some, beta-catenin
Low-grade fibromyxoid sarcoma	Skin, deep soft tissue, limbs/girdles	Fibromatosis-like areas, swirling fibromyxoid transitions, cellular myxoid areas without pleomorphism. Some nuclei are lozenge shaped, no nucleoli. Giant collagenous rosettes.	Occasionally SMA+, EMA+, claudin-1+ in some Nuclear beta-catenin usually negative. t(7;16)(q34;p11) *FUS-CREB3L2I* or *FUS-CREB3L1* fusion
Fibromatosis–desmoid type	Deep in limbs, head and neck, body cavities	Parallel myofibroblasts evenly dispersed in collagen, slit-like and thick-walled small-caliber vessels, perivascular and interstitial mast cells	SMA+, nuclear beta-catenin+, CD34–
Fibromatosis–superficial	Palm, sole, penis; infiltrative plaque	Variably cellular nodules in dense collagen. Cells are parallel aligned, lack atypia. Mast cells	SMA+, nuclear beta-catenin+ occasionally, CD34–
Palisaded encapsulated neuroma	Small nodule on face, adults	Thinly encapsulated, Schwann cells associated with axons, perineurial cell "capsule." Similar to schwannoma but more axons.	S100pr+ (Schwann cells), EMA+ (perineurial cells), NF+ (axons)
Schwannoma	Any location, nerve of origin. Encapsulated (except in GI tract, nose, bone) Cellular, plexiform, myxoid, epithelioid, and melanotic variants	Antoni A areas with palisading and Verocay bodies, Antoni B areas with spindle cells in myxoid stroma Cyst formation, thick-walled vessels, thrombi, hemosiderin	S100 protein+ diffusely, EMA+ in peripheral perineurial cells, CD34+, GFAP+, CK+ occasionally

(Continued)

TABLE 9.1 **Differential Diagnosis of Nerve Sheath Tumors (continued)**

	Typical Clinical Features	Microscopic Features	Ancillary Investigations
Schwannoma, cellular	F > M, Middle age. Paravertebral in retroperitoneum or pelvis can erode bone. Also submucosal in nose, stomach, or intestine (no capsule).	Thick capsule, subcapsular lymphoid aggregates. Fascicles of cells with eosinophilic cytoplasm, focal pleomorphism, occasional mitoses. Lacks Antoni A and B areas. Lymphocytes, clusters of foamy cells, thick-walled vessels, hemosiderin	S100 protein+ diffusely CD34 focal, GFAP focal, occasional CK+, CD117.
Ganglioneuroma	Retroperitoneum, mediastinum	Schwann cell background with ganglion cells of variable maturity	S100 protein+ in spindle cells, NSE+, CD56+, NF+ in ganglion cells.
Malignant peripheral nerve sheath tumor.	M > F. In NF1 or sporadic, axial, or in limbs. Origin in nerve or neurofibroma.	Variably cellular and myxoid, fascicular pattern. Nuclei wavy, buckled or lanceolate, with one blunt end. Palisading, neuroid whorls, vascular wall involvement, rare small collagenous "rosettes." Heterologous elements–rhabdomyosarcoma, angiosarcoma, epithelial glands	S100 protein+ (65%), occasional GFAP+, CK+ (but not usually CK7 or CK19).

NEUROMAS

Neuromas are disorderly benign proliferations of nerves, which display all the component cell types in conventional relationship to each other. This can be demonstrated by antibodies to S100 protein, EMA, and neurofilaments. The principal clinical types are traumatic neuroma, mucosal neuromas, pacinian neuroma, and palisaded encapsulated neuroma. Ganglioneuroma, considered below, is a predominantly Schwann cell neoplasm related to neuroblastoma (see Chapter 14).

TRAUMATIC NEUROMA

Clinical Features

This forms a painful or tender nodule following surgery or other trauma, and is continuous with the damaged nerve.

Pathologic Features

Microscopically traumatic neuroma is composed of normally constituted nerve bundles irregularly dispersed in scar tissue (Fig. 9.1, e-Figs. 9.5 and 9.6). The lesion is nonencapsulated and differs from neurofibroma in cellular architecture and composition and in the absence of collagen bundles and mast cells.

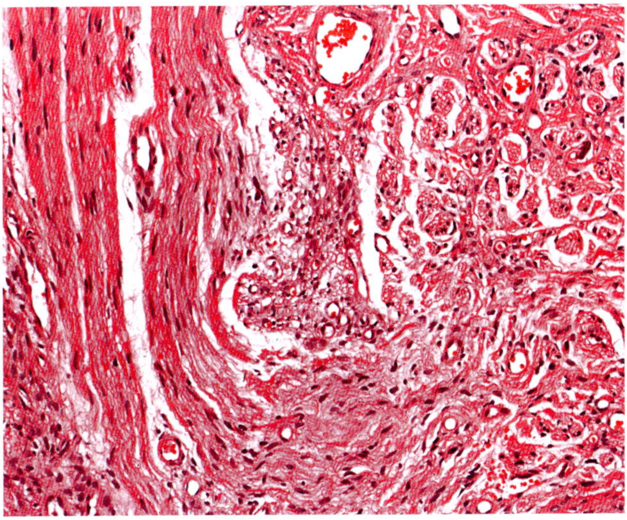

FIGURE 9.1 **Traumatic Neuroma.** Proliferating small nerve bundles in fibrous tissue are seen adjacent to and contiguous with a nerve trunk.

MUCOSAL NEUROMA

Clinical Features

Mucosal neuroma is a clinical marker for patients with multiple endocrine neoplasia (MEN) type IIB, in which medullary carcinoma of thyroid, adrenal pheochromcytoma, and parathyroid hyperplasia are associated. The neuromas occur most often in younger subjects beneath the surface epithelium of oral cavity (including inner aspect of lips), eyelids, and small and large intestine, where (in MEN type IIB) there is also increase of all neural elements in the autonomic plexuses.

Pathologic Features

Each neuroma is a noncircumscribed cluster of uniform nerve bundles (Fig. 9.2, e-Fig. 9.7), with distinct perineurium and focal myxoid change.

Ancillary Investigations

Diagnosis of this lesion should prompt further clinical assessment including measurement of the serum calcitonin.

PACINIAN NEUROFIBROMA

Clinical Features

This is a rare lesion that normally presents to the dermatologist as a tender small mass on the finger.

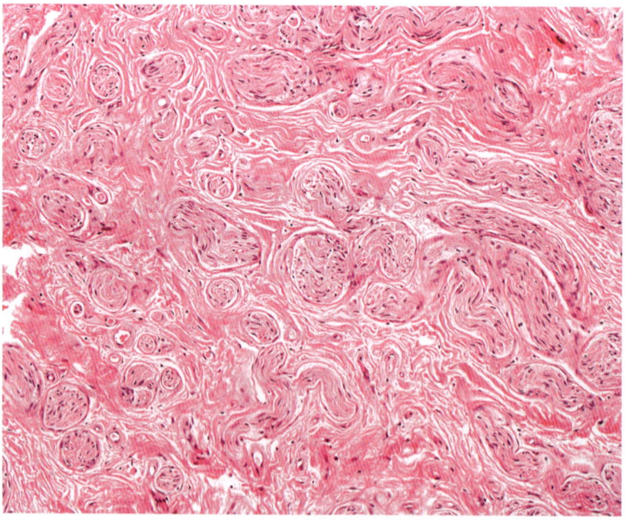

FIGURE 9.2 **Mucosal Neuroma.** Medium-sized nerve bundles are randomly orientated within connective tissue. Note prominent perineurial cell layer.

Pathologic Features

Microscopically, this is composed of several enlarged pacinian corpuscles, each of which has concentric lamellae of perineurial cells around a central axon (e-Fig. 9.8).[7]

Ancillary Investigations

The perineurial cells are EMA-positive and the central axon can be demonstrated with antibodies to neurofilament proteins.

PALISADED ENCAPSULATED NEUROMA

Clinical Features

Palisaded encapsulated neuroma (also termed solitary circumscribed neuroma) is a painless nodule 2 to 6 mm in diameter, usually on the face, in middle-aged adults.

Pathologic Features

Microscopically, this neuroma is a dermal or subcutaneous, thinly encapsulated nodule (sometimes multiple) composed of Schwann cells (rarely with nuclear palisading) associated with axons, and a perineurial outer layer that forms the "capsule" (Fig. 9.3, e-Figs. 9.9–9.12). A contiguous nerve is sometimes seen, as in schwannoma, but the axons, demonstrable by immunostaining for neurofilaments, are dispersed throughout (e-Fig. 9.12) and closely associated with the Schwann cells. Fortunately, the distinction is not clinically significant.

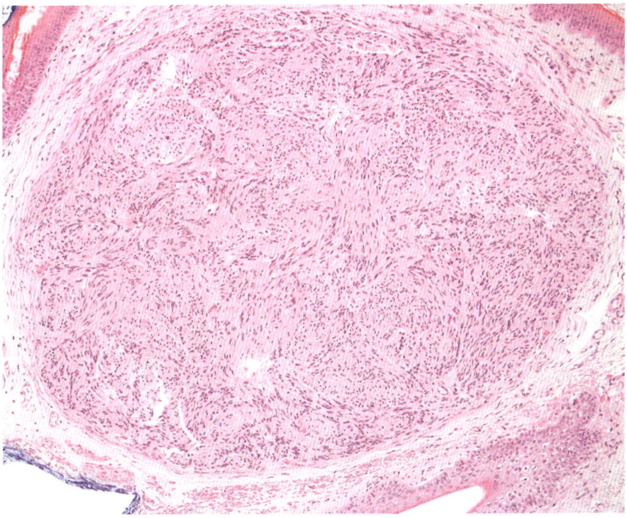

FIGURE 9.3 **Palisaded Encapsulated Neuroma.** This is a subcutaneous circumscribed lesion composed of closely packed nerve bundles.

Ancillary Investigations

The lesional cells are S100 protein–positive (e-Fig. 9.11) and EMA highlights the perineurial cells at the periphery. Electron microscopy shows mostly nonmyelinated axons only partially enveloped by Schwann cells.

Dermal nerve sheath myxoma (neurothekeoma) is considered in Chapter 20.

NEUROFIBROMA

Clinical Features

Localized neurofibroma is a sporadic lesion of young adults without neurofibromatosis, usually presenting as a cutaneous nodule, but sometimes involving a larger nerve. Malignant change in solitary localized neurofibroma is exceptionally rare. Less commonly, these lesions can be massive or multiple in patients with neurofibromatosis type 1 (NF1, von Recklinghausen neurofibromatosis), an autosomal dominant disease with variable penetrance, which is more common in males. NF-1 is additionally characterized by cutaneous café-au-lait macules, pigmented iris hamartomas (Lisch nodules), skeletal abnormalities (including intraosseous cysts), increased incidence of malignant peripheral nerve sheath and other soft tissue tumors, and an association with gastrointestinal (GI) stromal tumors, pheochromocytoma, and leukemia.[8]

Diffuse neurofibroma, which is sometimes associated with NF1, arises predominantly in the head and neck in children and young adults, and forms a plaque-like thickening within subcutis.

Plexiform neurofibromas, which occur only in NF1, arise in childhood and enlarge slowly, so that large lesions can be found in young adults. They form large tortuous masses of expanded nerves in any area, and in a limb can cause hypertrophy with laxity of overlying skin.

Pathologic Features

A typical localized neurofibroma is circumscribed or, in a larger nerve, encapsulated, with a firm white cut surface, often with myxoid areas. Microscopically, it comprises bland wavy elongated spindle cells in a variably collagenous and myxoid stroma with mast cells (Fig. 9.4, e-Figs. 9.13–9.15). The collagen fibers are wavy and form discrete bundles, which are sometimes prominent ("shredded carrot" pattern) (e-Fig. 9.13). Focal nuclear enlargement and hyperchromasia (without nucleoli) can be seen (e-Fig. 9.16), but significant mitotic activity and necrosis are absent.

Diffuse neurofibroma is an infiltrative tumor composed of uniform short slightly curved spindle cells, distributed within a finely collagenous stroma (Fig. 9.5, e-Figs. 9.16–9.18). A characteristic feature is the presence of Wagner-Meissner bodies, which are rounded, laminated eosinophilic masses with scattered cells (e-Figs. 9.19–9.22). The appearances vary somewhat according to the plane of section and the stage of development

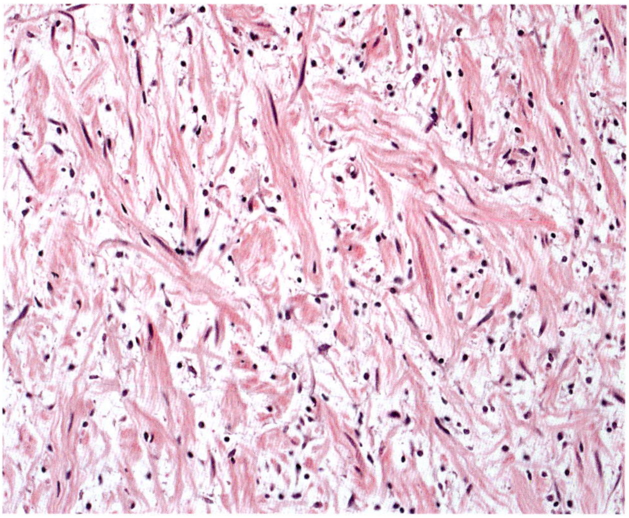

FIGURE 9.4 **Neurofibroma—Regular.** A typical neurofibroma has wavy spindle cells, some with hyperchromatic nuclei, dispersed between collagen bundles with focally myxoid stroma.

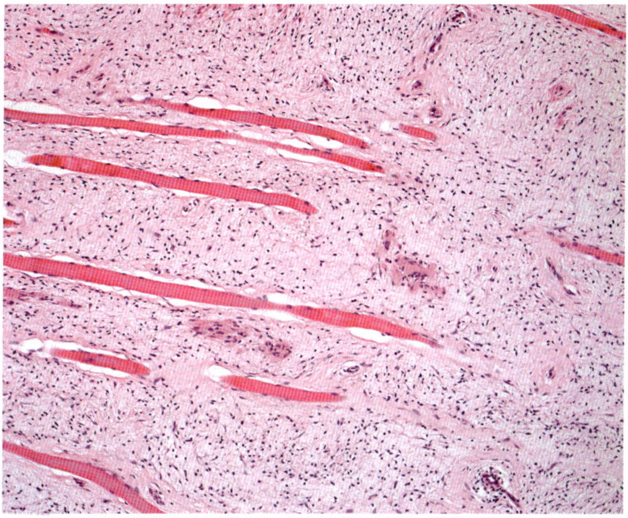

FIGURE 9.5 **Neurofibroma—Diffuse.** Loosely cellular sheets of cells with short slightly wavy nuclei infiltrate between and separate skeletal muscle bundles.

of the structure. Some diffuse neurofibromas have an angiomatous or adipose component (increased over that of the normal subcutaneous fat). The neurofibromatous tissue infiltrates the subcutis along interlobular septa, surrounds adnexa, and sometimes extends into adjacent organs such as salivary gland.

Plexiform neurofibroma comprises a bundle of expanded nerves that is continuous at either end with normal nerve. The expansion is due initially to increased myxoid stroma, with subsequent increase in cellular components, which can extend outside the nerve and resemble diffuse neurofibroma. This is considered further and illustrated in Chapter 22.

Ancillary Investigations

Many of the spindle cells in regular neurofibromas express S100 protein (e-Figs. 9.14, 9.18, and 9.22), and axons can often be demonstrated with antibodies to neurofilaments. The pattern differs from that in schwannoma as not every cell is S100 protein–positive. EMA is usually negative in the intervening spindle cells, but CD34 is focally positive. Diffuse neurofibroma is composed purely of Schwann cells and is diffusely S100 protein–positive (e-Fig. 9.18), as are the Wagner-Meissner bodies (e-Fig. 9.22). Ultrastructurally, regular neurofibromas comprise a mixture of Schwann cells (some associated with axons) and fibroblast-like cells that display rough endoplasmic reticulum and no external lamina. NF1 is characterized genetically by abnormalities in the *NF1* gene, a tumor suppressor gene located on chromosome 17. This encodes the protein neurofibromin which is expressed in neural tissues and has a role in cell growth and differentiation.[9]

CRITERIA OF MALIGNANCY IN NEUROFIBROMA WITH ATYPICAL NUCLEI

Neurofibromas can have degenerate nuclear atypia, with irregularly shaped, bizarre, or multinucleated cells, which is not by itself an indicator of malignancy. Although published criteria vary,[10,11] tumors with marked hypercellularity with "back to back" cells, and diffuse atypia (with or without mitotic activity) should be regarded as low-grade MPNST (e-Fig. 9.23).[11] A lesion with increased cellularity and an occasional mitosis but lacking diffuse atypia can be termed cellular neurofibroma or neurofibroma with atypical features.[12] In the absence of other criteria, minimum mitotic counts for malignancy have not been defined, but neurofibromas with more than 1 mitosis in 10 hpf should be regarded as suspicious.[12] In reality, malignant change in neurofibroma, and especially in plexiform neurofibroma, is often a gradual process, with variable cellularity in different parts of the lesion. It can therefore be difficult, particularly in a core biopsy, to define the precise point at which a lesion should be designated as malignant, and the pathologist's report should indicate that the findings might not be representative and must be interpreted in the clinical context.

VARIANTS

Pigmented neurofibroma occurs in patients with NF1 and is a diffuse or occasionally plexiform neurofibroma with foci of dendritic or epithelioid melanocytes which can involve dermis, subcutis, or skeletal muscle

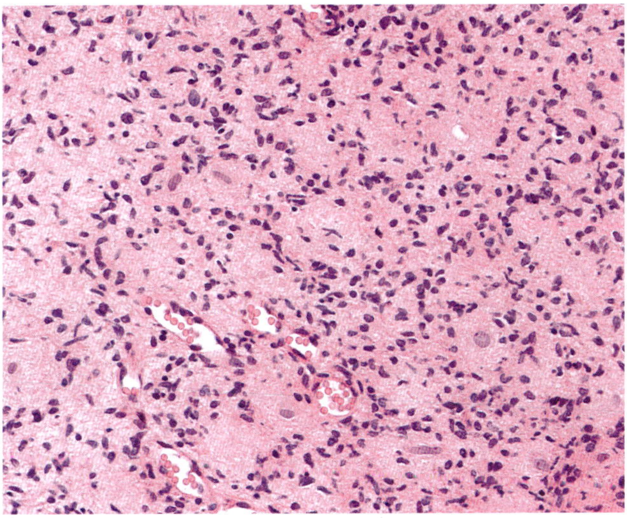

FIGURE 9.6 **Dendritic Cell Neurofibroma.** Small darkly staining cells surround fibrillary rosette-like structures with scattered larger nuclei.

(e-Fig. 9.24).[13] There is immunoreactivity for both S100 protein and melanocytic markers.

Epithelioid neurofibroma is a rare variant (see chapter 22).

Dendritic cell neurofibroma with pseudorosettes is a rare variant of cutaneous neurofibroma in which small darkly staining lymphocyte-like cells surround larger, pale-staining cells in a rosette-like fashion (Fig. 9.6, e-Figs. 9.25 and 9.26).[14] The lesional cells are S100 protein–positive with a peripheral rim of EMA-positive perineurial cells.

PERINEURIOMA

Clinical Features

Perineurioma is a benign tumor of perineurial cells, which arises most often in skin or subcutis in male or female adults, in almost any location, as a circumscribed painless mass with a mean diameter of about 4 cm but occasionally reaching a large size.[15] Perineurioma differs from neurofibroma in being composed of one cell type, although hybrid examples with features of both occasionally occur.[16] Perineuriomas rarely recur and have not been reported to metastasize regardless of atypical histologic features. Malignant perineurial cell tumor with overtly sarcomatous features is considered as a variant of MPNST. The differential diagnosis of perineurioma in the head and neck can include ectopic meningioma, which also has a whorled architecture and can be positive for EMA and claudin-1. However, this usually occurs in a highly specific setting in the nasal region in soft tissue or bone[17] (and very rarely in lung or mediastinum[18]). Similar considerations apply to heterotopic glial tissue and soft tissue ependymoma.

Pathologic Features

Soft tissue perineurioma is a mostly circumscribed but occasionally infiltrative solid tumor with a mean diameter of 4 cm (though some tumors reach 20 cm), which can occasionally ossify. A nerve of origin is not usually evident. Microscopically, perineurioma is a variably cellular tumor composed of elongated cells with slender nuclei and long, bipolar cytoplasmic processes, arranged in streaming fascicles, sometimes with storiform architecture and meningothelial-like perivascular whorls (Fig. 9.7, e-Figs. 9.27–9.30). The stroma is usually collagenous, but there can be focal or predominant myxoid change. Some cases have focal nuclear atypia, mitotic activity, or infiltrative margins, but these features appear to have no prognostic significance. Plexiform architecture is seen in rare examples.[19]

Ancillary Investigations

Electron microscopy shows characteristic slender elongated cell processes with focal pinocytotic vesicles and continuous external lamina, which can be revealed by immunostaining for collagen type IV, and to a lesser extent laminin. Immunohistochemistry shows positivity for EMA (e-Fig. 9.31) but usually only focally, and about two thirds of cases express CD34 (e-Fig. 9.32). Claudin-1 (e-Fig. 9.33) and GLUT1 are additional markers of perineurial cell differentiation. Very occasional tumors also display focal

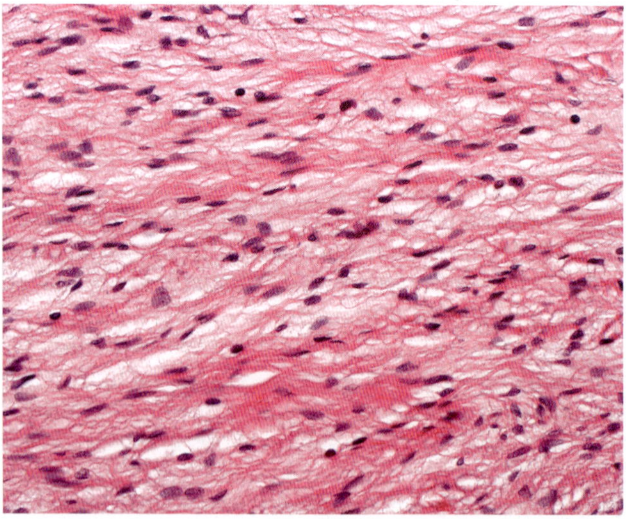

FIGURE 9.7 **Perineurioma.** Elongated spindle cells with slender, slightly wavy nuclei and terminal cytoplasmic processes are dispersed in a fibrous stroma.

positivity for SMA or S100 protein, some of the latter perhaps representing hybrid nerve sheath tumors. Abnormalities in chromosome 22, including mutations in the NF2 tumor suppression gene, have been described in perineurial cell tumors, which rarely occur in neurofibromatosis type 2.[20] Some perineuriomas, especially in the skin, can resemble low-grade fibromyxoid sarcoma which can also express EMA and claudin-1.[21] The latter, however, has a diagnostic translocation t(7;16)(q34;p11).

VARIANTS

Intraneural perineurioma is a benign condition that causes a fusiform expansion of a nerve, over a length of several centimeters, in children or young adults.[22] It shows increased nerve fascicles surrounded by "onion-bulb"-like concentric layers of EMA-positive perineurial cells (Fig. 9.8, e-Figs. 9.34 and 9.35). Clonal abnormalities of chromosome 22 have been reported,[23,24] indicating a neoplastic rather than reactive nature. The term localized hypertrophic neuropathy has been used synonymously but possibly represents a separate entity, characterized by Schwann cell proliferation.

Sclerosing perineurioma is a benign tumor found in the hands (fingers, thumb, palm) in young adults aged 20 to 40 years and more commonly in males.[25] It is a slowly growing, circumscribed, firm dermal or subcutaneous nodule that rarely exceeds 2 cm in diameter. Reported examples have not recurred. The lesional cells are rounded or epithelioid,

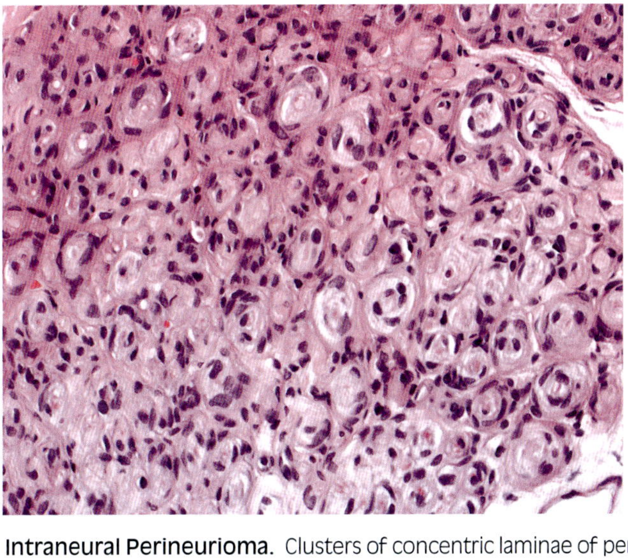

FIGURE 9.8 **Intraneural Perineurioma.** Clusters of concentric laminae of perineurial cells around axons are characteristic of this lesion (from a slide courtesy of Prof T Revesz).

and are arranged in cords, files, or perivascular whorls, in a collagenous stroma (e-Figs. 9.36–9.38). The cells are uniform, and mitotic activity is minimal. Electron microscopy confirms perineurial differentiation. Immunohistochemistry is positive for EMA (e-Fig. 9.38), GLUT1, and collagen IV, with occasional expression of actins or cytokeratin. Genetically, there are abnormalities of 10q, and NF2 deletions, similar to usual-type perineurioma.[24,26]

Reticular perineurioma is a rare variant that occurs mostly in adult females (median age: 43 years), and has a predilection for the arm and hand.[19] The tumors, located in subcutaneous tissue, range between 1.5 and 10 cm in diameter, are not associated with nerves, although a focally retiform intraneural perineurioma has been reported.[27] They are usually circumscribed and show perineurial cells arranged in a predominantly laciform or reticular growth pattern (Fig. 9.9, e-Figs. 9.39 and 9.40) within a collagenous or focally myxoid stroma, sometimes with cyst formation. Multinucleated cells are occasionally seen, but mitoses are absent. The reported examples all showed diffuse immunoreactivity for EMA.

Intestinal perineuriomas are a subset of perineuriomas that occur predominantly in females and are mostly found incidentally at colonoscopy.[28] They are mostly polypoid intramucosal or occasionally submucosal tumors of colon or rarely jejunum which are circumscribed or occasionally infiltrative, with a collagenous or myxoid stroma (e-Figs. 9.41 and 9.42). Tumors termed polypoid fibroblastic polyps of the colon that are reactive to perineurial cell markers are in fact perineuriomas.[29]

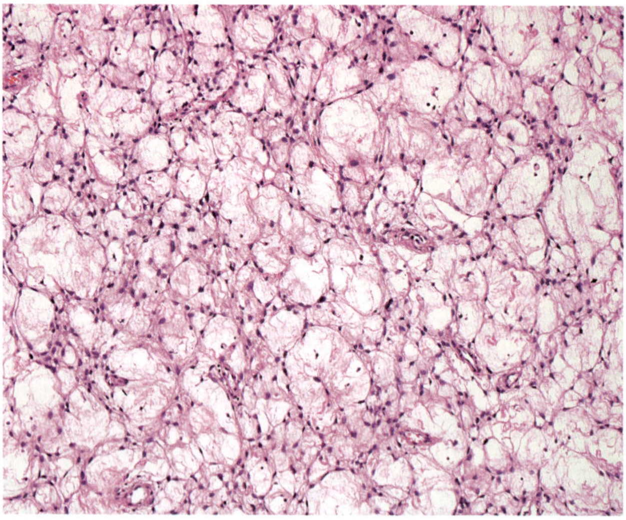

FIGURE 9.9 **Reticular Perineurioma.** Anastomosing cords of long slender spindle cells are arranged in a myxoid stroma.

SCHWANNOMA

Clinical Features

This is a benign neoplasm of Schwann cells that usually arises sporadically in superficial or deep locations as a slowly growing, well-defined tumor. Schwannomas can present as a mass, with symptoms related to neural compression, or be found incidentally. They occur most commonly in adults up to 50 years of age, and arise in cranial, spinal, peripheral, or autonomic nerves especially in the head and neck and limbs, but also in retroperitoneum, posterior mediastinum (sometimes as a dumbbell mass that is partially located within the spinal canal), and GI sites.[30,31] Multiple schwannomas, including bilateral acoustic nerve lesions, are a feature of neurofibromatosis type 2 (NF2). This is an autosomal dominant condition that manifests in childhood and adolescence, in association with multiple meningiomas (sometimes also a feature of NF2, as are other central nervous system tumors including ependymomas and gliomas), and in schwannomatosis.[8] The latter is rarely familial, is distinct from NF2, and has been proposed as a third type of neurofibromatosis.[8] It is characterized by multiple painful lesions. Usual-type schwannomas, unlike cellular schwannomas, do not recur after excision, and malignant change is extremely rare.

Pathologic Features

Schwannomas typically have a fibrous capsule, sometimes with peripheral lymphoid aggregates (Fig. 9.10). This is usually lacking in the GI tract (e-Fig. 9.43) and sinonasal area (e-Fig. 9.44), where the infiltrative and locally erosive margin and hypercellularity can lead to overdiagnosis of malignancy.[32] A nerve of origin is sometimes seen attached to the tumor.

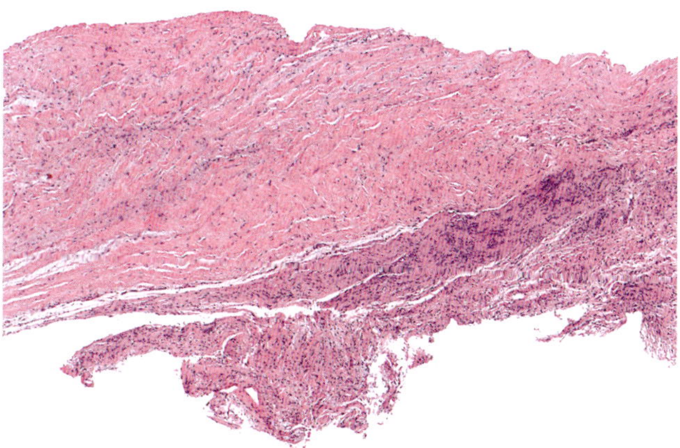

FIGURE 9.10 **Schwannoma.** This core biopsy has sampled the thick capsule with a fragment of attached schwannomatous tissue in lower part of field showing Antoni A pattern with discernible nuclear palisading.

The size varies, with deeply seated lesions sometimes growing to 20 cm in diameter before causing symptoms. The cut surface is moderately firm or soft and pale (e-Fig. 9.44), and can show myxoid or cystic areas (e-Fig. 9.45–9.47), old or fresh hemorrhage, or calcification. The lesions are composed of short wavy spindle cells with darkly staining nuclei, with two predominant patterns (e-Fig. 9.48) in varying proportion. In Antoni A areas, the cells are arranged in palisades, with two files of nuclei enclosing foci of eosinophilic fibrillary or amorphous material that represent Schwann cell processes and external lamina (Verocay bodies) (Fig. 9.11, e-Figs. 9.49 and 9.50). Antoni B areas have spindle or rounded cells within a stroma which is myxoid, contains fine collagen fibers and inflammatory cells, or is hyalinized (e-Fig. 9.51). These areas are more difficult to recognize as schwannoma, but diagnostic clues include the waviness of the cells, and the presence of clusters of dilated vessels with hyalinized walls, containing thrombi with associated xanthoma cells and siderophages (e-Figs. 9.52 and 9.53). Antoni A architecture can sometimes be revealed by cutting further into the block. In the GI tract, schwannoma can occur in the submucosa, especially in the stomach, or in muscularis propria (e-Fig. 9.42). The tumors are circumscribed but the capsule is lacking; however, the cells are often arranged in cords or trabeculae (e-Fig. 9.54) and the peripheral lymphoid cuff, sometimes with adjacent fibrosis, remains as a useful diagnostic feature.

Ancillary Investigations

Schwannomas are diffusely immunoreactive for S100 protein in nuclei and cytoplasm (e-Fig. 9.55), and many express glial fibrillary acidic protein (GFAP) (e-Fig. 9.56) and CD34. Cytokeratin positivity is also seen

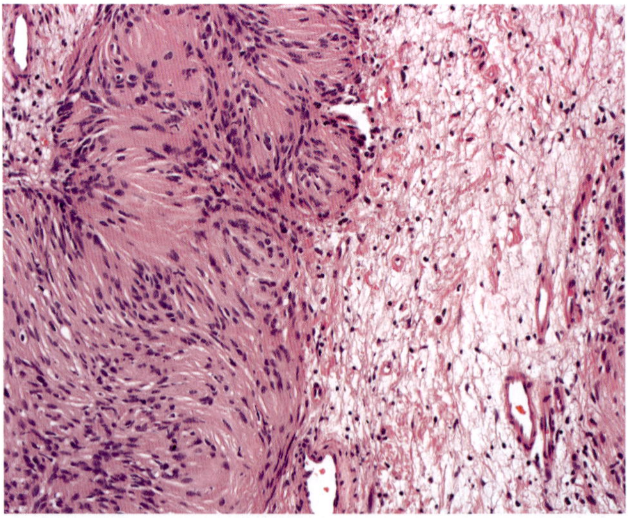

FIGURE 9.11 **Schwannoma.** Typical Antoni A area with Verocay bodies is present (left) adjacent to Antoni B area (right).

focally in some cases, including those in retroperitoneum (e-Fig.9.56A). A peripheral rim of perineurial cells is immunoreactive for EMA (e-Fig. 9.57), and immunostaining for neurofilaments reveals axons in 55% of conventional schwannomas and 75% of cellular schwannomas.[33]

In NF-2, there are germline inactivating mutations in the *NF2* gene on chromosome 22, which encodes the protein schwannomin (merlin), an inhibitor of cell proliferation and cell cycle progression by repressing cyclin D1 expression.[34] Schwannomatosis, however, is associated with abnormalities in a different gene located on chromosome 22 proximal to the *NF2* gene,[35] although nonactivating mutations in the *NF2* gene have also been found in schwannomatosis.[36] GI schwannomas usually have *NF1* rather than *NF2* mutations, and in this respect are more like neurofibromas.[37]

Criteria of Malignancy

A common finding is so-called degenerative or ancient change, with spindle cells displaying larger hyperchromatic nuclei containing pseudoinclusions but no nucleoli (e-Fig. 9.58). This is often associated with hemorrhage, cyst formation, and calcification, and should not be misinterpreted: when the lesion is clearly encapsulated and displays diffuse immunoreactivity for S100 protein the presence of focal pleomorphism, mitoses, and even necrosis does not usually indicate malignancy. Such findings are more difficult to assess in a core biopsy which does not include the capsule, but (a) in spindle cell MPNST immunoreactivity for S100 protein is usually focal rather than diffuse, and (b) malignant change in schwannoma is exceptionally rare and usually takes the form of epithelioid MPNST.[38] Observation of plump enlarged epithelioid cells with prominent nucleoli in an otherwise typical schwannoma suggests early malignant change.[39] Angiosarcoma arising in schwannoma has also been reported[40] and usually has an epithelioid component.[41]

VARIANTS

Cellular schwannoma mostly arises in deep soft tissue. Distinct clinicopathologic settings are on spinal nerve roots, in the presacral space, and in the retroperitoneum and mediastinum, when erosion of adjacent vertebrae can be identified on imaging.[42] This tumor can recur, especially if incompletely excised, but does not metastasize. Cellular schwannoma has a thick fibrous capsule, with subcapsular lymphoid aggregates (e-Figs. 9.59–9.63), and is composed of short or herringbone fascicles of elongated cells with eosinophilic cytoplasm and generally uniform tapered nuclei, resembling the Antoni A pattern but lacking typical Verocay bodies (Fig. 9.12, e-Fig. 9.64). These appearances are distinctive in core biopsies although demonstration of S100 protein positivity can sometimes be required to be certain that one is not dealing with a smooth muscle tumor. Additional features include clusters of foamy macrophages (Fig. 9.13, e-Fig. 9.65), scattered lymphocytes and thick walled vessels. Mitotic activity and necrosis can be seen but do not indicate malignancy if the lesion is encapsulated,

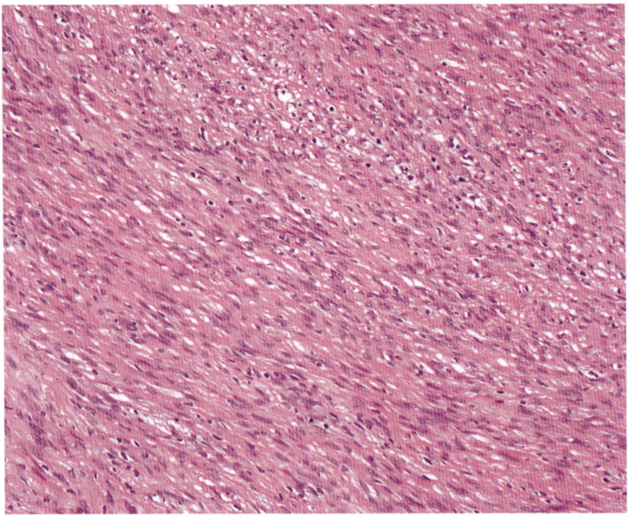

FIGURE 9.12 **Cellular Schwannoma.** Spindle cells with eosinophilic cytoplasm are arranged in a well-defined fascicular pattern. The nuclei are relatively plump but have pointed rather than blunt ends. Note the patchy infiltrate of lymphocytes and mast cells.

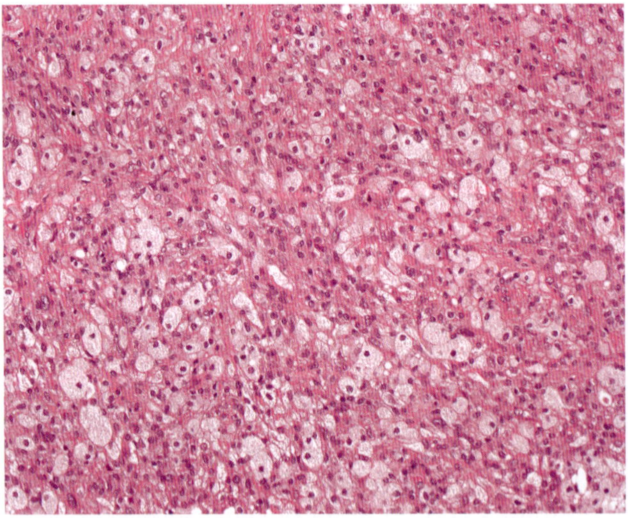

FIGURE 9.13 **Cellular Schwannoma.** Foamy macrophages, dispersed singly and in clusters or sheets, are frequently seen in this tumor.

lacks frank anaplasia, and shows diffuse strong positivity for S100 protein (e-Fig. 9.66) (a particularly useful finding in core specimens).

Melanotic (pigmented) schwannoma is associated with Carney complex (but not with the neurofibromatoses) that includes cardiac and

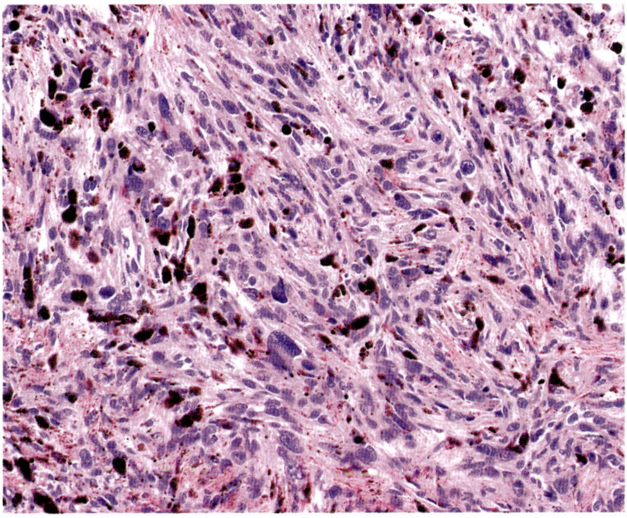

FIGURE 9.14 **Melanotic Schwannoma.** This is a cellular tumor with focal nuclear hyperchromasia, and variable amounts of melanin pigmentation in coarse granules within tumor cells.

cutaneous myxomas, dermal pigmented lesions, and adrenal and pituitary hyperactivity and neoplasia.[43,44] These tumors can recur locally and metastasize, sometimes after a long interval. Melanotic schwannomas can be multiple and commonly involve spinal nerve roots or autonomic nerves but also occur in superficial or deep soft tissue around the midline, and in viscera. The tumor is usually heavily pigmented and often appears dark brown or black. Microscopically, there is both schwannian and melanocytic differentiation with fascicles or whorls of epithelioid or short spindle cells containing variable amounts of melanin pigment (Fig. 9.14, e-Figs. 9.67–9.69). This is reflected at ultrastructural level where there are features of Schwann cells (intertwining cytoplasmic processes with continuous external lamina containing melanosomes at varying stages of formation), and by immunohistochemistry, since the tumor cells express both S100 protein and melanocytic antigens such as HMB45. Occasional psammoma bodies are seen in many cases (Fig. 9.15, e-Fig. 9.70), allowing the alternative designation of psammomatous melanotic schwannoma. There can also be a component of differentiated fat. Metastasis can occur in cases without significant atypia, but those with frequent mitoses should be regarded as potentially malignant. The presence of marked nuclear atypia with nucleoli, or necrosis also raises concern about malignant potential, and additionally makes it difficult to exclude metastatic melanoma. In the usual case, the lack of marked or widespread atypia and mitoses as well as the presence of psammoma bodies can aid this distinction.

Schwannoma with epithelial elements (benign glands) is extremely rare. In some cases involving the dermis or subcutis, the glandular structures

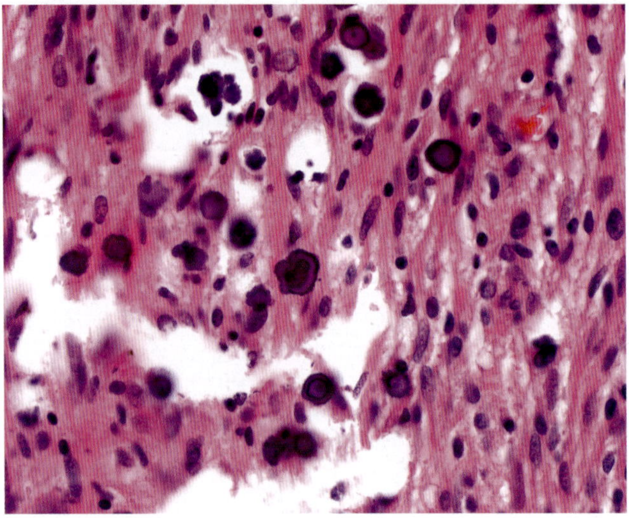

FIGURE 9.15 **Psammomatous Schwannoma.** Psammoma bodies can be very sparse or focally abundant as in this example.

might represent entrapped adnexa.[45] The cysts are usually solitary and lined by a single layer of columnar or cuboidal epithelium. Pseudoglandular schwannoma is a schwannoma with microcystic spaces that are lined by Schwann cells rather than epithelium (e-Fig. 9.71); Immunostaining is positive for S100 protein (e-Fig. 9.72) and negative for cytokeratins.

Epithelioid and plexiform variants of schwannoma are described in chapters 11 and 22, respectively.

Neuroblastoma-like schwannoma (neurilemmoma) is a rare lesion that presents as a small, firm nodule in the subcutis in limbs, trunk, or head and neck.[46] It is a benign schwannoma composed mainly of small rounded cells with darkly staining rounded nuclei and little cytoplasm. The distinctive feature is the presence of collagenous "giant rosettes," surrounded by more rounded cells, giving a vaguely resemblance to neural rosettes, in a background of epithelioid or spindled Schwann cells that are S100 protein–positive (Fig. 9.16, e-Figs. 9.73 and 9.74). Hyaline rosettes are also seen in regular schwannomas on occasion, and must not be confused with the giant rosettes of low-grade fibromyxoid sarcoma which, apart from its other morphologic features, lacks immunoreactivity for S100 protein.

Ganglioneuroma is the differentiated form of neuroblastoma (Chapter 14). It occurs in mediastinum or retroperitoneum and morphologically resembles neurofibroma with variable numbers of ganglion cells (e-Figs. 9.75 and 9.76). These are immunoreactive for CD56, neuron-specific enolase (NSE), and chromogranin and negative for S100 protein. **Ganglioneuromatosis** is a rare condition of the colon or small intestine that is associated with MEN syndrome, type IIb. Its occurrence in neurofibromatosis, in which the large intestine is usually affected, is much rarer. It

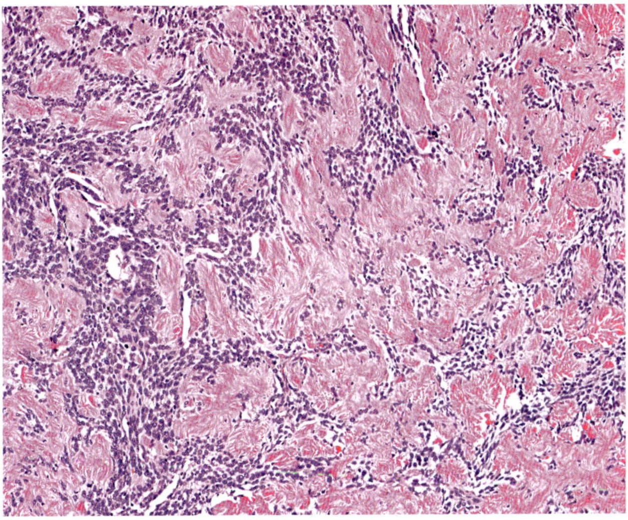

FIGURE 9.16 **Neuroblastoma-like Neurilemmoma.** Small darkly staining Schwann cells are arranged around eosinophilic fibrillary structures resembling rosettes.

is characterized by increased numbers of ganglion cells and Schwann cells within the mucosa and submucosa of the bowel (e-Fig. 9.77).[47]

HYBRID BENIGN PERIPHERAL NERVE SHEATH TUMORS

It can on occasion be difficult to decide whether a nerve sheath tumor is a neurofibroma or a schwannoma and hybrid forms with features of both have been described.[48] Immunohistochemistry might be contributory in that S100 protein is less widespread in neurofibroma, and calretinin[49] and GFAP are reportedly positive in schwannoma and negative in neurofibroma. Conversely, neurofibroma is often immunoreactive for CD57, which is usually lacking in schwannoma. Schwannoma and neurofibroma have also been described in combination, with the components being discrete (e-Fig. 9.78)[50] or intermingled (e-Figs. 9.79 and 9.80),[51] as demonstrated by immunostaining for both S100 protein and EMA (e-Figs. 9.81 and 9.82). The latter are noncircumscribed dermal or cutaneous lesions which can show nuclear atypia.

Lipoblastic nerve sheath tumors are benign nerve sheath tumors (usually schwannoma, but occasionally neurofibroma) with scattered signet-ring lipoblast-like cells (e-Figs. 9.83 and 9.84).[52] This feature is of no behavioral significance.

REFERENCES

1. Fanburg-Smith JC, Majidi M, Miettinen M. Keratin expression in schwannoma; a study of 115 retroperitoneal and 22 peripheral schwannomas. *Mod Pathol.* 2006;19:115–121.
2. Erlandson RA. The enigmatic perineurial cell and its participation in tumors and in tumorlike entities. *Ultrastruct Pathol.* 1991;15:335–351.

3. Perentes E, Nakagawa Y, Ross GW, et al. Expression of epithelial membrane antigen in perineurial cells and their derivatives. An immunohistochemical study with multiple markers. *Acta Neuropathol.* 1987;75:160–165.
4. Folpe AL, Billings SD, McKenney JK, et al. Expression of claudin-1, a recently described tight junction-associated protein, distinguishes soft tissue perineurioma from potential mimics. *Am J Surg Pathol.* 2002;26:1620–1626.
5. Hirose T, Tani T, Shimada T, et al. Immunohistochemical demonstration of EMA/Glut1-positive perineurial cells and CD34-positive fibroblastic cells in peripheral nerve sheath tumors. *Mod Pathol.* 2003;16:293–298.
6. Weiss SW, Nickoloff BJ. CD-34 is expressed by a distinctive cell population in peripheral nerve, nerve sheath tumors, and related lesions. *Am J Surg Pathol.* 1993;17:1039–1045.
7. Burgues O, Monteagudo C, Noguera R, et al. Cutaneous sclerosing Pacinian-like perineurioma. *Histopathology.* 2001;39:498–502.
8. McClatchey AI. Neurofibromatosis. *Annu Rev Pathol.* 2007;2:191–216.
9. Theos A, Korf BR. Pathophysiology of neurofibromatosis type 1. *Ann Intern Med.* 2006;144:842–849.
10. Scheithauer BW, Woodruff JM, Erlandson RA. *Tumors of the Peripheral Nervous System.* Washington, DC: American Registry of Pathology, 1999.
11. Weiss SW, Goldblum JR. Benign tumors of peripheral nerves. *Soft Tissue Tumors.* Philadelphia, PA: Mosby Elsevier, 2008;825–901.
12. Lin BT, Weiss LM, Medeiros LJ. Neurofibroma and cellular neurofibroma with atypia: a report of 14 tumors. *Am J Surg Pathol.* 1997;21:1443–1449.
13. Fetsch JF, Michal M, Miettinen M. Pigmented (melanotic) neurofibroma: a clinicopathologic and immunohistochemical analysis of 19 lesions from 17 patients. *Am J Surg Pathol.* 2000;24:331–343.
14. Michal M, Fanburg-Smith JC, Mentzel T, et al. Dendritic cell neurofibroma with pseudorosettes: a report of 18 cases of a distinct and hitherto unrecognized neurofibroma variant. *Am J Surg Pathol.* 2001;25:587–594.
15. Hornick JL, Fletcher CD. Soft tissue perineurioma: clinicopathologic analysis of 81 cases including those with atypical histologic features. *Am J Surg Pathol.* 2005;29:845–858.
16. Kazakov DV, Pitha J, Sima R, et al. Hybrid peripheral nerve sheath tumors: Schwannoma-perineurioma and neurofibroma-perineurioma. A report of three cases in extradigital locations. *Ann Diagn Pathol.* 2005;9:16–23.
17. Cummings TJ, George TM, Fuchs HE, et al. The pathology of extracranial scalp and skull masses in young children. *Clin Neuropathol.* 2004;23:34–43.
18. Falleni M, Roz E, Dessy E, et al. Primary intrathoracic meningioma: histopathological, immunohistochemical and ultrastructural study of two cases. *Virchows Arch.* 2001;439:196–200.
19. Mentzel T, Kutzner H. Reticular and plexiform perineurioma: clinicopathological and immunohistochemical analysis of two cases and review of perineurial neoplasms of skin and soft tissues. *Virchows Arch.* 2005;447:677–682.
20. Pitchford CW, Schwartz HS, Atkinson JB, et al. Soft tissue perineurioma in a patient with neurofibromatosis type 2: a tumor not previously associated with the NF2 syndrome. *Am J Surg Pathol.* 2006;30:1624–1629.
21. Thway K, Fisher C, Debiec-Rychter M, et al. Claudin-1 is expressed in perineurioma-like low-grade fibromyxoid sarcoma. *Hum Pathol.* 2009;40:1586–1590.
22. Boyanton BL Jr, Jones JK, Shenaq SM, et al. Intraneural perineurioma: a systematic review with illustrative cases. *Arch Pathol Lab Med.* 2007;131:1382–1392.
23. Emory TS, Scheithauer BW, Hirose T, et al. Intraneural perineurioma. A clonal neoplasm associated with abnormalities of chromosome 22. *Am J Clin Pathol.* 1995;103:696–704.

24. Brock JE, Perez-Atayde AR, Kozakewich HP, et al. Cytogenetic aberrations in perineurioma: variation with subtype. *Am J Surg Pathol.* 2005;29:1164–1169.
25. Fetsch JF, Miettinen M. Sclerosing perineurioma: a clinicopathologic study of 19 cases of a distinctive soft tissue lesion with a predilection for the fingers and palms of young adults. *Am J Surg Pathol.* 1997;21:1433–1442.
26. Sciot R, Cin PD, Hagemeijer A, et al. Cutaneous sclerosing perineurioma with cryptic NF2 gene deletion. *Am J Surg Pathol.* 1999;23:849–853.
27. de La Jarte-Thirouard AS, Jacquier I, de Saint-Maur PP. Intraneural reticular perineurioma of the neck. *Ann Diagn Pathol.* 2003;7:120–123.
28. Hornick JL, Fletcher CD. Intestinal perineuriomas: clinicopathologic definition of a new anatomic subset in a series of 10 cases. *Am J Surg Pathol.* 2005;29:859–865.
29. Groisman GM, Polak-Charcon S. Fibroblastic polyp of the colon and colonic perineurioma: 2 names for a single entity? *Am J Surg Pathol.* 2008;32:1088–1094.
30. Daimaru Y, Kido H, Hashimoto H, et al. Benign schwannoma of the gastrointestinal tract: a clinicopathologic and immunohistochemical study. *Hum Pathol.* 1988;19:257–264.
31. Miettinen M, Shekitka KM, Sobin LH. Schwannomas in the colon and rectum: a clinicopathologic and immunohistochemical study of 20 cases. *Am J Surg Pathol.* 2001;25:846–855.
32. Hasegawa SL, Mentzel T, Fletcher CD. Schwannomas of the sinonasal tract and nasopharynx. *Mod Pathol.* 1997;10:777–784.
33. Nascimento AF, Fletcher CD. The controversial nosology of benign nerve sheath tumors: neurofilament protein staining demonstrates intratumoral axons in many sporadic schwannomas. *Am J Surg Pathol.* 2007;31:1363–1370.
34. Xiao GH, Gallagher R, Shetler J, et al. The NF2 tumor suppressor gene product, merlin, inhibits cell proliferation and cell cycle progression by repressing cyclin D1 expression. *Mol Cell Biol.* 2005;25:2384–2394.
35. MacCollin M, Willett C, Heinrich B, et al. Familial schwannomatosis: exclusion of the NF2 locus as the germline event. *Neurology.* 2003;60:1968–1974.
36. Jacoby LB, Jones D, Davis K, et al. Molecular analysis of the NF2 tumor-suppressor gene in schwannomatosis. *Am J Hum Genet.* 1997;61:1293–1302.
37. Lasota J, Wasag B, Dansonka-Mieszkowska A, et al. Evaluation of NF2 and NF1 tumor suppressor genes in distinctive gastrointestinal nerve sheath tumors traditionally diagnosed as benign schwannomas: s study of 20 cases. *Lab Invest.* 2003;83:1361–1371.
38. Woodruff JM, Selig AM, Crowley K, et al. Schwannoma (neurilemoma) with malignant transformation. A rare, distinctive peripheral nerve tumor. *Am J Surg Pathol.* 1994;18:882–895.
39. McMenamin ME, Fletcher CD. Expanding the spectrum of malignant change in schwannomas: epithelioid malignant change, epithelioid malignant peripheral nerve sheath tumor, and epithelioid angiosarcoma: a study of 17 cases. *Am J Surg Pathol.* 2001;25:13–25.
40. Ruckert RI, Fleige B, Rogalla P, et al. Schwannoma with angiosarcoma. Report of a case and comparison with other types of nerve tumors with angiosarcoma. *Cancer.* 2000;89:1577–1585.
41. Lee FY, Wen MC, Wang J. Epithelioid angiosarcoma arising in a deep-seated plexiform schwannoma: a case report and literature review. *Hum Pathol.* 2007;38:1096–1101.
42. White W, Shiu MH, Rosenblum MK, et al. Cellular schwannoma. A clinicopathologic study of 57 patients and 58 tumors. *Cancer.* 1990;66:1266–1275.
43. Carney JA. Psammomatous melanotic schwannoma. A distinctive, heritable tumor with special associations, including cardiac myxoma and the Cushing syndrome. *Am J Surg Pathol.* 1990;14:206–222.

44. Carney JA. The Carney complex (myxomas, spotty pigmentation, endocrine overactivity, and schwannomas). *Dermatol Clin.* 1995;13:19–26.
45. Woodruff JM, Christensen WN. Glandular peripheral nerve sheath tumors [see comments]. *Cancer.* 1993;72:3618–3628.
46. Goldblum JR, Beals TF, Weiss SW. Neuroblastoma-like neurilemoma. *Am J Surg Pathol.* 1994;18:266–273.
47. Thway K, Fisher C. Diffuse ganglioneuromatosis in small intestine associated with neurofibromatosis type 1. *Ann Diagn Pathol.* 2009;13:50–54.
48. Feany MB, Anthony DC, Fletcher CD. Nerve sheath tumours with hybrid features of neurofibroma and schwannoma: a conceptual challenge. *Histopathology.* 1998;32:405–410.
49. Fine SW, McClain SA, Li M. Immunohistochemical staining for calretinin is useful for differentiating schwannomas from neurofibromas. *Am J Clin Pathol.* 2004;122:552–559.
50. Michal M, Kazakov DV, Belousova I, et al. A benign neoplasm with histopathological features of both schwannoma and retiform perineurioma (benign schwannoma-perineurioma): a report of six cases of a distinctive soft tissue tumor with a predilection for the fingers. *Virchows Arch.* 2004;445:347–353.
51. Hornick JL, Bundock EA, Fletcher CD. Hybrid schwannoma/perineurioma: clinicopathologic analysis of 42 distinctive benign nerve sheath tumors. *Am J Surg Pathol.* 2009;33:1554–1561.
52. Plaza JA, Wakely PE Jr, Suster S. Lipoblastic nerve sheath tumors: report of a distinctive variant of neural soft tissue neoplasm with adipocytic differentiation. *Am J Surg Pathol.* 2006;30:337–344.

10

SPINDLE CELL SARCOMAS

INTRODUCTION

Spindle cell sarcomas are a large group of tumors that can occur in many different locations and have morphologic similarities. They can usually be distinguished by the clinical setting and morphologic clues, notably the low-power patterns and nuclear features (Table 10.1), as well as the use of immunohistochemistry and molecular diagnostic techniques. Sarcomas that are encountered most frequently within the abdomen (e.g., inflammatory myofibroblastic tumor, gastrointestinal stromal tumor, dedifferentiated liposarcoma, follicular dendritic cell sarcoma) are presented in Chapter 5, tumors with smooth muscle differentiation in Chapter 6, and predominantly myxoid sarcomas (e.g., low-grade myxofibrosarcoma, myxoinflammatory fibroblastic sarcoma, extraskeletal myxoid chondrosarcoma) in Chapter 21. Some of the entities included in this chapter are additionally discussed in other chapters. It should also be remembered that spindle cell carcinoma, especially in relation to epithelial structures and viscera, can mimic sarcomas, and similar considerations apply to melanoma and some types of lymphoma. The differential diagnosis is summarized in Tables 10.2 and 10.3.

MALIGNANT PERIPHERAL NERVE SHEATH TUMOR

Clinical Features

Malignant peripheral nerve sheath tumor (MPNST) can show differentiation toward one of the cell types of the nerve sheath, although such differentiation is usually incomplete. It represents about 6% of adult soft tissue sarcomas and a smaller proportion in childhood. MPNST can arise sporadically, following irradiation, or in patients with neurofibromatosis type 1 (NF-1). The incidence of malignant change in NF-1 is about 4.6%, and individual patients have at least a 10% lifetime risk of developing a malignant neoplasm.[1] The tumors mostly originate in neurofibromas (especially the plexiform type) or in a nerve trunk in proximal extremities, trunk, head and neck region, mediastinum, or retroperitoneum. They

TABLE 10.1 **Nuclear Features of Selected Spindle Cell Sarcomas**

Tumor Type	Nuclear Morphology
MPNST	Wavy, buckled, arrowhead shape (tapered at one end)
Synovial sarcoma	Short, oval, darkly staining, apparently overlapping
Leiomyosarcoma	Elongated, nontapered (parallel sided), blunt ended
Myofibrosarcoma	Oval or tapered, small distinct nucleolus
Fibrosarcoma	Tapered at both ends

manifest as a painful mass, or as a rapid enlargement of a pre-existing neurofibroma with neurologic symptoms and signs. Compared with sporadic examples, in NF-1 MPNST develops at a younger age (with a peak in the fourth decade), is more frequent in males, occurs in axial rather than peripheral sites, is more aggressive, and is more likely to show divergent differentiation.

The prognosis relates to grade, tumor size, and presence of tumor at surgical resection margins, but this is generally a high-grade sarcoma of which 40% recur and 65% metastasize with 5-year survival of 44%.[2]

Pathologic Features

Most MPNSTs are large, deep-seated tumors arising in a nerve trunk or neurofibroma (e-Figs. 10.1 and 10.2). The tumor forms a mass that expands the nerve and, because of its tendency for intraneural spread, has ill-defined margins. The cut surface is solid and can display focal necrosis, hemorrhage, or myxoid change (e-Fig. 10.3). Microscopically, MPNST can manifest spindled, epithelioid, pleomorphic or rarely small round cell morphology, and a small proportion of high-grade tumors additionally have heterologous elements representing divergent differentiation. The usual spindled tumor is of intermediate to high grade, and displays a fibrosarcoma-like parallel or herringbone pattern of highly cellular fascicles (Fig. 10.1, e-Fig. 10.4). Typically, there are cellular and myxoid zones in an alternating pattern with occasional nuclear palisading (e-Figs. 10.5 and 10.6). Other architectural clues to the diagnosis include infiltration of tumor cells into vessel walls (e-Fig. 10.7), neuroid whorls (e-Fig. 10.8), and the occasional presence of small or large collagenous nodules or rosettes (e-Fig. 10.9). The cells are elongated, with scanty cytoplasm and nuclei which are wavy, serpiginous, buckled, or lanceolate, with one end pointed and the other blunt; in its extreme form the nucleus can appear triangular (Fig. 10.2, e-Fig. 10.10). Pleomorphic or small round cell areas can occur, and mitoses and necrosis are usual. Some MPNSTs are histologically low grade (neurofibroma-like) and less cellular, though more cellular than neurofibroma and with focal nuclear atypia and mitotic activity

TABLE 10.2 Differential Diagnosis of Spindle Cell Sarcomas

	Typical Clinical Features	Microscopic Features	Ancillary Investigations
Malignant peripheral nerve sheath tumor	M > F. In NF-1 or sporadic, axial or in limbs. Origin in nerve or neurofibroma	Variably cellular and myxoid, fascicular pattern. Nuclei wavy, buckled or lanceolate with one blunt end. Palisading, neuroid whorls, vascular wall involvement, collagenous "rosettes"	S100 protein+ (65%), occasional GFAP+, CK+ (but not usually CK7 or CK19)
Cellular schwannoma	F > M. Middle age. Paravertebral in retroperitoneum or pelvis, can erode bone. Also submucosal in nose, stomach, or intestine	Thick capsule, subcapsular lymphoid aggregates. Fascicles of cells with eosinophilic cytoplasm, focal pleomorphism, occasional mitoses. Lacks Antoni A and B areas. Lymphocytes, clusters of foamy cells, thick-walled vessels, hemosiderin	S100 protein diffusely+, CD34 focal, GFAP focal, occasional CK+, CD117–
Clear cell sarcoma	Extremities especially lower limb, young adults. Subcutaneous or deep soft tissue, related to tendons or aponeuroses	Nests of rounded or spindled cells, round nuclei with central nucleolus, clear or granular cytoplasm. Occasional multinucleated cells, melanin pigment in some	S100 protein+, HMB45+ and melan A+, other markers negative t(12;22)(q13;q12) *EWSR1-ATF1* fusion
PEComa	Intra-abdominal, uterine, extremities (rarely)	Nests of ovoid or spindled cells with clear or granular cytoplasm, delicate fibrous septa. Malignant variants often epithelioid	SMA+, HMB45+, melan-A+, desmin+ in some CD117+ in some, S100 protein+ rarely

(Continued)

TABLE 10.2 **Differential Diagnosis of Spindle Cell Sarcomas (Continued)**

	Typical Clinical Features	Microscopic Features	Ancillary Investigations
Synovial sarcoma	Slowly growing mass, any location but mostly around knee	Sheets of uniform short spindle cells with ovoid nuclei and minimal cytoplasm so that nuclei appear to overlap. Many mast cells. Poorly differentiated SS is a small round cell tumor	CK, EMA, CD99, S100pr focally+, bcl-2+, TLE1+, CD34–, CD117– t(X;18)(p11;q11) *SS18-SSX* fusions
SETTLE	Adolescents or young adults, in or adjacent to thyroid. Can metastasize	Biphasic pattern with mucous glands in spindle cell component. Can resemble synovial sarcoma	CK5/6+, CK7+, CK20–, bcl-2+, CD99+, TLE1+ rarely Genetic features of synovial sarcoma absent
Spindle cell (sarcomatoid) carcinoma	Related to epithelial surface or viscus. Previous carcinoma at same site	Pleomorphic spindled tumor cells in sheets, sometimes areas of epithelial morphology or overlying dysplasia. Nested reticulin pattern. Rare osteochondroid or skeletal muscle differentiation	CK+, EMA+, CD34–, SMA+ in some, desmin–, h-caldesmon–
Sarcomatoid mesothelioma	Sheet-like mass involving peritoneal surface or omentum. Can present as metastasis. History of asbestos exposure	Fascicles of pleomorphic spindle cells, tapered nuclei, scanty cytoplasm, mitoses, necrosis. Desmoplastic or hyalinized stroma. Epithelioid component in some	CK focal+, calretinin+ EMA+ occasionally, D2-40+ occasionally, CD34–, bcl-2–

Solitary fibrous tumor	Circumscribed mass in subcutis, deep soft tissue, abdomen, retroperitoneum, thorax, viscera	Circumscribed, not usually encapsulated, Distinct cellular and fibrous areas, focal myxoid stroma, patternless short spindle cells. Hemangiopericytomatous pattern focally. Malignant variant has hypercellularity, mitoses >4 per 10 hpf, necrosis	CD34+, bcl-2+, CD99+
Adult fibrosarcoma	Older adults, rare. Deep soft tissue, pelvis retroperitoneum	Herringbone fascicles of spindle cells with tapered nuclei	Some subsets CD34+, other markers negative.
Infantile fibrosarcoma	Mostly first year, <4 y. Deep soft tissue, rapid growth	Sheets or fascicles of ovoid cells, hemangiopericytomatous pattern, hemorrhage	SMA+. Occasional CK+, ALK–. t(12;15)(p13;q25) *ETV6-NTRK3* fusion
Inflammatory myofibroblastic tumor	Mesentery, retroperitoneum, lung, other sites	Fascicular, myxoid, sclerosing patterns, mostly bland myofibroblasts, occasional atypical polygonal cells.	SMA+, ALK+ 55%
		Marked inflammation, especially plasma cells, often present in clumps	ALK gene rearrangements
Low-grade myofibrosarcoma	Head and neck, extremities, retroperitoneum, bone, infiltrative mass, recurs	Cellular fascicles infiltrate muscle. Myofibroblastic morphology, mostly uniform, but focal nuclear atypia is diagnostic. Occasional necrosis in higher grade tumors	SMA+, desmin±, h-caldesmon–

(Continued)

TABLE 10.2 Differential Diagnosis of Spindle Cell Sarcomas (Continued)

	Typical Clinical Features	Microscopic Features	Ancillary Investigations
Leiomyosarcoma	F > M. Limbs, head and neck, retroperitoneum, bowel wall or wall of vessel including IVC, renal vein.	Fascicles at right angles. Cells elongated with eosinophilic cytoplasm and nontapered nuclei. Paranuclear vacuoles. Myxoid change, fibrosis	SMA+, desmin+, h-caldesmon+, Occasional CK+ (dot)
Low-grade fibromyxoid sarcoma	Skin, deep soft tissue, limbs/girdles	Fibromatosis-like areas, swirling fibromyxoid transitions, cellular myxoid areas without pleomorphism. Some nuclei lozenge shaped, no nucleoli. Giant collagenous rosettes	Occasionally SMA+, or CD34+, mostly lacks markers t(7;16)(q34;p11) *FUS-CREB3L2* or *FUS-CREB3L1* fusion
Fibromatosis - desmoid type	Deep soft tissue, limbs, head and neck, body cavities	Parallel myofibroblasts evenly dispersed in uniform collagen, slit-like and thick-walled vessels, mast cells. Normal mitoses acceptable but not nuclear atypia or necrosis	SMA+, nuclear beta-catenin+, CD34–
Perineurioma	Skin, subcutis, most locations. Subset in colon. Intraneural, sclerosing, reticular, and plexiform variants	Spindle cells with long thin nuclei and very long slender terminal processes, in fascicles or perivascular whorls. Fibrous or myxoid stroma. Usually no atypia	EMA+, claudin-1+, CD34+ in some, beta-catenin–

Sclerosing epithelioid fibrosarcoma	Deep soft tissue, limbs/girdles, head and neck. Can involve or arise in bone	Multinodular, focal calcification. Cellular islands in dense fibrosis, Nests of ovoid cells, clear cytoplasm, or single files simulating carcinoma. Fibrosarcoma-like spindle cell areas in many cases	Occasional and variable expression of bcl-2, EMA, CK, S100 protein. No specific immunophenotype. Some have genetic features of low-grade fibromyxoid sarcoma
Spindle cell rhabdomyosarcoma	Children and adolescents in neck or paratestis. More aggressive subset in adults	Fascicles of spindle cells resembling smooth muscle, scattered rhabdomyoblasts. In adults, high-grade spindle cell sarcoma in fascicles with variable myoid differentiation	Desmin+, myogenin+ (nuclear), MyoD1+ (nuclear). H-caldesmon–.
Follicular dendritic cell sarcoma	Omentum, GI tract, liver, spleen, soft tissue	Sheets, whorls, and fascicles of ovoid cells. Prominent nuclear membranes, speckled chromatin. Intimate admixture of lymphocytes. Rarely giant cells, pleomorphism, necrosis	CD21/35+, CD23+, S100 protein±, EMA+, D2-40+, fascin+, clusterin+, desmoplakin+, CD45–
Angiosarcoma	Older adults, head and neck, deep soft tissue	Infiltrative, variably cellular nodules, focal vasoformation, epithelioid areas, hemorrhage.	CD31+, CD34+, FLI-1+ (nuclear), HHV8–.
Kaposi sarcoma	Skin, soft tissue, lymph nodes, viscera	Curved fascicles, mild pleomorphism. Intercellular hemorrhage, hyaline globules	HHV8+ (nuclear), CD31+, CD34+, D2-40+, CD117+

(Continued)

TABLE 10.2 **Differential Diagnosis of Spindle Cell Sarcomas (Continued)**

	Typical Clinical Features	Microscopic Features	Ancillary Investigations
Intranodal myofibroblastoma	Inguinal lymph node, rarely submandibular node. Very rarely recurs	Rim of lymph node. Solid, hemorrhagic cut surface. Cellular fascicles of slender spindle cells with nuclear palisading. Hyaline-walled vessels, amianthoid fibers, hemorrhage, hemosiderin	SMA+, other markers negative
Intimal sarcoma	Older adults. Pulmonary trunk or artery, thoracic or abdominal aorta	Undifferentiated pleomorphic sarcoma. Spindle and polygonal cells. Myxoid change. Can show myoid, endothelial, or osseous differentiation	SMA+ focally, other markers according to differentiation

TABLE 10.3 Immunohistochemistry of Selected Malignant Spindle Cell Tumors

	SS	MPNST	Leiomyosarcoma	Rhabdomyosarcoma	Angiosarcoma	Spindle Cell Carcinoma	Melanoma
CK (pan)	+	+[a]	+[a]	–[a]	±	+	–
EMA	+	+[a]	+[a]	–	–	+	–
S100	±	±	+[a]	–	–	–	+
CD34	–	±	–	–	+	–	–
CD31	–	–	–	–	+	–	–
CD99	+	±	–	–	–	–	–
Bcl-2	+	–	–	–	–	±	–
Desmin	–	–	+	+	–	–	+[a]
SMA	–	–	+	–	–	–	–
h-caldesmon	–	–	+	–	–	–	–
Myogenin	–	–	–	+	–	–	–
P63	–	–		–	–	+	–
TLE1	+	±	–	–	–	–	–

[a]Rarely.

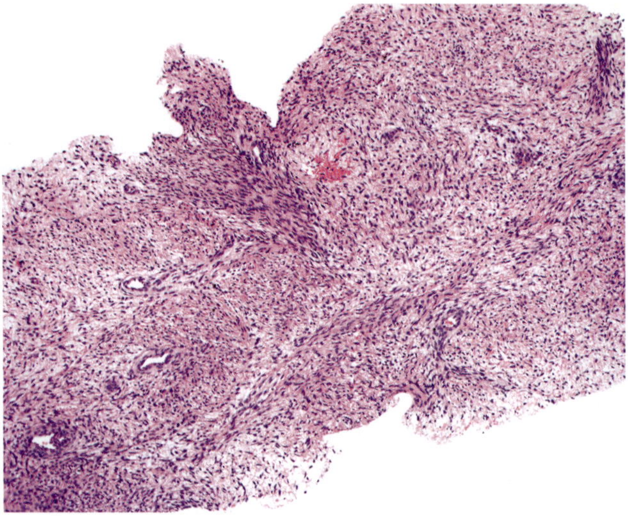

FIGURE 10.1 **Malignant Peripheral Nerve Sheath Tumor.** Core biopsy showing cellular fascicles alternating with myxoid zones.

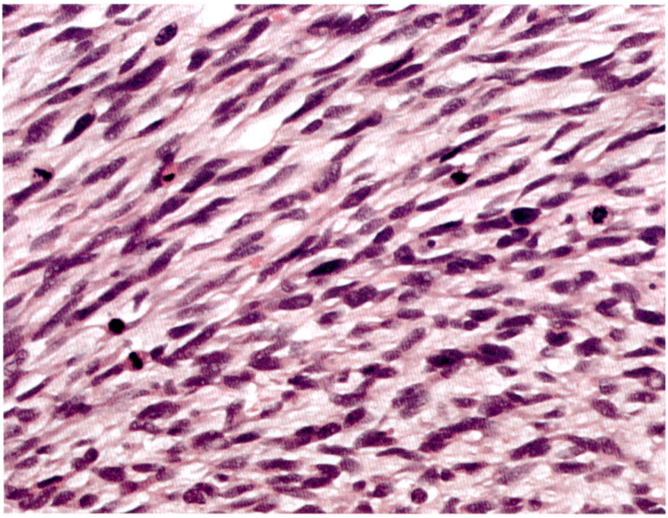

FIGURE 10.2 **Malignant Peripheral Nerve Sheath Tumor.** Cells have nuclei that are wavy, buckled, diamond shaped, or pointed at one end. Mitoses are evident.

(e-Fig. 10.11). The presence of hyaline nodules or "rosettes" should not be misinterpreted as indicating low-grade fibromyxoid sarcoma, which is less cellular than MPNST, has fibromatosis-like areas with collagen "cracking," is nonpleomorphic, and differs in nuclear morphology. Unusually

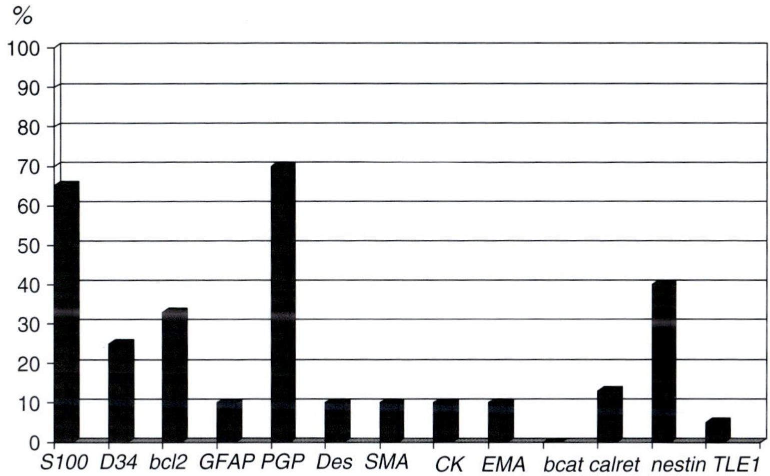

FIGURE 10.3 Immunophenotype of MPNST.

TABLE 10.4 Ancillary Investigations in SS and MPNST

	CK7	CK19	EMA	S100 Protein	CD99	CD34	Bcl-2	TLE1	t(X;18)
SS	+	+	+	+	+	–	D	D	+
MPNST	–	–	–	+	+	+	F	F, rare	–

+, positive in some cases; –, negative in nearly all cases; D, diffuse; F, focal.

among sarcomas, MPNST can infiltrate within and expand nerve bundles (e-Figs. 10.12 and 10.13) and thereby extend proximally, and on occasion into the spinal cord.

Ancillary Investigations

The immunophenotype is summarized in Figure 10.3. About 65% of all spindled MPNSTs express S100 protein, usually focally in scattered single cells (e-Figs. 10.14 and 10.15). Other markers sometimes seen in benign nerve sheath tumors such as GFAP are negative or inconsistently expressed, and neuron-specific enolase (NSE) and PGP 9.5 are too nonspecific to be of diagnostic use. Epithelial antigens are occasionally demonstrable in MPNST, but CK7 and CK19, seen in most monophasic synovial sarcomas (SSs), are negative (Table 10.4). Unlike in SS, CD34 is positive in about 25% of MPNST, and bcl-2 is negative or only focally rather than diffusely positive. Additionally, absence of t(X;18) or *SS18-SSX* fusion gene products on genetic analysis favors MPNST over SS.

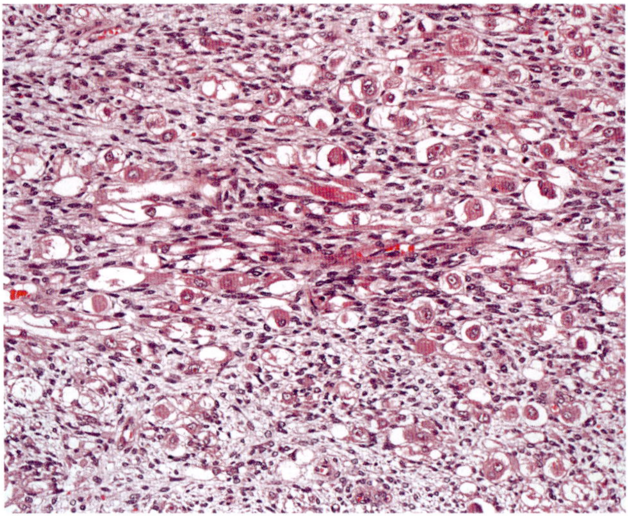

FIGURE 10.4 **Malignant Peripheral Nerve Sheath Tumor.** Focal rhabdomyoblastic differentiation (Triton tumor) is manifested by rounded rhabdomyoblasts. In some cases, this is a spindle cell component that is best seen by immunostaining for desmin and myogenin.

Genetic features of MPNST include inactivation of the tumor suppressor gene *NF1* gene in both sporadic cases and those arising in NF-1,[3] p53 gene mutations, deletion of *INK4A* gene (encoding p16, an inhibitor of CDK4 and CDK6 that affect pRB phosphorylation) on chromosome 9p21,[4] and changes to other chromosomes including 17p. Electron microscopy shows a spectrum of Schwann cell differentiation with interdigitating cytoplasmic processes and external lamina in S100 protein–positive cases. Such features can be focally present in S100 protein–negative MPNSTs, which can be useful in diagnosis.

VARIANTS

Malignant Peripheral Nerve Sheath Tumor with Divergent Differentiation

Heterologous elements can be found in MPNST arising in NF-1 and rarely in spontaneous examples. These tumors occur mostly in the head and neck region and trunk, and can show mesenchymal (osteochondroid or skeletal muscle) differentiation or rarely an epithelial component. MPNST with divergent skeletal muscle differentiation is termed *malignant Triton tumor*, and manifests foci of spindled or rounded rhabdomyoblasts (Fig. 10.4, e-Figs. 10.16 and 10.17). These are often sufficiently differentiated to show cross-striations but can readily be demonstrated with immunostaining for desmin (in cytoplasm) and myogenin (in nuclei) (e-Figs. 10.18 and 10.19). The extremely rare malignant glandular Triton tumor additionally contains mucin-secreting glands that can be bland or resemble adenocarcinoma (e-Fig. 10.20) or SS. Glandular elements can also be seen without accompanying rhabdomyoblastic differentiation, and can show goblet cells and focal neuroendocrine differentiation, suggesting intestinal differentiation. Angiosarcoma can also occur rarely as a focal component of MPNST (e-Fig. 10.21).

The heterologous elements lie in a background of high-grade spindle cell sarcoma, which displays focal S100 protein positivity but not desmin or cytokeratins (CKs). This allows distinction from pure rhabdomyosarcoma and carcinosarcoma respectively.

Malignant perineurial cell tumor is a very rare malignant neoplasm composed of elongated bipolar cells in which the nuclei have prominent nucleoli and mitotic activity.[5] Most are of high-grade malignancy (e-Figs. 10.22 and 10.23). The cells are focally epithelial membrane antigen (EMA)-positive and have ultrastructural features of perineurial cell differentiation. In theory, other perineurial cell markers (claudin-1, GLUT1) might be expressed.

SYNOVIAL SARCOMA

Clinical Features

SS is a translocation sarcoma that is unrelated to synovium in origin or differentiation.[6] A few cases have arisen postirradiation for other lesions. It is a tumor typically of young adults with a mean age of 34 years, and nearly half the cases arise in patients younger than 30 years. Examples have been described, however, at any age, with a slight predominance in males. SS arises in connective tissue adjacent to joints, but very rarely within them, and has now been reported in virtually all anatomic locations.[6] The most common is the lower limb, especially around the knee joint, followed by upper limb and head and neck, notably in parapharyngeal tissues. The majority occurs in deep soft tissues, but occasional SSs arise in subcutis or skin. The tumor forms a painful or painless mass, with clinical features related to the location. SS can be slowly growing with a very long history and can attain a large size. Most, however, are <10 cm in maximum dimension. Very small tumors (<1 cm) are sometimes seen.[7] Imaging reveals focal calcification in up to 20% of cases.

SS is generally an aggressive tumor with metastases, to lung bone and occasionally lymph node in up to 50% of cases.[8] The survival after 5 years is 36% to 76% and at 10 years 20% to 63%.[9] Adverse prognostic factors include high disease stage and grade, male sex, age >40 years, tumor size >5 cm, poorly differentiated histology, and proximal location. Favorable indicators include young age (childhood), very small size, distal location, and ossifying histology. It has been suggested that SS with SSX2 gene rearrangement have a better outcome,[8] but this not been confirmed as a factor independent of grade.

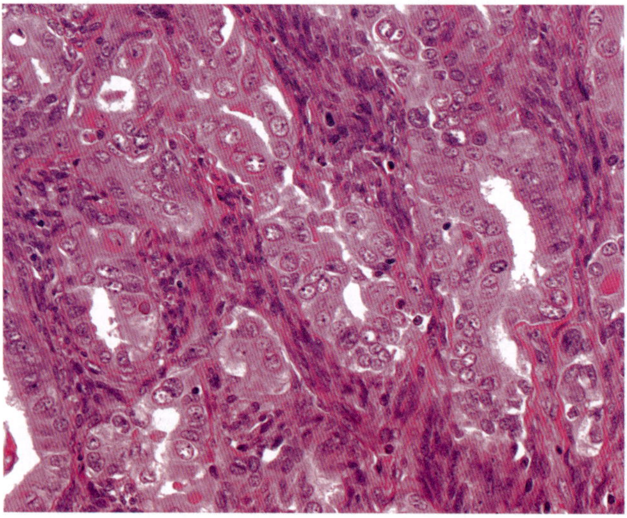

FIGURE 10.5 **Synovial Sarcoma, Biphasic.** Glandular epithelial elements are interspersed with bundles of sarcomatous spindle cells.

Pathologic Features

SS usually forms a circumscribed, pseudoencapsulated soft white or tan tumor, sometimes with cystic change and with hemorrhage and necrosis in poorly differentiated examples. This sarcoma can display a range of microscopic appearances which give rise to a wide differential diagnosis. Biphasic, monophasic spindle cell, poorly differentiated, calcifying/ossifying, and myxoid subtypes have been described.

The typical distinctive biphasic pattern, containing glandular or solid epithelial elements, is readily recognized (Fig. 10.5). The glands have cuboidal cells with uniform nuclei (e-Fig. 10.24) and intraluminal (rarely intracellular) epithelial-type mucin which stains with mucicarmine, PASD, and Alcian blue. There is sometimes a papillary pattern, but the papillary cores contain spindled tumor cells rather than collagenous stroma (e-Fig. 10.25). The glandular element can be predominant, with enlarged, sometimes dilated glands and a sparse spindle cell component which can easily be overlooked (e-Figs. 10.26 and 10.27). Rarely, there is squamous metaplasia with keratinization (e-Figs. 10.28). In the neck, biphasic SS should not be confused with spindle cell carcinoma.

The spindle cell component comprises uniform short spindle cells with ovoid vesicular nuclei which, because of the very scanty cytoplasm, appear focally to overlap. In the monophasic variant (Fig. 10.6, e-Fig. 10.29–10.31), the spindle cells are identical to those in biphasic tumors but can vary in shape from rounded to longer and more spindled. Mitotic activity varies and is sometimes minimal, but pleomorphism is absent

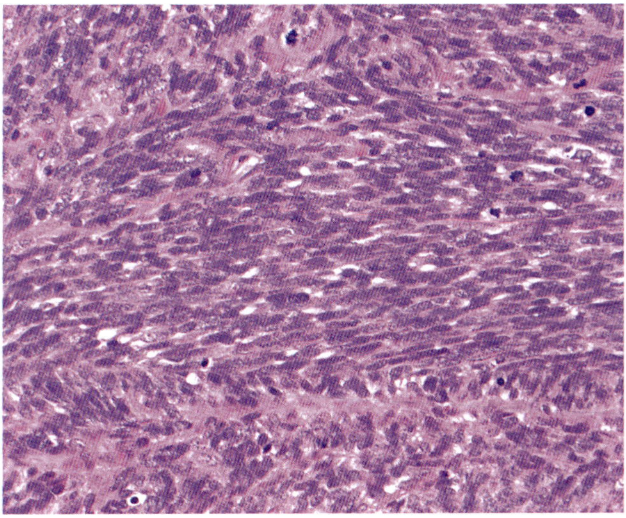

FIGURE 10.6 **Synovial Sarcoma, Monophasic.** Cellular fascicles of uniform spindle cells with darkly staining nuclei and very scanty cytoplasm. Nuclei appear to overlap. There is minimal intercellular stroma.

except following radiation therapy or chemotherapy. Mast cells are often numerous (e-Figs. 10.32 and 10.33).

There is minimal intercellular stroma in most cases, but some monophasic SSs have characteristic bands of hyalinized collagen, and more widespread fibrosis is a feature in SS recurring in sites of therapeutic irradiation. Small myxoid foci, separating individual cells, are common, with diffuse myxoid change (involving >50% of the tumor) in rare cases (e-Fig. 10.34). SS can display a prominent hemangiopericytomatous pattern (e-Fig. 10.35), and also focal nuclear palisading (e-Fig. 10.36). Focal intratumoral calcification is common in SS (e-Fig. 10.37), and a subset of extensively calcified or ossified tumors (Fig. 10.7) occurs mainly in the extremities. When mineralization is anticipated from imaging studies, the tissue should be decalcified before processing. Sometimes, however, it is an unexpected finding in a core biopsy, and the calcified material can fragment during sectioning. This makes interpretation more difficult, especially in ossifying SS. In this, and in other monophasic SS with prominent stromal changes, the lesional cells are often sparse and deceptively bland. Diagnosis in a core biopsy can sometimes be made by examination of multiple levels in an attempt to detect an epithelial component, but immunohistochemistry for epithelial markers is often required, with the addition of genetic analysis where available.

Ancillary Investigations

These are required mostly for monophasic SS and poorly differentiated synovial sarcoma (PDSS). Reticulin staining, unlike in most sarcomas, is not pericellular but displays a pattern of small nests (e-Fig. 10.43).

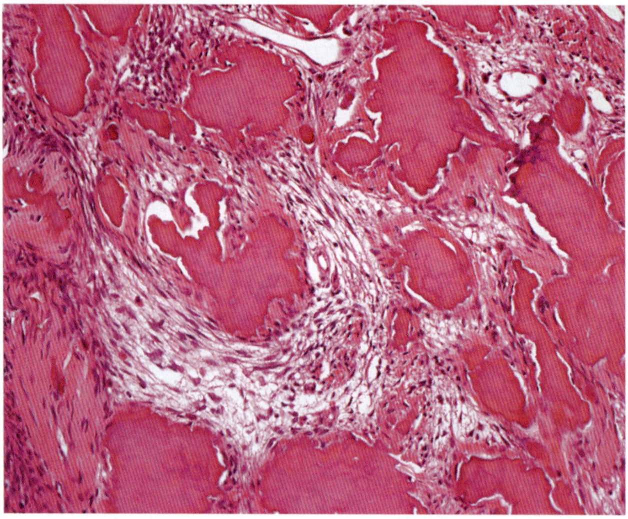

FIGURE 10.7 **Synovial Sarcoma, Ossifying.** Metaplastic bone formation. The spindle cells are neoplastic and can be highlighted by immunostaining for CKs, EMA, or TLE1.

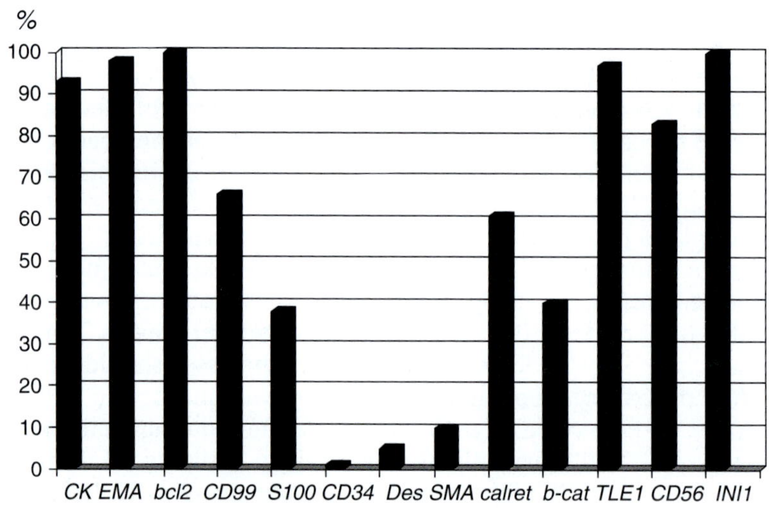

FIGURE 10.8 **Immunophenotype of SS.**

Electron microscopy can reveal features of incomplete epithelial differentiation, including intercellular junctions and fragments of external lamina. The immunophenotype is summarized in Figure 10.8. With immunohistochemistry, SS shows epithelial marker (CK and EMA) positivity in over 90% of cases (e-Figs. 10.44 and 10.45). In PDSS, a smaller proportion is CK-positive and EMA is more sensitive. The staining is typically multifocal in single cells or small groups rather than diffuse. Among keratin subtypes, CK7 and CK19 are expressed, unlike in MPNST and Ewing sarcoma, as well as CK8/18 (antibody CAM5.2). Bcl-2 (e-Fig. 10.38) is usually diffusely positive, and CD99, S100 protein, CD56, and calponin at least focally so in many cases. TLE1, a marker derived from gene profiling studies, is a highly sensitive nuclear marker for SS (e-Fig. 10.39), but not wholly specific since some examples of MPNST and solitary fibrous tumor are also focally positive.[10] However, a spindle cell sarcoma lacking TLE1 is unlikely to be SS. CD34 is almost always negative in SS and can therefore be a useful marker of exclusion. One example of this is ectopic hamartomatous thymoma (see Chapter 7), which occurs in the neck in young adult males and can resemble SS, but expresses both CKs and CD34.[11] Among other markers, beta catenin and calretinin are also sometimes detectable in tumor cell nuclei. An antibody derived from fusion gene products[12] has also proved to be sensitive for SS but demonstrates weak immunoreactivity in a variety of other soft tissue tumors.

More than 90% of SS have a balanced reciprocal nonrandom translocation t(X;18)(p11;q11), with fusion of *SSX* and *SS18* (SYT) genes.[13] The *SSX* gene has 5 subtypes, of which types 1 and 2 (commonly) and 4 (rarely) participate in rearrangements. Variant and additional rearrangements continue to be described in single cases and rarely translocations involving other chromosomes. The rearrangements or fusion gene products can be detected by fluorescence *in situ* hybridization or Polymerase chain reaction, respectively, which is of considerable diagnostic use since the same genetic changes are found in all types of SS but not in other morphologically similar tumor types, such as MPNST or spindle epithelial tumor with thymus-like differentiation (SETTLE).[14] The genetic findings have clinical correlations in that the M:F ratios of fusion types SSX1 and SSX2 are 1:1 and 1:2, respectively, and tumors with *SS18-SSX1* rearrangements occur in limbs more often than elsewhere.[15] Genetic data do not correlate directly with morphology, except that the *SSX2* gene is rarely rearranged in biphasic SS.

Poorly Differentiated Synovial Sarcoma

PDSS has increased mitotic activity and necrosis and the cells can be rounded (Fig. 10.9, e-Figs. 10.40 and 10.41). Poorly differentiated areas can be seen in otherwise typical biphasic or monophasic SS, but when they are widespread PDSS resembles Ewing sarcoma or other small round cell tumors. PDSS can usually be distinguished from CK-positive Ewing sarcoma by its prominent hemangiopericytomatous pattern (Fig. 10.10), by its immunoreactivity for CD56 and TLE1, and by genetic analysis since the tumor types have different translocations. The reticulin pattern can also be

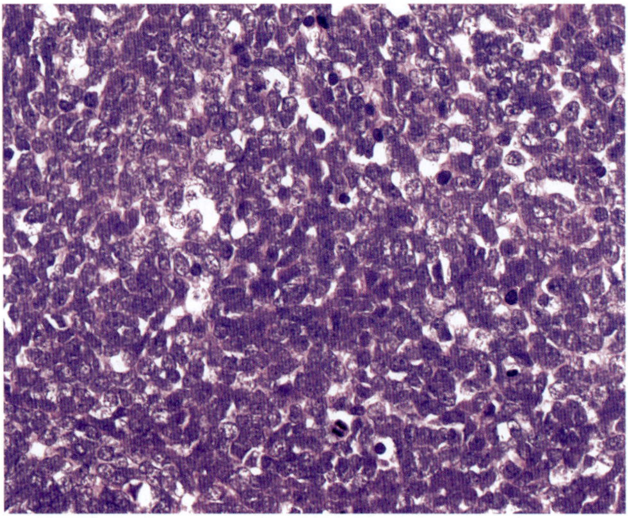

FIGURE 10.9 **Synovial Sarcoma, Poorly Differentiated.** This is a small round cell tumor, with focally overlapping nuclei, and mitoses.

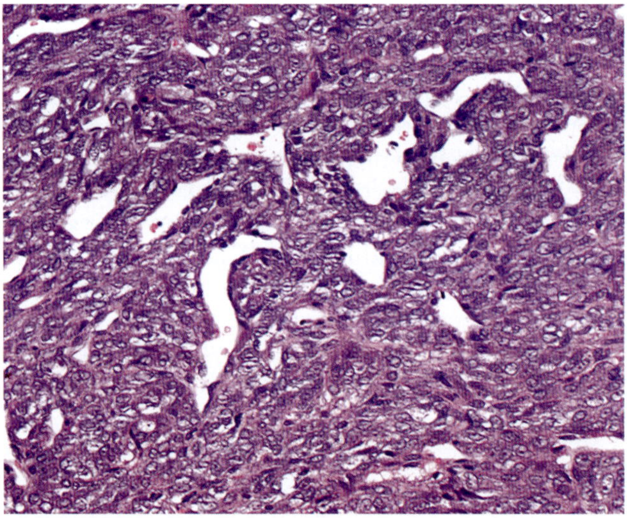

FIGURE 10.10 **Synovial Sarcoma, Poorly Differentiated.** A hemangiopericytomatous pattern is often seen.

helpful since intercellular reticulin is often absent in Ewing sarcoma. The differential diagnosis is considered further in Chapter 14. Less commonly, PDSS has larger cells with epithelioid morphology, resembling carcinoma or closely packed elongated spindle cells superficially resembling fibrosarcoma (e-Fig. 10.42).

ADULT-TYPE FIBROSARCOMA

With the multiple techniques now available, spindle cell sarcomas with a fascicular pattern and varying degrees of intercellular collagen are nearly always diagnosable as synovial sarcoma, MPNST, leiomyosarcoma, or other specific sarcoma subtype. Those without morphologic or immunohistochemical indication of a definite lineage are sometime called *fibrosarcoma* by exclusion. Strictly speaking, this diagnosis should be made not only by failure to identify specific differentiation or genetic abnormality, but also by the positive demonstration that the lesional cells are fibroblasts. This requires electron microscopy, which is rarely done for this purpose. Also, pleomorphic sarcomas with fibroblastic differentiation are currently classified as pleomorphic undifferentiated sarcomas or malignant fibrous histiocytomas. Thus, unspecified types of fibrosarcoma in adults have become increasingly rare and difficult to define. Examples remain which can be termed *fibrosarcoma*, which recur and have metastatic potential, especially when arising in deep soft tissue, with a 5-year survival of 39% to 54% in older series. However, previous clinical and pathological studies have most likely comprised a heterogeneous set of neoplasms.

Clinical Features

Fibrosarcoma in adults is most common in deep soft tissue, where it usually presents as a mass especially in the thigh but also the arm and trunk. A subset of subcutaneous fibrosarcomas has the same genetic changes as fibrosarcoma arising in dermatofibrosarcoma,[16] and conceivably arises by a similar mechanism (translocation) but without manifesting the dermatofibrosarcoma component. Fibrosarcoma can arise postirradiation and rarely in scar tissue due to burns sustained many years previously.

Pathologic Features

Typically, this is a cellular tumor composed of relatively long spindle cells arranged in parallel or herringbone fascicles (Fig. 10.11, e-Fig. 10.46). The cells have tapered relatively featureless nuclei and inconspicuous cytoplasm, with variable mitotic activity. Most fibrosarcomas are relatively uniform, though there can be variable pleomorphism; highly pleomorphic sarcomas are classified as undifferentiated sarcomas or malignant fibrous histiocytomas. Intercellular collagen also varies but most tumors have closely packed cells at least focally. There can be hemorrhage and necrosis in higher grade neoplasms.

Ancillary Investigations

With immunohistochemistry, fibrosarcomas do not express specific antigens. The cells are immunoreactive for vimentin, and focal positivity for smooth muscle actin (SMA) can be seen. Widespread actin expression prompts consideration of low-grade myofibrosarcoma. Some fibrosarcomas

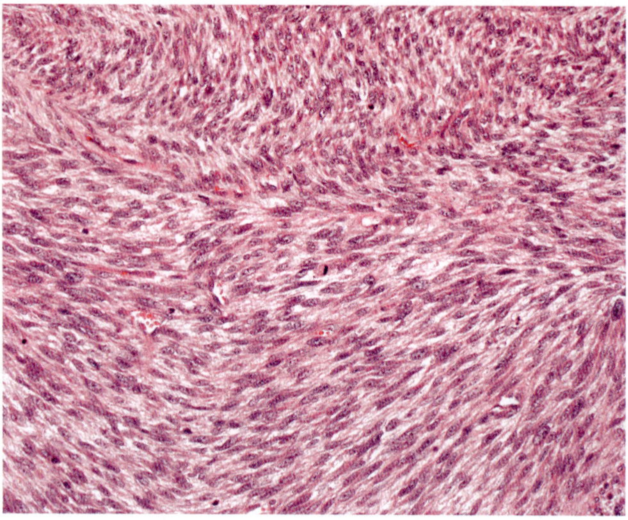

FIGURE 10.11 **Adult Fibrosarcoma.** Intersecting fascicles of spindle cells in a herringbone pattern. The cells are slender and elongated and have scanty cytoplasm.

are CD34-positive; of these some represent malignant solitary fibrous tumors, and some superficial examples show *PDGFRB1-COL1A1* fusion gene transcripts as in dermatofibrosarcoma (but without a typical component) (see Chapter 4). Electron microscopy identifies fibroblasts with abundant rough endoplasmic reticulum and absence of intercellular junctions or external lamina. The cytoplasmic filament pattern is usually nonspecific, though stress fibers suggesting focal myofibroblastic differentiation are occasionally seen. Other than in the specific fibrosarcoma subtypes, there are no characteristic genetic findings.

INFANTILE FIBROSARCOMA

Clinical Features

This tumor occurs predominantly in the first 4 years of life, with a peak incidence in the first 3 months, and presents as a rapidly growing mass which can reach a large size. It arises in deep soft tissue, in limbs, where it can erode bone, and less commonly involves the trunk or head and neck region. Unlike adult fibrosarcoma, this is a tumor of intermediate malignancy: about a third of cases recur but very few (0% to 5%) metastasize,[17] and the 5-year survival exceeds 90%. Cases treated with preoperative chemotherapy,[17] or with chemotherapy alone,[18] have done well. Axial tumors seem to behave more aggressively but there are no histological predictors of behavior. Most deaths from this disease are due to local complications.

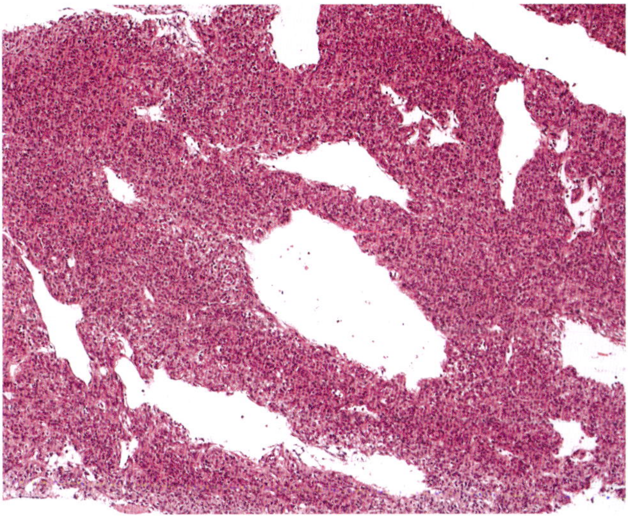

FIGURE 10.12 **Infantile Fibrosarcoma.** This is a highly cellular tumor composed of fascicles of short spindle cells, with a prominent hemangiopericytomatous pattern.

Pathologic Features

Infantile fibrosarcoma forms a circumscribed mass, sometimes with hemorrhage and necrosis. The tumor is composed of uniform ovoid spindle cells arranged in sheets or herringbone fascicles (Fig. 10.12, e-Figs. 10.47 and 10.48). The cells are mitotically active but, as with other translocation sarcomas, cytologic atypia and pleomorphism are typically absent. A more primitive-looking round cell component is, however, sometimes a feature. The stroma can be scanty, collagenous, or myxoid, and the vasculature can be angiomatous or display a hemangiopericytomatous pattern, and some cases have foci resembling infantile myofibroma; composite forms with features of both entities have been described.

Ancillary Investigations

A proportion of cases show positivity for SMA or desmin, with occasional expression of CK, CD34, and S100 protein in reported examples. Infantile fibrosarcoma has a specific translocation t(12;15)(p13;q25) leading to fusion of *ETV6* and *NTRK3* genes[19] Identical findings have been reported in the cellular variant of congenital mesoblastic nephroma, a microscopically similar tumor of the kidney[20] (and also in secretory carcinoma of breast[21] and acute myelogenous leukemia[22]). If genetic techniques are not available, the distinction from other sarcomas (especially SS and MPNST) can be made by careful attention to morphology and demonstration of the relevant immunophenotype.

Inflammatory myofibroblastic tumor most commonly arises at intra-abdominal sites and is considered in Chapter 5. Similar tumors have been described in the lung, a subset arise in the urinary tract, notably in the bladder, and soft tissue sites are occasionally affected.

LOW-GRADE MYOFIBROSARCOMA

Clinical Features

Low-grade sarcomas with myofibroblastic differentiation occur in children or adults (range: 9–75, mean: 40 years) with a slight male predominance.[23] They arise most commonly in deep soft tissue, with a predilection for head and neck sites, including tongue, oral cavity and jawbones, as well as extremities, including the hand. Examples have also been reported in retroperitoneum, trunk, and other bones. They are slowly growing and form discrete but infiltrative masses which can vary from 1.5 to 17 cm in size. This tumor is categorized as intermediate (rarely metastasizing) in the WHO 2002 Classification. A third or more of the cases recur, especially if incompletely excised, and occasional examples metastasize or transform to a higher grade sarcoma.[24] Low-grade myofibrosarcoma is usually managed by surgical excision.

Pathologic Features

The tumors are circumscribed or infiltrative and usually solid with infrequent hemorrhage or necrosis. They are variably cellular and composed of spindle cells with ovoid nuclei, often with a single nucleolus, and variable amounts of eosinophilic or amphophilic cytoplasm (Fig. 10.13,

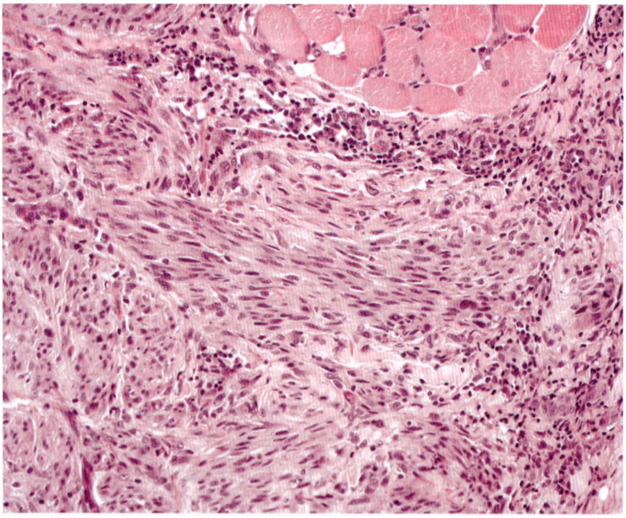

FIGURE 10.13 **Low-grade Myofibrosarcoma.** This is a cellular tumor arranged in fascicles, here infiltrating skeletal muscle. The cells have mostly uniform nuclei, but there is focal pleomorphism.

e-Figs. 10.49–10.52). The latter is less abundant and eosinophilic than in smooth muscle tumors. The nuclei are mostly uniform, but there is mitotic activity and almost always focal (or very focal) nuclear enlargement or hyperchromasia. Necrosis can occasionally be seen, including in cytologically bland areas. The cells are arranged in sweeping, nonalternating fascicles which infiltrate fat or between the fibers of skeletal muscle. There is little intercellular collagen. Sometimes, there is a loose storiform pattern, with focal myxoid change, and a scanty lymphocytic infiltrate, imparting a resemblance to nodular fasciitis (e-Fig. 10.52). However, an infiltrative growth pattern, nuclear atypia, and necrosis are not seen in nodular fasciitis.

Ancillary Investigations

Like other myofibroblastic lesions, the cells are positive for SMA (with peripheral "tram-track" accentuation) (e-Fig. 10.53) and calponin. Less often there is focal immunoreactivity for desmin (with a lower incidence in cases confirmed by electron microscopy, suggesting that some desmin-positive cases are misinterpreted smooth muscle tumors) but h-caldesmon,[25] smooth muscle myosin, S100 protein, and CD34 are negative. Electron microscopy shows relatively abundant rough endoplasmic reticulum, subplasmalemmal stress fibers, and very rarely a fibronexus structure. In common with some other low-grade sarcomas, changes in 12p11 and 12q13–q22 regions, with multiple ring chromosomes, have been reported.[26]

LEIOMYOSARCOMA

Criteria for malignancy in smooth muscle tumors and features of leiomyosarcoma are discussed in detail in Chapter 6. Leiomyosarcomas have a characteristic pattern of fascicles intersecting abruptly at right angles, and their cells are nontapered with blunt-ended nuclei (often showing nuclear pleomorphism which is disproportionate to the mitotic activity) and brightly eosinophilic cytoplasm. The diagnosis can be confirmed by demonstration of immunoreactivity for SMA, desmin, and h-caldesmon. It should be noted that the expression of SMA alone is more indicative of myofibroblastic than of smooth muscle differentiation.

LOW-GRADE FIBROMYXOID SARCOMA

Clinical Features

This fibrosarcoma variant presents as a well-defined mass in deeper soft tissues of extremities (especially the thigh), trunk, and rarely other locations, including viscera, in young adults of either sex.[27,28] Examples located superficially have a higher incidence in childhood.[29] Low-grade fibromyxoid sarcoma (LGFMS) is a histologically low-grade sarcoma with metastatic potential, and some examples present as metastatic disease, usually in the

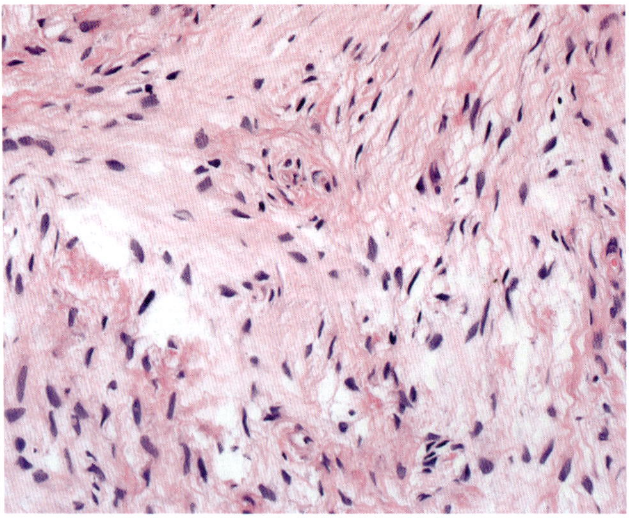

FIGURE 10.14 **Low-grade Fibromyxoid Sarcoma.** Swirling pattern of fibrous and myxoid areas. The nuclei are homogeneous and often square ended, and lack the ovoid shape and punctate nucleoli of myofibroblasts.

lungs, especially in patients with a history of apparent fibromatosis many years earlier. Deep lesions have multiple recurrences and some eventually metastasize (predominantly to lung), typically over a long period. Reported rates of recurrence and metastasis were high in the early reports,[27] which were retrospective studies of cases previously diagnosed as other tumors, with long follow-up. More recent studies indicate recurrence rates of 9% to 21%.[28,30] In one large series, metastasis occurred in about 6% of cases,[28] but this might relate to short follow-up since, in genetically confirmed cases with a metastatic rate of 27%, more than 80% of metastases appeared after 9 years.[30] The finding at presentation of foci of higher grade sarcoma appears not to be prognostically adverse. Superficial examples have a lower recurrence rate of 12% and none has been reported to metastasize.[29]

Pathologic Features

Macroscopically, LGFMS is a circumscribed tumor with firm whorled cut surface. Histologically, the neoplasm shows predominantly fibrous and focally myxoid areas with a swirling or loosely whorled growth pattern (Fig. 10.14). An abrupt transition to myxoid whorls is characteristic. The fibrous areas resemble fibromatosis, with low to moderate cellularity and bland spindle cells with minimal pleomorphism and rare mitoses (e-Figs. 10.54–10.56). The nuclei, unlike those in fibromatosis, are not tapered but are ovoid or rectangular, and lack the distinctive small nucleolus seen in myofibroblasts. The stroma is not markedly vascular, but tumor cells sometimes aggregate around vessels and a plexiform vascular pattern is occasionally seen in myxoid areas. This can be distinguished from

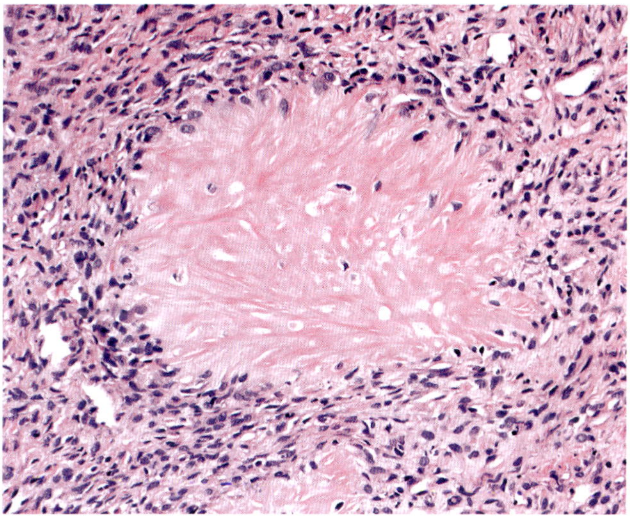

FIGURE 10.15 **Low-grade Fibromyxoid Sarcoma.** Hyaline "giant" rosette, in a more cellular area of the tumor.

myxofibrosarcoma by the lack of nuclear pleomorphism in most cases, though some are identical. Recurrences can show grade progression, with increased cellularity and mitotic activity, and ultimately pleomorphism. A distinctive feature in 15% to 30% of cases is the presence of large rosette-like collagenous structures bordered by more epithelioid or rounded cells (Fig. 10.15, e-Fig. 10.57). The rosettes are usually found within foci of dense hyalinization, often with "cracking" artifact in the collagen. A portion of a rosette can sometimes be seen at the edge of a core biopsy and must not be mistaken for necrosis. This variant was originally termed *hyalinizing spindle cell tumor with giant rosettes* but is now known to be genetically identical to LGFMS.[31] A relationship between LGFMS and sclerosing epithelioid fibrosarcoma (SEF) has been suggested.[30]

Ancillary Investigations

The spindle cells are immunoreactive in some examples for EMA and rarely for SMA and S100 protein. These must be distinguished from perineurioma which has a mostly superficial location, elongated spindle cells with extended bipolar processes, perivascular whorls, and immunoreactivity for claudin-1, GLUT1 and often CD34, as well as a characteristic ultrastructure. However, both EMA and claudin-1 can be positive in LGFMS[32] so that genetic analysis can be required to make the diagnosis. The epithelioid cells around the rosettes can express S100 protein NSE and Leu 7 (11/13), and rarely CD34. Ultrastructurally, both cell types appear fibroblastic[33] with very rare myofibroblastic differentiation. A consistent chromosomal translocation, t(7;16)(q34;p11) with fusion gene *FUS-CREB3L2* (also known as *BBF2H7*), or *FUS-CREB3L1* in some cases, has been described in both

LGFMS and hyalinizing spindle cell tumor with giant rosettes,[31,34] and this is of diagnostic value in paraffin-embedded material.

SCLEROSING EPITHELIOID FIBROSARCOMA

Clinical Features

First described in 1995,[35] SEF is a rare tumor that presents in adults (mean age: 40–45 years) with a slight female predominance. SEF presents as a deep-seated mass in lower limb and limb girdle, shoulder, trunk and neck, and rarely in visceral sites. The tumor sometimes involves underlying bone[36] and rarely is primary in bone. It is a circumscribed neoplasm that can exceed 20 cm in diameter. In the initial series,[35] the tumor was described as low grade with 75% 5-year survival and a proliferation index (Ki67) of <5%, but 53% persisted or recurred and 43% metastasized to lung or bone. Furthermore, follow-up of cases in a subsequent report[36] showed persistent disease or local recurrence in 50% and metastasis in 86%, so that this is clearly an aggressive neoplasm.

Pathologic Features

Macroscopically, SEF is a hard, multinodular, and sometimes cystic or grossly calcified mass. Microscopic examination shows a densely sclerosed stroma with cellular islands composed of nests and cords of polygonal cells, which often have ovoid angulated nuclei and clear cytoplasm and therefore simulate carcinoma cells within scirrhous stroma (Fig. 10.16, e-Figs. 10.57–10.59). The cells are mostly uniform but can be focally pleomorphic;

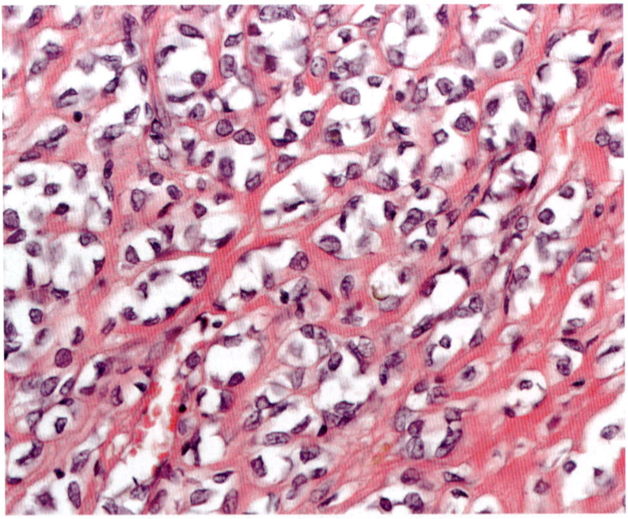

FIGURE 10.16 **Sclerosing Epithelioid Fibrosarcoma.** Nests of rounded cells with vesicular nuclei and clear cytoplasm are separated by thick hyaline collagen bands.

although the mitotic index is usually low, focal necrosis is sometimes seen. Areas of more typical fibrosarcoma, with spindle cells in fascicles can be present elsewhere in the tumor. The stroma is hyalinized or exhibits myxohyaline change, with calcification and osteochondroid metaplasia, and the vasculature is often focally pericytomatous. SEF has been described combined with other patterns of fibrosarcoma, notably LGFMS[30] and adult-type fibrosarcoma.[35]

Ancillary Investigations

This tumor has a varied and nonspecific immunophenotype. All are positive for vimentin and beta catenin (in cytoplasm), but these are nonspecific fibroblastic markers. Most are bcl-2–positive, and around half of the tumors show focal reactivity for EMA. Occasional cases are focally immunoreactive for CKs or S100 protein. The ultrastructure of both epithelioid and spindle cells is interpreted as fibroblastic. Amplification of 12q13 and 12q15 sequences and rearrangements of 10p11 have been described, and SEF-like components have been observed in genetically confirmed examples of LGFMS.[30]

RHABDOMYOSARCOMA

This can assume spindle cell morphology in childhood or adults, as either embryonal or spindle cell types. Alveolar rhabdomyosarcoma is considered with other small round cell tumors in Chapter 14. It should be remembered that apart from its pure forms rhabdomyosarcoma can be present as a component of other sarcoma types, such as MPNST, dedifferentiated sarcomas especially liposarcoma and chondrosarcoma, and ectomesenchymoma, and also nonmesenchymal tumors such as Wilms tumor, germ cell tumors, pleuropulmonary blastoma, and medulloblastoma. Rhabdomyosarcomas can undergo maturation following therapy so that a biopsy can show cells which more closely resemble skeletal muscle at myotube stage, with cross-striations, or even simulate rhabdomyoma.

EMBRYONAL RHABDOMYOSARCOMA

Clinical Features

This is predominantly a tumor of childhood, in which it is the commonest sarcoma especially in the first 5 years, but examples also occur in adult life. There is a slight male predominance. The commonest sites are head and neck (orbit, middle ear, paranasal sinuses, pharynx) pelvis, especially genitourinary sites (paratestis, bladder, prostate), and bile duct, but other viscera can also be affected. The tumor presents as a rapidly growing mass, or with mass effects according to location. In the botryoid form, the tumor can protrude into visceral lumina as a multinodular, often myxoid, lesion, Favorable prognostic factors are young age, orbital or paratesticular location, botryoid morphology, spindle cell histology (in childhood but not in adults), and low stage.

Pathologic Features

The tumor is variably cellular and myxoid. It is composed of small darkly staining spindle and stellate cells with ovoid nuclei, and variable mitotic activity (Fig. 10.17, e-Figs. 10.60 and 10.61). The cytoplasm is scanty in primitive tumors, and increases with differentiation, so that strap or tadpole cells can be seen, sometimes with cross-striations. Necrosis is common, and in subepithelial tumors there can be prominent myxoid change, with condensation of cells beneath the epithelial surface ("cambium" layer). Foci of immature cartilage or rarely bone formation are occasionally seen, especially in tumors of cervix. Pleomorphism is unusual; it can be focal or diffuse and indicates categorization as the anaplastic variant of embryonal rhabdomyosarcoma, which is prognostically unfavorable.[37] The distinction from myxoid (immature) fetal rhabdomyoma can be difficult in a small biopsy especially when the tumor is in an unusual location. However, apart from the absence of pleomorphism and necrosis, rhabdomyoma usually lacks mitotic activity. Therapy can result in variable maturation towards skeletal musule with reduced mitoses.

Ancillary Investigations

Except for very primitive tumors, embryonal rhabdomyosarcoma is immunoreactive for desmin in the cytoplasm and myogenin and myoD1 in nuclei. CD56 is also usually positive. CK or S100 protein positivity is sometimes seen but not without expression of muscle antigens. Embryonal rhabdomyosarcoma has no specific chromosomal translocation, but there can be

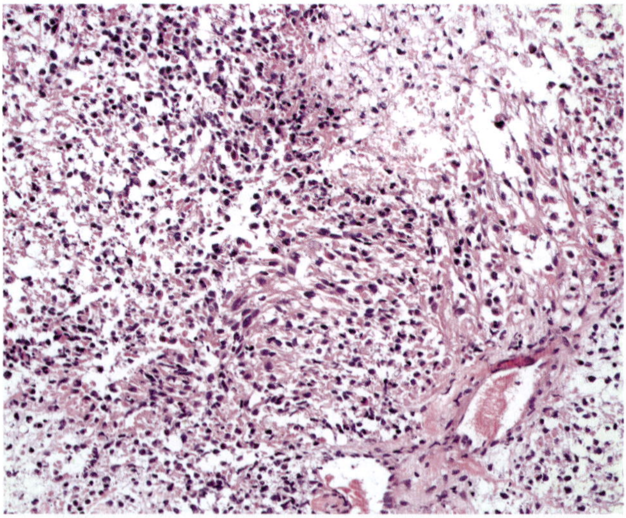

FIGURE 10.17 **Embryonal Rhabdomyosarcoma.** The tumor has cellular and myxoid areas and focal necrosis.

rearrangement of 1p11q and often 11p15 deletion, which is heritable in Beckwith-Wiedemann syndrome.

SPINDLE CELL RHABDOMYOSARCOMA

Clinical Features

This is a rare variant of rhabdomyosarcoma mostly occurring in children and adolescents which is categorized as a variant of embryonal rhabdomyosarcoma in the 2002 WHO classification. It is placed in the superior prognosis category of the International Prognostic Classification of Pediatric Rhabdomyosarcoma; in contrast to other types of rhabdomyosarcoma, the 5-year survival is over 95%.[38] Typically, this arises in males as a mass in the paratesticular region and less commonly in the head and neck. About 16% of cases have been reported to metastasize to lymph nodes.[39] Spindle cell rhabdomyosarcoma also occurs rarely in adults, in various locations including head and neck region, when it is a more aggressive neoplasm which recurs and metastasizes to lungs.[40] Spindle cell foci can be seen in other embryonal rhabdomyosarcoma subtypes, but the presence of an alveolar component excludes the diagnosis.

Pathologic Features

Macroscopically, this forms a poorly circumscribed firm mass with whorled cut surface. Microscopically, in the pediatric variant, there are fascicles or occasionally storiform whorls of relatively uniform elongated tapered spindle cells with focally blunt-ended nuclei, resembling smooth muscle cells. However, the cytoplasm is often highly eosinophilic, cross-striations

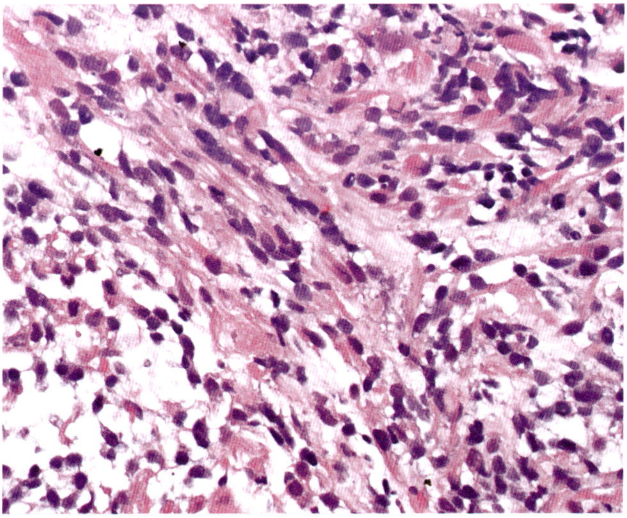

FIGURE 10.18 **Spindle Cell Rhabdomyosarcoma.** This shows fascicles of spindle cells with eosinophilic cytoplasm and occasional more rounded rhabdomyoblast-like cells.

may be seen, and scattered large rounded rhabdomyoblasts are sometimes present (Fig. 10.18, e-Figs. 10.62 and 10.63). According to the amount of intercellular collagen, the tumors can be regarded as either "collagen-rich," resembling fibrosarcoma, or "collagen-poor," resembling leiomyosarcoma; this grouping is without prognostic significance. Adult cases are cellular fibrosarcoma-like spindle cell sarcomas with atypia, frequent mitoses, scanty cytoplasm, and variable numbers of rhabdomyoblasts. Necrosis, pleomorphic areas, and foci resembling sclerosing pseudovascular rhabdomyosarcoma[41] can be seen in some cases. The tumor can be differentiated from the juvenile (intermediate) variant of fetal rhabdomyoma by the presence of mitoses, pleomorphism, and necrosis as well as the clinical picture.

Ancillary Investigations

Spindle cell rhabdomyosarcomas are immunoreactive for desmin, titin, and troponin D, and in nuclei for myogenin and MyoD1 (cytoplasmic staining with anti-MyoD1 is of no diagnostic significance). Some also express SMA focally, but h-caldesmon is absent and this, as well as the diffuse expression of desmin and myogenin, enables the distinction from leiomyosarcoma.

SCLEROSING (PSEUDOVASCULAR) RHABDOMYOSARCOMA

Clinical Features

This is a variant of rhabdomyosarcoma with abundant stroma that occurs mostly in adults of either sex, in deep soft tissue of limbs or head and neck, or in bone (especially sacrum), forming a mass up to 12 cm in diameter. Some reported cases have behaved aggressively, but there are few cases with long-term follow-up.[42]

Pathologic Features

The tumor is composed of "pseudovascular" cords and nests of predominantly small round cells without distinct pattern in a densely hyalinized stroma with osteoid or chondroid appearances (e-Figs. 10.64–10.66). Mitoses are frequent but rhabdomyoblastic differentiation including strap cells is rarely seen. Mitotic activity was >20 mitotic figures per 20 hpf in three of four cases.

Ancillary Investigations

Immunohistochemically, desmin is diffusely or more often focally positive, with a dot distribution (e-Fig. 10.66). MyoD1 is diffusely positive and myogenin focally so. Genetically, gene fusions associated with alveolar rhabdomyosarcoma have not been found. Using comparative genomic hybridization, losses of 10q22 and Y chromosomes, and trisomy 18 were detected in one case.[43].

ANGIOSARCOMA

This tumor can assume spindle cell morphology (see Chapter 18) and resemble other spindle cell sarcomas, which can be a problem particularly in the skin. (e-Figs. 10.67 and 10.68) Diagnostic clues include areas of vasoformation, foci of epithelioid angiosarcoma, and the presence of marked stromal hemorrhage. Immunoreactivity for CD34, CD31, and FLI1 (in nuclei) can help the diagnosis, and absence of HHV8 excludes Kaposi sarcoma (KS).

KAPOSI SARCOMA

This is discussed in detail in Chapter 17. In the plaque stage of cutaneous lesions, in lymph nodes, in generalized KS, and in visceral lesions, there is increased cellularity with a fibrosarcoma-like proliferation. This is composed of tapered slender spindle cells with mildly pleomorphic nuclei and mitoses, disposed in curved fascicles and interspersed with extravasated red blood cells (e-Figs. 10.69–10.74). In cross section, there is a sieve-like pattern, with dilated vascular spaces peripherally. Hyaline globules can be found (e-Fig. 10.72), but there is minimal intercellular collagen. Occasionally, in aggressive KS, more pleomorphic tumors develop or appear de novo (especially in endemic African KS), or resemble angiosarcoma, sometimes with lymphangioma-like areas. KS is immunoreactive for CD31 (e-Fig. 10.673), CD34 and FLI-1, and for podoplanin (D2-40), a marker of lymphatic endothelium. In addition, nuclear immunostaining for HHV8 is seen in KS of all types and stages (e-Fig. 10.74). This can be focal or diffuse, and is extremely useful for diagnosis since other endothelial lesions, including spindle cell hemangioma, Kaposiform hemangioendothelioma, angiosarcoma, and intranodal vascular transformation of sinuses, are nonimmunoreactive. It is of particular value in identifying the earliest lesions, in skin in which both the spindle cells and the flat endothelial-lining cells are HHV8-positive,[44] and in the subtle subcapsular and sinusoidal dilatation of vessels in early intranodal KS.

INTIMAL SARCOMA

Clinical Features

This is a rare neoplasm that can arise in large arterial vessels, including pulmonary trunk and artery from which they can involve pulmonary valve or right ventricle. Less frequently, the tumor occurs in descending thoracic or lower abdominal aorta. Intimal sarcomas arise in older adults of either sex, although pulmonary intimal sarcomas are slightly more common in females. They form obstructing masses with high metastatic potential due to the tendency to embolize, to lung, or to lymph nodes, liver, and bone in the case of intra-abdominal lesions. This is often the presenting feature, but many cases are discovered incidentally at autopsy. In one series of

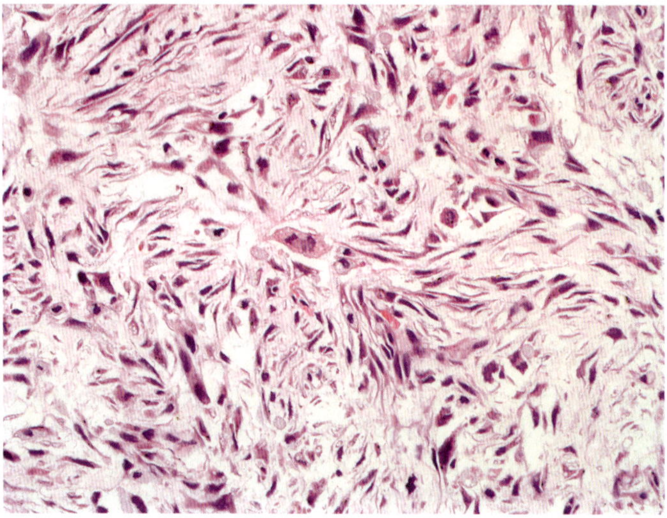

FIGURE 10.19 **Intimal Sarcoma.** Pleomorphic spindle cells are arranged in ill-defined fascicles or loose storiform whorls in a myxoid stroma.

systemic intimal tumors diagnosed in life, 78% died in an average period of 11 months after diagnosis.[45]

Pathological Features

Intimal sarcoma forms an intravascular polypoid lesion adherent to and extending along vessel wall. Microscopically, this is usually an undifferentiated pleomorphic spindle and polygonal cell sarcoma with cellular and myxoid areas (Fig. 10.19, e-Figs. 10.75 and 76). Focal rhabdomyoblastic, osteosarcomatous, or angiosarcomatous differentiation can be seen, especially in pulmonary arterial tumors.

Ancillary Investigations

Undifferentiated sarcomas frequently show focal immunoreactivity for SMA, indicating myofibroblastic differentiation. Relevant antigens can be detected in areas with specific differentiation. Genetically, a complex karyotype with amplification of *MDM2, CDK4,* and *SAS* genes has been described.[46]

REFERENCES

1. Ferner RE. Neurofibromatosis 1. *Eur J Hum Genet.* 2007;15:131–138.
2. Wanebo JE, Malik JM, VandenBerg SR, et al. Malignant peripheral nerve sheath tumors. A clinicopathologic study of 28 cases. *Cancer.* 1993;71:1247–1253.
3. Bottillo I, Ahlquist T, Brekke H, et al. Germline and somatic NF1 mutations in sporadic and NF1-associated malignant peripheral nerve sheath tumours. *J Pathol.* 2009;217:693–701.

4. Sabah M, Cummins R, Leader M, et al. Loss of p16 (INK4A) expression is associated with allelic imbalance/loss of heterozygosity of chromosome 9p21 in microdissected malignant peripheral nerve sheath tumors. *Appl Immunohistochem Mol Morphol.* 2006;14:97–102.
5. Hirose T, Scheithauer BW, Sano T. Perineurial malignant peripheral nerve sheath tumor (MPNST). A clinicopathologic, immunohistochemical, and ultrastructural study of seven cases. *Am J Surg Pathol.* 1998;22:1368–1378.
6. Fisher C. Synovial sarcoma. *Ann Diagn Pathol.* 1998;2:401–421.
7. Michal M, Fanburg-Smith JC, Lasota J, et al. Minute synovial sarcomas of the hands and feet: a clinicopathologic study of 21 tumors less than 1 cm. *Am J Surg Pathol.* 2006;30:721–726.
8. Ladanyi M, Antonescu CR, Leung DH, et al. Impact of SYT-SSX fusion type on the clinical behavior of synovial sarcoma: a multi-institutional retrospective study of 243 patients. *Cancer Res.* 2002;62:135–140.
9. Spillane AJ, A'Hern R, Judson IR, et al. Synovial sarcoma: a clinicopathologic, staging, and prognostic assessment. *J Clin Oncol.* 2000;18:3794–3803.
10. Kosemehmetoglu K, Vrana JA, Folpe AL. TLE1 expression is not specific for synovial sarcoma: a whole section study of 163 soft tissue and bone neoplasms. *Mod Pathol.* 2009;22:872–878.
11. Kushida Y, Haba R, Kobayashi S, et al. Ectopic hamartomatous thymoma: a case report with immunohistochemical study and review of the literature. *J Cutan Pathol.* 2006;33:369–372.
12. He R, Patel RM, Alkan S, et al. Immunostaining for SYT protein discriminates synovial sarcoma from other soft tissue tumors: analysis of 146 cases. *Mod Pathol.* 2007;20:522–528.
13. Ladanyi M. Fusions of the SYT and SSX genes in synovial sarcoma. *Oncogene.* 2001;20:5755–5762.
14. Folpe AL, Lloyd RV, Bacchi CE, et al. Spindle epithelial tumor with thymus-like differentiation: a morphologic, immunohistochemical, and molecular genetic study of 11 cases. *Am J Surg Pathol.* 2009;33:1179–1186.
15. Ladanyi M. Correlates of SYT-SSX fusion type in synovial sarcoma: getting more complex but also more interesting? *J Clin Oncol.* 2005;23:3638–3639; author reply 3639–3640.
16. Sheng WQ, Hashimoto H, Okamoto S, et al. Expression of COL1A1-PDGFB fusion transcripts in superficial adult fibrosarcoma suggests a close relationship to dermatofibrosarcoma protuberans. *J Pathol.* 2001;194:88–94.
17. Loh ML, Ahn P, Perez-Atayde AR, et al. Treatment of infantile fibrosarcoma with chemotherapy and surgery: results from the Dana-Farber Cancer Institute and Children's Hospital, Boston. *J Pediatr Hematol Oncol.* 2002;24:722–726.
18. Surico G, Muggeo P, Daniele RM, et al. Chemotherapy alone for the treatment of congenital fibrosarcoma: is surgery always needed? *Med Pediatr Oncol.* 2003;40:268–270.
19. Knezevich SR, McFadden DE, Tao W, et al. A novel ETV6-NTRK3 gene fusion in congenital fibrosarcoma. *Nat Genet.* 1998;18:184–187.
20. Knezevich SR, Garnett MJ, Pysher TJ, et al. ETV6-NTRK3 gene fusions and trisomy 11 establish a histogenetic link between mesoblastic nephroma and congenital fibrosarcoma. *Cancer Res.* 1998;58:5046–5048.
21. Tognon C, Knezevich SR, Huntsman D, et al. Expression of the ETV6-NTRK3 gene fusion as a primary event in human secretory breast carcinoma. *Cancer Cell.* 2002;2:367–376.
22. Eguchi M, Eguchi-Ishimae M, Tojo A, et al. Fusion of ETV6 to neurotrophin-3 receptor TRKC in acute myeloid leukemia with t(12;15)(p13;q25). *Blood.* 1999;93:1355–1363.
23. Fisher C. Myofibroblastic malignancies. *Adv Anat Pathol.* 2004;11:190–201.
24. Eyden B, Banerjee SS, Shenjere P, et al. The myofibroblast and its tumours. *J Clin Pathol.* 2009;62:236–249.

25. Perez-Montiel MD, Plaza JA, Dominguez-Malagon H, et al. Differential expression of smooth muscle myosin, smooth muscle actin, h-caldesmon, and calponin in the diagnosis of myofibroblastic and smooth muscle lesions of skin and soft tissue. *Am J Dermatopathol.* 2006;28:105–111.
26. Lestou VS, O'Connell JX, Ludkovski O, et al. Coamplification of 12p11 and 12q13 approximately q22 in multiple ring chromosomes in a spindle cell sarcoma resolved by novel multicolor fluorescence in situ hybridization analysis. *Cancer Genet Cytogenet.* 2002;139:44–47.
27. Evans HL. Low-grade fibromyxoid sarcoma. A report of 12 cases. *Am J Surg Pathol.* 1993;17:595–600.
28. Folpe AL, Lane KL, Paull G, et al. Low-grade fibromyxoid sarcoma and hyalinizing spindle cell tumor with giant rosettes: a clinicopathologic study of 73 cases supporting their identity and assessing the impact of high-grade areas. *Am J Surg Pathol.* 2000;24:1353–1360.
29. Billings SD, Giblen G, Fanburg-Smith JC. Superficial low-grade fibromyxoid sarcoma (Evans tumor): a clinicopathologic analysis of 19 cases with a unique observation in the pediatric population. *Am J Surg Pathol.* 2005;29:204–210.
30. Guillou L, Benhattar J, Gengler C, et al. Translocation-positive low-grade fibromyxoid sarcoma: clinicopathologic and molecular analysis of a series expanding the morphologic spectrum and suggesting potential relationship to sclerosing epithelioid fibrosarcoma: a study from the French Sarcoma Group. *Am J Surg Pathol.* 2007;31:1387–1402.
31. Reid R, de Silva MV, Paterson L, et al. Low-grade fibromyxoid sarcoma and hyalinizing spindle cell tumor with giant rosettes share a common t(7;16)(q34;p11) translocation. *Am J Surg Pathol.* 2003;27:1229–1236.
32. Thway K, Fisher C, Debiec-Rychter M, et al. Claudin-1 is expressed in perineurioma-like low-grade fibromyxoid sarcoma. *Hum Pathol.* 2009;40:1586–1590.
33. Lindberg GM, Maitra A, Gokaslan ST, et al. Low grade fibromyxoid sarcoma: fine-needle aspiration cytology with histologic, cytogenetic, immunohistochemical, and ultrastructural correlation. *Cancer.* 1999;87:75–82.
34. Mertens F, Fletcher CD, Antonescu CR, et al. Clinicopathologic and molecular genetic characterization of low-grade fibromyxoid sarcoma, and cloning of a novel FUS/CREB3L1 fusion gene. *Lab Invest.* 2005;85:408–415.
35. Meis-Kindblom JM, Kindblom LG, Enzinger FM. Sclerosing epithelioid fibrosarcoma. A variant of fibrosarcoma simulating carcinoma. *Am J Surg Pathol.* 1995;19:979–993.
36. Antonescu CR, Rosenblum MK, Pereira P, et al. Sclerosing epithelioid fibrosarcoma: a study of 16 cases and confirmation of a clinicopathologically distinct tumor. *Am J Surg Pathol.* 2001;25:699–709.
37. Qualman S, Lynch J, Bridge J, et al. Prevalence and clinical impact of anaplasia in childhood rhabdomyosarcoma: a report from the Soft Tissue Sarcoma Committee of the Children's Oncology Group. *Cancer.* 2008;113:3242–3247.
38. Parham DM, Ellison DA. Rhabdomyosarcomas in adults and children: an update. *Arch Pathol Lab Med.* 2006;130:1454–1465.
39. Leuschner I, Newton WA, Jr., Schmidt D, et al. Spindle cell variants of embryonal rhabdomyosarcoma in the paratesticular region. A report of the Intergroup Rhabdomyosarcoma Study. *Am J Surg Pathol.* 1993;17:221–230.
40. Nascimento AF, Fletcher CD. Spindle cell rhabdomyosarcoma in adults. *Am J Surg Pathol.* 2005;29:1106–1113.
41. Mentzel T, Kuhnen C. Spindle cell rhabdomyosarcoma in adults: clinicopathological and immunohistochemical analysis of seven new cases. *Virchows Arch.* 2006;449: 554–560.

42. Folpe AL, McKenney JK, Bridge JA, et al. Sclerosing rhabdomyosarcoma in adults: report of four cases of a hyalinizing, matrix-rich variant of rhabdomyosarcoma that may be confused with osteosarcoma, chondrosarcoma, or angiosarcoma. *Am J Surg Pathol.* 2002;26:1175–1183.

43. Kuhnen C, Herter P, Leuschner I, et al. Sclerosing pseudovascular rhabdomyosarcoma-immunohistochemical, ultrastructural, and genetic findings indicating a distinct subtype of rhabdomyosarcoma. *Virchows Arch.* 2006;449:572–578.

44. Dupin N, Fisher C, Kellam P, et al. Distribution of human herpesvirus-8 latently infected cells in Kaposi's sarcoma, multicentric Castleman's disease, and primary effusion lymphoma. *Proc Natl Acad Sci U S A.* 1999;96:4546–4551.

45. Sebenik M, Ricci A, Jr., DiPasquale B, et al. Undifferentiated intimal sarcoma of large systemic blood vessels: report of 14 cases with immunohistochemical profile and review of the literature. *Am J Surg Pathol.* 2005;29:1184–1193.

46. Zhang H, Macdonald WD, Erickson-Johnson M, et al. Cytogenetic and molecular cytogenetic findings of intimal sarcoma. *Cancer Genet Cytogenet.* 2007;179:146–149.

11

EPITHELIOID TUMORS OF SOFT TISSUE

INTRODUCTION

Many spindle cell or pleomorphic tumors of soft tissue can assume at least focally an epithelioid appearance, in which the cells become rounded with discernible, often abundant cytoplasm, and additional clear cell or granular cell variation in some cases. These include tumors of nerve sheath, endothelium and smooth muscle, gastrointestinal stromal tumor, myxofibrosarcoma, and pleomorphic liposarcoma. Diagnosis is relatively easy when this component is small, though it may be more of a challenge when it is predominant in a core biopsy.

Soft tissue tumors composed primarily of epithelioid cells include epithelioid sarcoma, extraskeletal myxoid chondrosarcoma, epithelioid mesothelial proliferations, and sclerosing epithelioid fibrosarcoma, as well as carcinoma, melanoma, plasmacytoma, and chordoma involving soft tissue. *Rhabdoid cells* are epithelioid cells with prominent cytoplasm displacing the nucleus. They can be seen in malignant rhabdoid tumor (MRT), as well as on occasion in epithelioid sarcoma, extraskeletal myxoid chondrosarcoma, mesothelioma, synovial sarcoma, and melanoma.

Those sarcomas in which other features such as spindle cells or myxoid stroma are generally prominent are dealt with principally in other chapters. This chapter concerns those in which epithelioid cell morphology is the dominant feature. The differential diagnosis is summarized in Tables 11.1 and 11.2.

EPITHELIOID SARCOMA

Epithelioid sarcoma is a mesenchymal tumor that has prominent epithelial differentiation as well as demonstrating myofibroblastic and other lineages.[1] It can therefore mimic carcinoma, epithelioid angiosarcoma, synovial sarcoma, and mesothelioma and also resemble melanoma and rhabdomyosarcoma. The principal subtypes are the classic and proximal variants, though each can occur in both proximal and distal sites and both patterns can, rarely, coexist in the same tumor.

TABLE 11.1 Differential Diagnosis of Epithelioid Soft Tissue Tumors

	Typical Clinical Features	Microscopic Features	Ancillary Investigations
Epithelioid sarcoma	Nonhealing ulcerated nodules, typically on hand or forearm, mainly first two decades. Proximal variant in young adults, in limb girdles, or axial in perineum, chest wall, pelvis, mediastinum	Centrally necrotic granuloma-like lesions, mainly polygonal cells with mildly pleomorphic nuclei and abundant eosinophilic cytoplasm Proximal variant has large cells with vesicular nuclei and prominent nucleoli, focal rhabdoid appearance	CK+, EMA+, CD34+ (50%),SMA focal, INI1– in most cases, S100 protein–, desmin–
Extrarenal malignant rhabdoid tumor	Children, young adults, head and neck, mediastinum, paraspinal, vulva, perineum	Multinodular, central necrosis, sheets or cords of polygonal cells, vesicular nucleoli, large nucleoli, eccentric cytoplasm. Occasional fibrosis or myxoid stroma	CK+, EMA+, CD34–, INI1–
Epithelioid angiosarcoma	Usually deep, mostly adults. Can arise in immunosuppression, or in course of other tumor, e.g., hemangioma, schwannoma, MPNST	Sheets of polygonal cells, rounded vesicular nuclei, prominent nucleoli. Focal vasoformation, intracytoplasmic lumina. Geographic necrosis, old and recent hemorrhage	CD31+, CD34+, FLI1+, CK+ in some, EMA+ in some, D240 in some, S100 protein–, desmin–, nuclear INI1+
Epithelioid hemangioendothelioma	Deep lesions of soft tissues, lungs, and liver of adults	Epithelioid cells in a chondromyxoid background, sometimes associated with a vessel. The cells infiltrate singly, in cords or small nests and do not form vascular channels, but individual cells can have intracytoplasmic lumina	CD34+, CD31 +, Fli-1+, CK+ in some, VEGFR-3– nuclear INI1+

(Continued)

TABLE 11.1 Differential Diagnosis of Epithelioid Soft Tissue Tumors (Continued)

	Typical Clinical Features	Microscopic Features	Ancillary Investigations
Epithelioid hemangioma	Adults (20–40 y), head-neck region, single or multiple smooth papules or plaques (superficial). Benign but can locally recur	Lobular vascular proliferation surrounded by lymphoid cuff, often associated with damaged artery. Vessels lined by epithelioid endothelial cells, background eosinophils	CD34+, CD31+ in epithelioid cells
Epithelioid sarcoma-like hemangioendothelioma	Rare tumors of young adults Extremities or trunk, in subcutis or deep soft tissue. Indolent behavior with local or regional recurrence	Sheets, ill-defined nodules, fascicles of deeply eosinophilic cells in desmoplastic stroma but no overt vascular channel formation. Occasional cells with intracytoplasmic vacuoles suggesting vascular lumen formation	CK+, CD31+, Fli-1 +, CD34–, nuclear INI1+
Epithelioid malignant peripheral nerve sheath tumor	Adults, F > M. Subcutaneous or deep, the latter usually associated with a nerve	No capsule, Nodules of cells in cords, nests or sheets. Cells have large nucleoli, eosinophilic cytoplasm, with occasional rhabdoid or clear cell change. Pleomorphism is rare. Spindle cell component is common.	S100 protein+, CD34+ in some, INI1+ (in about 50%). HMB45–, melan A–, desmin–
Epithelioid schwannoma	Adults, superficial soft tissue of digits, ear, thigh, and on VIII cranial nerve	Circumscribed, encapsulated. Cords of rounded cells, focal hyperchromatic nuclei, rare mitoses, thick-walled vessels. Epithelioid change can be focal in regular schwannoma	S100 protein+ (diffuse), GFAP+, CK+ in some. Rim of EMA+ perineurial cells

Epithelioid neurofibroma	Very rare focal feature in typical neurofibroma in NF-1	Clusters and cords of plump epithelioid Schwann cells	S100 protein+, CK–
Sclerosing perineurioma	M > F, affects fingers, thumb, palm	Cords and whorls of rounded or epithelioid cells in dense stroma, without atypia	EMA+, claudin-1+, CD34+ in some. CK–, beta-catenin–, INI1+
Epithelioid smooth muscle tumor	Female genital tract, skin, subcutis especially head and neck, usually <2.5 cm	Sheets of cells with distinct cell membranes, rounded nuclei, and eosinophilic, granular, or clear cytoplasm. Atypia, mitoses, necrosis, vascular invasion in epithelioid leiomyosarcoma	SMA+, desmin+, h-caldesmon+, occasional CK+ (dot)
Epithelioid gastrointestinal stromal tumor	Related to wall of any part of alimentary tract (most commonly stomach, small intestine), Also, in retroperitoneum, omentum	Sheets of epithelioid or clear cells often a spindle component. Organoid pattern, occasional plasmacytoid, or rhabdoid change	CD117+, DOG1+, CD34+, h-caldesmon+, SMA variable, desmin+ rarely, S100 protein+ rarely. CK+ in some after therapy. *KIT* or *PDGFRA* mutations
Epithelioid pleomorphic liposarcoma	Deep soft tissue, extremities, rarely retroperitoneum, rarely subcutis	Sheets of clear or granular cells, admixed with pleomorphic lipoblasts. Usually focal, more typical tumor elsewhere	S100 protein+, AE1/3 +, melan-A+, SMA+
Angiomatoid fibrous histiocytoma	Children, young adults, deep dermis or subcutis of upper limb, antecubital fossa, axilla, head and neck, trunk, groin	Circumscribed, fibrous, and lymphoplasmacytoid cuff with germinal centers. Sheets of bland ovoid cells with scanty cytoplasm. Variable cystic blood-filled spaces without endothelial lining	Desmin+ (60%), h-caldesmon+, EMA+, CD99+, CD68+, S100 protein–. t(2;22)(q33;q12) (*EWS-CREB1*), t(12;22)(q13;q12) (*EWS-ATF1*) or t(12;16)(q13;p11)(*FUS-ATF1*)

(Continued)

TABLE 11.1 Differential Diagnosis of Epithelioid Soft Tissue Tumors (Continued)

	Typical Clinical Features	Microscopic Features	Ancillary Investigations
Epithelioid myxofibrosarcoma	Most subcutaneous, some subfascial. Extremities, M = F	Epithelioid cells with prominent nucleoli in myxoid stroma, pattern of short curved vessels	CK negative, EMA negative, desmin negative, S100 protein negative
Extraskeletal myxoid chondrosarcoma	Deep soft tissues of extremities, slight male predominance	Cords, sheets, and reticular pattern of uniform rounded cells with eosinophilic cytoplasm in hypovascular myxoid background	S100 protein+, neuroendocrine markers+ in a subset. t(9;22)(q22;q12) *EWSR1-NR4A3*, t(9;17)(q22;q11) *TAF1168-NR4A3*, or t(9;15)(q22;q21) *TCF12-R4A3*
Sclerosing epithelioid fibrosarcoma	Deep soft tissue, limbs/girdles, head and neck. Can involve or arise in bone	Multinodular, focal calcification. Cellular islands in dense fibrosis, Nests of ovoid cells, clear cytoplasm, or single files simulating carcinoma. Fibrosarcoma-like spindle cell areas in many cases.	Occasional and variable expression of bcl-2, EMA, CK, S100 protein. No specific immunophenotype. Some have genetic features of low-grade fibromyxoid sarcoma
Carcinoma	Usually metastatic deposit in skin or subcutis	Cords and sheets of epithelioid cells with variable pleomorphism, sometimes with focal glandular formation	CK+, EMA+, nuclear INI1+, CD34– Other markers as indicated: PSA, thyroglobulin, calcitonin, hepar-1, CD56, chromogranin, WT1, GCDFP15, TTF-1, ER, PgR, etc.

Epithelioid mesothelioma	Pleural, peritoneal, paratesticular solitary or multiple masses or sheet-like proliferation. Can infiltrate organs	Sheets of epithelioid cells, adenopapillary formations, necrosis	CK5/6+, calretinin+, thrombomodulin+, D2-40+, desmin+ in some, CD34 and bcl2–, BerEP4 and CEA–, nuclear INI1+
Melanoma	Primary or metastatic	Plump epithelioid cells in sheets, often with prominent nucleoli. Cytoplasm eosinophilic, sometimes rhabdoid. Anisocytosis and nuclear pleomorphism can be prominent, unlike in most epithelioid soft tissue tumors	S100 protein+, melan-A+, HMB45+, INI1+, CK rare
PEComa	Intra-abdominal, soft tissue or gynecologic locations	Monotypic epithelioid type has sheets of granular or epithelioid cells. Malignant variants also have pleomorphism, multinucleation, and abnormal.	SMA+, HMB45+, melan-A+, desmin+ in some, CD117+ in some, S100 protein+ rarely, TFE3+ in some
Anaplastic large cell lymphoma	Skin or soft tissue involvement, the latter usually associated with advanced nodal disease	Sheets of polygonal cells, prominent nucleoli, multinucleated forms. Can be spindled	CD30+, ALK+ (or –), CD43+, CD45+, CD3+, TIA1+, t(2;5)(p23;q35),*TMP3-ALK* fusion
Histiocytic sarcoma	Very rare tumor occurring in skin, lymph nodes, GI tract	Sheets of epithelioid cells with eosinophilic cytoplasm and prominent nucleoli, binucleated or giant cells, necrosis. Marked neutrophilic or lymphocytic infiltrate	CD45+, CD45RO+, CD68+, CD4+, lysozyme+, CD31+

(Continued)

TABLE 11.1 Differential Diagnosis of Epithelioid Soft Tissue Tumors (Continued)

	Typical Clinical Features	Microscopic Features	Ancillary Investigations
Rhabdomyoma	Extracardiac lesions occur in larynx, oral cavity, neck, female genital tract	Adult type has large polygonal cells with voluminous granular cytoplasm, some with cross striations. Fetal type is myxoid or cellular with spindle cells and variable myotube formation, and some with cross striation.	Desmin+, myogenin+ (nuclear), MyoD1+ (nuclear)
Granular cell tumor	Skin, head and neck sites (tongue), viscera	Infiltrative, cords and nests of cells with small nuclei, large amounts of coarsely granular cytoplasm, and distinct cell margins.	S100 protein+, CEA+, melanocytic and myoid markers negative

TABLE 11.2 Immunohistochemistry of Selected Malignant Epithelioid Tumors

	Epithelioid Sarcoma	Epithelioid Angiosarcoma	Epithelioid MPNST	Pleomorphic Rhabomyosarcoma	Carcinoma	Melanoma	Anaplastic Large Cell Lymphoma
CK (pan)	+	+[a]	–[a]	+[a]	+	+*	+[a]
EMA	+	+[a]	–[a]	–	+	–	+
S100	–	–	+	–	±	+	–
CD34	+	+	–	–	–	–	–
CD31	–	–	–	–	–	–	–
Desmin	–	–	–	+	–	–	–
SMA	+	–	–	–	–	–	–
INI1 (n)	–	+	±	+	+	+	+
Myogenin (n)	–	–	–	+	–	–	–
P63 (n)	–	–	–	–	+	–	–
CD30	–	–	–	–	+[b]	–	+
CD45	–	–	–	–	–	–	+

[a]rarely; [b]+ in some germ cell tumors (embryonal carcinoma) n, nuclear.

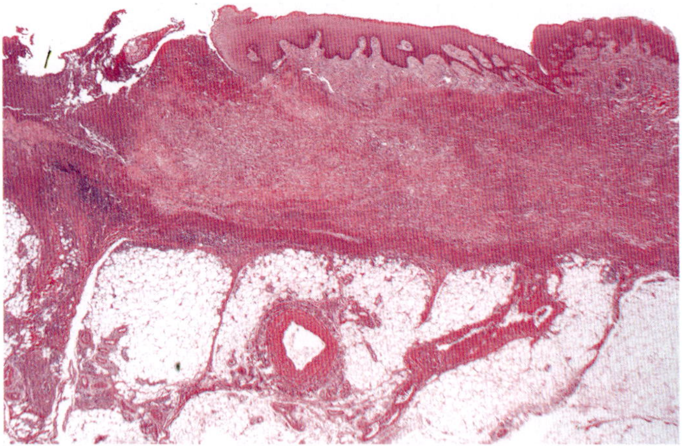

FIGURE 11.1 **Epithelioid Sarcoma.** This is the typical appearance of a dermal lesion of epithelioid sarcoma with ulceration and central necrosis within a peripheral ring of eosinophilic tumor cells. The margins of the lesion are indistinct. Note the epidermal hyperplasia adjacent to the ulcer.

Clinical Features

This tumor arises at any age but mostly in the second and the third decades, and more often in males than females. The commonest site is the forearm and hand, but any site can be affected. The proximal variant (see below) predilects for the midline of trunk and the proximal limbs and limb girdles. Usual epithelioid sarcoma typically arises in dermis and subcutis, but can also involve and extend along tendon sheaths and, rarely, bone. It often presents as a slowly growing nodule, which forms a nonhealing ulcer. Multiple lesions can appear, extending proximally, during the course of the disease. The recurrence rate is very high at over 70%, and over 40% metastasize, to lymph nodes (in 34%) and remote sites, including scalp (22%) and lungs (51%).[2] Epithelioid sarcoma is an aggressive sarcoma that can have a protracted course, with a 5-year survival of about 70% and a 10-year survival of 42% to 62%.[2,3] Treatment is essentially surgical, that is, excision of lesions, which sometimes requires amputation, although isolated limb perfusion might have a role.[4]

Pathologic Features

The classic lesion of epithelioid sarcoma is an ulcerating dermal or subcutaneous nodule with central necrosis, surrounded by plump epithelioid cells with relatively uniform nuclei and abundant, markedly eosinophilic cytoplasm (Figs. 11.1 and 11.2, e-Figs. 11.1–11.3). The cells are sometimes rhabdoid, although this is more common in the proximal variant. At the periphery of the nodules, the neoplastic cells can assume a spindled shape,

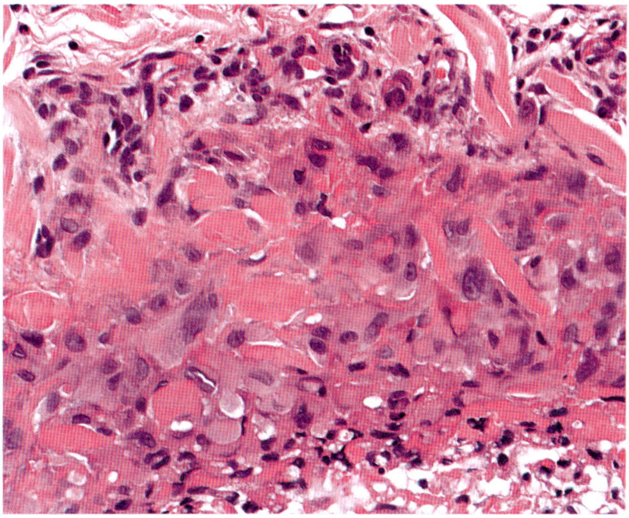

FIGURE 11.2 **Epithelioid Sarcoma.** The tumor cells have markedly eosinophilic cytoplasm and mildly pleomorphic, ovoid vesicular nuclei.

by gradual transition; the tumor is not truly biphasic. Mitoses are variable, but abnormal forms are rare. The stroma can be sclerosed, with neoplastic cells in carcinoma-like files (e-Figs. 11.4 and 11.5) or forming spindle cells with storiform pattern (fibroma-like variant) (e-Fig. 11.6) or modified by hemorrhage (angiomatoid or angiosarcoma-like variant) (e-Fig. 11.7) or, very rarely, myxoid change(e-Fig. 11.8).[5] There is often increased desmoplasia in recurrent lesions. Multinucleated giant cells, calcification, and osteochondroid metaplasia are occasionally seen.

Ancillary Investigations

Almost all epithelioid sarcomas express cytokeratins (Fig. 11.3, e-Fig. 11.9), with diffuse cytoplasmic distribution, and epithelial membrane antigen (EMA), mostly on cell membranes. Among cytokeratin subtypes, CK8, CK19, and CK14 are demonstrable in the majority of cases, whereas CK7, CK20, and (in contrast to cutaneous carcinomas[6]) CK5/6 are infrequently expressed. About half of epithelioid sarcomas are positive for CD34 (e-Fig. 11.10); this is useful in excluding carcinomas, which almost always lack this marker. Claudin-1 is also positive,[7] and reactivity for smooth muscle actin (SMA) is found in about 40% of cases, especially in the spindle cells. Diagnostically relevant negative markers are desmin and S100 protein, assisting the distinction from rhabdomyosarcoma, melanoma, or epithelioid malignant peripheral nerve sheath tumor (MPNST).[1] Also, FLI1 and CD31 are negative in epithelioid sarcoma but positive in epithelioid angiosarcoma and epithelioid sarcoma-like hemangioendothelioma (both of which can also express cytokeratins). Recently, INI1 has

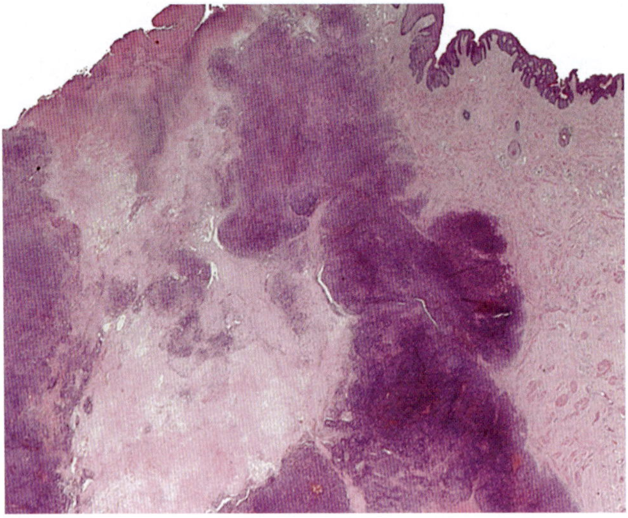

FIGURE 11.3 **Epithelioid Sarcoma, Proximal Variant.** Highly cellular multinodular tumor surrounds an ulcerated area of geographic necrosis.

been shown to be negative in up to 93% of epithelioid sarcomas, which is of diagnostic use since almost all carcinomas and epithelioid endothelial neoplasms, and 50% of malignant epithelioid schwannomas, display nuclear immunoreactivity for this otherwise ubiquitous antigen.[8] Ultrastructurally, epithelioid sarcomas show features of epithelial, fibrohistiocytic, and myofibroblastic differentiation. The cytoplasm contains whorls of intermediate filaments, mainly of vimentin and cytokeratin subtypes, with peripheral myofilaments in the spindle cells. Genetically, epithelioid sarcoma shows deletion of 22q, or abnormalities involving 22q11 or 18q11, and there is associated inactivation of a tumor suppressor gene SMARCB1/INI1 located at 22q11.[8] A rearrangement t(8;22)(q22;q11) has been described in one case,[9] but in contrast to synovial sarcoma, no consistent translocation has been reported.

VARIANTS

Proximal aggressive epithelioid sarcoma is mainly located in proximal extremities, perineum, chest wall, and mediastinum,[10] and is a highly malignant neoplasm with metastases in up to 75% of cases and 35% survival.[11] It forms a subcutaneous or deep-seated irregular infiltrating tumor which is often multinodular with foci of necrosis (Figs. 11.4 and 11.5, e-Fig. 11.11). The cells are generally large, featuring round vesicular nuclei, large nucleoli, and frequently display rhabdoid morphology, with voluminous eosinophilic cytoplasm that displaces the nucleus to one side (e-Fig. 11.12). Rarely, classical and proximal-type patterns are found in the

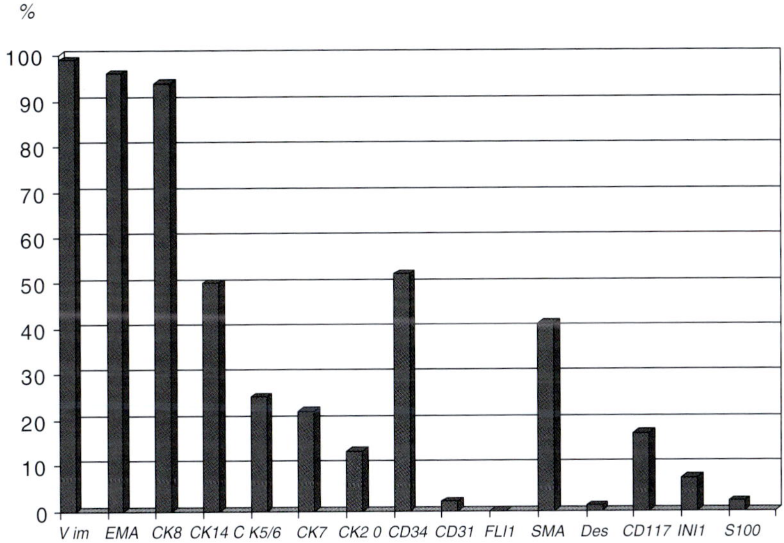

FIGURE 11.4 **Immunophenotype of Epithelioid Sarcoma.**

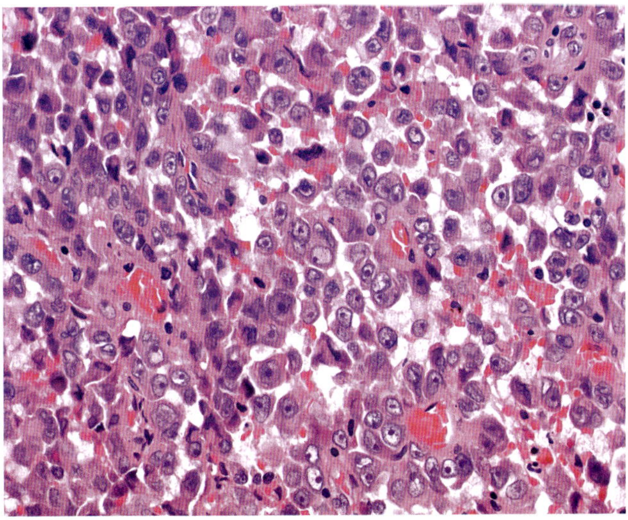

FIGURE 11.5 **Epithelioid Sarcoma, Proximal Variant.** Discohesive sheets of large polygonal cells with rounded vesicular nuclei and distinct nucleoli.

same tumor.[12] The immunoprofile is similar to that of classical epithelioid sarcoma (e-Fig. 11.13), although focal immunoreactivity for S100 protein[11] and HMB45[10] has been observed. In such cases, the coexpression of cytokeratins, EMA, and CD34 indicates the diagnosis, although some are indistinguishable from melanoma. Genetic abnormalities are also similar to typical examples of epithelioid sarcoma, with the addition of t(10;22) found in two cases of proximal epithelioid sarcoma.[13] However, fewer cases show loss of SMARCB1/INI1 protein expression (e-Fig. 11.14) compared with the classical variant.[14]

EXTRARENAL MALIGNANT RHABDOID TUMOR

This tumor is recognized in infants and children in kidney and central nervous system but is less well defined in adults because rhabdoid cells can be seen in numerous specific tumor types.[15] These include epithelioid sarcoma, poorly differentiated synovial sarcoma, extraskeletal myxoid chondrosarcoma, desmoplastic small round cell tumor, Ewing sarcoma, epithelioid MPNST, mesothelioma, carcinoma, melanoma, and rhabdomyosarcoma itself. The existence of MRT as a separate entity has been questioned.[16] There remains, however, a group of tumors with diffuse rhabdoid morphology that cannot be specifically categorized. Many of these closely resemble proximal epithelioid sarcoma, of which MRT might simply be a variant. However, sufficient differences are currently recognized by some workers to allow continued recognition of MRT as a distinct entity.

Clinical Features

Extrarenal MRT occurs congenitally, in children or young adults, and rarely in middle age.[17,18] It usually arises in deep soft tissue in central (axial) locations, including head and neck, mediastinum, paraspinal regions, vulva and perineum, and less often in extremities. This is a rapidly growing and aggressive neoplasm, which is prone to local recurrence and metastasis to lymph node or lung and has a very poor prognosis with mortality of up to 85% after 5 years.[17,19] There is no specific therapy although, based so far on in vitro studies, novel approaches involving use of etodolac, a selective cyclooxygenase-2 inhibitor,[20,21] or trastuzumab, a monoclonal antibody against human epidermal growth factor receptor-2, have been suggested.

Pathologic Features

MRT forms a poorly circumscribed, irregularly infiltrative multinodular mass with central or geographic necrosis. The tumors rarely exceed 5 cm in diameter, but more superficial examples can ulcerate through the skin. Microscopically, these are cellular tumors composed of sheets and cords of polygonal cells with rounded vesicular nuclei which usually contain a single large eosinophilic nucleolus (Figs. 11.6 and 11.7, e-Figs. 11.15 and 11.16). The cells are plasmacytoid or rhabdoid and have abundant eosinophilic cytoplasm, often with an eccentric nucleus displaced to one side of the cell. Small lipid droplets are sometimes seen beneath the cell membrane. Fibrosis (e-Fig. 11.17) and myxoid change (e-Figs. 11.18 and 11.19) can occasionally occur.

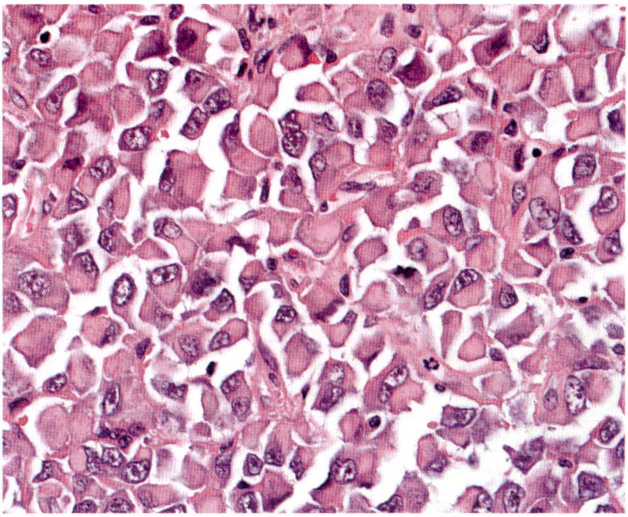

FIGURE 11.6 **Malignant Rhabdoid Tumor.** This neoplasm is composed predominantly of cells with prominent eosinophilic cytoplasm that can indent the nucleus and displace it eccentrically. The cells are often disposed in discohesive sheets.

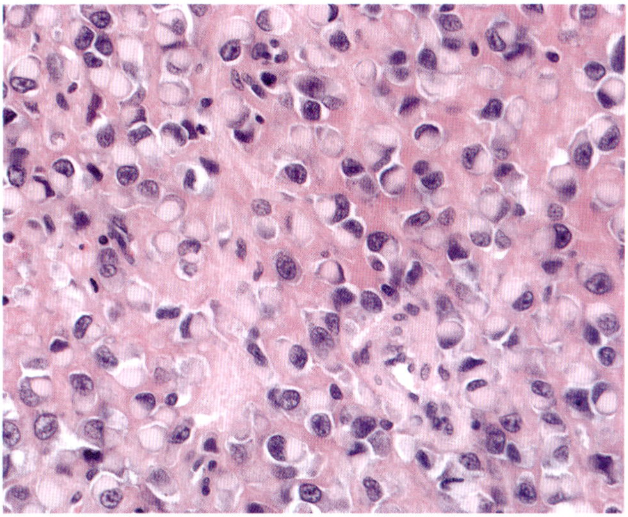

FIGURE 11.7 **Malignant Rhabdoid Tumor.** The nuclei here show prominent indentation, with a "signet-ring" appearance.

Ancillary Investigations

Most MRT express cytokeratins (e-Fig. 11.20) and vimentin, often in a dot-like pattern, as well as EMA on cell membrane; about 80% express at least one epithelial marker. Immunohistochemical staining is negative for CD34 and also for INI1, which helps to exclude carcinoma and melanoma.

Immunoreactivity for CD99, S100 protein, synaptophysin, NSE, and neurofilament has been reported in some cases, suggesting possible neural or neuroendocrine differentiation.[17] However, diffuse S100 protein positivity indicates diagnosis of melanoma or epithelioid MPNST. The presence of desmin suggests rhabdomyosarcoma and indicates further immunohistochemistry for myogenin and MyoD1.

Genetically, deletions and alterations involving chromosome 22q have been described in MRT,[22] with 1;22 translocations,[23] as well as deletions in the SMAR-CB1 (INI1) gene, a tumor suppressor gene that is part of the SWI/SNF chromatin remodeling complex located on chromosome 22q11.[24] These findings, as well as the CK/EMA-positive and INI1-negative immunophenotype, are similar to those in many epithelioid sarcomas. However, there are clinical differences, the pattern of cytokeratin staining in MRT is more dot-like, CD34 is usually absent, and the frequency of SMARCB1/INI1 gene alteration at the DNA level is significantly higher in MRT than in proximal-type epithelioid sarcoma.[14]

EPITHELIOID ANGIOSARCOMA

Angiosarcoma is discussed in detail in Chapters 17 and 18. Predominantly, epithelioid angiosarcoma comprises 70% of deep soft tissue angiosarcomas. Epithelioid angiosarcoma rarely arises in the skin.

Clinical Features

The tumor can arise spontaneously, following irradiation, during immunosuppression, in association with long-standing implants of foreign material, or in a disused arteriovenous fistula placed for hemodialysis.[25] Angiosarcoma arising in other benign or malignant neoplasms, such as vascular malformations, schwannoma, or MPNST, often displays epithelioid morphology.[26] It forms an infiltrative, hemorrhagic tumor mass and is clinically a very aggressive neoplasm.[27]

Pathologic Features

Epithelioid angiosarcoma is composed of sheets of relatively uniform mitotically active polygonal cells with prominent central nucleoli and moderate amounts of eosinophilic cytoplasm, rarely with rhabdoid morphology (Figs. 11.8 and 11.9, e-Figs. 11.21–11.25). Foci of vascular channel formation and of spindling can be seen, often at the periphery of the lesion, and intracytoplasmic lumen formation is sometimes a feature. Recent and old hemorrhage and geographic necrosis are commonly present.

Ancillary Investigations

Immunohistochemistry shows positivity for CD31 (e-Fig. 11.26), FLI-1 and INI1 (in nuclei), and more variably for CD34 and FVIIIRAg (which is less sensitive). Podoplanin (D2-40) can be positive in tumors with lymphatic endothelial differentiation. A variable proportion of epithelioid

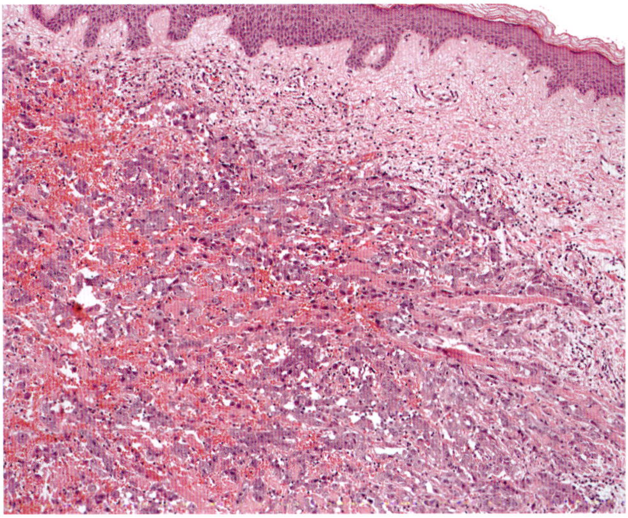

FIGURE 11.8 **Epithelioid Angiosarcoma.** Cords of epithelioid cells infiltrate the dermis accompanied by diffuse hemorrhage. The tumor is not circumscribed.

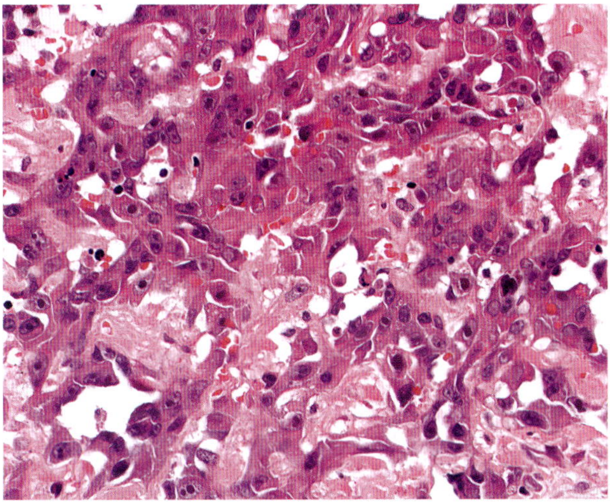

FIGURE 11.9 **Epithelioid Angiosarcoma.** The cells have eosinophilic cytoplasm, and there is attempted vasoformation.

angiosarcomas express cytokeratins, usually focally and, in fewer cases, EMA, but S100 protein is negative. There are no specific genetic findings; a variety of complex changes have been described including loss of Y chromosome.

Epithelioid hemangioma is discussed in Chapter 17. Epithelioid hemangioendothelioma and epithelioid sarcoma-like hemangioendothelioma are discussed in Chapter 18.

EPITHELIOID NERVE SHEATH TUMORS

Both benign and MPNSTs can assume predominantly epithelioid cell morphology. Most of the benign lesions can be categorized as schwannoma or neurofibroma, based on their additional features including a spindle component. In some, however, the diagnosis is not conclusive for either subtype, and these have been termed benign epithelioid peripheral nerve sheath tumors.[28]

EPITHELIOID SCHWANNOMA

Clinical Features

Epithelioid schwannoma is a rare entity that has been described in superficial soft tissue,[29] in GI tract,[30] urinary bladder,[29] and arising from nerve in various locations including acoustic nerve.[31] Soft tissue examples occur in adults between third and eighth decades, and reported sites of occurrence include digits, thigh, and ear.[29] They are generally small, not exceeding 4.5 cm in diameter, and present in a similar fashion to regular schwannoma in the same locations. Reported examples have not recurred or undergone malignant change. However, epithelioid malignant change has been reported in regular schwannomas.[32]

Pathologic Features

These tumors are located in subcutis and circumscribed and often encapsulated. They are composed of nests, cords, and trabeculae of rounded cells with distinct cell margins and mostly uniform nuclei (Fig. 11.10,

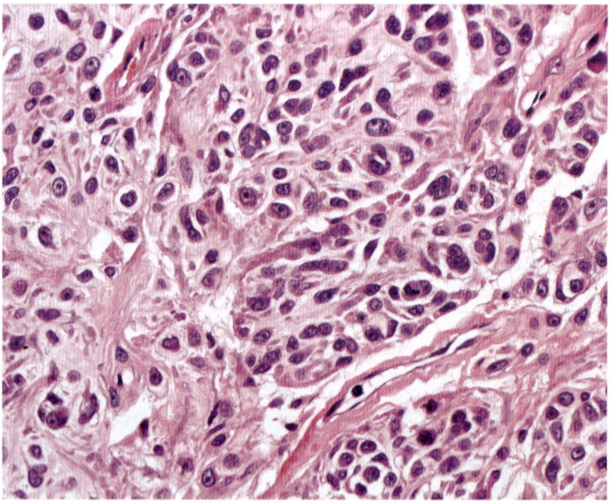

FIGURE 11.10 **Epithelioid Schwannoma.** Cords and nests of rounded schwannoma cells without pleomorphism. This often a focal phenomenon, with the tumor elsewhere demonstrating the more usual spindle cell morphology.

e-Figs. 11.27 and 11.28). Focally, however, there can be large hyperchromatic nuclei with inclusions, but mitoses do not exceed 1 per 10 hpf. Stromal myxoid change and thick-walled vessels with hyalinization can be found, and areas of typical schwannoma coexist in some examples. There is some morphologic overlap with neuroblastoma-like schwannoma (see Chapter 9).

Ancillary Investigations

The lesional cells are diffusely positive for S100 protein and focally so for glial fibrillary acidic protein (GFAP). As with regular schwannoma, a rim of EMA-positive perineurial cells can be seen at the periphery. Ultrastructurally, cells have interdigitating cytoplasmic processes and prominent external lamina.

Epithelioid neurofibroma is a very rare lesion in which clusters and cords of epithelioid Schwann cells are found within typical neurofibroma (e-Figs. 11.29 and 11.30), usually in a patient with neurofibromatosis type 1.[28] This has no prognostic significance. Exceptionally rarely, benign mucous glands are found.

EPITHELIOID MALIGNANT PERIPHERAL NERVE SHEATH TUMOR

Clinical Features

This is a rare variant of MPNST that occurs mostly in third to sixth decades with a slight female predominance.[33,34] Only a small proportion of cases are associated with neurofibromatosis type 1, but some examples arise as malignant change in schwannoma, which is an extremely rare phenomenon.[35] Epithelioid MPNST comprises two clinicopathologic groups: those originating in subcutis and deeply located lesions that often arise from a major nerve in the proximal extremities or spinal nerve root. Superficial tumors have a more favorable outcome with 12.5% of cases resulting in metastasis, compared with 30% to 50% of deeply located examples.[33,34]

Pathologic Features

This is a nonencapsulated tumor composed of variably cellular nodules of epithelioid cells arranged in cords, small nests, or sheets. The cells have rounded nuclei with large nucleoli, and abundant eosinophilic cytoplasm (Figs. 11.11 and 11.12, e-Figs. 11.31 and 11.32), and rhabdoid or clear cell change can be a feature. The cells are usually fairly uniform with variable mitotic activity, but rarely there is nuclear pleomorphism. Many examples have a small spindle malignant component with transitions between the two patterns, and residual neurofibroma was present in one case.[33] Malignant change in schwannoma usually takes the form of epithelioid MPNST, and a possible precursor lesion, designated epithelioid malignant change, has been described, comprising large epithelioid

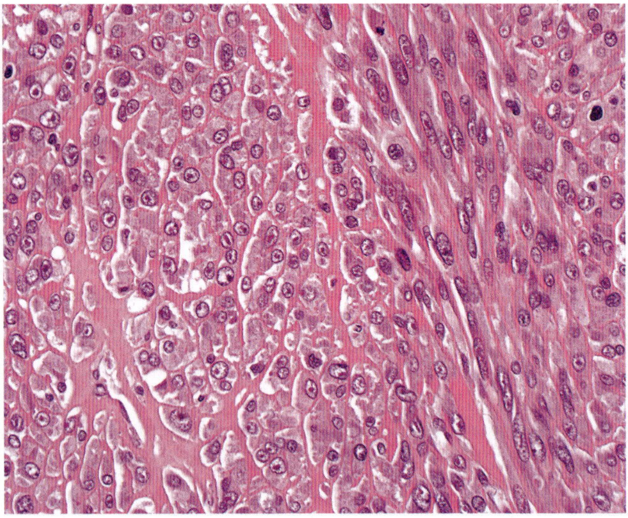

FIGURE 11.11 **Epithelioid MPNST.** This tumor has mainly epithelioid morphology with nests of cells and foci of transitional spindle cells with increased cytoplasm.

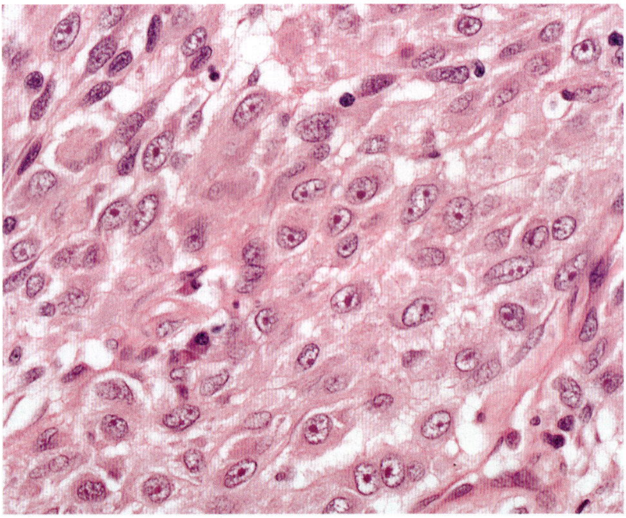

FIGURE 11.12 **Epithelioid MPNST.** The cells have nuclei with distinct nuclear membranes and prominent eosinophilic nucleoli.

MPNST-like cells scattered singly, in clusters, or as small nodules, throughout the schwannoma.[32]

Ancillary Investigations

Unlike spindled MPNST, epithelioid MPNST is usually diffusely positive for S100 protein (e-Fig. 11.33). Melanocytic markers, including HMB45, melan-A, and MiTF, are negative, helping to exclude melanoma. However, distinction from melanomas that fail to express these antigens can be difficult or impossible. A small number of cases have focal positivity for cytokeratins, but finding the latter warrants investigation for carcinoma. Only 50% of cases are immunohistochemically positive for INI1 (e-Fig. 11.34).[36] This marker is negative in most epithelioid sarcomas, but as they are S100 protein–negative there should be no diagnostic confusion with the subset of epithelioid MPNST that fail to express INI1.

EPITHELIOID SMOOTH MUSCLE TUMORS

Smooth muscle tumors with predominant epithelioid cytomorphology were formerly relatively common in the gastrointestinal tract, but most such cases are now diagnosed as epithelioid gastrointestinal stromal tumors (see Chapter 5). Partial or predominant epithelioid change is now most frequently seen in benign or malignant smooth muscle neoplasms of the female genital tract, especially in those involving the vulva (epithelioid leiomyoma) or the uterus (epithelioid leiomyoma and leiomyosarcoma) (e-Figs. 6.29 and 6.30). Single examples of epithelioid leiomyoma have been reported in other sites including breast, bladder, and larynx. Epithelioid leiomyosarcomas arising in somatic soft tissue are rare, and mostly originate in skin or subcutis (e-Fig. 6.35).[37] Cases have also been described in paratesticular region, thigh, larynx and breast, as well as bone.[38] However, examples with a complete smooth muscle immunophenotype or convincing ultrastructural evidence of smooth muscle differentiation are very rare.[39]

Clinical Features

These tumors present in a similar fashion to regular smooth muscle tumors. In skin and subcutaneous tissue, epithelioid leiomyosarcomas mostly affect the head and neck region in older adults, and are usually small (<2.5 cm).[40] They have a tendency to recur, on occasion with progression to high-grade malignancy.[40]

Pathologic Features

In many cases, there is a diagnostic component of spindle cells which facilitates diagnosis. In those examples composed mostly of epithelioid cells, the nuclei are rounded, with variably prominent nucleoli and cytoplasm that can vary from granular through eosinophilic to clear, with distinct cell membranes (e-Figs. 11.35 and 11.36). In epithelioid leiomyosarcoma, there is variable nuclear atypia, mitotic activity, necrosis, and vascular invasion.

Ancillary Investigations

There is variable and often incomplete expression of smooth muscle antigens. Actins are most commonly positive, often in a peripheral rim, but many cases lack desmin. There have been few studies of the frequency of expression of h-caldesmon, but its presence supports the diagnosis of smooth muscle differentiation. In addition, cytokeratins and EMA can be found, usually focally. Epithelioid smooth muscle tumors of female genital tract, including cases with clear cell morphology, sometimes display positivity for HMB45, which in this location should not lead to misinterpretation as PEComa in the absence of the appropriate morphologic and ancillary features.

MESOTHELIAL PROLIFERATIONS

Reactive, benign, and malignant mesothelial proliferations can enter the differential diagnosis of pleural, pericardial, chest wall, and intra-abdominal epithelioid neoplasms, as well as metastatic tumors. General features of mesothelioma and sarcomatoid mesothelioma are discussed in Chapter 5.

Mesothelial cysts are lined by a single layer of cuboidal mesothelium (e-Fig. 11.37). **Multicystic peritoneal mesothelioma** occurs mostly in adult females and often is associated with abdominal surgery, pelvic inflammatory disease, or endometriosis.[41] It comprises multiple thin-walled cysts lined by cuboidal or flattened mesothelial cells which are positive for cytokeratin and calretinin. **Adenomatoid tumor** is a benign mesothelial lesion that occurs mainly in genital organs of both males (epididymis, spermatic cord, tunica) and females (uterus, fallopian tube, ovary). It is composed of gland-like spaces or thin-walled spaces lined by plump, cuboidal, or flattened mesothelial cells (Fig. 11.13, e-Figs. 11.38–11.40), set in a fibrous or smooth muscle stroma. **Reactive mesothelial hyperplasia**

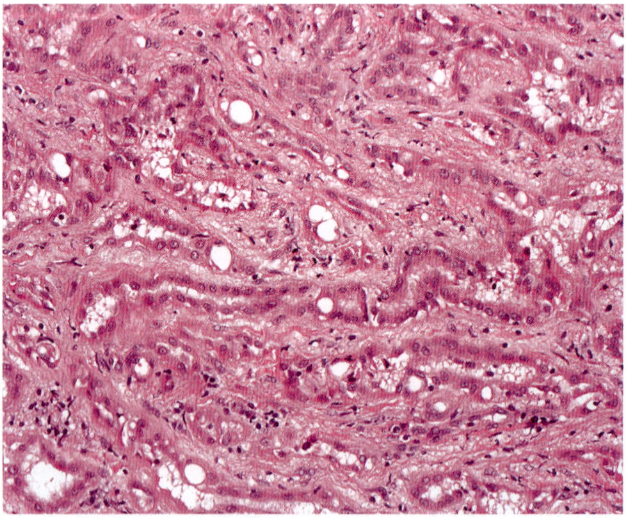

FIGURE 11.13 **Adenomatoid Tumor.** Elongated tubular (gland-like) cords of mesothelial cells. There are inflammatory cells within the fibromyxoid stroma.

can be multicentric and manifests as multiple layers of usually uniform polygonal mesothelial cells, or papillary tufts that lack fibrovascular cores (Fig. 11.14). There are usually no atypical cytologic features and no invasion of underlying stroma (e-Figs. 11.41 and 11.42). The latter can sometimes be more easily demonstrated by immunohistochemistry for cytokeratins. However, entrapment or mesothelial inclusions, which often form a linear pattern or elongated clefts, should not be mistaken for invasion.[42] It should also be noted that mesothelial inclusions can be seen in mediastinal or pelvic lymph nodes. **Atypical mesothelial hyperplasia** has a single cell layer or multiple layers of at least focally atypical cells (e-Fig. 11.43). This is probably part of a spectrum with mesothelioma,[42] and such cases should be examined carefully for features of invasion. Clinical and radiologic correlation is also important, since the presence of a definite tumor mass or masses favors malignancy. Some examples of reactive mesothelial hyperplasia have eventuated in frank mesothelioma, so close follow-up is indicated after making this diagnosis.

Well-differentiated papillary mesothelioma can occur at any mesothelial surface, with equal sex incidence in pleural lesions and a female predominance in peritoneal tumors.[43] Although generally benign, multiple lesions can be progressive and rarely there is recurrence as mesothelioma. The tumor has a papillary architecture with fibrous cores covered by usually a single layer of cuboidal cells (e-Fig. 11.44)

Epithelioid malignant mesothelioma is composed of plump rounded epithelioid cells with abundant cytoplasm, arranged in sheets, nests, or papillary formations (Figs. 11.15 and 11.16, e-Figs. 11.45–11.47), sometimes

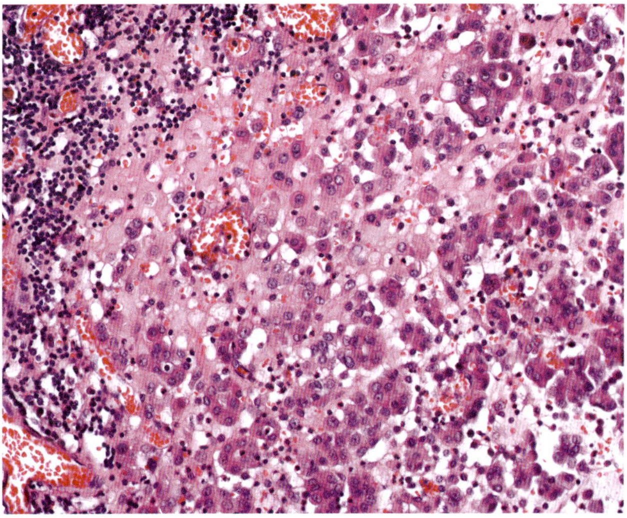

FIGURE 11.14 **Reactive Mesothelial Hyperplasia.** The cells form sheets and pseudopapillary tufts, with chronic inflammatory response. There is no significant nuclear pleomorphism, and no necrosis is seen.

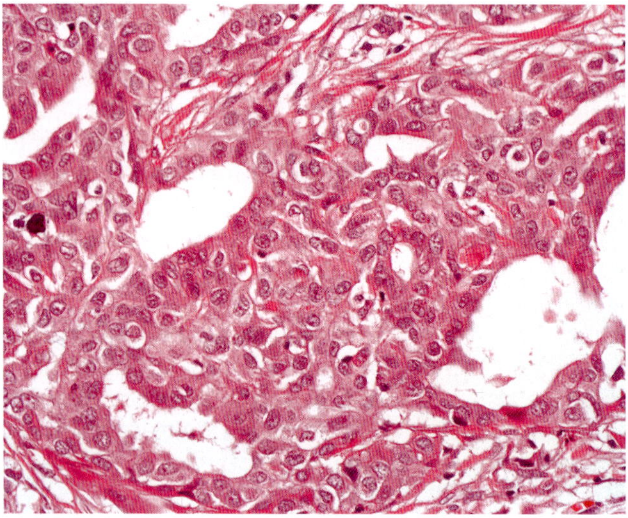

FIGURE 11.15 **Epithelioid Malignant Mesothelioma.** Gland-like and solid formations of epithelioid mesothelial cells.

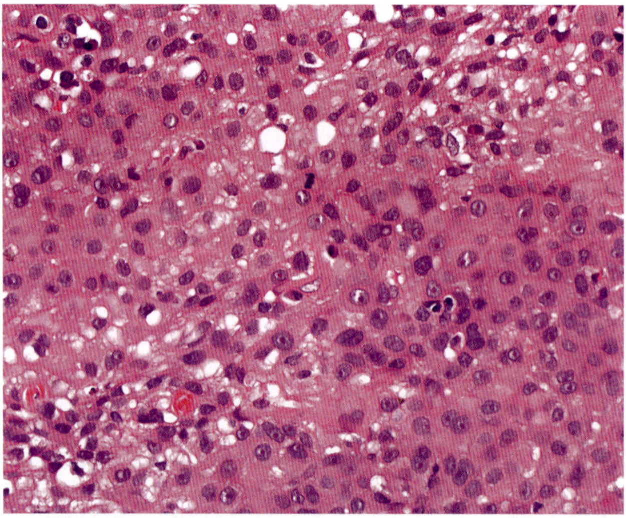

FIGURE 11.16 **Epithelioid Malignant Mesothelioma.** This tumor forms a solid sheet of malignant epithelioid cells, with prominent nucleoli and mitotic activity.

with psammoma bodies. Variable features include mitotic activity and the presence of necrosis. Mesothelioma can be distinguished from reactive mesothelial hyperplasia by the presence of pleomorphism, abnormal mitoses and necrosis, and by detection of invasion into submesothelial adipose or fibrous tissue (e-Figs. 11.48 and 11.49) or viscera.[44]

Ancillary Investigations

With immunohistochemistry, all forms of mesothelial tumor demonstrate positivity to a variable extent for pancytokeratins (e-Fig. 11.49), CK7, CK5/6, INI1, calretinin, thrombomodulin, D2-40, HBME1, WT1, and INI1. EMA is more often negative in reactive mesothelial cells than in mesothelioma, but this is not wholly sensitive or specific. Mesotheliomas sometimes express desmin. They are usually negative for CK20, CEA, BerEP4, MOC31, CD34, bcl-2, and ER (which is useful in the distinction from ovarian or peritoneal serous carcinoma).[45,46] Electron microscopy can demonstrate long slender microvilli in sufficiently differentiated mesothelial proliferations.

REFERENCES

1. Fisher C. Epithelioid sarcoma of Enzinger. *Adv Anat Pathol.* 2006;13:114–121.
2. Chase DR EF. Epithelioid sarcoma. Diagnosis, prognostic indicators and treatment. *Am J Surg Pathol.* 1985;9:241–263.
3. Baratti D, Pennacchioli E, Casali PG, et al. Epithelioid sarcoma: prognostic factors and survival in a series of patients treated at a single institution. *Ann Surg Oncol.* 2007;14:3542–3551.
4. de Visscher SA, van Ginkel RJ, Wobbes T, et al. Epithelioid sarcoma: Still an only surgically curable disease. *Cancer.* 2006;107:606–612.
5. Fadare O. Myxoid epithelioid sarcoma: clinicopathologic analysis of 2 cases. *Int J Surg Pathol.* 2009;17:147–152.
6. Lin L, Skacel M, Sigel JE, et al. Epithelioid sarcoma: an immunohistochemical analysis evaluating the utility of cytokeratin 5/6 in distinguishing superficial epithelioid sarcoma from spindled squamous cell carcinoma. *J Cutan Pathol.* 2003;30:114–117.
7. Smith ME, Awasthi R, O'Shaughnessy S, et al. Evaluation of perineurial differentiation in epithelioid sarcoma. *Histopathology.* 2005;47:575–581.
8. Modena P, Lualdi E, Facchinetti F, et al. SMARCB1/INI1 tumor suppressor gene is frequently inactivated in epithelioid sarcomas. *Cancer Res.* 2005;65:4012–4019.
9. Cordoba JC, Parham DM, Meyer WH, et al. A new cytogenetic finding in an epithelioid sarcoma, t(8;22)(q22;q11). *Cancer Genet Cytogenet.* 1994;72:151–154.
10. Guillou L, Wadden C, Coindre JM, et al. "Proximal-type" epithelioid sarcoma, a distinctive aggressive neoplasm showing rhabdoid features. Clinicopathologic, immunohistochemical, and ultrastructural study of a series. *Am J Surg Pathol.* 1997;21:130–146.
11. Hasegawa T, Matsuno Y, Shimoda T, et al. Proximal-type epithelioid sarcoma: a clinicopathologic study of 20 cases. *Mod Pathol.* 2001;14:655–663.
12. Rakheja D, Wilson KS, Meehan J, et al. "Proximal-type" and classic epithelioid sarcomas represent a clinicopathologic continuum: case report. *Pediatr Dev Pathol.* 2005;8:105–114.
13. Lualdi E, Modena P, Debiec-Rychter M, et al. Molecular cytogenetic characterization of proximal-type epithelioid sarcoma. *Genes Chromosomes Cancer.* 2004;41:283–290.
14. Kohashi K, Izumi T, Oda Y, et al. Infrequent SMARCB1/INI1 gene alteration in epithelioid sarcoma: a useful tool in distinguishing epithelioid sarcoma from malignant rhabdoid tumor. *Hum Pathol.* 2009;40:349–355.
15. Tsuneyoshi M, Daimaru Y, Hashimoto H, et al. The existence of rhabdoid cells in specified soft tissue sarcomas. Histopathological, ultrastructural and immunohistochemical evidence. *Virchows Arch A Pathol Anat Histopathol.* 1987;411:509–514.

16. Wick MR, Ritter JH, Dehner LP. Malignant rhabdoid tumors: a clinicopathologic review and conceptual discussion. *Semin Diagn Pathol.* 1995;12:233–248.
17. Fanburg-Smith JC, Hengge M, Hengge UR, et al. Extrarenal rhabdoid tumors of soft tissue: a clinicopathologic and immunohistochemical study of 18 cases. *Ann Diagn Pathol.* 1998;2:351–362.
18. Brand A, Covert A. Malignant rhabdoid tumor of the vulva: case report and review of the literature with emphasis on clinical management and outcome. *Gynecol Oncol.* 2001;80:99–103.
19. Parham DM, Weeks DA, JB B. The clinicopathologic spectrum of putative extrarenal rhabdoid tumors: an analysis of 42 cases studied with immunohistochemistry or electron microscopy. *Am J Surg Pathol.* 1994;18:1010–1029.
20. Hakozaki M, Hojo H, Kikuchi S, et al. Etodolac, a selective cyclooxygenase-2 inhibitor, induces apoptosis by activating caspases in human malignant rhabdoid tumor cells (FRTK-1). *Oncol Rep.* 2007;17:169–173.
21. Katsumi Y, Kuwahara Y, Tamura S, et al. Trastuzumab activates allogeneic or autologous antibody-dependent cellular cytotoxicity against malignant rhabdoid tumor cells and interleukin-2 augments the cytotoxicity. *Clin Cancer Res.* 2008;14:1192–1199.
22. White FV, Dehner LP, Belchis DA, et al. Congenital disseminated malignant rhabdoid tumor: a distinct clinicopathologic entity demonstrating abnormalities of chromosome 22q11. *Am J Surg Pathol.* 1999;23:249–256.
23. Simons J, Teshima I, Zielenska M, et al. Analysis of chromosome 22q as an aid to the diagnosis of rhabdoid tumor: a case report. *Am J Surg Pathol.* 1999;23:982–988.
24. Biegel JA, Tan L, Zhang F, et al. Alterations of the hSNF5/INI1 gene in central nervous system atypical teratoid/rhabdoid tumors and renal and extrarenal rhabdoid tumors. *Clin Cancer Res.* 2002;8:3461–3467.
25. Wehrli BM, Janzen DL, Shokeir O, et al. Epithelioid angiosarcoma arising in a surgically constructed arteriovenous fistula: a rare complication of chronic immunosuppression in the setting of renal transplantation. *Am J Surg Pathol.* 1998;22:1154–1159.
26. Ruckert RI, Fleige B, Rogalla P, et al. Schwannoma with angiosarcoma. Report of a case and comparison with other types of nerve tumors with angiosarcoma. *Cancer.* 2000;89:1577–1585.
27. Fletcher CDM, Beham A, Bekir S, et al. Epithelioid angiosarcoma of deep soft tissue: a distinctive tumour readily mistaken for an epithelial neoplasm. *Am J Surg Pathol.* 1991;15:915–924.
28. Laskin WB, Fetsch JF, Lasota J, et al. Benign epithelioid peripheral nerve sheath tumors of the soft tissues: clinicopathologic spectrum of 33 cases. *Am J Surg Pathol.* 2005;29:39–51.
29. Kindblom LG, Meis-Kindblom JM, Havel G, et al. Benign epithelioid schwannoma. *Am J Surg Pathol.* 1998;22:762–770.
30. Ples R, Lazure T, Dimet S, et al. Epithelioid schwannoma of the colon. Report of two cases. *Ann Pathol.* 2007;27:243–246.
31. Kroh H, Matyja E, Marchel A. Epithelioid schwannomas of the acoustic nerve. *Folia Neuropathol.* 2000;38:23–27.
32. McMenamin ME, Fletcher CD. Expanding the spectrum of malignant change in schwannomas: epithelioid malignant change, epithelioid malignant peripheral nerve sheath tumor, and epithelioid angiosarcoma: a study of 17 cases. *Am J Surg Pathol.* 2001;25:13–25.
33. Lodding P, Kindblom LG, Angervall L. Epithelioid malignant schwannoma. A study of 14 cases. *Virchows Arch A Pathol Anat Histopathol.* 1986;409:433–451.
34. Laskin WB, Weiss SW, Bratthauer GL. Epithelioid variant of malignant peripheral nerve sheath tumor (malignant epithelioid schwannoma). *Am J Surg Pathol.* 1991;15:1136–1145.

35. Woodruff JM, Selig AM, Crowley K, et al. Schwannoma (neurilemoma) with malignant transformation. A rare, distinctive peripheral nerve tumor. *Am J Surg Pathol.* 1994;18:882–895.
36. Hornick JL, Dal Cin P, Fletcher CDM. Loss of INI1 Expression Is Characteristic of Both Conventional and Proximal-Type Epithelioid Sarcoma. *Mod Pathol.* 2007;20:16A.
37. Suh KS, Jang MS, Chae YS, et al. Epithelioid leiomyosarcoma of the skin. *J Dermatol.* 1998;25:121–125.
38. Marshman LA, Pollock JR, King A, et al. Primary extradural epithelioid leiomyosarcoma of the cervical spine: case report and literature review. *Neurosurgery.* 2005;57:E372; discussion E372.
39. Eyden B. Epithelioid leiomyosarcoma of the external deep soft tissue. *Arch Pathol Lab Med.* 2003;127:402–404; author reply 404.
40. Suster S. Epithelioid leiomyosarcoma of the skin and subcutaneous tissue. Clinicopathologic, immunohistochemical, and ultrastructural study of five cases. *Am J Surg Pathol.* 1994;18:232–240.
41. Weiss SW, Tavassoli FA. Multicystic mesothelioma. An analysis of pathologic findings and biologic behavior in 37 cases. *Am J Surg Pathol.* 1988;12:737–746.
42. Cagle PT, Churg A. Differential diagnosis of benign and malignant mesothelial proliferations on pleural biopsies. *Arch Pathol Lab Med.* 2005;129:1421–1427.
43. Hoekstra AV, Riben MW, Frumovitz M, et al. Well-differentiated papillary mesothelioma of the peritoneum: a pathological analysis and review of the literature. *Gynecol Oncol.* 2005;98:161–167.
44. Butnor KJ. My approach to the diagnosis of mesothelial lesions. *J Clin Pathol.* 2006;59:564–574.
45. Ordonez NG. Immunohistochemical diagnosis of epithelioid mesothelioma: an update. *Arch Pathol Lab Med.* 2005;129:1407–1414.
46. Ordonez NG. Value of estrogen and progesterone receptor immunostaining in distinguishing between peritoneal mesotheliomas and serous carcinomas. *Hum Pathol.* 2005;36:1163–1167.

12

SOFT TISSUE LESIONS WITH CLEAR OR GRANULAR CELLS

INTRODUCTION

Clear cell change can be seen in some examples of myoepithelioma (Chapter 6), smooth muscle tumors (Chapter 7), atypical fibroxanthoma (Chapter 13), Ewing sarcoma (Chapter 14), rhabdomyosarcoma (Chapter 14), and gastrointestinal stromal tumor (Chapter 5). Tumors in which clear cell change can be predominant include glomus tumor (Chapter 7), alveolar soft part sarcoma, clear cell sarcoma, PEComa, and paraganglioma, as well as metastases from other organs including carcinomas. Lesions with lipoblastic and pseudolipoblastic differentiation can also enter the differential diagnosis and are discussed in Chapter 15. *Granular cell or oncocytic change* is seen in granular cell tumor, and in some examples of hibernoma (Chapter 15), myoepithelioma (Chapter 7), smooth muscle tumors (Chapter 6), nerve sheath tumors (Chapter 9), dermatofibroma (Chapter 4), dermatofibrosarcoma protuberans (Chapter 4), atypical fibroxanthoma (Chapter 13), and benign and malignant PEComas. Finally, reactive and neoplastic histiocytic proliferations can present in soft tissue as clear or granular cell tumors. The differential diagnoses are summarized in Tables 12.1 and 12.2.

CLEAR CELL SARCOMA OF SOFT TISSUE

Clinical Features

This is a tumor of young adults (more often in females) that arises predominantly in the extremities, especially the foot and rarely in trunk or head and neck sites as a slowly growing firm mass. The usual location is deep subcutaneous or subfascial tissue, often with involvement of tendon sheath or aponeurosis. This is an aggressive neoplasm that metastasizes to lymph node, lung and bone, with survival rates of 67%, 33%, and 10% after 5, 10, and 15 years, respectively.[1,2] A genetically distinct subset of clear cell sarcoma arises in the gastrointestinal tract, where it presents with obstruction, bleeding, or mass effect. Neither subtype is related to clear cell sarcoma of kidney.

TABLE 12.1 Differential Diagnosis of Clear Cell and Granular Cell Tumors

	Typical Clinical Features	Microscopic Features	Ancillary Investigations
Clear cell cutaneous fibrous histiocytoma	Raised firm nodule on extremities, young adults	Epidermal hyperplasia, areas of typical dermatofibroma, peripheral collagen bundles	CK–, SMA–, desmin–, S100 protein–
Clear cell atypical fibroxanthoma	Sun-exposed areas, elderly patients	Sheets of clear cells with pleomorphic nuclei, and prominent cell membranes	CD10+ in some cases, S100 protein–, HMB45–, melan-A–, desmin–, AE1/3–
Ossifying fibromyxoid tumor	Subcutaneous well-demarcated nodule, any age	Partial shell of bone in many, thick fibrous capsule, cords of rounded glomus-like or occasionally spindled cells, fibromyxoid stroma. Atypical variant can have increased cellularity, mitoses, intralesional osteoid	S100 protein+, GFAP+, desmin/SMA+ in some, rarely CK+
Clear cell sarcoma (soft tissue)	Extremities especially lower limb, young adults. In subcutis or deeper tissue, it involves tendons. Subset in GI tract	Nested pattern, round nuclei with central nucleolus, clear or granular cytoplasm, sometimes spindling, multinucleated cells, melanin pigment. No junctional activity	S100 protein+, HMB45+ and melan-A+ (except in GI tract), other markers negative t(12;22)(q13;q12), *EWSR1-ATF1* *or* t (2;22)(q33;q12), *EWSR1-CREB1* (mostly GI cases)
Granular cell tumor	Subcutaneous in adults, especially in head and neck sites. Also in various organs	Infiltrative sheets and cords of large polygonal cells, coarsely granular cytoplasm. Clear cell areas often present also	S100 protein+, CD68+, CEA+

(Continued)

TABLE 12.1 **Differential Diagnosis of Clear Cell and Granular Cell Tumors (Continued)**

	Typical Clinical Features	Microscopic Features	Ancillary Investigations
Granular cell dermatofibrosarcoma	Like typical dermatofibrosarcoma	Sheets of granular cells involving dermis and superficial subcutis. Areas of typical dermatofibrosarcoma usually present, with transitional forms	CD34+, S100 protein–
Granular cell leiomyoma	Rare focal change in smooth muscle tumors of soft tissue or gynecologic origin	Granular cell areas within epithelioid or spindle cell smooth muscle tumor	SMA+, desmin+, h-caldesmon+, S100 protein–
Paraganglioma	In locations of paraganglia–carotid body, base of skull, mediastinum, retroperitoneum. Some are functional–hypertension, vagal symptoms	Nests of ovoid cells with clear or granular cytoplasm and variable nuclear pleomorphism. Prominent or sinusoidal thin-walled blood vessels, sometimes fibrosis	CD56+, NF+, SYN+, CG+. S100 protein+ in sustentacular cells
Paraganglioma-like dermal melanocytic tumor	Adult females, extremities, dermal nodule	Circumscribed or infiltrative, can extend into subcutis. Nests of cells within slender fibrous septa, uniform rounded nuclei, small nucleoli, abundant clear or amphophilic cytoplasm	S100 protein+, HMB45+, melan-A±
Alveolar soft part sarcoma	Childhood or adult. Single mass or multicentric. Mesenteric, retroperitoneal, other sites	Nests of large polygonal cells with uniform vesicular nuclei and clear or finely granular cytoplasm. A solid pattern of closely packed nests is sometimes seen especially in childhood cases	TFE3+, desmin+ t(X;11)(p11;q25) *TFE3-ASPL*

Rhabdomyoma	Adult or fetal (median: 4 y) type in head and neck, or (mostly female) genital tract locations. Also cardiac rhabdomyoma (adult type)	Sheets of large polygonal cells with abundant eosinophilic cytoplasm. Fetal rhabdomyoma has long spindle cells in myxoid stroma (immature type) or spindled and round cells with variable skeletal muscle differentiation (intermediate type)	Desmin+, myogenin+ (in nuclei), MyoD1+ (in nuclei)
PEComa (other than organ-specific subtypes)	Intra-abdominal, soft tissue or gynecologic locations	Nests of ovoid or spindled cells with clear or granular cytoplasm, delicate fibrous septa. Malignant variants often epithelioid with large polygonal cells, pleomorphism, mitoses, necrosis	SMA+, HMB45+, melan-A+, desmin+ in some, CD117+ in some, S100 protein+ rarely, TFE3+ in some, Cathepsin-K in some
Chordoma	Mainly in sacrum/coccyx, or skull base, rarely other vertebrae. Can extend into adjacent tissues as tumor mass	Cords and nests of polygonal cells with eosinophilic cytoplasm, resembling adenocarcinoma. Larger vacuolated (physaliferous) cells. Can have areas of dedifferentiation	S100 protein+, CK+, EMA+, brachyury+
Epithelioid leiomyosarcoma	F > M. Gynecologic sites. Retroperitoneum, bowel wall or wall of vessel including IVC, renal vein	Sheets of polygonal cells with clear or finely granular cytoplasm. Not usually pleomorphic. Typical spindle cell areas can coexist	SMA+, desmin+, h-caldesmon+, CD117−. Some HMB45+
Epithelioid gastrointestinal stromal tumor	Related to wall of any part of alimentary tract (most commonly stomach, small intestine), Also, in retroperitoneum, omentum	Sheets of clear or epithelioid cells often with a focal spindle component. Organoid pattern, plasmacytoid or rhabdoid change can be seen	CD117+, DOG1+, CD34+, h-caldesmon+. SMA variable, desmin+ rarely, S100 protein+ rarely. CK sometimes+ after therapy. *KIT* or *PDGFRA* mutations

(*Continued*)

TABLE 12.1 Differential Diagnosis of Clear Cell and Granular Cell Tumors (Continued)

	Typical Clinical Features	Microscopic Features	Ancillary Investigations
Epithelioid pleomorphic liposarcoma	Deep soft tissue, extremities, rarely retroperitoneum, rarely subcutis	Sheets of clear or granular cells, pleomorphic lipoblasts. Usually focal, more typical pleomorphic liposarcoma elsewhere	S100 protein+, AE1/3+, melan-A+, SMA+
Renal cell carcinoma	Origin in kidney, can present as metastasis	Clear or granular cells in sheets, or adenopapillary formations Variable nuclear grade. Can have sarcomatoid change with divergent differentiation	CK+, EMA+, RCC-positive, CD117 (oncocytoma), vimentin (chromophobe carcinoma)
Adrenal cortical carcinoma	Origin in adrenal gland. Can be functioning or nonfunctioning	Sheets of clear or granular cells with small nuclei and occasional pleomorphism. Lacks sinusoidal vascular pattern	Inhibin+, melan-A+, CD56+, CK usually negative

TABLE 12.2 Differential Diagnosis of Histiocytic Tumors in Soft Tissue

	Typical Clinical Features	Microscopic Features	Ancillary Investigations
Juvenile xanthogranuloma, cutaneous	Infants, head and neck, trunk, proximal limbs. Yellow-brown plaque or nodule	Infiltrative dermal lesion. Sheets of histiocytes. Older lesions have more foamy cells and more Touton giant cells	CD68+, CD163+, S100 protein−, CD1a−
Juvenile xanthogranuloma, deep	Infants or young children, trunk, intramuscular	Monotonous sheets of macrophages, occasional foamy or multinucleated cells	CD68+, S100 protein−, CD1a−
Xanthoma	Skin or subcutis, rarely associated with tendon sheath or joint synovium. Hyperlipidemia or normolipidemia	Circumscribed or diffuse, sheets of foamy lipid-laden macrophages, variable admixture of siderophages, cholesterol clefts with giant cells, fibrosis	
Reticulohistiocytoma	Solitary cutaneous or multicentric reticulohistiocytosis affecting skin and synovium of joints	Multinucleated giant cells predominate, with plump histiocytes and mixed inflammatory cells	PAS+ (diastase resistant) CD68+, CD163+, MiTF+ (nuclear) in some
Epithelioid benign cutaneous fibrous histiocytoma	Dermal nodule, extremities or trunk, young adults	Overlying epidermal hyperplasia, bland plump cells, sometimes spindle component, peripheral collagen bundles, lymphocytic infiltrate	SMA+, CD34−, S100 protein−, desmin−
Rosai-Dorfman disease	Children or young adults. Lymph node or soft tissue mass	Large cells with abundant clear cytoplasm, phagocytosis of lymphocytes, mild or moderate focal nuclear enlargement and hyperchromasia. Admixed plasma cells, lymphocytes	S100 protein+, CD68+, CD1a−

(Continued)

TABLE 12.2 Differential Diagnosis of Histiocytic Tumors in Soft Tissue (Continued)

	Typical Clinical Features	Microscopic Features	Ancillary Investigations
Langerhans cell histiocytosis	Bone, lung, lymph node, spleen, pituitary, or other affected. Occasionally seen in a biopsy for suspected soft tissue tumor	Sheets of ovoid cells with folded or grooved nuclei, no nucleoli Admixed eosinophils	S100 protein+, CD1a+, langerin+ CD68+ in some. Birbeck granules on EM
Silicone granuloma	History of injection or implant, with recent change. Lumpy swelling	Foamy lipoblast-like cells, foreign body giant cells, birefringent material, fibrosis	CK–, S100 protein–
Malakoplakia	History of urinary tract infection. Can form perinephric mass	Sheets of discohesive polygonal cells with eosinophilic cytoplasm and dot-like inclusions (Michaelis-Gutmann)	Von Kossa stain+, CD68+
Granular histiocytic reaction	Related to surgery, often hip joint replacement	Nodules and sheets of histiocytes with granular, eosinophilic cytoplasm infiltrate fat. Sometimes adjacent amorphous foreign material	CD68+, S100 protein–, epithelial markers negative
Polyvinylpyrrolidone storage disease	Following IV plasma expander, exposure to some cosmetics or drugs containing PVP	Sheets of macrophages containing bubbly mucin-like material	Mucicarmine+, CD68+, CK–, EMA–, S100 protein–
Crystal-storing histiocytosis	Associated with B cell lymphoma or myeloma, rarely other causes	Cells expanded by cytoplasmic rod-like crystals	CD68+, S100 protein–
Mycobacterial spindle cell pseudotumor	HIV-positive patients, in lymph nodes, skin, spleen, lung, bone marrow, brain. Mycobacteria often atypical species	Sheets of spindle cells with storiform pattern and plump epithelioid macrophages, foamy and multinucleated cells	Ziehl-Neelsen stain for acid-fast bacilli is positive

Pathologic Features

This is a firm white tumor that can appear lobulated or multinodular (e-Fig. 12.1) and can be focally necrotic. Melanin pigmentation is rarely seen on gross examination. Histologically, the tumor is typically composed of uniform nests, separated by delicate connective tissue septa, of round cells with clear or finely granular eosinophilic cytoplasm and centrally located rounded nuclei each with a single basophilic nucleolus (Figs. 12.1 and 12.2, e-Figs. 12.2–12.9). Cells can be spindled with a fascicular architecture in some cases (e-Fig. 12.5), but pleomorphism is rare and mitotic activity often low. Multinucleated giant cells are seen in some examples (e-Fig. 12.4), and rarely there is myxoid change (e-Fig. 12.6). The intestinal subtype can have osteoclast-like giant cells. Melanin pigment is seen in tumor cells in about half of the soft tissue cases.

Ancillary Investigations

Reticulin staining shows a pattern of small nests (e-Fig. 12.10). Histochemical stains for melanin pigment (e.g., Fontana Masson) can sometime reveal it when unapparent on H and E, and melanosomes can be found with electron microscopy in many cases. Immunohistochemistry is diffusely positive for S100 protein (e-Fig. 12.11) and usually for HMB45 (e-Fig. 12.12) and melan-A. The latter two, however, are negative in the intestinal subtype. Neural markers and rarely cytokeratin have been reported in occasional cases. CD117 is usually negative in contrast to some cases of melanoma, but because many of the latter are also negative this is of limited value for diagnosis.

Genetically, clear cell sarcoma of soft parts is characterized by t(12;22)(q13;q12) with fusion of *EWS* and *ATF1* genes, as well as additional

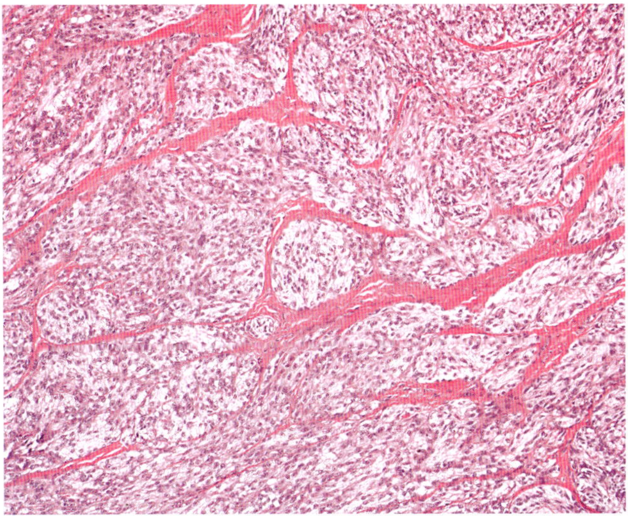

FIGURE 12.1 **Clear Cell Sarcoma.** Uniform tumor cells form variably sized nests separated by fibrous septa of varying thickness.

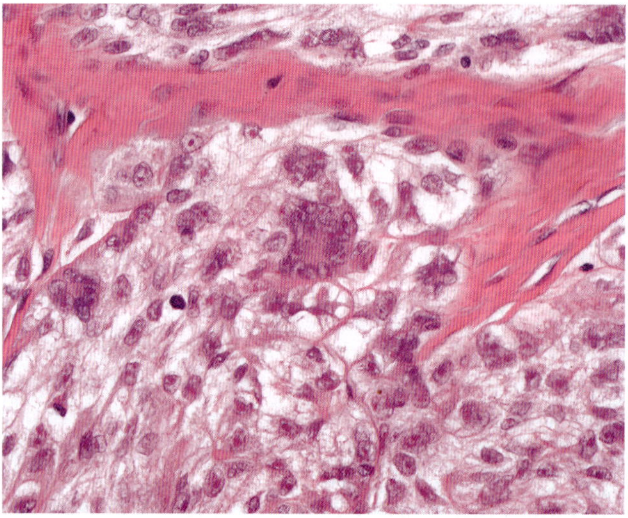

FIGURE 12.2 **Clear Cell Sarcoma.** The cells have round nuclei, distinct nucleoli, and moderate amounts of amphophilic cytoplasm. The multinucleated cell shown here is a frequent feature of these tumors in soft tissue.

aberrations.[3] The intestinal variant, though morphologically similar, has a different translocation, t(2;22)(q33;q12), which results in the EWS-CREB1 gene fusion. The subtypes are not wholly distinct since both fusion genes have been identified in examples of both.[4] These two translocations are identical to the genetic rearrangements in some examples of angiomatoid fibrous histiocytoma, a morphologically and immunophenotypically different entity (see Chapter 17).[5,6]

PARAGANGLIOMA

Clinical Features

Tumors of paraganglia arise in a variety of locations, of which the principal ones are carotid, mediastinal, retroperitoneal (from aorticosympathetic paraganglia or organ of Zuckerkandl), jugulotympanic, and vagal. Rarer sites are larynx, orbit, nasopharynx, heart, and cauda equina. Although the chromaffin reaction has fallen into disuse, the terminology extra-adrenal paraganglia is sometimes used for chromaffin-positive tumors, which are presumed to be similar to pheochromocytoma of adrenal medulla, and can cause raised amounts of urinary catecholamines, whereas those of chemoreceptor (branchiomeric) type are chromaffin-negative and usually nonfunctional.

Paragangliomas usually present with symptoms due to a mass, and are sometimes multifocal, especially in familial examples. Some, such as glomus jugulare tumors, can have functional effects, including on blood pressure, and vagal paragangliomas can affect cranial nerves at the base of the

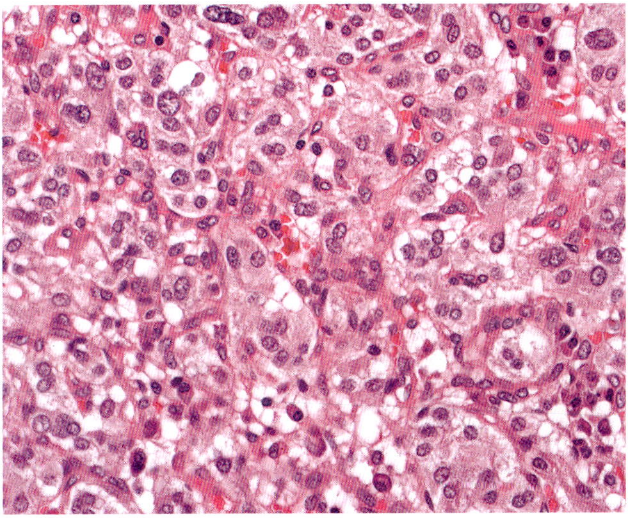

FIGURE 12.3 **Paraganglioma.** Cells in nested pattern. The cells are arranged in discrete nests, separated by delicate fibrovascular septa. The cells have rounded nuclei with small nucleoli. The variation in nuclear size and staining is typical and does not indicate malignant potential.

skull. Mediastinal tumors, arising from aortic arch or pulmonary artery paraganglia (anterior mediastinum) or sympathetic paraganglia (posterior mediastinum), can be part of Carney triad. Most paragangliomas are benign, but those in retroperitoneum or mediastinum tend to be more aggressive. Malignant examples can metastasize to lymph nodes and lung or bone.[7]

Pathologic Features

These tumors are usually encapsulated and are composed of round or polygonal cells with central nucleoli and finely granular, clear or sometimes vacuolated cytoplasm, arranged in nests or cords within a vascular stroma (Fig. 12.3, e-Figs. 12.13–12.16). The cells are larger than normal and nuclei can show pleomorphism. The nests are surrounded to a variable extent by sustentacular cells with elongated cytoplasmic processes. A more syncytial pattern can be found in retroperitoneal paragangliomas. Nuclear variation and hyperchromasia are not uncommon (e-Fig. 12.15), and the cells can display clear cytoplasm (e-Fig. 12.16). The stroma can be focally hyalinized[8] (e-Fig. 12.17), and the vessels can be hemangiopericytomatous (e-Fig. 12.18), with both features coexisting in some examples. Features suggestive of malignancy include marked nuclear pleomorphism, mitotic activity, necrosis, vascular invasion. However, none is reliably predictive of behavior, and tumors without these features have metastasized.

Ancillary Investigations

The lesional cells are immunoreactive for chromogranin, synaptophysin, and neurofilament proteins and CD56 (e-Fig. 12.19), and the sustentacular cells are S100 protein–positive (e-Fig. 12.20). Electron microcopy shows dense core neuroendocrine granules 100 to 200 nm in diameter.

VARIANT

Gangliocytic paraganglioma is a rare submucosal tumor of the second part of the duodenum and periampullary area that is usually benign or locally recurrent and rarely metastasizes.[9] Similar tumors rarely occur in other locations. It is an infiltrative tumor composed of rounded carcinoid-like plump cells in paraganglioma-like nests, Schwann cell–like spindle cells, and ganglion cells (e-Figs. 12.21 and 12.22). The cells in the nests are positive for somatostatin, the spindle cells for S100 protein, and the ganglion cells for chromogranin and synaptophysin.

PARAGANGLIOMA-LIKE DERMAL MELANOCYTIC TUMOR

Clinical Features

This is a rare lesion that arises in the skin of the extremities mostly in adult females, usually as a small nodule.[10] Reported cases have not recurred.

Pathologic Features

The tumor is circumscribed or, less often, infiltrative and composed of closely packed but clearly delineated nests of cells separated by delicate fibrous septa (Fig. 12.4, e-Figs. 12.23 and 12.24). The cells are oval with minimal nuclear atypia, inconspicuous nucleoli, infrequent mitoses, and abundant clear or amphophilic cytoplasm.

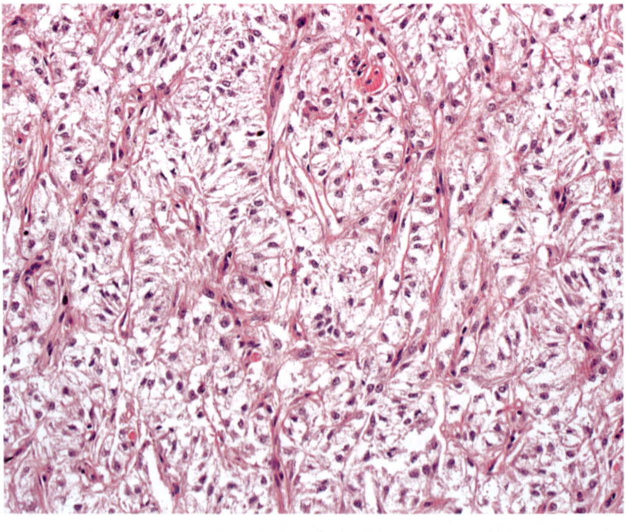

FIGURE 12.4 **Paraganglioma-like Melanocytic Tumor.** Well-defined nests of cells with clear cytoplasm. The cells are immunoreactive for S100 protein and melanocytic markers.

Ancillary Investigations

The cells are melanocytic and express S100 protein (e-Fig. 12.25) and HMB45, and melan-A (e-Fig. 12.26) in about half of the cases. Epithelial and myoid markers are negative. A rearrangement involving the EWSR1 gene has not been found in this entity, unlike in clear cell sarcoma, with which it can be confused.

GRANULAR CELL TUMOR

Clinical Features

This tumor, regarded as showing Schwann cell differentiation, is most common in adult females, and arises in skin (as a sometimes painful nodule), head and neck (especially tongue), and occasionally in viscera including upper aerodigestive tract, biliary tract, and posterior pituitary gland. Intraneural examples have been reported. Multiple granular cell tumors occur in 10% to 20% of patients. Most cases are benign; malignant variants, which are more often deeply located, are characterized by large size, rapid growth, ulceration, and metastasis to lymph nodes. Nonneural granular cell tumors of skin have also been described.[11]

Pathologic Features

The tumor is usually small (<3 cm in diameter) and poorly defined and infiltrates dermis, subcutis, nerves, and occasionally skeletal muscle (e-Fig. 12.27). The neoplastic cells are large and polygonal with abundant, finely or coarsely granular, eosinophilic cytoplasm with small, round, centrally located nuclei which can show occasional enlargement (e-Fig. 12.28). The granules are rounded and of variable size, eosinophilic, and sometime have a surrounding clear zone or halo (Fig. 12.5). The stroma is sometimes sclerosed (e-Fig. 12.29). The overlying epithelium can show pseudoepitheliomatous hyperplasia (e-Fig. 12.30) and care should be taken, especially in biopsies from tongue, not to misdiagnose squamous cell carcinoma by overlooking the granular cell tumor lying beneath. Atypical features include pleomorphism, prominent nucleoli, high nuclear to cytoplasmic ratio, spindling, more than two mitoses per ten high-power fields (at 200× magnification), and necrosis (Fig. 12.6). Tumors with three or more of these features have been regarded as histologically malignant, those with one or two features as atypical, and those that display only focal pleomorphism as benign.[12]

Ancillary Investigations

The intracytoplasmic granules are PAS-positive (diastase resistant). Lesional cells are positive for S100 protein (e-Fig. 12.31), NSE, and CD68; and nuclear immunoreactivity for TFE3 has been reported in rare examples. Ultrastructurally, the granules are secondary lysosomes of various types (e-Figs. 12.32 and 12.33).

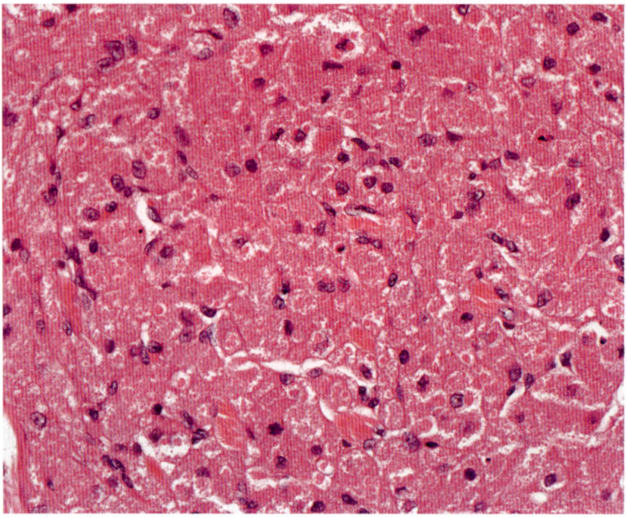

FIGURE 12.5 **Granular Cell Tumor.** Sheets of tumor cells with rounded small nuclei and abundant granular cytoplasm. The granules are derived from lysosomes and vary in size.

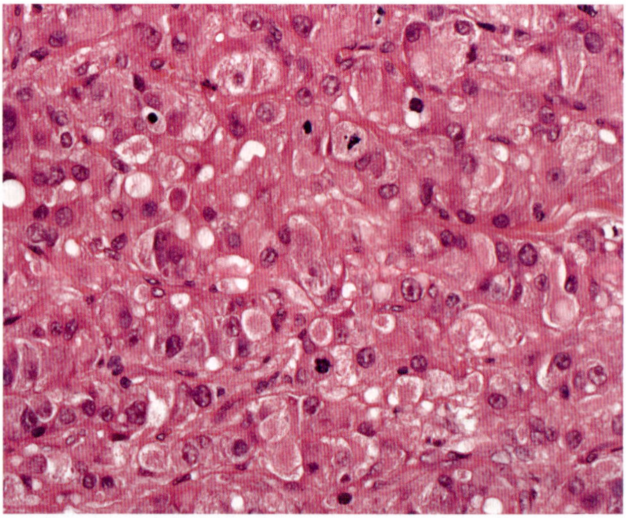

FIGURE 12.6 **Malignant Granular Cell Tumor.** Compared with Figure 12.5, the cells have a higher nuclear-cytoplasmic ratio, more prominent nucleoli and mitotic figures.

ALVEOLAR SOFT PART SARCOMA

Clinical Features

Alveolar soft part sarcoma is rare, accounting for fewer than 1% of soft tissue sarcomas,[13] and typically arising in second to fourth decades and more frequently in females. The most common sites are quadriceps and other thigh muscles, with occasional examples in other locations including bladder,[14] cervix, vagina, uterus, mediastinum, heart,[15] and GI tract. In children, the tumor more commonly originates in head and neck sites, notably tongue and orbit. It forms a large mass, often with necrosis, and is an aggressive sarcoma that metastasizes to lung, brain, and bone. Patients with metastases at presentation have a median survival of 40 months and a 5-year survival of 20%,[16] but those with localized disease can fare better, with survival figures of 77% at 2 years, 60% at 5 years, 38% at 10 years, and 15% at 20 years (median: 6 years).[17]

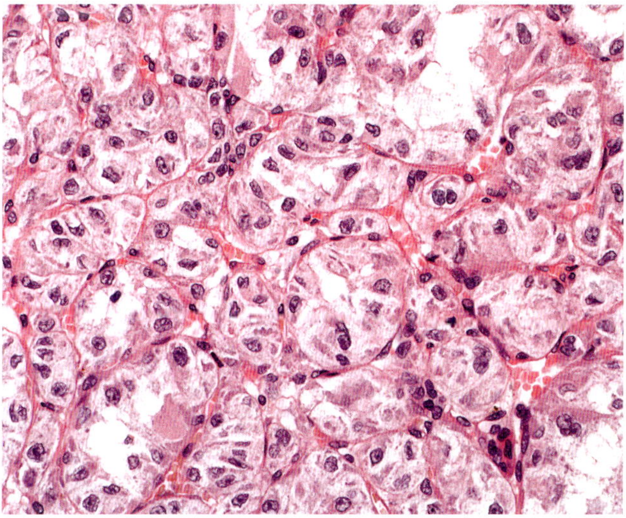

FIGURE 12.7 **Alveolar Soft Part Sarcoma.** Typical organoid pattern of large polygonal cells.

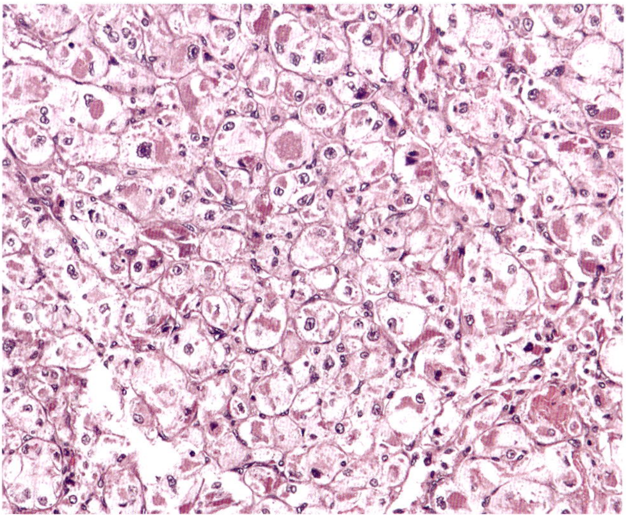

FIGURE 12.8 **Alveolar Soft Part Sarcoma.** Solid pattern with "single cell nests." This is more commonly seen in childhood examples.

Favorable prognostic factors are young age (especially for head and neck tumors) and small tumor size.[10]

Pathologic Features

Microscopically, there is a characteristic pattern of cell nests separated by thin fibrous septa with thin-walled blood vessels (Fig. 12.7, e-Figs. 12.34 and 12.35). The tumor cells are large and rounded with uniform vesicular nuclei and clear or finely granular cytoplasm. A more solid pattern of closely packed nests is sometimes seen (Fig. 12.8) especially in childhood cases. The two patterns are genetically identical.

Ancillary Investigations

Needle-like cytoplasmic crystals can be seen on PASD staining (e-Fig. 12.36). Ultrastructurally, these are well-defined, membrane-bound rhomboidal crystals with lattice-like filaments 4 to 6 nm in diameter with a periodicity of 10 nm (e-Fig. 12.37). Most alveolar soft part sarcomas show nuclear immunoreactivity with an antibody to TFE3 (also seen in Xp11 translocation-associated renal cell carcinomas and in some PEComas and granular cell tumors), and sometimes diffuse cytoplasmic positivity for desmin, but none for myogenin or h-caldesmon. Genetically, this tumor is characterized by an unbalanced (nonreciprocal) translocation, der(17) t(X;17)(p11;q25) resulting in the fusion gene *TFE3-ASPL*.[11] The fusion protein can be demonstrated using an antibody to TFE3.[13]

PECOMA

PEComas are mesenchymal tumors composed of histologically and immunohistochemically distinctive perivascular epithelioid cells. The nature of the cell is, however, conjectural since no normal counterpart has been described. The PEComa "family" now includes angiomyolipoma (AML), clear cell "sugar" tumor of lung, primary extrapulmonary sugar tumor, lymphangioleiomyomatosis (LAM), clear cell myomelanocytic tumor of the falciform ligament/ligamentum teres (CCMMT)[18] and similar tumors, and abdominopelvic sarcoma of perivascular epithelioid cells.[19,20] There is an association between some PEComas and tuberous sclerosis complex (TSC).[21] CCMMT, clear cell 'sugar' tumor, and epithelioid AML show considerable morphologic overlap, supporting the view that they are variants of a single entity. Nonetheless, the age, sex, presentation, and gross and microscopic appearances are different for each of these lesions. Some cases are not epithelioid, some are not perivascular, and some are not associated with TSC. It is, therefore, appropriate for the present to retain the individual terms to reflect not only morphologic but significant clinical differences as well.

Clinical Features

Most of the specific subtypes of PEComas have occurred in females. PEComas at soft tissue sites are extremely uncommon and are very rarely associated with TSC. One group comprises an entity initially termed "clear cell myomelanocytic tumor of the falciform ligament/ligamentum teres" (CCMMT).[18] The original report of CCMMT included seven tumors, six in females, with a mean age at diagnosis of 11 years (range: 3–21 years).[14] The tumors involved or were adjacent to the falciform ligament or ligamentum teres. Most patients remained free of disease, but one had a radiologically presumed lung metastasis. Similar cases have subsequently been described in soft tissue[15,16] in the urinary bladder,[22] and prostate,[23] liver[24] or common bile duct,[25] and in other locations. A large subset occurs in the female genital tract, especially the uterus. PEComas can grow to a large size and present with mass effects related to the anatomic location. The majority of soft tissue PEComas are benign, but clinically and histologically malignant examples are increasingly recognized.[26] One variant is abdominopelvic sarcoma of PEC,[20] in four females aged 19 to 41 years, who presented with a mass involving the serosa of the ileum, uterus, or pelvis. Lymphovascular invasion was present in all, lymph node metastasis in two cases, and metastasis to the ovary in one. Two patients developed widespread metastatic disease at 10 and 28 months. One patient had features of TSC.

Pathologic Features

The cells in PEComas are typically arranged in fascicular or nested patterns and disposed around and infiltrate the muscle walls of small to medium-sized blood vessels (Fig. 12.9, e-Figs. 12.38–12.43). CCMT and soft tissue lesions predominantly comprise moderately sized spindle cells with small, centrally located round to oval nuclei, small distinct nucleoli, and faintly eosinophilic to clear cytoplasm, the latter sometimes manifesting

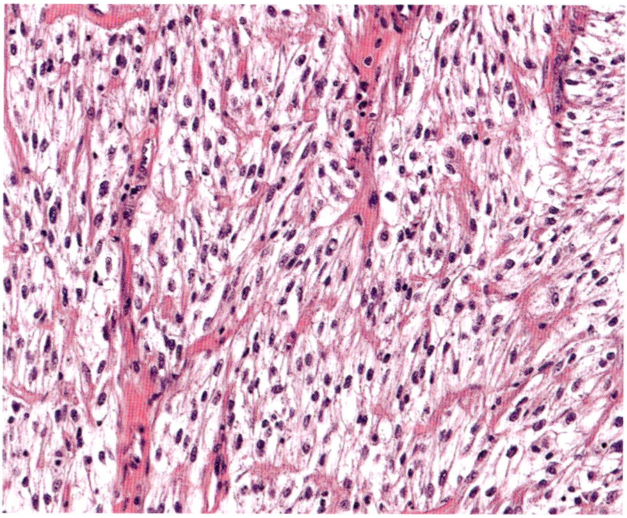

FIGURE 12.9 **PEComa.** Nests of cells with clear cytoplasm, delineated by slender fibrous septa.

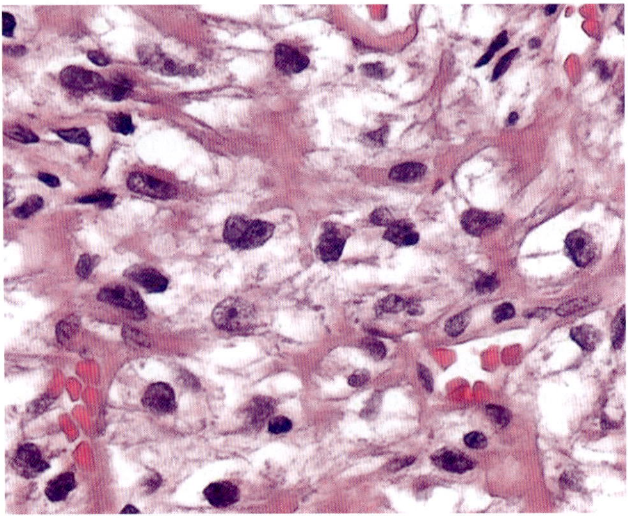

FIGURE 12.10 **PEComa.** The cells have clear cytoplasm and uniform rounded nuclei with small central nucleoli.

a perinuclear eosinophilic zone (Fig. 12.10). There is sometimes focally marked nuclear atypia, but mitotic activity is low. Periluminal cells are more frequently epithelioid and the more peripheral cells spindle shaped. Fatty change can be seen, especially in the peripheral cells, so that cells mimic lipoblasts. The differential diagnosis can therefore include carcinomas, smooth muscle tumors, clear cell sarcoma, and adipocytic tumors. A sclerosing variant has been described (e-Fig. 12.41).

PEComas displaying any combination of infiltrative growth, marked hypercellularity, nuclear enlargement and hyperchromasia, high mitotic activity, atypical mitotic figures, and coagulative necrosis should be regarded as malignant (e-Figs. 12.44–12.46). Predictors for malignancy include size >7 cm, mitoses >1 per 50 hpf, and necrosis,[27] and large size might also be an adverse prognostic factor. Abdominopelvic PEComas have overlapping features of clear cell "sugar" tumor of the lung and epithelioid angiomyolipoma, displaying sheets of large polygonal cells with glycogen-rich cytoplasm and moderately pleomorphic nuclei, a delicate vasculature, necrosis, and occasional mitotic figures.

Ancillary Investigations

PEComas coexpress melanocytic markers HMB-45 (in a granular pattern in cytoplasm), melan-A, tyrosinase, and microphthalmia transcription factor (MiTF) (in nuclei) (e-Figs. 12.47 and 12.48) and also muscle markers, such as smooth muscle actin, panmuscle actin, muscle myosin, calponin, and sometimes h-caldesmon. Desmin is less often positive. The spindle cells tend to express smooth muscle differentiation, whereas melanocytic differentiation is more frequently found in cells with epithelioid morphology.

The most sensitive melanocytic markers for the diagnosis of PEC are HMB45 (in about 80% of AML), melan-A, and MiTF. About a third of PEComas also express S100 protein, usually focally; this is in contrast to melanoma that usually has diffuse immunoreactivity for S100 protein and is generally more pleomorphic. Some PEComas are immunoreactive for TFE3.[27] Among other markers, cytokeratin positivity can occasionally be seen, and CD117 is expressed in some examples, predominantly in the cytoplasm of both spindle and epithelioid cells, with strong perinuclear staining in vacuolated clear epithelioid cells.[27] Cathepsin-K positivity has also been found in some PEComas[28] and Xp11.2 translocation carcinomas.[29] Ultrastructurally, PEComas have cytoplasmic glycogen and lipid droplets, and rare premelanosomes or stage II melanosomes. They lack junctions, microlumina, and microvilli, but external lamina has been described.[30]

The genes involved in TSC are TSC1 on chromosome 9q34 and TSC2 on chromosome 16p13.3. LOH mainly at the TSC2-containing region has been found in both sporadic and TSC-associated AML,[31] and allelic alterations in the same region in PEComa.[32] These genes relate to enzymes involved in catecholamine metabolism and melanin formation. A small number of CCMMT have also been shown to lack tuberin expression. One case studied cytogenetically disclosed a t(3;10) rearrangement.[18]

VARIANT

Uterine PEComas occur in middle-aged patients (mean: 54 years), and two microscopic types have been described.[33] Group A tumors, composed of cells with clear to pale granular cytoplasm, demonstrated a tongue-like growth pattern resembling low-grade endometrial stromal sarcoma and were diffusely positive for HMB-45 and SMA. Group B tumors were composed of epithelioid cells, smaller numbers of which were HMB-45–positive. They also featured extensive SMA and a lesser degree of the endometrial stromal sarcoma-like growth pattern. Two of the four patients with group B tumors had pelvic lymph nodes involved by LAM, and one of these patients had TSC. These PEComas and epithelioid smooth muscle tumors were parts of a continuous histologic spectrum. A similar possible continuum between epithelioid smooth muscle tumors and PEComas has been suggested by Silva et al.[34] Notwithstanding their morphology, these tumors appear unrelated to endometrial stromal sarcoma.

CHORDOMA

Clinical Features

Chordoma is a tumor that arises in adult life in notochordal remnants in the vertebral column at sites from base of skull to sacrum and coccyx, with predominance at either end. Examples can present in soft tissue in the lower back or pelvis, with a mass, constipation, or neural symptoms. Head and neck examples can cause pain or cranial nerve damage, and

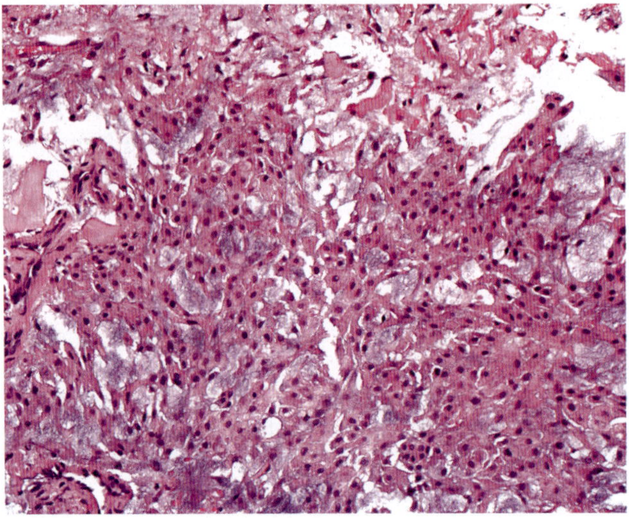

FIGURE 12.11 **Chordoma.** Cords and sheets of cells with eosinophilic cytoplasm and extracellular mucin secretion. There is minimal nuclear pleomorphism and mitotic activity.

sphenooccipital tumors can present as a mass in the nose or paranasal sinuses. Chordomas can metastasize to lymph nodes, lung, bone, and soft tissue sites. Some tumors express PDGFRB and have responded to therapy with the receptor tyrosine kinase inhibitor imatinib.[27]

Pathologic Features

The tumor forms a lobulated, circumscribed mass. It is composed of sheets or cords of tumor cells with vacuolated eosinophilic cytoplasm and variable nuclear atypia, in myxoid stroma (Fig. 12.11, e-Figs. 12.49 and 12.50). The tumor can resemble adenocarcinoma, and can resemble chondrosarcoma (chondroid chordoma), especially in sphenooccipital tumors. Rarely, chordomas undergo dedifferentiation, forming high-grade undifferentiated pleomorphic sarcoma in a demarcated focus contiguous with the typical chordoma (e-Fig. 12.51).[35]

Ancillary Investigations

The tumor cells are immunoreactive for epithelial antigens (cytokeratins, EMA) (e-Fig. 12.52) and S100 protein (e-Fig. 12.53). Cathepsin-K positivity can help distinguish chordoma from chondrosarcoma.[36] Immunoreactivity with an antibody to brachyury appears to be specific for chordoma and is negative in adenocarcinomas and chondrosarcoma.[37]

RHABDOMYOMA

Clinical Features

This is a benign tumor showing skeletal muscle differentiation, which can arise in the heart or in extracardiac locations. The adult type occurs mainly in the sixth and seventh decades, and the fetal type is more common in the first years of life. The commonest sites are in the head and neck region (larynx, oral cavity, pharynx, neck), more often in males, or female genital tract (vagina, vulva, and rarely cervix). It presents as a painless mass that is frequently an incidental finding, although lesions involving the airway can be symptomatic. Most lesions do not recur after surgical excision. Rhabdomyomatous mesenchymal hamartoma is a very rare benign lesion composed of a mixture of rhabdomyoblasts, adipose tissue, and fibrous tissue. Nearly all cases are congenital and occur in the head and neck region, though occasional examples have been reported in adults.[38]

Pathologic Features

The lesions are small and usually solitary. Adult-type rhabdomyomas[39] are composed of large rounded or epithelioid-like cells with large amounts of eosinophilic cytoplasm, sometimes vacuolated (spider cells) (Fig. 12.12). Cross striations may be found. The nuclei are small and bland, though some have prominent nucleoli, and mitoses are rare or absent. Fetal rhabdomyomas[40] are classified as immature or intermediate. The immature (myxoid) type has bland spindle cells with eosinophilic cytoplasm, some of which have striations, in a myxoid stroma, without mitoses, pleomorphism, or necrosis (unlike in embryonal rhabdomyosarcoma). Intermediate or juvenile fetal rhabdomyoma is characterized by bundles of spindle cells with variable skeletal muscle differentiation including strap cells (with cross-striations), smooth-muscle like cells, and scattered rhabdomyoblast-like cells (e-Fig. 12.54). Mitoses, significant atypia, and necrosis are absent (unlike in spindle cell rhabdomyosarcoma). The stroma is fibrous rather than myxoid.

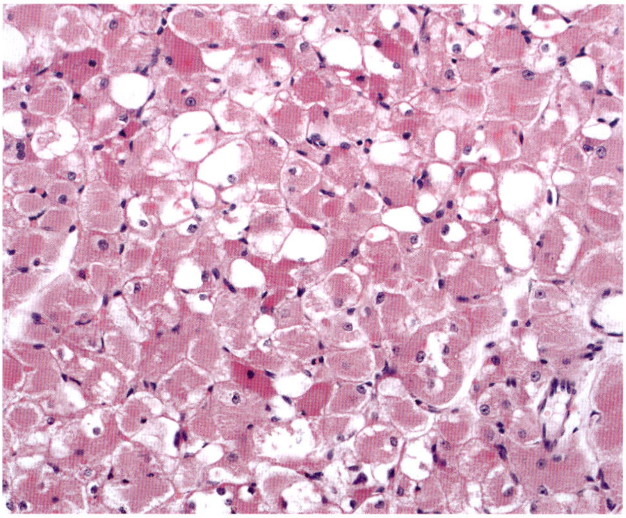

FIGURE 12.12 **Rhabdomyoma, Adult Type.** Large cells with abundant cytoplasm and vacuolated "spider" cells are features of this tumor.

Ancillary Investigations

The lesional cells are diffusely positive for desmin and display nuclear immunoreactivity for myogenin and MyoD1.

LESIONS OF HISTIOCYTES

A number of soft tissue tumors are composed predominantly of histiocytes or histiocyte-like cells, and others are formed of histiocytes with various types of included material. These are considered below, and the differential diagnosis is summarized in Table 12.2.

JUVENILE XANTHOGRANULOMA

Clinical Features

This can be cutaneous or rarely deep. Cutaneous juvenile xanthogranuloma is a tumor predominantly of the first year of life, although examples can be seen in adults. There is an increased incidence in neurofibromatosis type 1, and an association with juvenile myelomonocytic leukemia. The common sites are head and neck, trunk and proximal limbs, presenting as a yellow-brown plaque or nodule. Deep lesions occur in infants and young children as solitary intramuscular lesions mainly in the trunk.[41] Childhood lesions usually regress, but adult lesions can persist. Erdheim-Chester disease is a related lipid-storing condition that usually occurs in adults in soft tissue, bone, and lung.[42]

Pathologic Features

Cutaneous juvenile xanthogranuloma has epidermal thinning (with slender elongated rete ridges) over a dense dermal infiltrate of polygonal or spindled histiocytes with eosinophilic, finely vacuolated cytoplasm

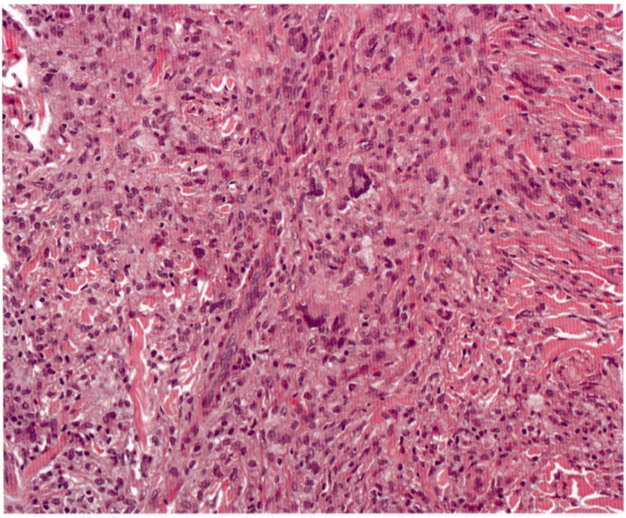

FIGURE 12.13 **Juvenile Xanthogranuloma.** There is a mixture of histiocyte, inflammatory cells, and multinucleated giant cells with variable fibrosis.

(Fig. 12.13, e-Figs. 12.55–12.58). There is a sprinkling of mixed inflammatory cells including eosinophils. Touton-type giant cells with wreath-like nuclei are a characteristic feature but are not always present in early lesions. Older lesions have more foamy cells and eventually fibrosis (e-Fig. 12.58). Deep juvenile xanthogranuloma is a rare infiltrative lesion, confined to infants and young children composed of sheets of uniform histiocyte-like cells, with few multinucleated or foamy cells, with occasional mitoses (e-Figs. 12.59–12.61).

Ancillary Investigations

The histiocytes in both cutaneous and deep forms are positive for CD68 and CD163[43] and negative for S100 protein and CD1a.

ROSAI-DORFMAN DISEASE

Clinical Features

This is a proliferation of histiocytes that affects lymph nodes, especially in children and young adults, but can also arise as solitary or multiple lesions in skin, extranodal soft tissue, or viscera.[44] It presents as a firm, usually ill-defined mass. The disease is benign and self-limiting, and often regresses without intervention.

Pathologic Features

The appearances are usually less distinctive in soft tissue than in lymph nodes. The lesional cell is polygonal, but can also be spindled with an ill-defined storiform pattern (e-Fig. 12.62). The nuclei are usually uniform but can be enlarged and hyperchromatic, or multinucleated. The cytoplasm is abundant and clear, and typically contains phagocytosed lymphocytes (emperipolesis) (e-Fig. 12.63). Additional features include plasma cells, lymphocytes, and collagen formation.

Ancillary Investigations

The lesional cells are positive for S100 protein in nuclei and cytoplasm, showing in the latter a characteristic pattern of diffuse positivity (e-Fig. 12.64). CD68 and CD163[43] are also positive and CD1a and langerin are negative.

LANGERHANS CELL HISTIOCYTOSIS (EOSINOPHILIC GRANULOMA, HISTIOCYTOSIS X)

This usually involves bone, lymphoid tissue, lung, pituitary, or other organs but can occasionally appear in a biopsy as a suspected soft tissue tumor. It is composed of Langerhans cells that are large polygonal cells with vesicular, grooved ("coffee-bean") or folded nuclei, without nucleoli (e-Figs. 12.65 and 12.66). There are variable numbers of admixed eosinophils. The lesional cells are immunoreactive for S100, CD1a, CD163, langerin, and sometimes CD68, and electron microscopy shows characteristic Birbeck granules.

HISTIOCYTIC INCLUSION DISORDERS

Xanthomas are aggregates of lipid-containing histiocytes that can develop in normolipidemic patients or in the course of primary or secondary hyperlipidemia. They usually arise in skin or subcutis but are sometimes are associated with tendon sheaths or synovium. They appear as yellow or brown nodules, and are sometimes infiltrative. Microscopically, there are sheets of foamy histiocytes (e-Fig. 12.67) with variable amounts of hemosiderin, cholesterol clefts with giant cells and fibrosis. A plexiform variant is described (see Chapter 22).

Silicone granuloma is considered in Chapter 15. Awareness of the clinical history of silicone injection can prevent misdiagnosis. **Malakoplakia** can involve soft tissues especially of retroperitoneum by extension from the renal pelvis. It has characteristic eosinophilic macrophages (e-Fig. 12.68) with Michaelis-Gutmann bodies which can be highlighted by a von Kossa or Alizarin Red stain for calcium (e-Fig. 12.69). **Granular histiocytic reaction** is a term applied to aggregates of histiocytes with granular cytoplasm that form, usually in the abdomen or pelvis, at sites of surgical trauma, such as hip arthroplasty.[45] The lesional cells are CD68-positive and lack epithelial markers. **Polyvinylpyrrolidone (PVP) storage disease** affects skin and also bone marrow and lung, with accumulations of histiocytes containing PVP. This was formerly employed as a plasma expander but is now used in various products including cosmetics, adhesives, and some medications. The cells contain characteristic bubbly bluish material (e-Figs. 12.70 and 12.71) which stains positively with mucicarmine and also with stains for amyloid such as Congo red. An adjacent giant cell granulomatous reaction can also be seen.[46] The lesional cells can be mistaken for signet ring cells of adenocarcinoma, but lack atypia and on immunohistochemistry are negative for cytokeratins and EMA. **Crystal storing histiocytosis** is a rare condition that is mostly associated with B cell lymphoid neoplasia, especially plasma cell proliferations, MALT lymphoma and marginal zone lymphoma, in which there is cytoplasmic accumulation of immunoglobulins in macrophages in viscera, skin, or soft tissue (e-Fig. 12.72).[47] A similar phenomenon has been reported in eosinophilic colitis, where the inclusions resembled Charcot-Leyden crystals, and following clofazimine therapy for leprosy. The cytoplasm of the affected cells is expanded by abundant rod-like or rectangular crystalline material. The cells are CD68-positive and S100 protein–negative. **Mycobacterial spindle cell pseudotumor** occurs in HIV-positive patients and affects lymph nodes, skin,[48] and, occasionally, other sites such as spleen, lung, bone narrow, and brain. It results from the concentration within macrophages of *Mycobacterium tuberculosis* or atypical mycobacteria such as *Mycobacterium avium intracellulare*. The lesion is composed of sheets of spindled and epithelioid histiocytes (e-Figs. 12.73 and 12.74), focally in a storiform pattern, with foam cells and multinucleated giant cells. A stain for acid-fast bacilli (Ziehl-Neelsen) reveals the cells to be packed with organisms (e-Fig. 12.75).

REFERENCES

1. Lucas DR, Nascimento AG, Sim FH. Clear cell sarcoma of soft tissues. Mayo Clinic experience with 35 cases. *Am J Surg Pathol.* 1992;16:1197–1204.
2. Clark MA, Johnson MB, Thway K, et al. Clear cell sarcoma (melanoma of soft parts): the Royal Marsden Hospital experience. *Eur J Surg Oncol.* 2008;34:800–804.
3. Hisaoka M, Ishida T, Kuo TT, et al. Clear cell sarcoma of soft tissue: a clinicopathologic, immunohistochemical, and molecular analysis of 33 cases. *Am J Surg Pathol.* 2008;32:452–460.
4. Wang WL, Mayordomo E, Zhang W, et al. Detection and characterization of EWSR1/ATF1 and EWSR1/CREB1 chimeric transcripts in clear cell sarcoma (melanoma of soft parts). *Mod Pathol.* 2009;22:1201–1209.
5. Thway K. Angiomatoid fibrous histiocytoma: a review with recent genetic findings. *Arch Pathol Lab Med.* 2008;132:273–277.
6. Rossi S, Szuhai K, Ijszenga M, et al. EWSR1-CREB1 and EWSR1-ATF1 fusion genes in angiomatoid fibrous histiocytoma. *Clin Cancer Res.* 2007;13:7322–7328.
7. Wasserman PG, Savargaonkar P. Paragangliomas: classification, pathology, and differential diagnosis. *Otolaryngol Clin North Am.* 2001;34:845–862, v–vi.
8. Plaza JA, Wakely PE Jr, Moran C, et al. Sclerosing paraganglioma: report of 19 cases of an unusual variant of neuroendocrine tumor that may be mistaken for an aggressive malignant neoplasm. *Am J Surg Pathol.* 2006;30:7–12.
9. Garbrecht N, Anlauf M, Schmitt A, et al. Somatostatin-producing neuroendocrine tumors of the duodenum and pancreas: incidence, types, biological behavior, association with inherited syndromes, and functional activity. *Endocr Relat Cancer.* 2008;15:229–241.
10. Deyrup AT, Althof P, Zhou M, et al. Paraganglioma-like dermal melanocytic tumor: a unique entity distinct from cellular blue nevus, clear cell sarcoma, and cutaneous melanoma. *Am J Surg Pathol.* 2004;28:1579–1586.
11. Lazar AJ, Fletcher CD. Primitive nonneural granular cell tumors of skin: clinicopathologic analysis of 13 cases. *Am J Surg Pathol.* 2005;29:927–934.
12. Fanburg-Smith JC, Meis-Kindblom JM, Fante R, et al. Malignant granular cell tumor of soft tissue: diagnostic criteria and clinicopathologic correlation. *Am J Surg Pathol.* 1998;22:779–794.
13. Folpe AL, Deyrup AT. Alveolar soft-part sarcoma: a review and update. *J Clin Pathol.* 2006;59:1127–1132.
14. Amin MB, Patel RM, Oliveira P, et al. Alveolar soft-part sarcoma of the urinary bladder with urethral recurrence: a unique case with emphasis on differential diagnoses and diagnostic utility of an immunohistochemical panel including TFE3. *Am J Surg Pathol.* 2006;30:1322–1325.
15. Luo J, Melnick S, Rossi A, et al. Primary cardiac alveolar soft part sarcoma. A report of the first observed case with molecular diagnostics corroboration. *Pediatr Dev Pathol.* 2008;11:142–147.
16. Portera CA Jr, Ho V, Patel SR, et al. Alveolar soft part sarcoma: clinical course and patterns of metastasis in 70 patients treated at a single institution. *Cancer.* 2001;91:585–591.
17. Lieberman PH, Brennan MF, Kimmel M, et al. Alveolar soft-part sarcoma. A clinicopathologic study of half a century. *Cancer.* 1989;63:1–13.
18. Folpe AL, Goodman ZD, Ishak KG, et al. Clear cell myomelanocytic tumor of the falciform ligament/ligamentum teres: a novel member of the perivascular epithelioid clear cell family of tumors with a predilection for children and young adults. *Am J Surg Pathol.* 2000;24:1239–1246.

19. Folpe AL, Kwiatkowski DJ. Perivascular epithelioid cell neoplasms: pathology and pathogenesis. *Hum Pathol.* 2010;41:1–15.
20. Bonetti F, Martignoni G, Colato C, et al. Abdominopelvic sarcoma of perivascular epithelioid cells. Report of four cases in young women, one with tuberous sclerosis. *Mod Pathol.* 2001;14:563–568.
21. Bonetti F, Pea M, Martignoni G, et al. The perivascular epithelioid cell and related lesions. *Adv Anat Pathol.* 1997;4:343–358.
22. Pan CC, Yu IT, Yang AH, et al. Clear cell myomelanocytic tumor of the urinary bladder. *Am J Surg Pathol.* 2003;27:689–692.
23. Pan CC, Yang AH, Chiang H. Malignant perivascular epithelioid cell tumor involving the prostate. *Arch Pathol Lab Med.* 2003;127:E96–E98.
24. Zimmermann A, von der Brelie C, Berger B, et al. Primary perivascular epithelioid cell tumor of the liver not related to hepatic ligaments: hepatic PEComa as an emerging entity. *Histol Histopathol.* 2008;23:1185–1193.
25. Sadeghi S, Krigman H, Maluf H. Perivascular epithelioid clear cell tumor of the common bile duct. *Am J Surg Pathol.* 2004;28:1107–1110.
26. Harris GC, McCulloch TA, Perks G, et al. Malignant perivascular epithelioid cell tumour ("PEComa") of soft tissue: a unique case. *Am J Surg Pathol.* 2004;28:1655–1658.
27. Folpe AL, Mentzel T, Lehr HA, et al. Perivascular epithelioid cell neoplasms (PEComas) of soft tissue and gynecologic origin: a clinicopathologic study of 24 cases. *Mod Pathol.* 2005;18:14A.
28. Chilosi M, Pea M, Martignoni G, et al. Cathepsin-k expression in pulmonary lymphangioleiomyomatosis. *Mod Pathol.* 2009;22:161–166.
29. Martignoni G, Pea M, Gobbo S, et al. Cathepsin-K immunoreactivity distinguishes MiTF/TFE family renal translocation carcinomas from other renal carcinomas. *Mod Pathol.* 2009;22:1016–1022.
30. Tanaka Y, Ijiri R, Kato K, et al. HMB-45/melan-A and smooth muscle actin-positive clear-cell epithelioid tumor arising in the ligamentum teres hepatis: additional example of clear cell "sugar" tumors. *Am J Surg Pathol.* 2000;24:1295–1299.
31. Henske EP, Neumann HP, Scheithauer BW, et al. Loss of heterozygosity in the tuberous sclerosis (TSC2) region of chromosome band 16p13 occurs in sporadic as well as TSC-associated renal angiomyolipomas. *Genes Chromosomes Cancer.* 1995;13:295–298.
32. Pan CC, Chung MY, Ng KF, et al. Constant allelic alteration on chromosome 16p (TSC2 gene) in perivascular epithelioid cell tumour (PEComa): genetic evidence for the relationship of PEComa with angiomyolipoma. *J Pathol.* 2008;214:387–393.
33. Vang R, Kempson RL. Perivascular epithelioid cell tumor ("PEComa") of the uterus: a subset of HMB-45-positive epithelioid mesenchymal neoplasms with an uncertain relationship to pure smooth muscle tumors. *Am J Surg Pathol.* 2002;26:1–13.
34. Silva EG, Deavers MT, Bodurka DC, et al. Uterine epithelioid leiomyosarcomas with clear cells: reactivity with HMB-45 and the concept of PEComa. *Am J Surg Pathol.* 2004;28:244–249.
35. Meis JM. "Dedifferentiation" in bone and soft-tissue tumors. A histological indicator of tumor progression. *Pathol Annu.* 1991;26(Pt 1):37–62.
36. Haeckel C, Krueger S, Kuester D, et al. Expression of cathepsin K in chordoma. *Hum Pathol.* 2000;31:834–840.
37. Oakley GJ, Fuhrer K, Seethala RR. Brachyury, SOX-9, and podoplanin, new markers in the skull base chordoma vs chondrosarcoma differential: a tissue microarray-based comparative analysis. *Mod Pathol.* 2008;21:1461–1469.
38. Brinster NK, Farmer ER. Rhabdomyomatous mesenchymal hamartoma presenting on a digit. *J Cutan Pathol.* 2009;36:61–63.

39. Cleveland DB, Chen SY, Allen CM, et al. Adult rhabdomyoma. A light microscopic, ultrastructural, virologic, and immunologic analysis. *Oral Surg Oral Med Oral Pathol.* 1994;77:147–153.
40. Kapadia SB, Meis JM, Frisman DM, et al. Fetal rhabdomyoma of the head and neck: a clinicopathologic and immunophenotypic study of 24 cases. *Hum Pathol.* 1993;24:754–765.
41. Nascimento AG. A clinicopathologic and immunohistochemical comparative study of cutaneous and intramuscular forms of juvenile xanthogranuloma. *Am J Surg Pathol.* 1997;21:645–652.
42. Wang CW, Colby TV. Histiocytic lesions and proliferations in the lung. *Semin Diagn Pathol.* 2007;24:162–182.
43. Nguyen TT, Schwartz EJ, West RB, et al. Expression of CD163 (hemoglobin scavenger receptor) in normal tissues, lymphomas, carcinomas, and sarcomas is largely restricted to the monocyte/macrophage lineage. *Am J Surg Pathol.* 2005;29:617–624.
44. Gaitonde S. Multifocal, extranodal sinus histiocytosis with massive lymphadenopathy: an overview. *Arch Pathol Lab Med.* 2007;131:1117–1121.
45. Hicks DG, Judkins AR, Sickel JZ, et al. Granular histiocytosis of pelvic lymph nodes following total hip arthroplasty. The presence of wear debris, cytokine production, and immunologically activated macrophages. *J Bone Joint Surg Am.* 1996;78:482–496.
46. Hizawa K, Inaba H, Nakanishi S, et al. Subcutaneous pseudosarcomatous polyvinylpyrrolidone granuloma. *Am J Surg Pathol.* 1984;8:393–398.
47. Pock L, Stuchlik D, Hercogova J. Crystal storing histiocytosis of the skin associated with multiple myeloma. *Int J Dermatol.* 2006;45:1408–1411.
48. Shiomi T, Yamamoto T, Manabe T. Mycobacterial spindle cell pseudotumor of the skin. *J Cutan Pathol.* 2007;34:346–351.

13

PLEOMORPHIC SOFT TISSUE TUMORS

INTRODUCTION

Many benign soft tissue tumors can occasionally show focal variation in size, shape, and staining properties of cells and particularly of nuclei. Nuclear pleomorphism, which relates to polyploidy, is not itself conclusive of malignancy and must be assessed in the overall clinical and morphologic context of individual cases. Thus, exclusion of malignancy in benign tumors with focal atypia is considered in the accounts of specific entities. These include pleomorphic fibroma (Chapter 4), atypical cutaneous fibrous histiocytoma (Chapter 4), symplastic leiomyoma (Chapter 6), nerve sheath tumors (Chapter 9), and atypical vascular proliferations (Chapter 17). Another group of lesions consistently show diffuse pleomorphism but do not metastasize. They include pleomorphic hyalinizing angiectatic tumor (PHAT) and atypical fibroxanthoma (AFX), and are considered in this chapter.

Pleomorphic sarcomas account for up to 15% of adult soft tissue sarcomas, and although often grouped together as high-grade sarcomas for management purposes, it is increasingly clear that, in many instances, the specific lineage or differentiation is predictive of behavior. This can often be very focal or detectable only by immunohistochemistry or other techniques. These tumors, therefore, require wide sampling and ancillary investigation. There remain up to 10% of pleomorphic sarcomas that appear to show no differentiation after using all available diagnostic methods. These tumors have historically been termed malignant fibrous histiocytoma, (MFH) but since its prescription in the 2002 WHO classification, the alternative designation of undifferentiated pleomorphic sarcoma (with modifiers according to epiphenomena) has gained favor. Undifferentiated carcinomas can also assume a pleomorphic sarcoma-like morphology, and many organ-based apparent sarcomas are really of epithelial origin. In the abdomen, most pleomorphic sarcomas are now considered to represent dedifferentiated liposarcoma (Chapters 5 and 16). The differential diagnosis of pleomorphic tumors is summarized in Table 13.1.

TABLE 13.1 Differential Diagnosis of Pleomorphic Soft Tissue Tumors

	Typical Clinical Features	Microscopic Features	Ancillary Investigations
Pleomorphic hyalinizing angiectatic tumor	Adults, solitary subcutaneous lesion, lower leg	Circumscribed, dilated vessels with fibrinoid or hyalinized walls, atypical spindle cells, nuclear inclusions, inflammation, hemosiderin, myxoid change. No mitoses or necrosis	CD34+ in many cases
Undifferentiated pleomorphic sarcoma (MFH)	Adults, deep soft tissue, proximal limbs. Intra-abdominal tumors are mostly dedifferentiated liposarcoma	Large tumor with hemorrhage and necrosis. Pleomorphic spindle, polygonal and multinucleated tumor cells, atypical mitoses. Variable inflammation and myxoid change. Residual myxofibrosarcomatous areas in some.	Focal SMA or desmin in some cases, rare CK+ cells, CD34+ in some. MDM2+, CDK4+ in intra-abdominal examples
Undifferentiated pleomorphic sarcoma with giant cells (giant cell MFH)	Adults, deep soft tissue, proximal limbs	As undifferentiated pleomorphic sarcoma with admixture of osteoclast-like giant cells in variable numbers, often associated with hemorrhage	Focal SMA or desmin in some cases, rare CK+ cells. CD34+ in some. Osteoclast-like giant cells are CD68+
Undifferentiated pleomorphic sarcoma with inflammatory cells (inflammatory MFH)	Adults, retroperitoneum and deep soft tissue of proximal limbs	Areas of typical undifferentiated pleomorphic sarcoma, sheets of foamy cells, some atypical, heavy infiltrate predominantly of neutrophils	Focal SMA or desmin in some cases. CD68+ in retroperitoneum many are dedifferentiated liposarcoma–MDM2+, CDK4+

(Continued)

TABLE 13.1 **Differential Diagnosis of Pleomorphic Soft Tissue Tumors (Continued)**

	Typical Clinical Features	Microscopic Features	Ancillary Investigations
Inflammatory well-differentiated liposarcoma	Adults, retroperit-oneum, groin	Scattered cells with large irregular hyperchromatic nuclei in dense lymphoid infiltrate. Areas of typical well-differentiated liposarcoma sometimes found	MDM2+, CDK4+
Pleomorphic myofibrosa-rcoma	Adults, deep soft tissue, proximal limbs	Pleomorphic spindle, polygonal and multinucleated tumor cells, atypical mitoses. Variable inflammation and myxoid change	SMA+ multifocally in subplasma lemmal “tram-track” pattern, desmin+ occasionally, h-caldesmon–
Atypical fibroxanthoma	Adults, head and neck, shoulder, superficial dome-shaped lesion with overlying epidermal thinning or ulceration. Dermal infiltrate is storiform, fascicular or patternless	Pleomorphic spindle and polygonal cells throughout, abnormal mitoses. Clear cell, spindle cell, and giant cell variants	SMA+ focally, CD10+
Myxofibros-arcoma	Subcutis, fascia, or deep soft tissue. Extremities, older adults. Recurrent	Multinodular, spindle cells in myxoid stroma, variable nuclear pleomorphism. Can merge with high-grade pleomorphic sarcomatous areas	CD34+ in many, SMA+ in pleomorphic areas

Myxoinflammatory fibroblastic sarcoma	Mostly extremities, adults. Cutaneous or subcutaneous, can involve tendons	Multinodular ill-defined myxoid foci with vacuolated fibroblasts, intervening cellular areas with Reed-Sternberg–like and atypical mononuclear cells, eosinophils, plasma cells, hemosiderin	CD34+ in some. Rare cases with t(1;10)(p22;q24)
Pleomorphic liposarcoma	Adults, deep soft tissue, limbs, rarely skin or subcutis	Undifferentiated pleomorphic sarcoma with variable numbers of pleomorphic lipoblasts, sometimes forming sheets. Rare epithelioid variant focally	S100 protein+, CK+ (epithelioid variant), melan-A+, (epithelioid variant)
Dedifferentiated liposarcoma	Older adults, large retroperitoneal tumor, recurrences frequent	Low-grade dedifferentiation: cellular fascicles with mild pleomorphism High-grade dedifferentiation: pleomorphic undifferentiated sarcoma, or myxofibrosarcoma-like. Heterologous osteochondroid or rhabdomyosarcomatous elements. Extensive sampling might show well	MDM2+, CDK4+, P16+ Desmin, SMA, CD34 all variably focally positive. FISH shows *MDM2* and *CDK4* amplification

(Continued)

TABLE 13.1 Differential Diagnosis of Pleomorphic Soft Tissue Tumors (Continued)

	Typical Clinical Features	Microscopic Features	Ancillary Investigations
		differentiated liposarcomatous component, but this can be absent especially in tumors in abdomen	
Dedifferentiated chondrosarcoma	Usually bony origin, can extend into soft tissue	Undifferentiated pleomorphic sarcoma with contiguous differentiated chondrosarcoma of varying grade	SMA+, S100 protein+ in chondroid area
Pleomorphic leiomyosarcoma	Older adults, limbs, abdomen, head and neck sites	At least two thirds of tumor is pleomorphic, but focally typical smooth muscle cells in fascicles are present. Pleomorphic component is undifferentiated pleomorphic sarcoma	SMA+, desmin+, h-caldesmon+ variably in both components but less frequent in undifferentiated component
Pleomorphic rhabdomyosarcoma	Rare, older adults M > F, proximal limbs, retroperitoneum, pelvis	Sheets of polygonal, round, or spindle cells with abundant eosinophilic cytoplasm, atypical mitoses, necrosis	Desmin+, myogenin+ (nuclei), MyoD1+ (nuclei), CD56+
Pleomorphic mesothelioma	Sheet-like mass involving pleura, peritoneal surface or omentum	Fascicles of pleomorphic spindle cells, tapered nuclei, scanty cytoplasm, mitoses, necrosis. Desmoplastic or hyalinized stroma	CK+ focally, calretinin+

Undifferentiated (sarcomatoid) carcinoma	Adults, visceral and soft tissue sites. History of primary carcinoma in some.	Pleomorphic spindle or epithelioid tumor cells in sheets, sometimes areas of epithelial morphology or overlying dysplasia	CK+, EMA+, CD34 negative, SMA+ in some, desmin negative, h-caldesmon–
Metastatic melanoma	Any age, history of primary melanoma	Pleomorphic spindle and epithelioid tumor cells, sometimes rhabdoid appearance. Melanin pigment rare.	S100 protein+ (diffuse), HMB45 and melan-A+ variably in epithelioid areas. Rare aberrant CK+ or desmin+
Anaplastic large cell lymphoma	Extranodal (soft tissue) involvement is usually associated with advanced nodal disease	Sheets of cells with prominent nucleoli, multinucleated forms	CD30+, ALK+, CD43+, CD45+, CD3+, TIA1+, t(2;5)(p23;q35), *TMP3-ALK* fusion

PLEOMORPHIC HYALINIZING ANGIECTATIC TUMOR

Clinical Features

This is a pseudosarcomatous lesion that arises mainly in adults (median: 50 years) of either sex in the ankle, foot or leg, and occasionally other sites, as a slowly growing, painless subcutaneous mass up to 19 cm in diameter (mean: 5 cm). Over a third of reported examples have recurred, so that adequate local excision with follow-up is indicated. Disease has sometimes persisted after resection, and in one example the recurrence resembled myxofibrosarcoma,[1] but none has metastasized.[2,3]

Pathologic Features

PHAT is circumscribed but nonencapsulated (e-Fig. 13.1), often with a hemorrhagic cut surface. The principal microscopic features (Fig. 13.1, e-Figs. 13.2–13.7) are (a) dilated blood vessels of varying size with subintimal and extravascular fibrinoid or collagenous material, extending into zones of stromal hyalinization, and (b) short spindle or ovoid cells, including many with hyperchromatic pleomorphic nuclei and often prominent nuclear pseudoinclusions (e-Figs. 13.6 and 13.7). Mitotic activity and necrosis are usually absent. Additional features include focal myxoid change, a variable component of fat, mast cells, foamy macrophages, and intracellular hemosiderin deposition.

Early lesions show an infiltrate of iron-laden spindle cells around vessels with myxoid change. This is followed by vascular ectasia and fibrin exudation, and subsequently increased cellularity and atypia with loss of fat.[3]

Ancillary Investigations

The lesional cells in the majority of PHAT display immunoreactivity for CD34 but are negative for S100 protein, which is helpful in the distinction

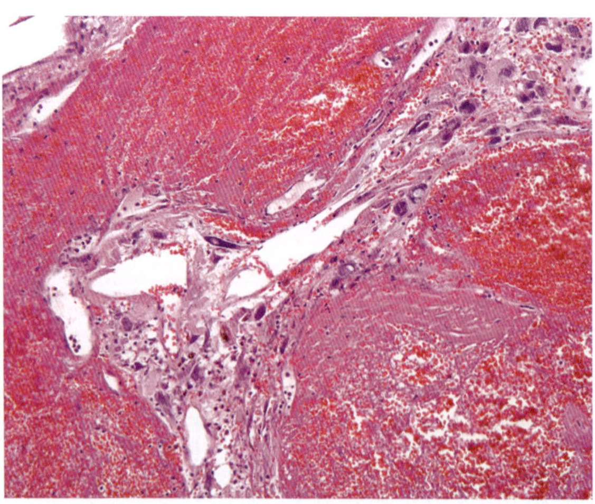

FIGURE 13.1 **Pleomorphic Hyalinizing Angiectatic Tumor.** Dilated and congested vessels with fibrinoid deposition in walls lie in a stroma containing cells with hyperchromatic pleomorphic nuclei and lymphocytes.

from schwannoma.[2,3] Electron microscopy does not reveal specific differentiation, but the cells are assumed to be fibroblastic.[2]

VARIANT

Hemosiderotic Fibrohistiocytic Lipomatous Lesion Early PHAT are very similar to cases that have been termed hemosiderotic fibrohistiocytic lipomatous lesion.[4–6] These are considered in more detail in Chapter 15. They occur mainly in females in fifth to seventh decades, in the ankle region with occasional examples at other sites. Most have a history of trauma and a correlation with venous stasis has been suggested.[7] Hemosiderotic fibrohistiocytic lipomatous lesions are circumscribed and composed of plump fibrohistiocytic-like cells (sometimes with intranuclear inclusions) in a septal and perivascular distribution in subcutaneous fat (e-Figs. 13.8 and 13.9). Other features include a focally myxoid stroma, aggregates of small vessels, and marked hemosiderin deposition. The lesional cells, as in PHAT, are immunoreactive for CD34 and also for calponin. About 50% recur.

PLEOMORPHIC SARCOMAS

These are generally high-grade neoplasms in which the common and predominant component is a mixture of undifferentiated spindle, polygonal or epithelioid, and multinucleated cells. Additional features include variable fibrosis, myxoid stroma, inflammatory infiltrate, hemorrhage, and necrosis. Many examples on detailed examination show foci of mesenchymal differentiation, such as lipoblastic or myoid cells, which allow specific categorization, and similar histological appearances can also be found in some undifferentiated carcinomas, melanomas, and mesotheliomas.

Prognostic factors in general include tumor size, grade, and location. Additionally, there is evidence that the presence of myoid differentiation, whether manifest morphologically or by immunohistochemistry, is an adverse prognostic factor.[8,9] Also, dedifferentiated liposarcoma in the abdomen has a better outcome than other pleomorphic sarcomas.[10] The pathologist should therefore attempt to subtype a pleomorphic sarcoma as far as possible to give maximum information for clinician and patient.

UNDIFFERENTIATED PLEOMORPHIC SARCOMA (MALIGNANT FIBROUS HISTIOCYTOMA)

The terminology of these tumors has been subject to repeated revisions. Until the 1960s, they were categorized as pleomorphic rhabdomyosarcoma, fibrosarcoma, or undifferentiated pleomorphic sarcoma. The term MFH was introduced in 1967, in the first AFIP fascicle on Soft Tissue Tumors, in the erroneous belief, based on tissue cultural studies of a mixed group of neoplasms, that they were composed of histiocytes that could demonstrate morphologic and functional properties of fibroblasts. A clinicopathologic series of MFH, published in 1972,[11] was followed by studies defining further morphologic types of MFH: giant cell,[12] inflammatory,[13] myxoid,[14] and angiomatoid.[15] MFH became the most common diagnosis among adult soft tissue sarcomas, and pleomorphic fibrosarcoma essentially disappeared. With the successive introduction of various diagnostic modalities, it became clear that many pleomorphic soft tissue tumors focally display specific differentiation at various levels. Immunohistochemistry showed absence of marrow-derived histiocytic antigens and presence of antigens associated with mesenchymal cells, including intermediate filaments.[16] Careful morphologic observation combined with immunohistochemical and genetic studies allow separation of other pleomorphic sarcomas such as pleomorphic liposarcoma or dedifferentiated liposarcoma (see Chapter 16), and of melanoma or poorly differentiated carcinoma.[17] The residual tumors are a genetically heterogeneous group of fascicular or storiform neoplasms composed of atypical spindle and polygonal cells which show no specific line of differentiation. The constituent cells are unrelated to histiocytes and, whether fusiform or plump and histiocyte-like, display ultrastructural features of fibroblasts that can sometimes manifest histiocytic properties including phagocytosis. In addition, many examples show at least focal myofibroblastic differentiation.

The original members of the MFH family have therefore been recategorized. Myxoid MFH is now regarded as myxofibrosarcoma, and the two patterns often coexist as low- and high-grade areas. Angiomatoid MFH, because of its low metastatic potential, has been downgraded to angiomatoid fibrous histiocytoma, but is in fact a translocation sarcoma with myoid differentiation and is unrelated to other "fibrohistiocytic" neoplasms. It is discussed in Chapter 17. Pleomorphic MFH is once again designated as undifferentiated pleomorphic sarcoma (some with giant or inflammatory cells), but being primarily composed of fibroblasts with or without myofibroblastic modulation, can be regarded as the pleomorphic form of fibrosarcoma.[18,19] The WHO 2002 classification allows the use of both the terms undifferentiated high-grade pleomorphic sarcoma (UPS) and MFH. Since the latter term, though inaccurate, is well established among clinicians, our current practice is to report them as undifferentiated pleomorphic sarcomas of MFH type.

Clinical Features

The majority of UPS arise in deep soft tissue in adults and predominantly in lower limb and trunk, with occasional cases in head and neck. Most similar tumors in the abdomen and retroperitoneum, and at least some of those in extremities,[20] represent dedifferentiated liposarcomas (see Chapters 5 and 16). UPS mostly occur in older adults after the sixth decade, with rare examples in childhood, and present as large, slowly growing masses with symptoms related to location. The course is one of local recurrence and metastasis.

Pathologic Features

Macroscopically, these are large, solid tumors with hemorrhage and necrosis (e-Fig. 13.10). Histologically, there are pleomorphic spindle and polygonal or large epithelioid cells with frequently abnormal mitotic activity, arranged in fascicular and storiform patterns (Figs. 13.2 and 13.3, e-Figs. 13.11–13.15). The polygonal cells can be multinucleated and often have abundant eosinophilic cytoplasm (e-Fig. 13.14). The stroma can show fibrosis, focal myxoid change (resembling myxofibrosarcoma) (e-Fig 13.15), necrosis, and variable infiltration by chronic inflammatory cells.

Ancillary Investigations

These tumors by definition do not show specific differentiation. There is often focal expression of smooth muscle actin (SMA), in a subplasmalemmal distribution (e-Fig. 13.16), indicating cells with myofibroblastic differentiation,[21] but widespread SMA positivity indicates classification as

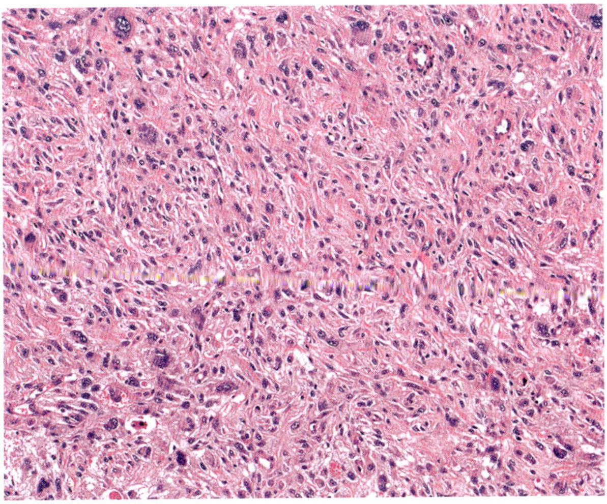

FIGURE 13.2 **Undifferentiated Pleomorphic Sarcoma.** Spindle and polygonal cells with variable pleomorphism are arranged in a vaguely storiform pattern in a fibrous stroma.

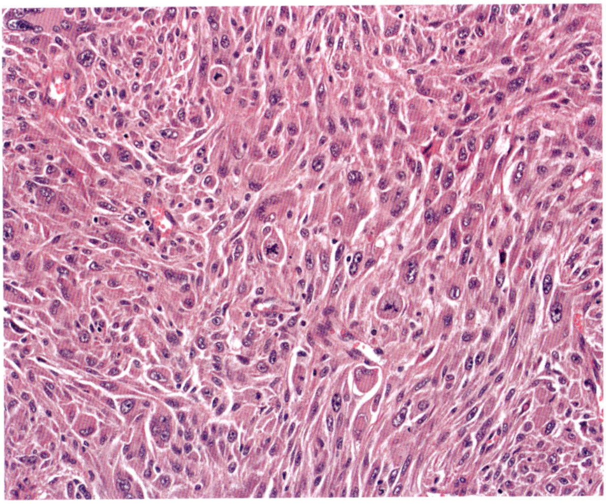

FIGURE 13.3 **Undifferentiated Pleomorphic Sarcoma.** Cells have variable amounts of eosinophilic cytoplasm and show abnormal mitotic figures.

pleomorphic myofibrosarcoma. Occasionally, scattered individual cells express desmin, or h-caldesmon, but a diagnosis of leiomyosarcoma should not be made in the absence of at least focal fascicular architecture and smooth muscle cytomorphology. Similarly, very focal aberrant expression of cytokeratins is well recognized in UPS,[16] but widespread immunoreactivity suggests a diagnosis of sarcomatoid carcinoma. The presence of any cytokeratin positivity should prompt further investigation for the latter, including exclusion of a primary tumor elsewhere. In this context, a reticulin stain can sometimes be useful in revealing a pattern of cell nests in carcinomas, unlike in sarcomas where the fibers are more often pericellular or disposed in parallel arrays. Similar considerations apply to sarcomatoid mesothelioma in the appropriate setting. Genetically, UPS are polyploid with no specific genetic rearrangements, and gene expression profiling shows a heterogeneous rather than a distinct group of tumors.[22]

UNDIFFERENTIATED PLEOMORPHIC SARCOMA WITH GIANT CELLS

This entity was originally described as giant cell tumor of soft tissue[12] and subsequently categorized as a giant cell variant of MFH.[23] It shows similar features to UPS with the addition of osteoclast-like giant cells.

Clinical Features

These tumors can be located in subcutaneous or deep soft tissue, but many superficial examples are now regarded as giant cell tumors of soft parts of low malignant potential. The prognosis relates to depth; about 65% of superficial tumors recur, and 0% to 15% metastasize, with corresponding figures for deeply located neoplasms of 40% and 50%. However, in one series, 50% of patients with superficial tumors and 57% of patients with deep-seated tumors died within 18 months of diagnosis.[24]

Pathologic Features

Microscopically, the tumor is multinodular, and composed of a background of pleomorphic spindle and polygonal cells with variable numbers of osteoclast-like giant cells, sometimes spindled and often in clusters (Fig. 13.4–13.5, e-Figs. 13.17–13.21). Foci of osteoid and bone formation can be seen, usually at the periphery (e-Fig. 13.21), but without atypical osteoblasts. The presence of malignant osteogenesis, however, indicates categorization as osteoclast-rich soft tissue osteosarcoma. UPS with osteoclast-like giant cells must be distinguished from (a) giant cell tumor of soft parts of low malignant potential, which lacks significant pleomorphism (but can also show mitotic activity and vascular invasion); (b) leiomyosarcoma with osteoclast-like giant cells (which shows focal fascicular architecture as well as expression of SMA, desmin, and h-caldesmon); and (c) undifferentiated carcinoma with osteoclast-like giant cells (which can arise at various sites, can show focal epithelial morphology, and usually expresses cytokeratins).

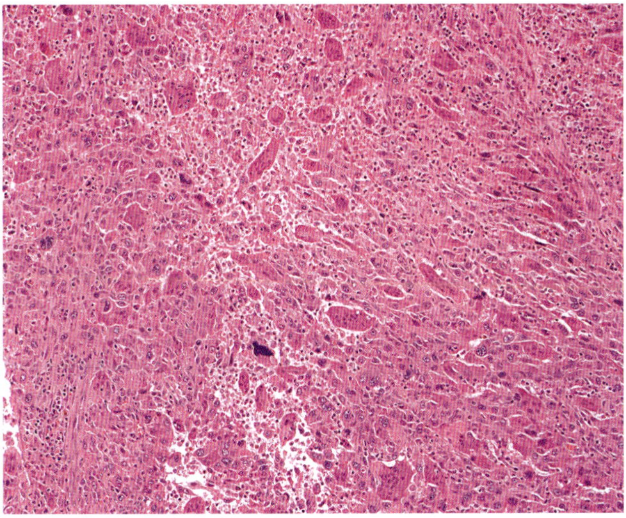

FIGURE 13.4 **Undifferentiated Pleomorphic Sarcoma with Giant Cells.** Osteoclastic giant cells are dispersed in a pleomorphic background.

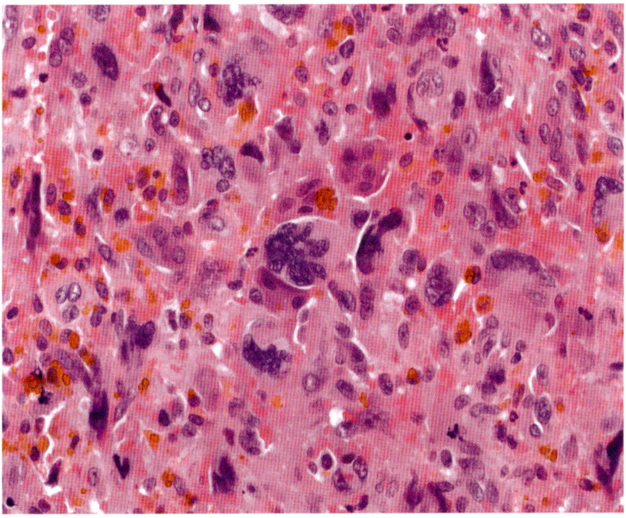

FIGURE 13.5 **Undifferentiated Pleomorphic Sarcoma with Giant Cells.** Multinucleated cells of both osteoclastic and malignant types coexist.

Undifferentiated Pleomorphic Sarcoma with Prominent Inflammation

Examples of this very rare tumor were first identified as retroperitoneal xanthogranuloma and subsequently classified as inflammatory MFH.[13] As with pleomorphic MFH, many cases can be reclassified after appropriate investigation as lymphoma or carcinoma. Furthermore, based on the

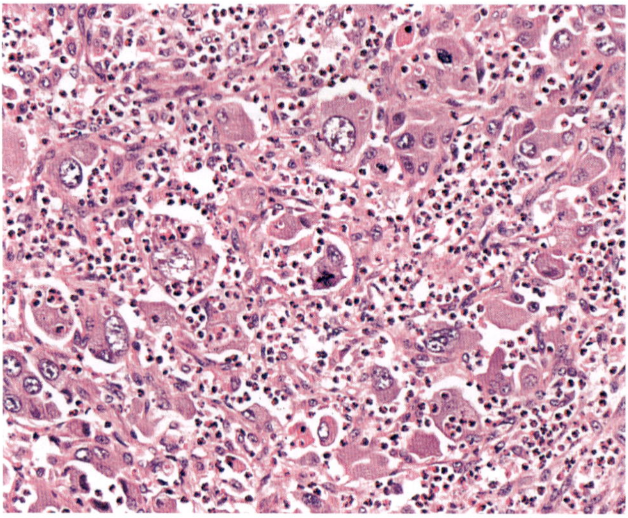

FIGURE 13.6 **Undifferentiated Pleomorphic Sarcoma with Prominent Inflammation.** This shows sheets of polygonal cells with plentiful cytoplasm and variably sized nuclei. There is a marked infiltrate of neutrophil polymorphonuclear leukocytes, some of which have been phagocytosed by tumor cells.

identification of adjacent foci of well-differentiated liposarcoma and ancillary studies, most of the remaining undifferentiated examples are now considered to represent dedifferentiated liposarcoma.[25]

CLINICAL FEATURES. This occurs predominantly in the retroperitoneum and presents like other sarcomas in this location as a mass or with related mechanical symptoms. Occasional examples arise in other parts of the abdomen or in deep somatic soft tissue. It can also be accompanied by systemic symptoms including fever and weight loss, and hematologic manifestations including eosinophilia and leukemoid reaction. It is an aggressive tumor that is prone to local recurrence and metastasis, with over 50% patients dying of tumor. However, there can be a relatively protracted clinical course; in a series of seven cases all patients died of disease, but the average survival was 53 months after diagnosis, and four patients survived over 5 years.[13]

PATHOLOGIC FEATURES. Macroscopically, there can be patchy yellow coloration (firmer than fat) if there is a large xanthomatous component. Microscopically, there are dispersed atypical polygonal cells with large pleomorphic nuclei and often abundant cytoplasm that can contain phagocytosed red or white blood cells (Fig. 13.6, e-Figs. 13.22–13.24). There is usually also a pleomorphic spindle cell component resembling usual-type UPS, with variable stromal fibrosis or hyalinization. The inflammatory cells are mixed, but neutrophils often predominate and sheets of xanthoma cells, focally with nuclear pleomorphism, are characteristic.

Ancillary investigations. The spindle cells can display focal immunoreactivity for CD34 or SMA. The atypical lesional cells also show immunoreactivity for MDM2 (in all cases) and CDK4 (in about 80%), and related gene amplification with corresponding supernumerary large marker and ring chromosomes especially in the 12q13 region. These findings, which are similar to those in WD liposarcoma, imply that most if not all UPS with prominent inflammation represent dedifferentiated liposarcoma.[25,26] The differential diagnosis includes (a) xanthogranulomatous pyelonephritis (which originates in the kidney and lacks nuclear atypia); (b) inflammatory myofibroblastic tumor (which lacks the marked atypia, and has a predominantly plasmacytic infiltrate, sclerosing areas and ALK1 positivity in over 50%); (c) inflammatory leiomyosarcoma (which displays smooth muscle cytomorphology and diffuse desmin positivity); and (d) lymphoma and carcinoma (which can be identified by their respective immunohistochemical markers).

PLEOMORPHIC MYOFIBROSARCOMA

Pleomorphic myofibrosarcomas are pleomorphic sarcomas that display only fibroblastic and myofibroblastic differentiation. They are morphologically indistinguishable from undifferentiated pleomorphic sarcoma, and immunohistochemistry or electron microscopy are required for their identification.[21] Their recognition has clinical relevance, however, since there is evidence that myofibroblastic differentiation in pleomorphic sarcomas is associated with more aggressive behavior.[8,9,21]

Clinical Features

Most pleomorphic myofibrosarcomas arise in deep soft tissue in adults and predominantly in lower limb and trunk, with occasional cases in head and neck including in childhood. Examples have also been reported in bony sites, including mandible, maxilla, humerus, and tibia. They usually arise de novo but low- or intermediate-grade myofibrosarcomas can recur as pleomorphic tumors.[27] Similar intra-abdominal or retroperitoneal tumors that display *MDM2* and *CDK4* amplification and immunoreactivity are now considered to represent dedifferentiated liposarcomas.[26] Pleomorphic myofibrosarcomas have a worse outcome than undifferentiated sarcomas with recurrence in a third of cases and metastases in up to 70%.[21]

Pathologic Features

The range of morphologic appearances is the same as for undifferentiated pleomorphic sarcoma. It is not possible to make the distinction on light microscopy alone.

Ancillary Investigations

Myofibroblastic differentiation is characterized by immunoreactivity for SMA which is focally expressed, in a typical subplasmalemmal distribution, in about half of the cases (e-Fig. 13.16), and desmin in 43%, though h-caldesmon is negative. This expression correlates with ultrastructural features of myofibroblastic differentiation, but can also be seen in cases lacking electron microscopic features of either myofibroblasts or smooth muscle cells. Myofibroblastic differentiation is therefore best confirmed by electron microscopy. Many of the lesional cells have the ultrastructural appearances of fibroblasts, some of which are plump and histiocyte-like, with abundant rough endoplasmic reticulum. A variable proportion, however, have additional features of myofibroblasts, including stress fibers and, very rarely, fibronexus structures.[28] These features can be seen in both polygonal and spindle cells, with an incidence related to diligence of search. There are no specific genetic data.

ATYPICAL FIBROXANTHOMA

Clinical Features

This is a superficial pleomorphic neoplasm of intermediate malignant potential which, though a distinct entity, is often regarded as the cutaneous counterpart of undifferentiated pleomorphic sarcoma (MFH). AFX occurs in elderly adults of either sex in areas exposed to sun or other forms of irradiation including scalp, other head and neck sites, and distal extremities. Genetic changes related to ultraviolet light exposure include p53 mutations[29] (also found in MFH[30]) and expression of Gadd45.[31] HRAS, KRAS, and NRAS gene mutations have been identified in MFH but not in AFX.[32] Tumors formerly regarded as AFX on limbs and limb girdles of younger adults probably represent atypical variants of cutaneous fibrous histiocytoma. AFX presents as a raised, dome-shaped nodule that grows slowly and can ulcerate. Lesions confined to dermis have a good prognosis following complete excision, with a recurrence rate of <7%.[33] Among strictly defined cases, metastasis is very rare, though occasional examples have behaved aggressively or metastasized. However, those tumors that extend significantly into subcutis have increased recurrence rate and metastatic potential, and should be diagnosed and managed as soft tissue sarcomas.

Pathologic Features

The lesions are relatively small and usually <2 cm in diameter, and the epidermis is thinned or occasionally ulcerated (Fig. 13.7). Typically, the dermis contains a dome-shaped, poorly demarcated cellular infiltrate of pleomorphic spindle and polygonal cells with frequent mitoses including abnormal forms (Fig. 13.8, e-Figs. 13.25–13.28). The tumor can be patternless or storiform, or arranged in fascicles. There is usually an admixture of chronic inflammatory cells, as well as actinic changes in adjacent collagen. As well as those infiltrating subcutis, AFX with necrosis, lymphovascular, and possibly perineurial invasion should be managed as pleomorphic sarcomas.

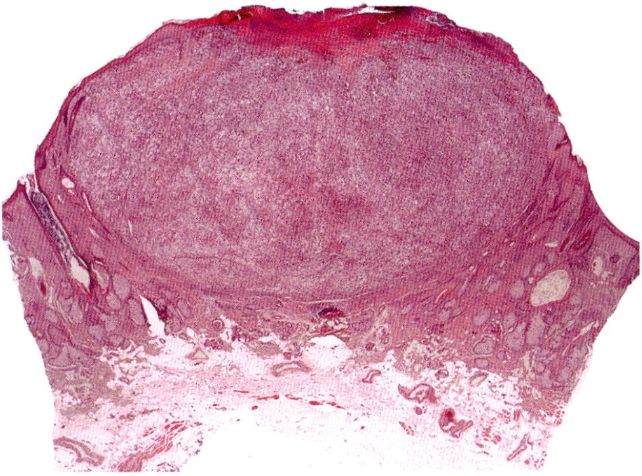

FIGURE 13.7 **Atypical Fibroxanthoma.** Typically, this is a dome-shaped dermal lesion with a well-defined lower border that does not extend into dermis. The surface is ulcerated.

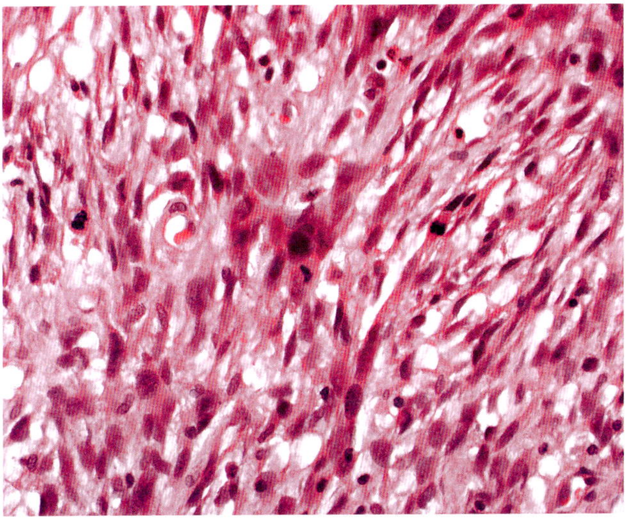

FIGURE 13.8 **Atypical Fibroxanthoma.** The lesion is composed of pleomorphic spindle and polygonal cells with mitoses and inflammatory cells.

Variants with pigment, osteoclast-like giant cells (sometimes with osteoid formation), nonpleomorphic spindle cells (e-Figs. 13.26 and 13.27), granular cells, or clear cells (e-Fig. 13.28) have been described. AFX differs from atypical cutaneous fibrous histiocytoma that typically features epidermal hyperplasia, peripheral collagen bundles, and only focal nuclear atypia.

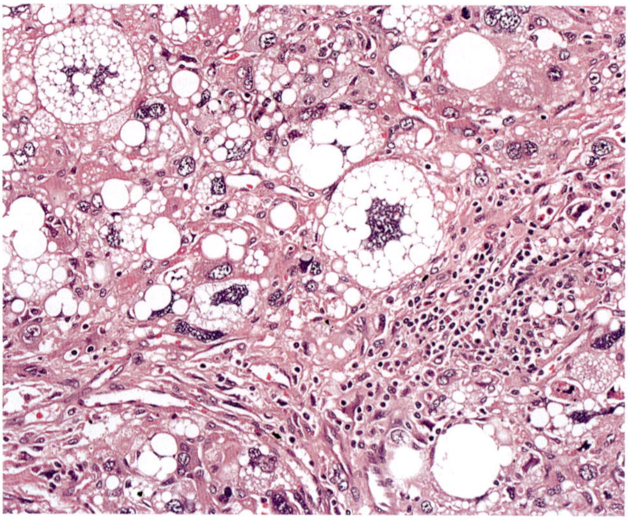

FIGURE 13.9 **Pleomorphic Liposarcoma.** This tumor is characterized by multivacuolated lipoblasts with indented hyperchromatic nuclei, in a background of undifferentiated pleomorphic sarcoma.

Ancillary Investigations

Immunostains are positive for SMA and CD99 in some cases, but cytokeratins, EMA, desmin, S100 protein, HMB45, CD34, and CD31 are typically negative, allowing distinction from undifferentiated carcinoma, melanoma, and cutaneous angiosarcoma, respectively.

PLEOMORPHIC LIPOSARCOMA

This is a high-grade, pleomorphic sarcoma with at least focal lipogenic differentiation.[34–36] This entity is discussed in detail in Chapter 16. Microscopically, the tumor usually resembles undifferentiated pleomorphic sarcoma with the addition of lipoblasts (Fig. 13.9, e-Figs. 13.29–13.31). These are univacuolated or multivacuolated and have enlarged hyperchromatic, multiply indented (scalloped) nuclei. They can be present multifocally in clusters or larger sheets (e-Fig. 13.31), or be extremely scanty and present only in an occasional block. A small number of examples show epithelioid change, with sheets of polygonal cells with clear cytoplasm, resembling adrenal cortical tissue (Fig. 13.10, e-Figs. 13.32–13.34).[37,38] A diagnostically helpful feature is the presence of transitional forms between lipoblasts and the epithelioid cells. An additional finding in pleomorphic liposarcoma is the presence in nonlipogenic multinucleated tumor cells of eosinophilic granular material (e-Fig. 13.35), but this can also be seen in other types of pleomorphic sarcoma. Divergent chondrosarcomatous differentiation has also been described.

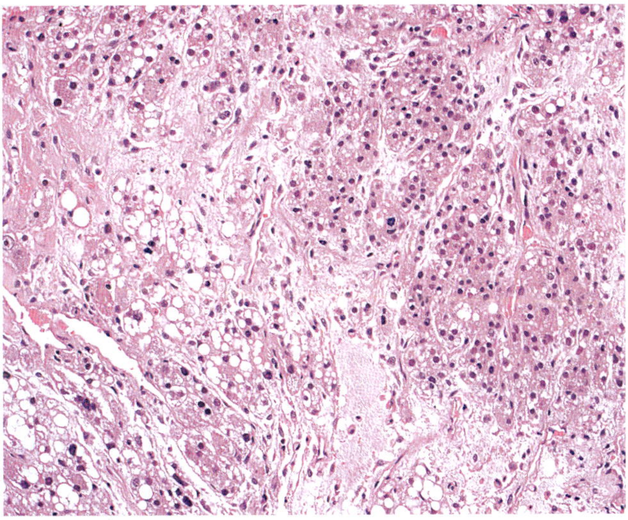

FIGURE 13.10 **Epithelioid Pleomorphic Liposarcoma.** This rare variant has areas of epithelioid cells resembling adrenal cortical carcinoma. Adjacent areas show lipoblastic differentiation.

The lipoblasts are immunoreactive for S100 protein. SMA, desmin, and cytokeratin can occasionally be positive in the pleomorphic background cells. In the epithelioid variant, focal immunoreactivity for cytokeratins (20%), melan-A (67%), or S100 protein (55%),[37,38] the former two enhancing the resemblance to metastatic adrenal cortical carcinoma, and the latter two suggesting metastatic melanoma. Inhibin is negative. As always, careful microscopic observation and consideration of the clinical picture can prevent a diagnostic error based on immunohistochemical findings. Pleomorphic liposarcomas are cytogenetically heterogeneous and do not have specific findings. Some pleomorphic liposarcomas and myxofibrosarcomas share genomic imbalances,[39] and array-based comparative genomic hybridization has shown that pleomorphic leiomyosarcoma and dedifferentiated liposarcoma are clearly separated by the genomic profiles.[40] An example of epithelioid pleomorphic liposarcoma has been found to have *FUS-CHOP (DDIT3)* transcripts,[41] which are normally a feature of myxoid-round cell liposarcoma.

PLEOMORPHIC LEIOMYOSARCOMA

The diagnosis of leiomyosarcoma is discussed in Chapter 6. Pleomorphic leiomyosarcoma has been defined as a pleomorphic undifferentiated sarcoma in which less than one third of the tumor shows smooth muscle differentiation with fascicular architecture (e-Fig. 13.36). In pleomorphic leiomyosarcoma, there is generally expression of the three muscle antigens (SMA, desmin, and h-caldesmon) in the pleomorphic areas but in fewer cells than in the fascicular component. Many other pleomorphic sarcomas also demonstrate focal expression of SMA and desmin (though rarely h-caldesmon), but this is insufficient for a diagnosis of leiomyosarcoma in the absence of the appropriate morphologic features. However, as noted above, this affects prognosis and such tumors should be reported as pleomorphic sarcomas with immunohistochemical evidence of myoid differentiation.

PLEOMORPHIC RHABDOMYOSARCOMA

Clinical Features

This tumor was formerly considered to be very rare but in recent years has been diagnosed with increasing frequency.[42,10] It occurs in adults generally over the age of 40 years (age range: 21–84) and predominantly in males, in deep soft tissue in proximal limbs (especially thigh), abdomen, pelvis, and head and neck region. Rare examples arise in the pediatric age group. Pleomorphic rhabdomyosarcoma is very aggressive with a 5-year survival rate of <30%.

Areas of rhabdomyoblastic differentiation resembling pleomorphic rhabdomyosarcoma can represent heterologous elements in malignant peripheral nerve sheath tumor, or divergent differentiation in sarcomatoid carcinomas (especially those of gynecologic or renal origin), malignant mesothelioma, or dedifferentiated liposarcoma. In fact, it has been suggested that any sarcoma with rhabdomyosarcomatous differentiation occurring in the internal trunk of adults represents dedifferentiated liposarcoma.[10] These possibilities should be borne in mind in the interpretation of core biopsies in the relevant clinical situations.

Pathologic Features

These tumors can reach 15 cm in diameter, and are characterized by variable numbers of large pleomorphic cells with abundant eosinophilic cytoplasm, in a background of smaller polygonal or spindle cell rhabdomyoblasts (Fig. 13.11, e-Figs. 13.37–13.39).[42] A high mitotic index and necrosis are typical features.

Ancillary Investigations

Most pleomorphic rhabdomyosarcomas are diffusely immunoreactive for desmin (e-Fig. 13.40), and show focal positivity in nuclei for myogenin (e-Fig. 13.41) and (less frequently) MyoD1. SMA is focally positive in about half of the cases,[42] which is a potential source of confusion unless a panel of myogenic markers, including myogenin and h-caldesmon (which is negative in rhabdomyosarcoma), is employed. Electron microscopy shows varying stages of sarcomeric differentiation. This tumor type has no specific or diagnostic genetic features although the *PAX3-FOXO1A* fusion gene, which is normally associated with alveolar rhabdomyosarcoma, has been identified in one case.[43]

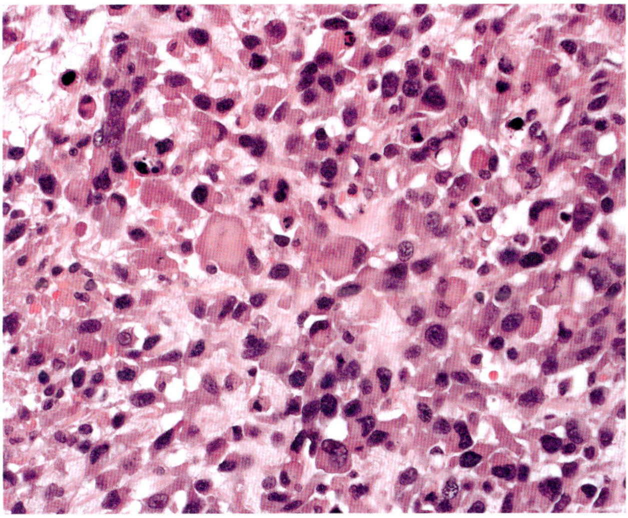

FIGURE 13.11 **Pleomorphic Rhabdomyosarcoma.** This tumor can have sheets of rhabdomyoblasts of varying size, in a background of darkly staining rounded or spindle cells.

REFERENCES

1. Kazakov DV, Pavlovsky M, Mukensnabl P, et al. Pleomorphic hyalinizing angiectatic tumor with a sarcomatous component recurring as high-grade myxofibrosarcoma. *Pathol Int.* 2007;57:281–284.
2. Smith ME, Fisher C, Weiss SW. Pleomorphic hyalinizing angiectatic tumor of soft parts. A low-grade neoplasm resembling neurilemoma. *Am J Surg Pathol.* 1996;20:21–29.
3. Folpe AL, Weiss SW. Pleomorphic hyalinizing angiectatic tumor: analysis of 41 cases supporting evolution from a distinctive precursor lesion. *Am J Surg Pathol.* 2004;28:1417–1425.
4. Marshall-Taylor C, Fanburg-Smith JC. Hemosiderotic fibrohistiocytic lipomatous lesion: ten cases of a previously undescribed fatty lesion of the foot/ankle. *Mod Pathol.* 2000;13:1192–1199.
5. Luzar B, Gasljevic G, Juricic V, et al. Hemosiderotic fibrohistiocytic lipomatous lesion: early pleomorphic hyalinizing angiectatic tumor? *Pathol Int.* 2006;56:283–286.
6. Browne TJ, Fletcher CD. Haemosiderotic fibrolipomatous tumour (so-called haemosiderotic fibrohistiocytic lipomatous tumour): analysis of 13 new cases in support of a distinct entity. *Histopathology.* 2006;48:453–461.
7. Kazakov DV, Sima R, Michal M. Hemosiderotic fibrohistiocytic lipomatous lesion: clinical correlation with venous stasis. *Virchows Arch.* 2005;447:103–106.
8. Deyrup AT, Haydon RC, Huo D, et al. Myoid differentiation and prognosis in adult pleomorphic sarcomas of the extremity: an analysis of 92 cases. *Cancer.* 2003;98:805–813.
9. Massi D, Beltrami G, Capanna R, et al. Histopathological re-classification of extremity pleomorphic soft tissue sarcoma has clinical relevance. *Eur J Surg Oncol.* 2004;30:1131–1136.
10. Binh MB, Guillou L, Hostein I, et al. Dedifferentiated liposarcomas with divergent myosarcomatous differentiation developed in the internal trunk: a study of 27 cases and comparison to conventional dedifferentiated liposarcomas and leiomyosarcomas. *Am J Surg Pathol.* 2007;31:1557–1566.

11. Kempson RL, Kyriakos M. Fibroxanthosarcoma of the soft tissues. A type of malignant fibrous histiocytoma. *Cancer.* 1972;29:961–976.
12. Guccion JG, Enzinger FM. Malignant giant cell tumor of soft parts. An analysis of 32 cases. *Cancer.* 1972;29:1518–1528.
13. Kyriakos M, Kempson RL. Inflammatory fibrous histiocytoma. An aggressive and lethal lesion. *Cancer.* 1976;37:1584–1606.
14. Weiss SW, Enzinger FM. Myxoid variant of malignant fibrous histiocytoma. *Cancer.* 1977;39:1672–1685.
15. Enzinger FM. Angiomatoid malignant fibrous histiocytoma: a distinct fibrohistiocytic tumor of children and young adults simulating a vascular neoplasm. *Cancer.* 1979;44:2147–2157.
16. Lawson CW, Fisher C, Gatter KC. An immunohistochemical study of differentiation in malignant fibrous histiocytoma. *Histopathology.* 1987;11:375–383.
17. Fletcher CD. Pleomorphic malignant fibrous histiocytoma: fact or fiction? A critical reappraisal based on 159 tumors diagnosed as pleomorphic sarcoma. *Am J Surg Pathol.* 1992;16:213–228.
18. Antonescu CR, Erlandson RA, Huvos AG. Primary fibrosarcoma and malignant fibrous histiocytoma of bone–a comparative ultrastructural study: evidence of a spectrum of fibroblastic differentiation. *Ultrastruct Pathol.* 2000;24:83–91.
19. Erlandson RA, Antonescu CR. The rise and fall of malignant fibrous histiocytoma. *Ultrastruct Pathol.* 2004;28:283–289.
20. Chung L, Lau SK, Jiang Z, et al. Overlapping features between dedifferentiated liposarcoma and undifferentiated high-grade pleomorphic sarcoma. *Am J Surg Pathol.* 2009;33:1594–1600.
21. Montgomery E, Fisher C. Myofibroblastic differentiation in malignant fibrous histiocytoma (pleomorphic myofibrosarcoma): a clinicopathological study. *Histopathology.* 2001;38:499–509.
22. Nielsen TO, West RB, Linn SC, et al. Molecular characterisation of soft tissue tumours: a gene expression study. *Lancet.* 2002;359:1301–1307.
23. Soule EH, Enriquez P. Atypical fibrous histiocytoma, malignant fibrous histiocytoma, malignant histiocytoma, and epithelioid sarcoma. A comparative study of 65 tumors. *Cancer.* 1972;30:128–143.
24. Angervall L, Hagmar B, Kindblom L-G, et al. Malignant giant cell tumor of soft tissues: a clinicopathologic, cytologic, ultrastructural, angiographic and microangiographic study. *Cancer.* 1981;47:736–747.
25. Coindre JM, Hostein I, Maire G, et al. Inflammatory malignant fibrous histiocytomas and dedifferentiated liposarcomas: histological review, genomic profile, and MDM2 and CDK4 status favour a single entity. *J Pathol.* 2004;203:822–830.
26. Coindre JM, Mariani O, Chibon F, et al. Most malignant fibrous histiocytomas developed in the retroperitoneum are dedifferentiated liposarcomas: a review of 25 cases initially diagnosed as malignant fibrous histiocytoma. *Mod Pathol.* 2003;16:256–262.
27. Montgomery E, Goldblum JR, Fisher C. Myofibrosarcoma: a clinicopathologic study. *Am J Surg Pathol.* 2001;25:219–228.
28. Watanabe K, Ogura G. Fibronexus in "malignant fibrous histiocytoma" of the bone: a case report of pleomorphic myofibrosarcoma. *Ultrastruct Pathol.* 2002;26:47–51.
29. Dei Tos AP, Maestro R, Doglioni C, et al. Ultraviolet-induced p53 mutations in atypical fibroxanthoma. *Am J Pathol.* 1994;145:11–17.
30. Sakamoto A, Oda Y, Itakura E, et al. Immunoexpression of ultraviolet photoproducts and p53 mutation analysis in atypical fibroxanthoma and superficial malignant fibrous histiocytoma. *Mod Pathol.* 2001;14:581–588.

31. Sakamoto A, Oda Y, Tsuneyoshi M, et al. Expression of the UV-induced molecule, Gadd45, in atypical fibroxanthoma. *Histopathology.* 2007;50:939–941.

32. Sakamoto A, Oda Y, Itakura E, et al. H-, K-, and N-ras gene mutation in atypical fibroxanthoma and malignant fibrous histiocytoma. *Hum Pathol.* 2001;32:1225–1231.

33. Mirza B, Weedon D. Atypical fibroxanthoma: a clinicopathological study of 89 cases. *Australas J Dermatol.* 2005;46:235–238.

34. Downes KA, Goldblum JR, Montgomery EA, et al. Pleomorphic liposarcoma: a clinicopathologic analysis of 19 cases. *Mod Pathol.* 2001;14:179–184.

35. Hornick JL, Bosenberg MW, Mentzel T, et al. Pleomorphic liposarcoma: clinicopathologic analysis of 57 cases. *Am J Surg Pathol.* 2004;28:1257–1267.

36. Gebhard S, Coindre JM, Michels JJ, et al. Pleomorphic liposarcoma: clinicopathologic, immunohistochemical, and follow-up analysis of 63 cases: a study from the French Federation of Cancer Centers Sarcoma Group. *Am J Surg Pathol.* 2002;26:601–616.

37. Miettinen M, Enzinger FM. Epithelioid variant of pleomorphic liposarcoma: a study of 12 cases of a distinctive variant of high-grade liposarcoma. *Mod Pathol.* 1999;12:722–728.

38. Huang HY, Antonescu CR. Epithelioid variant of pleomorphic liposarcoma: a comparative immunohistochemical and ultrastructural analysis of six cases with emphasis on overlapping features with epithelial malignancies. *Ultrastruct Pathol.* 2002;26:299–308.

39. Idbaih A, Coindre JM, Derre J, et al. Myxoid malignant fibrous histiocytoma and pleomorphic liposarcoma share very similar genomic imbalances. *Lab Invest.* 2005;85:176–181.

40. Fritz B, Schubert F, Wrobel G, et al. Microarray based copy number and expression profiling in dedifferentiated and pleomorphic liposarcoma. *Cancer Res.* 2002;62:2993–2998.

41. De Cecco L, Gariboldi M, Reid JF, et al. Gene expression profile identifies a rare epithelioid variant case of pleomorphic liposarcoma carrying FUS-CHOP transcript. *Histopathology.* 2005;46:334–341.

42. Furlong MA, Mentzel T, Fanburg-Smith JC. Pleomorphic rhabdomyosarcoma in adults: a clinicopathologic study of 38 cases with emphasis on morphologic variants and recent skeletal muscle-specific markers. *Mod Pathol.* 2001;14:595–603.

43. Gordon A, McManus A, Anderson J, et al. Chromosomal imbalances in pleomorphic rhabdomyosarcomas and identification of the alveolar rhabdomyosarcoma-associated PAX3-FOXO1A fusion gene in one case. *Cancer Genet Cytogenet.* 2003;140:73–77.

14

SMALL ROUND CELL TUMORS

INTRODUCTION

Small round cell tumors of soft tissue are a group of malignant neoplasms composed of monotonous undifferentiated cells with high nuclear-cytoplasmic ratio, which occur more frequently, although not exclusively, in childhood. They often share similar morphology and sometimes show immunophenotypic overlap. Many of them have characteristic genetic aberrations, including distinct chromosomal translocations that produce novel fusion genes resulting in disordered cellular function. Molecular genetic detection of the translocation (usually by fluorescence *in situ* hybridization [FISH]) or fusion gene (using reverse transcription-polymerase chain reaction [RT-PCR]) is therefore an essential part of the diagnostic workup of many of these tumors. Genetic studies also provide important prognostic information and have an increasing influence on clinical management.

The differential diagnosis includes poorly differentiated synovial sarcoma, soft tissue lymphoma (especially lymphoblastic lymphoma), leukemic deposits, and small cell carcinoma. These can be identified by their clinical setting and by the use of appropriate immunohistochemical panels. The differential diagnosis is summarized in Tables 14.1 and 14.2.

ALVEOLAR RHABDOMYOSARCOMA

Rhabdomyosarcomas are primitive malignant tumors that show incomplete differentiation toward skeletal muscle and are the most common soft tissue sarcomas in children. They constitute 7% of childhood cancers, although are much rarer in older adults. The most common subtype is embryonal rhabdomyosarcoma (ERMS) (see Chapter 10), which typically affects children younger than 10 years and shows a better response to established treatment regimens compared with alveolar rhabdomyosarcoma (ARMS). ARMS affects a slightly older population and accounts for approximately 31% of rhabdomyosarcomas.[1] It is an aggressive neoplasm that has been shown to have a 5-year event-free survival rate of 45% compared to 70% in ERMS, and distinguishing the two is crucial for treatment and prognostication. ARMS is consistently associated with

TABLE 14.1 **Differential Diagnosis of Small Round Cell Tumors**

	Typical Clinical Features	Microscopic Features	Ancillary Investigations
Alveolar rhabdomyosarcoma	Adolescents and young adults. Rapidly growing mass. Extremities, head and neck, trunk	Sheets and nests of cells with round nuclei of small to intermediate size and scant cytoplasm, separated by fibrous septa. Central necrosis and peripheral cellular preservation causing classic "alveolar" morphology. Solid variant lacks alveolar pattern. Rhabdomyoblasts in some cases	Desmin+, nuclear myogenin, and MyoD1+. FISH for *FOXO1* breakpoints and RT-PCR for *PAX3/7-FOXO1* fusion transcripts
Ewing sarcoma/primitive neuroectodermal tumor	Children and young adults, Extraskeletally in extremity deep soft tissue, paravertebral sites, retroperitoneum, thoracopulmonary region	Sheets of uniform cells with round nuclei, fine chromatin and scant cytoplasm. Sometimes rosette formation	Many tumors CD99+ (supporting diagnosis). Recurrent chromosomal translocations resulting in EWS-ETS family fusion oncoproteins, detectable by RT-PCR. *EWSR1* breakpoints detectable by FISH Minimal or absent intercellular reticulin
Poorly differentiated synovial sarcoma	Young adults. Any site, but most common in extremity deep soft tissue, especially around knee and adjacent to joints and tendons	Sheets of rounded to ovoid cells. More spindled cells may be seen focally. Mast cells	CK, EMA, CD99, S100 protein all focally+, bcl2+, TLE1+ (nuclear),CD34 and CD117–. Nested reticulin pattern t(X;18)(p11;q11), *SS18-SSX* fusion genes
Extraskeletal mesenchymal chondrosarcoma	Young adults. Head and neck, extremities. Exclude metastasis from extraosseous site	Biphasic morphology. Hypercellular sheets of primitive small cells with round, ovoid, or spindled nuclei. Interspersed islands of well-differentiated hyaline cartilage. Hemangiopericytic vascular pattern	Small cell component CD99+. Cartilaginous component S100 protein+

(Continued)

TABLE 14.1 Differential Diagnosis of Small Round Cell Tumors (Continued)

	Typical Clinical Features	Microscopic Features	Ancillary Investigations
Small cell osteosarcoma	All ages, but most frequently in second decade	Sheets of small, uniform, round to focally short spindled cells. Foci of malignant osteoid, and sometimes malignant cartilage	Variable focal S100 protein+. CD99–
Desmoplastic samll round cell tumor	Adolescents and young adults, particularly males. Abdomen or pelvis. Often widespread serosal involvement	Sheets of tightly packed monotonous cells with small nuclei and usually minimal cytoplasm. Striking desmoplastic stromal reaction which divides the tumor into sharply demarcated islands. Necrosis common	Nuclear expression of WT1 (carboxy terminal). Divergent differentiation with coexpression of desmin, cytokeratins and neural markers. t(11;22)(p13;q12) and *EWSR1-WT1* fusion gene
Neuroblastoma	Infants and children in first 2 years of life. Follow distribution of sympathetic ganglia, with majority arising in retroperitoneum (of which about half arise in adrenal gland)	Sheets and lobules of small to intermediate sized cells, with hyperchromatic round nuclei. Pale neurofibrillary matrix resembling neuropil. Cells may show rosette formation. May show small amounts of ganglionic differentiation	NSE+. Neurofilament+, NB84+. CD99–. Amplification of *MYCN* oncogene in approximately 25% of cases
Ganglioneuro-blastoma	Retroperitoneum, mediastinum	Neuroblastoma-like areas of primitive neuroblasts with areas of ganglioneuromatous stroma, subclassified according to arrangement and proportion of these areas	Ganglion cells NSE+, CD56+, NF+. Spindle Schwann cells S100 protein+

Olfactory neuroblastoma	Adults with bimodal peak (second and sixth decades). Roof of nasal fossa, maxillary and ethmoid sinuses, nasopharynx	Lobules and nests of uniform small cells with round vesicular nuclei and scanty cytoplasm, often within neurofibrillary background. Rosettes may be present	NSE+, NFP+ variably, synaptophysin+, chromogranin+. S100 protein+ in sustentacular-like cells that surround islands of tumor. CD99–
Ectomesen-chymoma	Children, M > F. Intracranial, nasal cavity, GU tract, and soft tissue	Neuroectodermal elements (usually ganglioneuroma or ganglioneuro-blastoma) and mesenchymal component, usually rhabdomyo-sarcoma	Appropriate immunoreactivity for each component
Small cell malignanat peripheral nerve sheath tumor	Deep soft tissue of trunk and limbs	Uniform, small, round cells with scanty cytoplasm. Sometimes foci of uniform, short, spindle-shaped tumor cells arranged in whorl-like patterns	S100 protein+ focally, occasional GFAP+. CD99–
Small cell carcinoma	Older adults. Usually lung, but can occur in many other primary sites	Sheets of small to medium round to fusiform cells with hyperchromatic nuclei. Nuclear molding, necrosis and frequent mitoses	CK+ (dot), many TTF1+, chromogranin+, synaptophysin+, CK20–, NF–
Merkel cell carcinoma	Older adults. Face and extremities	Tumor in dermis or subcutis. Monotonous round cells, multiple nucleoli	Low molecular weight CK+, CK20+ in perinuclear dot-like distributions. NSE, neurofilament+. TTF1–
Melanoma	Primary dermal lesion may be apparent	May have junctional component. Often in nested pattern. Melanin pigment	S100 protein+, HMB45+, melan-A+

(Continued)

TABLE 14.1 **Differential Diagnosis of Small Round Cell Tumors (Continued)**

	Typical Clinical Features	Microscopic Features	Ancillary Investigations
Lymphoma	May have lymphadenopathy	Cells have dispersed morphology, and tumor can have a more heterogeneous appearance with a mixed population of other inflammatory cells	CD45+, CD20, CD3+, TdT+ (lymphoblastic lymphoma)
Granulocytic sarcoma	Any site, including skin and lymph nodes. Patient may have underlying acute myeloid leukemia	Extramedullary tumor comprising immature myeloid (granulocytic or monocytic) cells	Lysozyme, CD43+, variably myeloperoxidase, CD117, CD13, CD33+
Round cell liposarcoma	Deep soft tissues of extremities of young adults. Often metastasizes to other soft tissue sites as well as to lungs	Monotonous small uniform rounded cells with minimal myxoid matrix, with some lipoblasts. Rich network of delicate vessels becomes inconspicuous in round cell liposarcoma	S100 protein+ in some cases, t(12;16)(q13;p11) or t(12;22)(q13;q12) with *FUS-DDIT3 or EWSR1-DDIT3* fusion genes
Endometrial stromal sarcoma	Females. Can arise in a focus of endometriosis or present as metastasis in abdomen or elsewhere	Short closely packed spindle cells, variable focal myoid differentiation. Thick-walled vessels	CD10+, SMA+, occasional des+, CK+ Nuclear beta catenin+ in 50% ER+, PgR + JAZF1-JJAZ1, JAZF1-PHF1, and EPC1-PHF1 fusion genes

TABLE 14.2 Immunohistochemistry of Selected Small Round Cell Tumors

	Alveolar RMS	ES	Desmoplastic SRCT	Neuroblastoma	PD SS	Small Cell Carcinoma	Lymphoma
Desmin	+	+[a]	+ dot	–	–	–	–
Myogenin	+	–	–	–	–	–	–
CD99	+[a]	+	–	–	±	–	±
CD56	+	–	+	+	+	+	±
NFP	–	±	+	+	±	–	–
Chromogranin	–	–	+[a]	+	–	±	–
Synaptophysin	–	–	±	+	–	±	–
CK	–	+[a]	+ dot	–	+	+ dot	–
EMA	–	–	–	–	+	–	–
Bcl-2	±	±	–	–	+	±	–
CD45	–	–	–	–	–	–	+
Others	MyoD1	FLI1	WT1	NB84	TLE1	TTF1	TdT (lymphoblastic)

[a] Rarely +, PDSS = poorly differentiated synovial sarcoma.
ES = Ewing sarcoma, SRCT = small round cell tumor, RMS = rhabdomyosarcoma.

characteristic translocations that result in chimeric transcription factors, which are hypothesized to generate novel transcriptional programs in an unknown target cell.[2]

Clinical Features

Although the age distribution is wide, ARMS predominantly affects adolescents and young adults and is rare in adults over 45 years. It typically presents as a rapidly growing mass in an extremity. Other sites include the head and neck and the trunk. ARMS often metastasizes early and can present primarily with widespread nodal or bony metastases. Tumors metastatic to marrow can present with leukoerythroblastic anemia. ARMS with *PAX7-FKHR (FOXO1)* fusion tend to remain localized and to be associated with longer survival than those with *PAX3-FKHR (FOXO1)* fusion,[3] and gene expression profiling can identify molecular risk groups, with outcome related to gene signatures.[4]

Pathologic Features

ARMS comprises nests and sheets of relatively small to intermediate cells with round to ovoid hyperchromatic nuclei and scanty cytoplasm (Figs. 14.1 and 14.2, e-Fig. 14.1), arranged in nests divided by thick fibrous septa. There is often central necrosis with cellular discohesion (e-Fig. 14.2), and peripheral preservation of cells creating an appearance resembling pulmonary alveoli. Tumor giant cells are fairly common, with abundant eosinophilic cytoplasm and nuclei arranged in peripheral or "wreath-like" distributions (Fig. 14.2, e-Fig. 14.2). The solid variant has the same cellular features

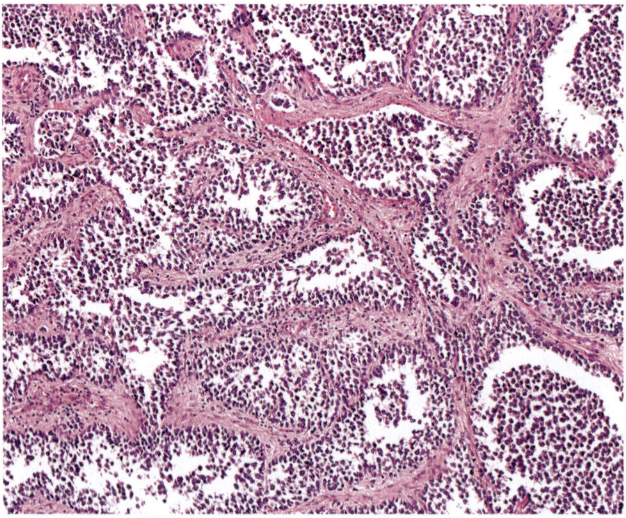

FIGURE 14.1 **Alveolar Rhabdomyosarcoma.** Central necrosis with peripheral preservation of cells creates an appearance resembling pulmonary alveoli. Thick fibrous septa traverse the tumor.

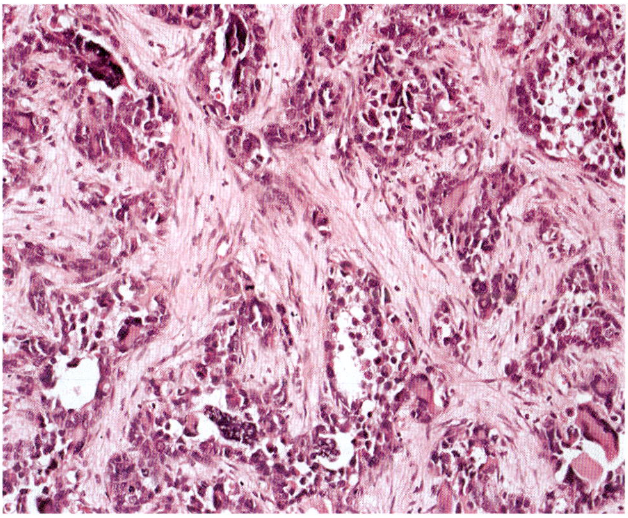

FIGURE 14.2 **Alveolar Rhabdomyosarcoma.** The tumor nests contain multinucleated wreath-like cells.

but lacks the characteristic architecture (Fig. 14.3, e-Figs. 14.3–14.8); however, small nests with typical appearances of ARMS may be found on thorough examination. In addition to the small cells, rhabdomyoblasts can be seen in some cases (Fig. 14.4, e-Fig. 14.7), although not as commonly as in ERMS. Rarely, tumors may show clear cell morphology due to cytoplasmic glycogen[5] (e-Fig. 14.9). These can mimic lipoblasts, but lack the characteristic nuclear scalloping of the latter. Although the tumor cells are generally fairly uniform in appearance, there can be focal pleomorphism (e-Figs. 14.10 and 14.11). Cellular spindling is usually lacking, in contrast to that seen in ERMS, but some tumors show mixed alveolar and embryonal histology, with foci of spindled cells in focally myxoid stroma. The presence of any alveolar pattern, however, usually indicates categorization as ARMS. Therapy can result in differentiation towards skeletal muscle, the extent of which relates to outcome.

Ancillary Investigations

Desmin positivity is strong and frequently present in the majority of cells (e-Figs. 14.12 and 14.13). Myogenin and MyoD1 are intranuclear myogenic transcriptional regulatory proteins that are expressed at early stages of skeletal muscle differentiation, and show strong nuclear positivity at least focally and often in a large proportion of nuclei (e-Figs. 14.14 and 14.15). Myogenin is more sensitive, and the proportion of cells with strong nuclear myogenin expression has been shown to be greater in ARMS than ERMS.[6,7] Additionally, there may be focal smooth muscle actin expression, and tumors can variably express neuroendocrine markers, particularly CD56 (e-Fig. 14.16). Immunostaining for myoglobin can give nonspecific positivity

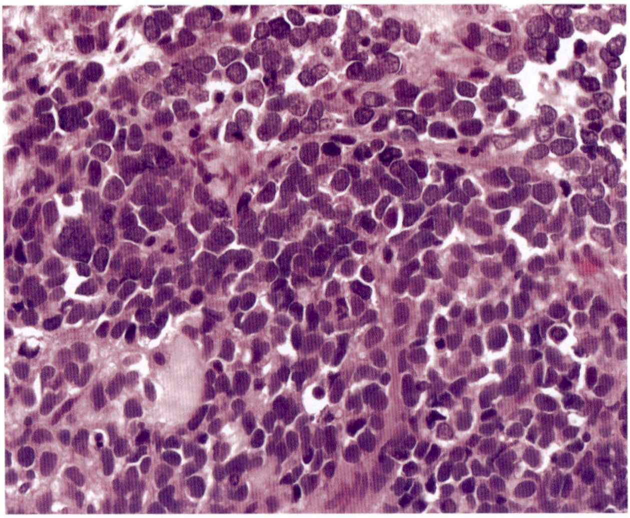

FIGURE 14.3 **Alveolar Rhabdomyosarcoma, Solid Variant.** There are sheets of small to intermediate sized cells with round hyperchromatic nuclei.

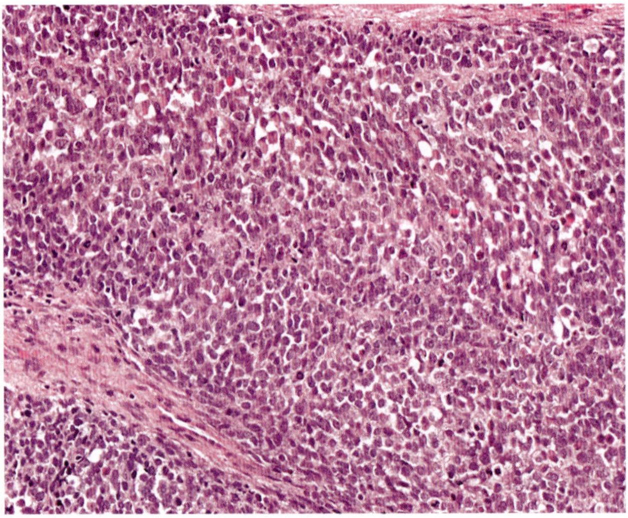

FIGURE 14.4 **Alveolar Rhabdomyosarcoma.** Some cells have discernible eosinophilic cytoplasm reflecting early rhabdomyoblastic differentiation.

in a variety of other tumor types and we no longer use this routinely. ALK is immunohistochemically positive in about half of ARMS.[8]

ARMS has two characteristic translocations that juxtapose the *PAX3* or *PAX7* genes on chromosomes 2 and 1, respectively, with the *FOXO1* gene on chromosome 13. The resultant fusion genes encode PAX3-FOXO1 and PAX7-FOXO1 chimeric proteins, which serve as potent transcriptional activators. The fusion transcripts can be detected by RT-PCR, and the genetic breakpoints by FISH. Also, it appears that immunostaining for PAX 5 can identify translocation-positive variants of either type.[9]

Approximately 20% of ARMS do not have a detectable *PAX-FOXO1* fusion, and these tend to be associated with a solid alveolar architecture.[10] Gene expression profiling can distinguish fusion-positive and fusion-negative tumors.[4]

EWING SARCOMA/PRIMITIVE NEUROECTODERMAL TUMOR

Ewing sarcoma (ES) and primitive neuroectodermal tumor (PNET), or Ewing family tumors, are a group of small round cell sarcomas that show common histologic and molecular findings, but varying degrees of neuroectodermal differentiation. They are characterized by recurrent balanced translocations involving the *EWSR1* gene on chromosome 22 and the *ETS* family of transcription factors, which lead to the formation of novel fusion oncogenes that contribute to pathogenesis. There is no known normal counterpart cell, but these tumors are considered as neuroectodermal with capacity for divergent differentiation detectable at various levels.[6,7] By convention, the term PNET is used for tumors with evidence of neuroectodermal differentiation by light or electron microscopy or immunohistochemistry, while ES is used for those lacking this. However, the tumors share overlapping features and it is unclear that their distinction has clinical impact.[11,12]

Clinical Features

Most patients with ES are adolescents or young adults younger than 30 years,[9] and ES/PNET is the second commonest pediatric sarcoma, after rhabdomyosarcoma. It can occur anywhere in the skeletal system but especially in long bones. Extraskeletally, it may arise at virtually every site, but common regions include extremity deep soft tissue, the paravertebral area, retroperitoneum, and thoracopulmonary region (Askin tumor). With modern chemotherapy, patients with localized disease can achieve 90% 5-year survival, but this falls to about 30% in patients who have metastatic disease at presentation.

Pathologic Features

Macroscopically, the tumors tend to be solid and friable with frequent hemorrhage and necrosis. Cyst formation is occasionally seen. Histologically, most ES/PNET are composed of sheets of uniform cells with round or ovoid vesicular nuclei with fine chromatin, small nucleoli, little cytoplasm (Fig. 14.5, e-Figs. 14.17–14.21) and indistinct cell borders. The nuclei appear evenly spaced with some overlapping (which is less in thin sections) but no molding. The cytoplasm is often clear (Fig. 14.6), owing to the presence of glycogen, which can be demonstrated with periodic acid

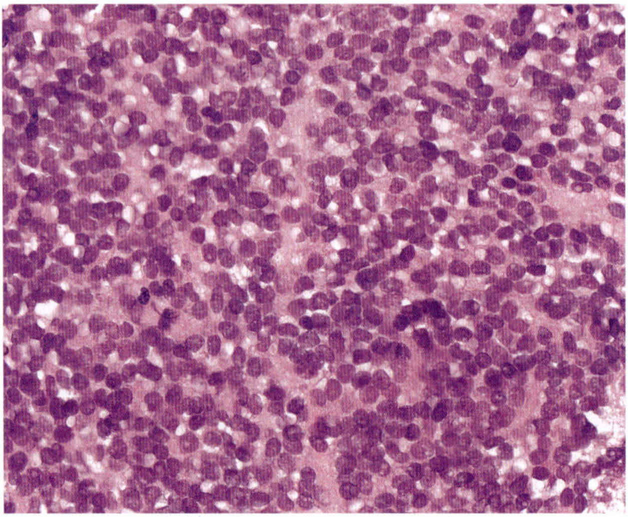

FIGURE 14.5 **Ewing Sarcoma/Primitive Neuroectodermal Tumor.** The tumor is composed of sheets of monotonous cells with round vesicular nuclei, finely distributed chromatin, and scant cytoplasm.

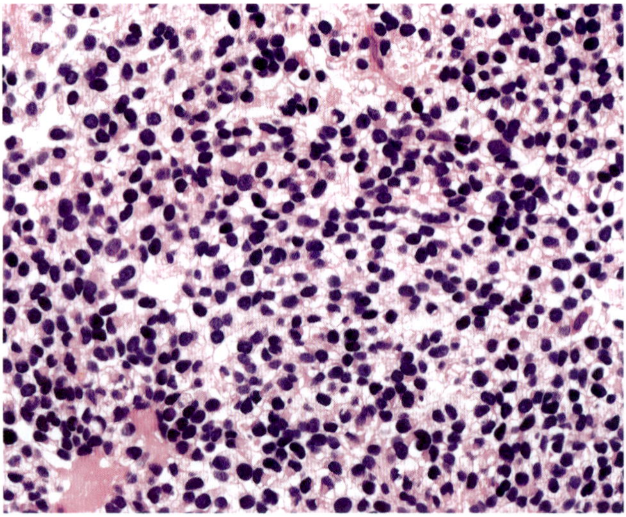

FIGURE 14.6 **Ewing Sarcoma/Primitive Neuroectodermal Tumor.** Cytoplasmic clearing is due to the presence of glycogen.

Schiff stain with and without diastase (e-Figs. 14.22 and 14.23), and may cause indentation of tumor nuclei. In some tumors, the cells are larger with moderately pleomorphic nuclei (e-Fig. 14.24) and often conspicuous nucleoli. These are referred to by some authors as large cell or atypical ES (e-Fig. 14.25).[13] Rarely, the cells focally assume a more spindled shape. Rosette

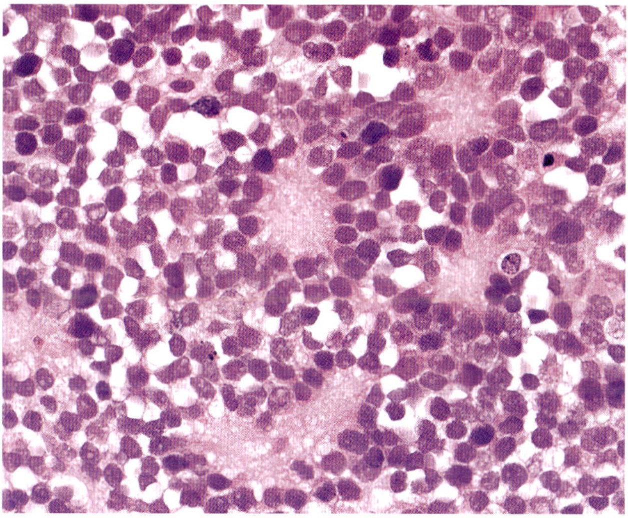

FIGURE 14.7 **Ewing Sarcoma/Primitive Neuroectodermal Tumor.** Rosettes can be prominent. These are of Homer Wright type, with cells arranged around central fibrillary cores.

formation can be present (e-Fig. 14.26), most commonly as circular distributions of cells with a central fibrillary core termed Homer-Wright rosettes (Fig. 14.7). Flexner-Wintersteiner rosettes, which contain a well-defined central lumen, are rarely seen. Fibrous septa may divide the cells into lobules. Tumors can also have a pseudoalveolar pattern (e-Fig. 14.27), and cystic change sometimes occurs (Fig. 14.8). Necrosis is common (and increased after therapy) with preservation of tumor islands around blood vessels.

Several rare morphologic variants of ES/PNET have been described. "Adamantinoma-like" ES has nests of moderately pleomorphic cells in a nested growth pattern with peripheral palisading and a prominent host desmoplastic response[11,12] and typically shows pancytokeratin expression.[12] Sclerosing ES is characterized by an abundant eosinophilic hyalinized matrix[12]; and spindle cell sarcoma-like ES has a greater degree of spindling than is typically seen in the usual ES, as well as a branching vasculature.[14] Divergent differentiation can sometimes be seen, including desmin expression that can lead to misinterpretation as rhabdomyosarcoma. These cases are particularly problematic for diagnosis and often require expert consultation.

Ancillary Investigations

Diffuse membranous positivity for CD99, a cell surface glycoprotein product of the *MIC2* gene, is present in over 90% of cases (Fig. 14.9, e-Figs. 14.28 and 14.29). This is supportive of a diagnosis of ES/PNET but not specific as it is found in a variety of similar tumors. About 70%

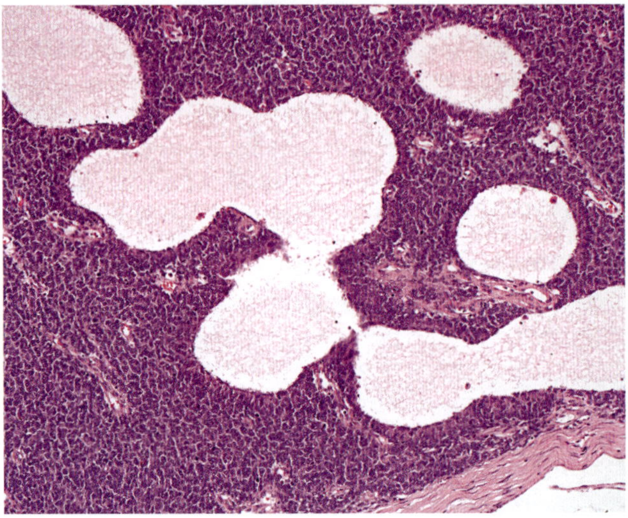

FIGURE 14.8 **Ewing Sarcoma/Primitive Neuroectodermal Tumor.** Microcystic change in the stroma.

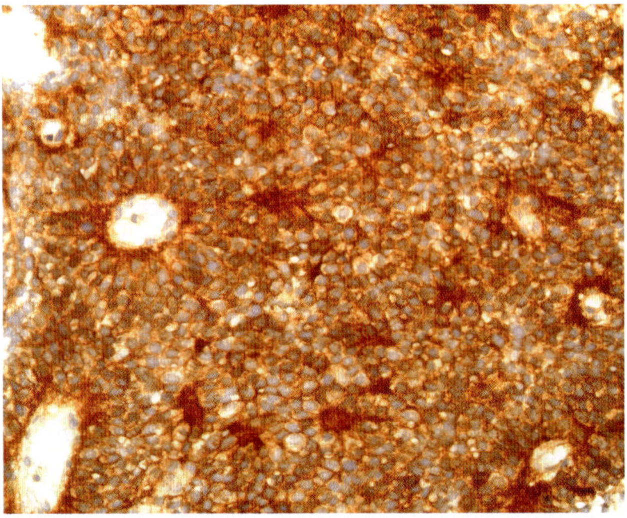

FIGURE 14.9 **Ewing Sarcoma/Primitive Neuroectodermal Tumor.** Diffuse membranous CD99 expression is a typical although not wholly specific finding. Immunoperoxidase.

show nuclear positivity for FLI1. ES/PNET can rarely express multiple lineage markers, including S100 protein (e-Fig. 14.30), cytokeratins (e-Fig. 14.31), CD117, and occasionally desmin.[15] However, CD56, TLE1, and myogenin are negative. PNET has variable expression of neural or neuroectodermal markers such as neuron-specific enolase (NSE), neurofilament (e-Fig. 14.32), chromogranin, synaptophysin, and CD56. Although there is a wide range of available antibodies, it has been reported that at least three of a panel composed of CD99, FLI-1, HNK1, and caveolin-1 show immunoreactivity in all cases with caveolin-1 being positive in CD99-negative cases.[16] Absence of reticulin fibers between tumor cells is characteristic for ES/PNET (e-Fig. 14.33) and contrasts with poorly differentiated synovial sarcoma which typically has a nested reticulin pattern.

All ES/PNET are characterized by recurrent chromosomal translocations resulting in EWS-ETS family fusion oncoproteins.[12] The most common of these is t(11;22)(q24;q12) with an *EWSR1-FLI1* fusion, found in approximately 85% of cases. Some 10% of tumors harbor a variant t(21;22)(q22;q12) with *EWSR1-ERG* fusion. These translocations can be routinely detected in paraffin-embedded material by FISH, using an *EWSR1*-specific break-apart probe that flanks the common *EWSR1* translocations, or the fusion transcripts can be identified by RT-PCR. However, because of the numerous variant translocations and fusions (see Chapter 1, Table 1.4), molecular investigation is sometimes negative in an otherwise typical Ewing family tumor.

The small cell component of extraskeletal mesenchymal chondrosarcoma (Chapter 19) closely resembles ES, and its typical islands of cartilage are not always present in a core biopsy. Since both tumors are CD99-positive, genetic analysis can be required for diagnosis.

DESMOPLASTIC SMALL ROUND CELL TUMOR

This is an aggressive small round cell tumor arising in children, adolescents, and young adults, with a male predominance.[17] The tumor is of uncertain lineage, but shows polyphenotypic differentiation, demonstrated by its immunoreactivity for epithelial, muscle, and neural markers. It is characterized by a t(11;22)(p13;q12) translocation, with formation of the *EWSR1-WT1* fusion gene.

Clinical Features

Desmoplastic small round cell tumor (DSRCT) presents in the abdomen or pelvis in most cases, often with widespread serosal involvement, but the tumor may present as an intrascrotal (paratesticular) tumor either in isolation or in continuity with the peritoneum via the processus vaginalis, Presentation in other sites is very rare but it has documented to arise within the thoracic cavity, head and neck, and brain. DSRCT is a high-grade neoplasm that responds poorly to chemotherapy.[18]

Pathologic Features

Macroscopically, DSRCT forms multiple firm, pale nodules on the peritoneal surface (e-Fig. 14.34), sometimes with hemorrhage and necrosis. Histologically, the tumor consists of variably sized nests of tightly packed, generally uniform cells with small, round vesicular or hyperchromatic nuclei, inconspicuous nucleoli, and minimal amounts of cytoplasm

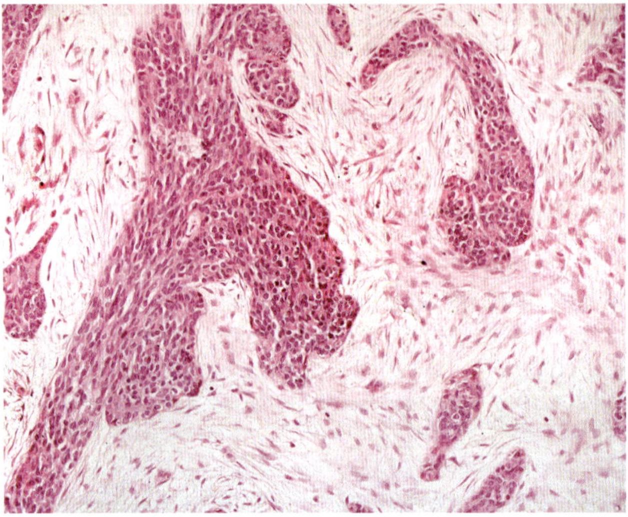

FIGURE 14.10 **Desmoplastic Small Round Cell Tumor.** Stromal desmoplasia is striking, and divides tumor into sharply defined nests and islands.

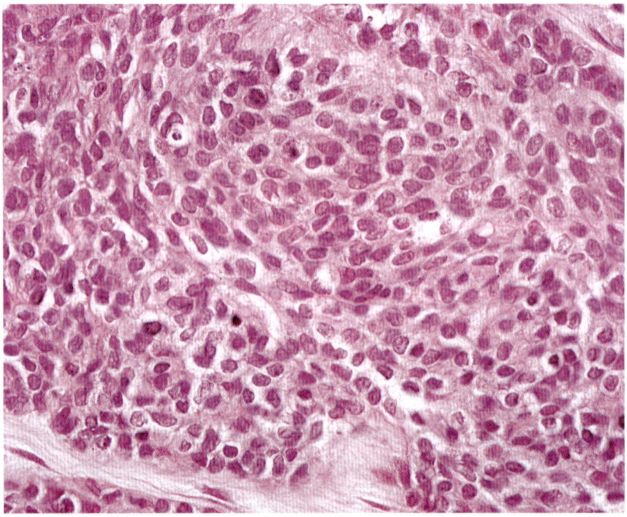

FIGURE 14.11 **Desmoplastic Small Round Cell Tumor.** Sheets of tightly packed cells with ovoid vesicular nuclei and scanty cytoplasm.

(Figs. 14.10 and 14.11, e-Figs. 14.35 and 14.36). Less often, the cytoplasm is more abundant, with clearing or vacuolation (e-Fig. 14.37). There can also be rosette formation (e-Fig. 14.38), and focally, tumor cells may have intracytoplasmic eosinophilic rhabdoid inclusions composed of bundles of intermediate filaments. There are numerous mitoses, and necrosis is common including in tumor islands and individual cells (e-Fig. 14.39).

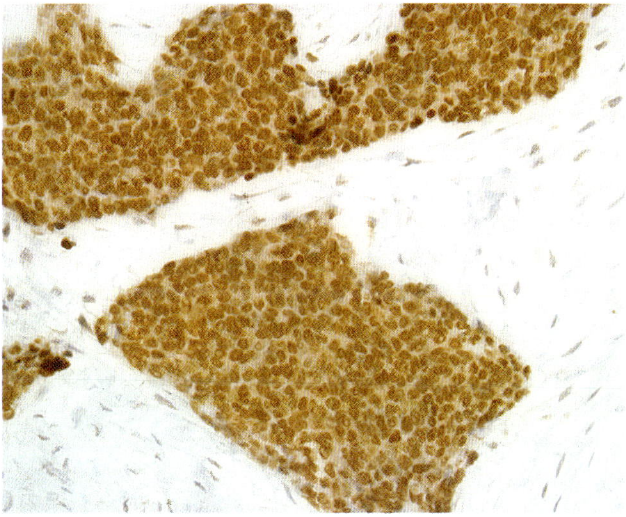

FIGURE 14.12 **Desmoplastic Small Round Cell Tumor.** The tumor shows nuclear immunoreactivity for antibodies directed to the carboxy terminus of WT1. Immunoperoxidase.

Typically, there is a striking desmoplastic stromal reaction that divides the tumor into sharply demarcated islands (Fig. 14.10, e-Figs. 14.40 and 14.41). This stroma is relatively cellular and contains of spindle-shaped fibroblasts and SMA-positive myofibroblasts (e-Figs. 14.42), sometimes with prominent vascularity. Some tumors show focal epithelial differentiation, with the presence of glands or pseudoglands, and single rows of cells may also be present within the stroma in a pattern reminiscent of lobular breast carcinoma (e-Fig. 14.43). Occasional examples show a greater amount of cytological atypia, with larger nuclei, and rarely, a tumor comprises predominantly cells with atypical nuclei or spindled morphology.[19]

Ancillary Investigations

DSRCT is immunoreactive for antibodies directed to the carboxy terminus of WT1 (Fig. 14.12).[17,20] In addition, the tumor is immunohistochemically polyphenotypic with coexpression of desmin (Fig. 14.13, e-Fig. 14.44), cytokeratins (e-Figs. 14.45 and 14.46) (but not CK5/6 or CK20) and neural markers (e-Fig. 14.47), including synaptophysin, chromogranin, neurofilament, CD56 and in some cases S100 protein.[19,21] The immunoreactivity to desmin (and sometimes the cytokeratin) is typically in a paranuclear dot distribution. However, not all of these antigens are expressed in every tumor. The rhabdomyoblastic nuclear antigens myogenin and MyoD1 are absent, and CD99 is usually negative, helping to distinguish this from ES. Occasional CD99-positive examples of DSRCT occur, and this should be evaluated with the other findings. However, the characteristic translocation of DSRCT can be detected in paraffin-embedded material by FISH, using a specific break-apart probe that

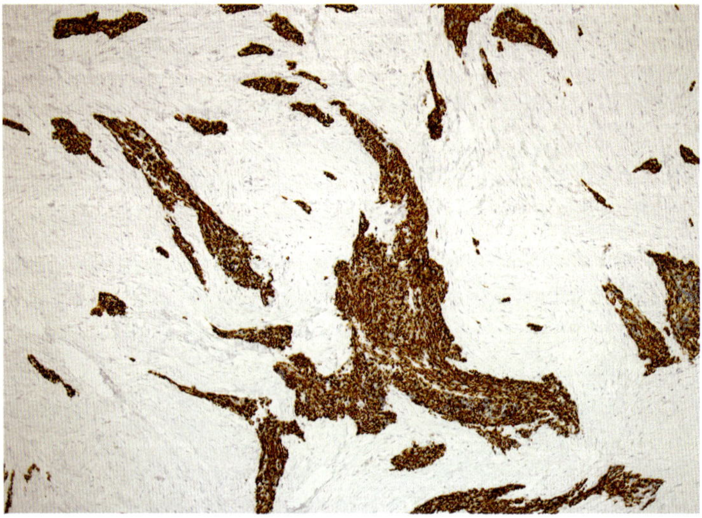

FIGURE 14.13 **Desmoplastic Small Round Cell Tumor.** There is often strong desmin expression, although the tumor is negative for myogenin and MyoD1. Immunoperoxidase.

flanks the common *EWSR1* translocations, or the *EWSR1-WT1* fusion transcript can be identified by RT-PCR.

NEUROBLASTIC TUMORS

Introduction

Neuroblastoma is a malignant tumor derived from embryonic neural crest cells that become a component of sympathetic ganglia including the adrenal medulla. It is composed of primitive neuroblasts that show a variable degree of ganglionic differentiation as ganglioneuroblastoma. These are mainly childhood neoplasms that, with ganglioneuroma, show a spectrum of differentiation and biologic behavior corresponding to points along the pathway of neuroblastic maturation. The terminology is complex. In the International Neuroblastoma Pathology Classification (based on the Shimada system), neuroblastoma is categorized as Schwannian stroma-poor (<50% of the tumor), and is further subdivided by degree of differentiation (see below). Ganglioneuroblastoma, which is less common, is classified as intermixed (stroma rich) or nodular (composite stroma rich/stroma dominant or stroma poor), and ganglioneuroma is recognized as a (stroma-dominant) maturing or mature stage.[22-24] It should be noted that the term stroma is used here to refer to Schwann cells rather than in its usual sense of a connective tissue component.

Risk estimation of each patient is necessary to decide the most appropriate therapy. Prognostic categories for neuroblastic tumors have been defined based on combinations of clinical and histological factors, including the mitosis-karyorrhexis index (MKI), which indicates the number of mitoses and karyorrhexes per 5,000 cells.[22-24] Favorable prognostic groups are (a) stroma rich, all ages, no nodular pattern; (b) stroma poor, age: 1.5 to 5 years, differentiated (i.e., with a ganglion cell component > 5%), MKI < 100; (c) stroma poor, age < 1.5 years, MKI < 200. Unfavorable prognostic groups are (a) stroma rich, all ages, nodular pattern; (b) stroma poor, age > 5 years; (c) stroma poor, age 1.5 to 5 years, undifferentiated; (d) stroma poor, age < 1.5 years, MKI > 200.

More recently, however, emphasis has been placed on the prognostic value of molecular abnormalities and the International Neuroblastoma Risk Group has developed a staging and risk classification that stratifies patients for clinical trials by both clinical and molecular parameters.[25-28] Favorable prognostic factors include young age, low stage, favorable histology, absence of *MYCN* amplification, and absence of loss in chromosome 1p. Conversely, allelic loss of chromosome 1p, *MYCN* amplification, and extra copies of chromosome 17q are significantly associated with unfavorable outcome. In a multivariate analysis, loss of chromosome 1p was the most powerful prognostic factor.[29] For more detailed information, the reader is referred to the literature,[22-28] to textbooks of pediatric pathology, and to the dedicated website of the National Cancer Institute in the United States (http://www.cancer.gov/cancertopics/pdq/treatment/neuroblastoma/HealthProfessional).

The pathologist should be cautious about assigning a histologic category in a small and possibly nonrepresentative biopsy, and the report should include a comment to that effect.

NEUROBLASTOMA

Clinical Features

Neuroblastoma is the third most common malignancy in childhood after hematolymphoid and central nervous system neoplasms. The peak age of presentation is approximately 18 to 21 months, and most cases are diagnosed by 5 years, although the tumor can rarely occur in adults. There is a slight excess in males.[30] Neuroblastic tumors mostly arise in the distribution of the sympathetic ganglia, with the majority of tumors originating in the retroperitoneum, including the adrenal medulla, and the organ of Zuckerkandl. Other sites include the mediastinum, cervical and sacral regions, and some examples occur in patients with other neoplasms including neurofibromatosis type 1 and translocation carcinomas of the kidney.

In addition to symptoms related to a mass, patients can present with a variety of systemic or local clinical features such as fever, anemia, and diarrhea, or unusual syndromes, including the "blueberry muffin baby" due to cutaneous tumor deposits, and "myoclonus-opsoclonus," suspected to be an autoimmune response against cross-reactive proteins of tumor and neuronal cells.[31] Patients often have elevated levels of urinary catecholamines and their metabolites. The clinical course of neuroblastoma is very variable, and can range from spontaneous regression to rapid progression and death. Neuroblastoma can also mature into ganglioneuroma, either spontaneously or following treatment (e-Fig. 14.48).

Pathologic Features

The tumor forms a nodular or multilobular mass, with a yellow to white cut surface or variable consistency. Hemorrhage and necrosis are common. Calcification is also a frequent finding, and there may be cyst formation. Microscopically, there are sheets, nested patterns, or lobules of tumor cells of medium to large size. The cells have rounded, ovoid, or elongated hyperchromatic nuclei (Fig. 14.14, e-Figs. 14.49 and 14.50), with evenly dispersed or clumped chromatin. There is minimal amphophilic cytoplasm and variable amounts of pale neurofibrillary matrix that resembles neuropil (Fig. 14.14). Artifactual crushing and streaking of tumor nuclei (e-Fig. 14.51) is common, and sometimes there is cytoplasmic clearing (e-Fig. 14.52). Rosette formation can be seen in varying degree from rudimentary cell clusters (e-Fig. 14.53) to well-formed Homer-Wright rosettes where neuritic processes of neuroblasts converge to a central point without a lumen. The large cell variant, composed of large neuroblasts with distinct nuclear membranes and multiple nucleoli, behaves particularly aggressively.[32] Spindled cells with features intermediate between neuroblastoma cells and Schwann cells are sometimes seen (e-Fig. 14.54). A pleomorphic (anaplastic) variant is also described, comprising cells with a striking

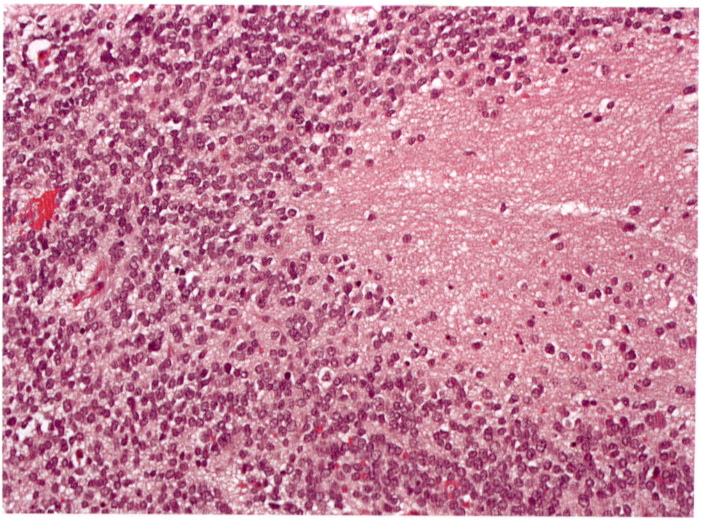

FIGURE 14.14 **Neuroblastoma.** The tumor comprises cells with round or ovoid nuclei, usually with minimal amounts of amphophilic cytoplasm. There is a variable amount of pale neurofibrillary matrix.

degree of cellular pleomorphism and anaplasia with bizarre forms, but this is of uncertain clinical significance.[33]

In tumors displaying ganglionic differentiation, the cells are polygonal and enlarged, with more obvious amphophilic or eosinophilic cytoplasm that with maturation increases in amount and is associated with round vesicular nuclei with prominent nucleoli (e-Fig. 14.55). Tumors are divided into undifferentiated, poorly differentiated and differentiating subtypes, according to the percentage of cells with ganglion cell differentiation. Undifferentiated neuroblastoma shows no ganglionic differentiation, while the poorly differentiated form shows <5% of differentiating cells and differentiating neuroblastoma displays >5%. Mitotic index and presence of calcification should also be recorded.

Ancillary Investigations

NSE is strongly expressed and was formerly advocated as a useful marker, but it is not specific and is often positive in other small round cell tumors. NB84 is a more specific antibody that recognizes an uncharacterized antigen in neuroblastoma cell lines (e-Fig. 14.56). Other markers that are consistently expressed include neurofilament protein (NFP) (e-Figs. 14.57 and 14.58), chromogranin, synaptophysin, and CD56. Neuroblastomas are negative for CD99, leukocytic and muscle markers, and cytokeratins. The cells of neuroblastoma can be particularly difficult to identify in bone marrow trephine biopsies, where they can closely resemble hematopoietic precursors, especially those of erythroid series, and are often subject to artifactual distortion (Fig. 14.15). This is particularly problematic when trying to identify small amounts of residual tumor following chemotherapy, and immunohistochemistry for neural markers and NB84 can be very helpful in identifying clusters of metastatic neuroblastoma. A panel including NB84, NSE, NFP, and CD56 gives a high degree of sensitivity for detecting residual tumor in this setting.

The *MYCN* oncogene is amplified in approximately a quarter of cases of neuroblastoma, and as mentioned its amplification is associated with advanced stage tumors and adverse outcomes. Loss of heterozygosity of chromosomes 1p36 and 11q23 is also found, with deletion of chromosome 1p being prognostically adverse.

GANGLIONEUROBLASTOMA

Ganglioneuroblastoma shows a degree of differentiation that is intermediate between neuroblastoma and ganglioneuroma (which is a fully differentiated tumor comprising Schwann cell stroma and mature ganglion cells, without immature elements). Ganglioneuroblastoma is composed of a mixture of ganglion cells, in varying stages of maturation, and immature neuroblasts. The proportions and arrangements of constituent cells vary, and the tumor has a range of morphology and behavior. Clinical stage and histological subtype are the major prognostic indicators.[34]

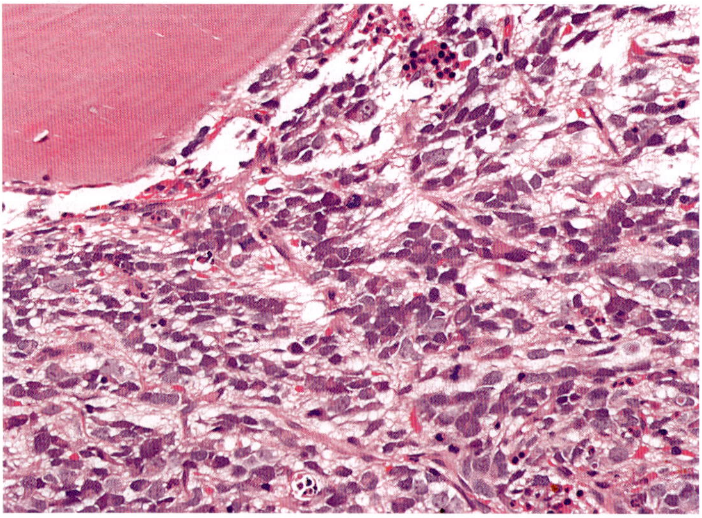

FIGURE 14.15 **Neuroblastoma.** The cells can be especially difficult to identify in bone marrow trephine biopsies, where they can resemble hemopoietic precursors, and there is often artifactual distortion. The tumor cells here have increased cytoplasm, reflecting differentiation.

Clinical Features

Most tumors occur in the retroperitoneum or mediastinum, with a distribution similar to that of ganglioneuroma.

Pathologic Features

The tumor is grossly circumscribed and lobulated. The cut surface is often heterogeneous, with soft hemorrhagic foci corresponding to neuroblastomatous areas, abutting firm, paler areas that represent the better-differentiated ganglioneuromatous areas. Gritty white areas of calcification are a common feature. Microscopically, the tumor displays neuroblastoma-like foci of primitive neuroblasts and areas of ganglioneuromatous spindle cell stroma (Fig. 14.16). Ganglioneuroblastoma is subclassified according to the arrangement and proportion of these areas. The nodular subtype (which can be Schwannian stroma rich, stroma poor or both) comprises defined, cellular nodules of neuroblastoma next to large areas of typical ganglioneuroma (Fig. 14.17). The intermixed subtype consists of microscopic nests of neuroblastoma within ganglioneuromatous stroma (Fig. 14.18). The stroma can vary from a delicate, eosinophilic fibrillary meshwork composed of tumor cell neurites (e-Figs. 14.59 and 14.60) to a Schwannian stroma that can be markedly collagenous, with large numbers of Schwann cells (e-Fig. 14.61). Ganglion cells are present, in varying stages of maturation (e-Fig. 14.62), and can appear atypical or dysplastic. The cells are polygonal, with moderate to abundant amphophilic cytoplasm, round to

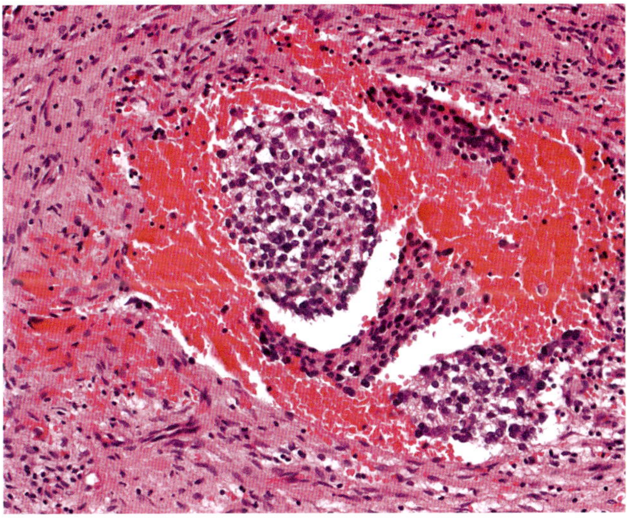

FIGURE 14.16 **Ganglioneuroblastoma.** The tumor comprises neuroblastoma-like areas of primitive neuroblasts along with areas of ganglioneuromatous stroma.

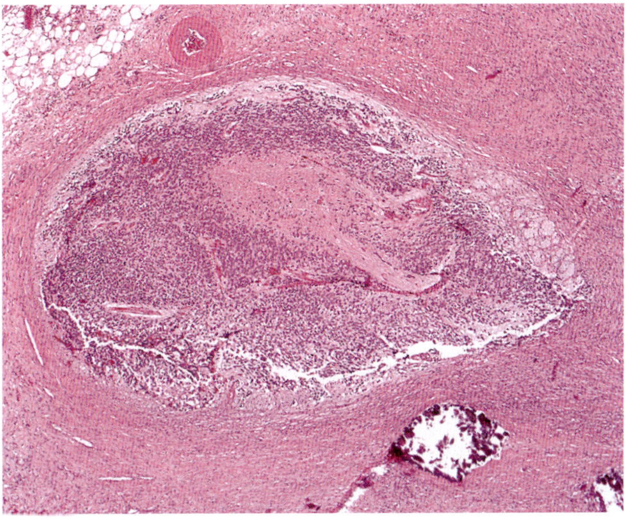

FIGURE 14.17 **Ganglioneuroblastoma.** The nodular subtype comprises well-defined nodules of neuroblastoma next to large areas of typical ganglioneuroma. Note the focal calcification.

ovoid vesicular nuclei, and prominent nuclei. Binucleate and sometimes trinucleate forms are often easily seen. Calcification can be prominent (e-Fig. 14.63). Rarely, ganglioneuroblastoma can be pigmented, with the pigment resembling neuromelanin.

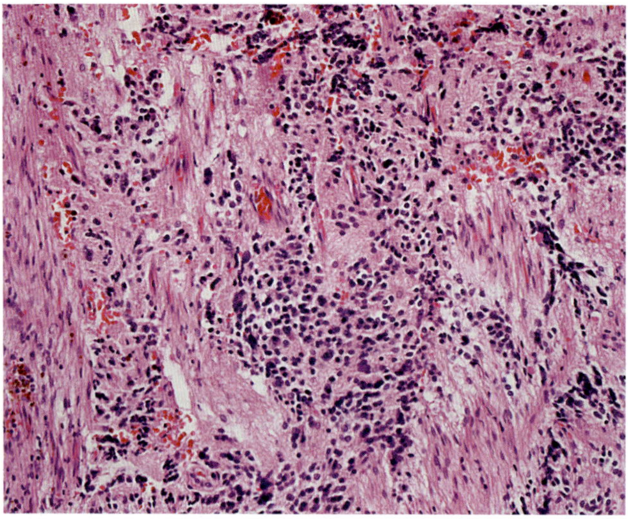

FIGURE 14.18 **Ganglioneuroblastoma.** The intermixed subtype consists of microscopic nests of neuroblastoma within ganglioneuromatous stroma.

Ancillary Investigations

The neuroblastic component expresses markers of neuroectodermal differentiation, and NB84 (e-Fig. 14.64). Ganglion cells express NSE, CD56, and neurofilament. S100 protein, although negative in ganglion cells, is positive within Schwann cells within the stroma. *In situ* hybridization and gene expression profiling[35] studies have shown that Schwann cells in maturing neuroblastomas differ genetically from neuronal cells. Additionally, the Schwann cells have been found to contain normal numbers of chromosomes, suggesting they are a reactive population of normal cells that invade the neuroblastoma.[36]

GANGLIONEUROMA (SEE ALSO CHAPTER 9)

Clinical Features

This is a differentiated neural tumor that occurs in older children and adults in the posterior mediastinum and retroperitoneum and, infrequently, in the adrenal gland. Ganglioneuromas can form large masses that present with pressure effects and sometimes with symptoms due to secretion of vasoactive peptides. Rare examples have been described in various other sites, including gastrointestinal tract, where diffuse infiltration is termed ganglioneuromatosis[37] (see Chapter 9).

Pathologic Features

This is a solid encapsulated lesion that can focally calcify. Histologically, there are fascicles of Schwann cells with variable numbers of ganglion cells, usually lacking satellite cells. A component of fat is sometimes present. Ganglioneuroma with pheochromocytoma has been described, sometimes in patients with neurofibromatosis type 1, or MEN type IIb, and several examples of malignant peripheral nerve sheath tumors (MPNSTs) arising in ganglioneuroma have also been reported.[38]

Ancillary Investigations

The ganglion cells express chromogranin, synaptophysin, NSE and CD56, whereas the Schwann cells are diffusely positive for S100 protein.

OLFACTORY NEUROBLASTOMA

Olfactory neuroblastoma (ON) is a malignant neuroectodermal tumor arising from the olfactory membrane of the sinonasal tract that represents approximately 2% to 3% of sinonasal tract neoplasms. It is also known as esthesioneuroblastoma and olfactory placode tumor, and appears to originate from the olfactory neuroepithelium found in the upper nasal septum, the cribriform plate, and the superior medial surface of the superior turbinate.[39] There are no known etiologic agents, and earlier suggestions that ON may belong to the ES/PNET family of tumors have been disproven in subsequent studies in which the *EWSR1-FLI1* fusion transcript or *EWSR1* rearrangement were unidentifiable by RT-PCR or FISH.[40,41]

Clinical Features

There is a slight female predominance and a wide age range, with bimodal peaks in the second and sixth decades of life.[42] The tumor typically occurs in the superior nasal cavity in the area of the cribriform plate. Similar tumors may also arise "ectopically," in the lower nasal cavity, within one of the paranasal sinuses or the nasopharynx. The main presenting symptoms are unilateral nasal obstruction and epistaxis. A sinonasal mass causing sinus opacification with or without bony erosion can be seen radiologically, and tumor calcifications may produce a speckled radiological appearance.[42]

Pathologic Features

Macroscopically, the tumor is soft and polypoid with hemorrhage and necrosis. There is a variety of histological patterns, as well as frequent morphological variation between tumors. The tumor is located submucosally (Fig. 14.19, e-Fig. 14.65), and the most common appearance is of cellular lobules, sheets and nests of uniform small cells with round vesicular nuclei, and scanty cytoplasm (e-Figs. 14.66 and 14.67). Small nucleoli may be conspicuous. The tumor cells can sometimes be larger

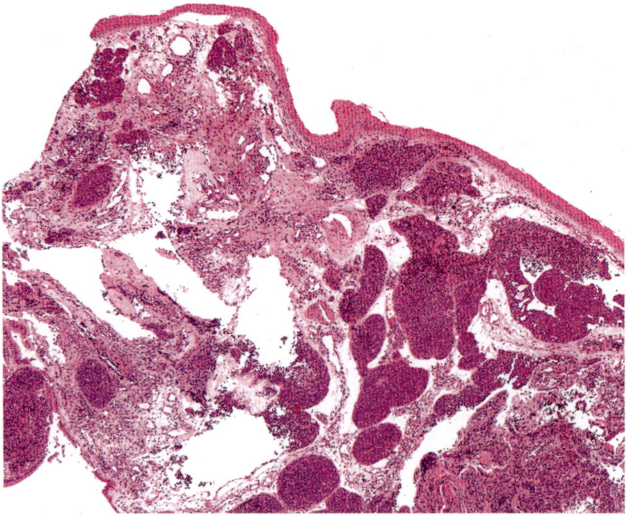

FIGURE 14.19 **Olfactory Neuroblastoma.** The tumor is located within the submucosa. The lobular appearance is easily discernible at low power.

and polygonal, with more abundant cytoplasm, and there is a spectrum of cellular atypia and mitotic activity. Sometimes, there is a neurofibrillary background (e-Fig. 14.67), similar to that seen in other neurogenic tumors such as ganglioneuroblastoma, but this can be sparse or absent. On occasion, there are rosettes of either Flexner-Wintersteiner (true neural rosettes) or Homer Wright-type (pseudorosettes) (e-Fig. 14.69), although ganglionic differentiation is a rare finding. The stroma is fibrovascular, and the vascular network can be prominent (e-Fig. 14.68). Calcification is often present.

Tumors are histologically graded into four categories as defined by Hyams.[43] Grade 1 tumors, the most differentiated, show a prominent lobular architecture (Fig. 14.20, e-Fig. 14.70). The constituent cells are uniform, with round nuclei, even chromatin (Fig. 14.20), and sometimes small nucleoli. Neurofibrillary matrix is prominent (e-Fig. 14.69), but mitotic figures and necrosis are not seen. In grade 2 tumors, the neoplastic cells show a greater degree of atypia, and there may be small numbers of mitotic figures (e-Fig. 14.70). In addition, the neurofibrillary matrix is less pronounced than in grade 1 tumors. Homer Wright rosettes may be noted in grade 1 and 2 tumors.

The higher grade neoplasms (grades 3 and 4) are markedly cellular, with greater cellular hyperchromasia and atypia (Fig. 14.21), as well as more solid growth with less obvious lobular architecture. Mitotic activity is more abundant and includes atypical forms, and there is often necrosis. The neurofibrillary component is generally only focal in grade 3 tumors and is usually absent in those of grade 4. True neural

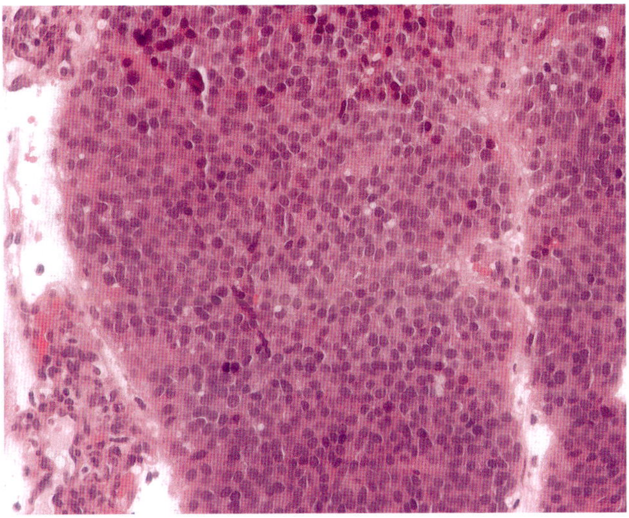

FIGURE 14.20 **Olfactory Neuroblastoma.** Grade 1 tumors are the most differentiated, showing a prominent lobular architecture.

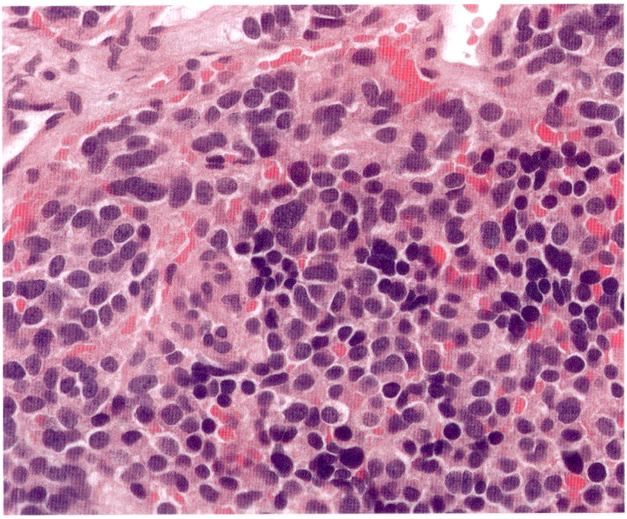

FIGURE 14.21 **Olfactory Neuroblastoma.** Higher grade neoplasms (grades 3 and 4) are markedly cellular, with greater hyperchromasia and atypia, and more solid growth with less pronounced lobular architecture.

(Flexner-Wintersteiner) rosettes can rarely be seen, but Homer-Wright rosettes, seen in better-differentiated tumors, are usually absent.[42] Histologically, lower grade tumors are reported to have a better 5-year survival than those of higher grade.[43]

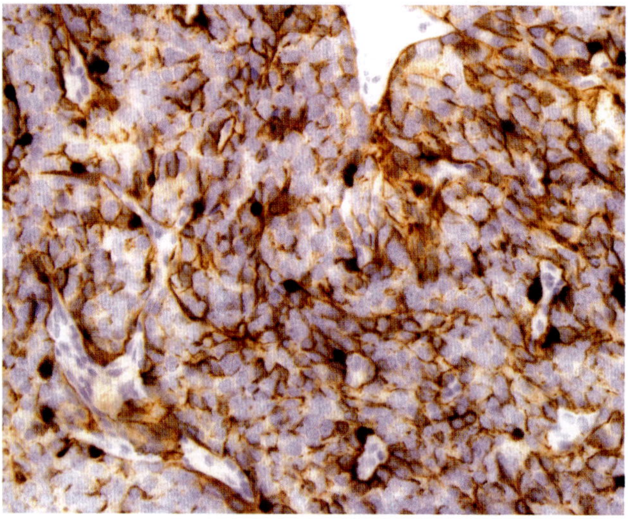

FIGURE 14.22 **Olfactory Neuroblastoma.** A network of S100 protein–positive cells surrounds small nests of lesional cells in a sustentacular-like pattern. Immunoperoxidase.

Ancillary Investigations

There is frequent variation in immunoprofile between tumors, but generally strong reactivity for NSE (e-Fig. 14.71), with variable expression of other neuroendocrine markers such as CD56, NFP, synaptophysin (e-Fig. 14.72), and chromogranin. A delicate network of S100 protein–positive cells often surrounds islands of lesional cells in a sustentacular-like pattern (Fig. 14.22), similar to that seen in paragangliomas. There can be focal expression of cytokeratins and EMA. The tumor does not express CD99, or leukocytic or muscle markers. Ultrastructurally, tumors display 80 to 230 nm diameter dense core neurosecretory granules.[44]

MELANOTIC NEUROECTODERMAL TUMOR OF INFANCY

This tumor arises mainly in the anterior maxilla and sometimes the mandible or skull of infants as an osteolytic lesion that can present intraorally. It is sometimes associated with elevated urinary excretion of vanillyl mandelic acid. Although many cases behave in a benign fashion, some recur and a small number metastasize so that early radical surgery with close follow-up is usually advised.[45] Histologically, the tumor is composed of large polygonal melanin-containing cells arranged around central smaller darkly staining cells with minimal pleomorphism but occasionally mitotic activity (e-Fig. 14.73). The tumor cells express neural markers such as synaptophysin and the larger pigmented cells additionally express cytokeratins and HMB45.

ECTOMESENCHYMOMA

This very rare malignant tumor occurs in childhood and mostly in males, in a variety of locations including intracranially, in the nasal cavity, in the genitourinary tract, and in soft tissue.[46] Rhabdomyosarcoma can also metastasize as ectomesenchymoma.[47] Histologically, it is composed of neuroectodermal elements, usually ganglioneuroma or ganglioneuroblastoma (e-Figs. 14.74 and 14.75), and a mesenchymal component, most commonly rhabdomyosarcoma of small round cell or spindle cell type. Other mesenchymal tissues are occasionally seen. Each component demonstrates appropriate immunoreactivity. Gene expression microarray analysis[48] has suggested that intracranial malignant ectomesenchymoma is more closely related to MPNST than to rhabdomyosarcoma.

OTHER SARCOMAS WITH SMALL ROUND CELL MORPHOLOGY

Poorly differentiated synovial sarcoma (see Chapter 10) can be diagnosed by the presence of more typical spindle cell or biphasic areas, by immunostaining for TLE1, and by demonstration of specific genetic features. **MPNST** (see Chapter 10) rarely has small cell morphology but needs to be considered especially in patients with neurofibromatosis type 1. This can be S100 protein–positive and in the absence of more typical morphologic features can require exclusion of other entities including melanoma. **Round cell liposarcoma** (see Chapter 16) has somewhat larger cells, and often there is a residual component of myxoid liposarcoma or lipoblastic differentiation. However, genetic investigation can sometimes be required.

NONMESENCHYMAL TUMORS

Small Cell Carcinoma

This can present as a metastasis in soft tissue, in the presence or absence of a known primary tumor in lung (where it can be very small) or elsewhere, and in a biopsy can be mistaken for a soft tissue small round cell tumor. The nuclei are darkly staining and often appear molded to each other, and cytoplasm is minimal (e-Figs. 14.76 and 14.77). There is often abundant apoptosis and areas of necrosis are common. Immunohistochemistry is diagnostic, with positivity for cytokeratin (often in dot pattern [e-Fig. 14.78]), chromogranin, NSE and TTF1 (in nuclei, e-Fig. 14.79), and none for other relevant markers including neurofilaments.

Lymphoma of Soft Tissue

Lymphomas can involve soft tissue by extranodal extension from adjacent nodes or as part of systemic involvement. Primary soft tissue lymphoma is rare and can arise in the proximal extremities or trunk in older adults.[49]

The majority are diffuse large B-cell lymphomas with occasional examples of other non-Hodgkin lymphomas. They can be diagnosed by relevant panels of lymphoid markers and by the absence of antigens expressed by cells of other lineages. Lymphoblastic lymphoma especially of B cell type can mimic other small round cell tumors and can be identified by immunostaining for TdT as well as CD10 and other B cell markers.

Tumors of Hemopoietic Cells

These rarely present as soft tissue tumors but can cause diagnostic difficulties. **Tumefactive extramedullary hemopoiesis** (see Chapter 15) occurs in some patients with extramedullary hemopoiesis from a variety of hematologic causes including severe anemias and myeloid metaplasia of bone marrow. It forms a soft tissue deposit containing a mixture of cells in which all three hemopoietic cell lines at various stages are usually represented (e-Fig. 14.80). A sclerosing variant is described (e-Fig. 14.81),which should not be confused with Hodgkin or non-Hodgkin lymphoma.[50] **Extramedullary myeloid tumor (granulocytic sarcoma)** can form a soft tissue mass known as chloroma in patients with acute or chronic myeloid leukemia. It can also be the presenting sign. The infiltrating cells form sheets or files of neutrophil (or sometimes eosinophil) myelocytes, with distinct nuclear membranes and small nucleoli (e-Fig. 14.82). They can be identified by immunohistochemistry for myeloperoxidase, CD117, CD43, CD68, and lysozyme. **Mastocytosis** can present in the skin or, exceptionally, as a soft tissue mass. There are usually admixed eosinophils. The mast cells can be identified with toluidine blue or by immunostaining for CD117.

REFERENCES

1. Newton WA Jr, Gehan EA, Webber BL, et al. Classification of rhabdomyosarcomas and related sarcomas. Pathologic aspects and proposal for a new classification–an Intergroup Rhabdomyosarcoma Study. *Cancer*. 1995;76:1073 - 1085.
2. Mercado GE, Barr FG. Fusions involving PAX and FOX genes in the molecular pathogenesis of alveolar rhabdomyosarcoma: recent advances. *Curr Mol Med*. 2007;7:47–61.
3. Sorensen PH, Lynch JC, Qualman SJ, et al. PAX3-FKHR and PAX7-FKHR gene fusions are prognostic indicators in alveolar rhabdomyosarcoma: a report from the children's oncology group. *J Clin Oncol*. 2002;20:2672–2679.
4. Davicioni E, Finckenstein FG, Shahbazian V, et al. Identification of a PAX-FKHR gene expression signature that defines molecular classes and determines the prognosis of alveolar rhabdomyosarcomas. *Cancer Res*. 2006;66:6936–6946.
5. Boman F, Champigneulle J, Schmitt C, et al. Clear cell rhabdomyosarcoma. *Pediatr Pathol Lab Med*. 1996;16:951–959.
6. Morotti RA, Nicol KK, Parham DM, et al. An immunohistochemical algorithm to facilitate diagnosis and subtyping of rhabdomyosarcoma: the Children's Oncology Group experience. *Am J Surg Pathol*. 2006;30:962–968.
7. Morgenstern DA, Rees H, Sebire NJ, et al. Rhabdomyosarcoma subtyping by immunohistochemical assessment of myogenin: tissue array study and review of the literature. *Pathol Oncol Res*. 2008;14:233–238.
8. Corao DA, Biegel JA, Coffin CM, et al. ALK expression in rhabdomyosarcomas: correlation with histologic subtype and fusion status. *Pediatr Dev Pathol*. 2009;12:275–283.

9. Sullivan LM, Atkins KA, LeGallo RD. PAX immunoreactivity identifies alveolar rhabdomyosarcoma. *Am J Surg Pathol.* 2009;33:775–780.
10. Parham DM, Qualman SJ, Teot L, et al. Correlation between histology and PAX/FKHR fusion status in alveolar rhabdomyosarcoma: a report from the Children's Oncology Group. *Am J Surg Pathol.* 2007;31:895–901.
11. Lazar A, Abruzzo LV, Pollock RE, et al. Molecular diagnosis of sarcomas: chromosomal translocations in sarcomas. *Arch Pathol Lab Med.* 2006;130:1199–1207.
12. Ordonez JL, Osuna D, Herrero D, et al. Advances in Ewing's sarcoma research: where are we now and what lies ahead? *Cancer Res.* 2009;69:7140–7150.
13. Nascimento AG, Unii KK, Pritchard DJ, et al. A clinicopathologic study of 20 cases of large-cell (atypical) Ewing's sarcoma of bone. *Am J Surg Pathol.* 1980;4:29–36.
14. Folpe AL, Goldblum JR, Rubin BP, et al. Morphologic and immunophenotypic diversity in Ewing family tumors: a study of 66 genetically confirmed cases. *Am J Surg Pathol.* 2005;29:1025–1033.
15. Parham DM, Dias P, Kelly DR, et al. Desmin positivity in primitive neuroectodermal tumors of childhood. *Am J Surg Pathol.* 1992;16:483–492.
16. Llombart-Bosch A, Machado I, Navarro S, et al. Histological heterogeneity of Ewing's sarcoma/PNET: an immunohistochemical analysis of 415 genetically confirmed cases with clinical support. *Virchows Arch.* 2009;455:397–411.
17. Gerald WL, Miller HK, Battifora H, et al. Intra-abdominal desmoplastic small round-cell tumor. Report of 19 cases of a distinctive type of high-grade polyphenotypic malignancy affecting young individuals. *Am J Surg Pathol.* 1991;15:499–513.
18. Stuart-Buttle CE, Smart CJ, Pritchard S, et al. Desmoplastic small round cell tumour: A review of literature and treatment options. *Surg Oncol.* 2008;17:107–112.
19. Ordonez NG. Desmoplastic small round cell tumor: I: a histopathologic study of 39 cases with emphasis on unusual histological patterns. *Am J Surg Pathol.* 1998;22:1303–1313.
20. Antonescu CR, Gerald WL, Magid MS, et al. Molecular variants of the EWS-WT1 gene fusion in desmoplastic small round cell tumor. *Diagn Mol Pathol.* 1998;7:24–28.
21. Ordonez NG. Desmoplastic small round cell tumor: II: an ultrastructural and immunohistochemical study with emphasis on new immunohistochemical markers. *Am J Surg Pathol.* 1998;22:1314–1327.
22. Shimada H, Ambros IM, Dehner LP, et al. Terminology and morphologic criteria of neuroblastic tumors: recommendations by the International Neuroblastoma Pathology Committee. *Cancer.* 1999;86:349–363.
23. Shimada H, Ambros IM, Dehner LP, et al. The International Neuroblastoma Pathology Classification (the Shimada system). *Cancer.* 1999;86:364–372.
24. Shimada H, Umehara S, Monobe Y, et al. International neuroblastoma pathology classification for prognostic evaluation of patients with peripheral neuroblastic tumors: a report from the Children's Cancer Group. *Cancer.* 2001;92:2451–2461.
25. Fischer M, Spitz R, Oberthur A, et al. Risk estimation of neuroblastoma patients using molecular markers. *Klin Padiatr.* 2008;220:137–146.
26. Mueller S, Matthay KK. Neuroblastoma: biology and staging. *Curr Oncol Rep.* 2009;11:431–438.
27. Ambros PF, Ambros IM, Brodeur GM, et al. International consensus for neuroblastoma molecular diagnostics: report from the International Neuroblastoma Risk Group (INRG) Biology Committee. *Br J Cancer.* 2009;100:1471–1482.
28. Cohn SL, Pearson AD, London WB, et al. The International Neuroblastoma Risk Group (INRG) classification system: an INRG Task Force report. *J Clin Oncol.* 2009;27:289–297.
29. Caron H, van Sluis P, de Kraker J, et al. Allelic loss of chromosome 1p as a predictor of unfavorable outcome in patients with neuroblastoma. *N Engl J Med.* 1996;334:225–230.

30. Stiller CA, Parkin DM. International variations in the incidence of neuroblastoma. *Int J Cancer*. 1992;52:538–543.
31. Korfei M, Fuhlhuber V, Schmidt-Woll T, et al. Functional characterisation of autoantibodies from patients with pediatric opsoclonus-myoclonus-syndrome. *J Neuroimmunol*. 2005;170:150–157.
32. Tornoczky T, Kalman E, Kajtar PG, et al. Large cell neuroblastoma: a distinct phenotype of neuroblastoma with aggressive clinical behavior. *Cancer*. 2004;100:390–397.
33. Cozzutto C, Carbone A. Pleomorphic (anaplastic) neuroblastoma. *Arch Pathol Lab Med*. 1988;112:621–625.
34. Burgues O, Navarro S, Noguera R, et al. Prognostic value of the International Neuroblastoma Pathology Classification in Neuroblastoma (Schwannian stroma-poor) and comparison with other prognostic factors: a study of 182 cases from the Spanish Neuroblastoma Registry. *Virchows Arch*. 2006;449:410–420.
35. Coco S, Defferrari R, Scaruffi P, et al. Genome analysis and gene expression profiling of neuroblastoma and ganglioneuroblastoma reveal differences between neuroblastic and Schwannian stromal cells. *J Pathol*. 2005;207:346–357.
36. Ambros IM, Zellner A, Roald B, et al. Role of ploidy, chromosome 1p, and Schwann cells in the maturation of neuroblastoma. *N Engl J Med*. 1996;334:1505–1511.
37. Thway K, Fisher C. Diffuse ganglioneuromatosis in small intestine associated with neurofibromatosis type 1. *Ann Diagn Pathol*. 2009;13:50–54.
38. de Chadarevian JP, MaePascasio J, Halligan GE, et al. Malignant peripheral nerve sheath tumor arising from an adrenal ganglioneuroma in a 6-year-old boy. *Pediatr Dev Pathol*. 2004;7:277–284.
39. Nakashima T, Kimmelman CP, Snow JB Jr. Structure of human fetal and adult olfactory neuroepithelium. *Arch Otolaryngol*. 1984;110:641–646.
40. Argani P, Perez-Ordonez B, Xiao H, et al. Olfactory neuroblastoma is not related to the Ewing family of tumors: absence of EWS/FLI1 gene fusion and MIC2 expression. *Am J Surg Pathol*. 1998;22:391–398.
41. Kumar S, Perlman E, Pack S, et al. Absence of EWS/FLI1 fusion in olfactory neuroblastomas indicates these tumors do not belong to the Ewing's sarcoma family. *Hum Pathol*. 1999;30:1356–1360.
42. Wenig BM. Undifferentiated malignant neoplasms of the sinonasal tract. *Arch Pathol Lab Med*. 2009;133:699–712.
43. Hyams. *Tumors of the Upper Respiratory Tract and Ear*. 2nd ed. Washington, DC: AFIP; 1988.
44. Hirose T, Scheithauer BW, Lopes MB, et al. Olfactory neuroblastoma. An immunohistochemical, ultrastructural, and flow cytometric study. *Cancer*. 1995;76:4–19.
45. Kruse-Losler B, Gaertner C, Burger H, et al. Melanotic neuroectodermal tumor of infancy: systematic review of the literature and presentation of a case. *Oral Surg Oral Med Oral Pathol Oral Radiol Endod*. 2006;102:204–216.
46. Mouton SC, Rosenberg HS, Cohen MC, et al. Malignant ectomesenchymoma in childhood. *Pediatr Pathol Lab Med*. 1996;6:607–624.
47. Edwards V, Tse G, Doucet J, et al. Rhabdomyosarcoma metastasizing as a malignant ectomesenchymoma. *Ultrastruct Pathol*. 1999;23:267–273.
48. Kleinschmidt-DeMasters BK, Lovell MA, Donson AM, et al. Molecular array analyses of 51 pediatric tumors shows overlap between malignant intracranial ectomesenchymoma and MPNST but not medulloblastoma or atypical teratoid rhabdoid tumor. *Acta Neuropathol*. 2007;113:695–703.
49. Lanham GR, Weiss SW, Enzinger FM. Malignant lymphoma. A study of 75 cases presenting in soft tissue. *Am J Surg Pathol*. 1989;13:1–10.
50. Remstein ED, Kurtin PJ, Nascimento AG. Sclerosing extramedullary hematopoietic tumor in chronic myeloproliferative disorders. *Am J Surg Pathol*. 2000;24:51–55.

15

BENIGN ADIPOSE TISSUE TUMORS

INTRODUCTION

Adipose tissue tumors and lesions resembling them are usually readily recognized as benign versus malignant, but there are a few pitfalls. These include fat necrosis, silicon granulomas, and tumefactive extramedullary hematopoiesis, all of which can be mistaken for well-differentiated liposarcoma. In general, superficial lesions are benign and deep ones are more likely to be liposarcomas (although intramuscular lipomas are more common than liposarcomas). The differential diagnosis is presented in Table 15.1.

FAT NECROSIS

Clinical Features

Fat necrosis is commonly a component in a host of lesions ranging from acute pancreatitis to operative sites or areas of trauma. However, liposarcomas can also be complicated by fat necrosis.

Pathologic Features

Fat necrosis is found in both normal and neoplastic fat (lipomas, omentum, subcutaneous tissues, and fat around organs) and shows damaged fat, mononuclear inflammatory cells, foamy macrophages, giant cells, and varying degrees of fibrosis. Often, fat necrosis involves a large expanse of tissue (Fig. 15.1, e-Figs. 15.1 and 15.2), but the pitfall is that many lipomas show a pattern of small foci of multinucleate histiocytes without sclerosis (Fig. 15.2, e-Fig. 15.3), which can be mistaken for atypical lipomatous tumor or well-differentiated liposarcoma (see Chapter 16). A clue in separating the two is found at low magnification. Note the appearance of the lipoma with focal fat necrosis depicted at 4× objective magnification in Figure 15.2 and compare it to Figure 15.3, which is a well-differentiated liposarcoma at the same magnification. The atypical nuclei of the latter are hyperchromatic compared to the multinucleated histiocytes in the lipoma with fat necrosis.

TABLE 15.1 Differential Diagnosis of Benign Tumors of Adipose Tissue

	Typical clinical features	Microscopic features	Ancillary investigations
Fat necrosis	No typical features; can be encountered in normal fat and in neoplasms with fat	Fat with necrosis and many foamy macrophages, some multinucleated	CD68+ in macrophages
Juxta-articular myxoma	Near large joints, especially knee, recurs locally but benign	Similar to intramuscular myxoma, but more infiltrative, with cysts and focal cellular areas, scattered mitoses	Can be CD34+, S100 protein–
Fat atrophy	Cachexia either from dieting, malignancy, or treatment for malignancy	Lobulated fat with adipocyte shrinkage, capillaries appear more prominent	
Tumefactive extramedullary hematopoiesis	Mass in patient with a myeloproliferative disorder, benign	Trilinear hematopoiesis with erythroid hyperplasia and fat	
Lipoma	Usually superficial well-circumscribed masses in adults (some intramuscular, rarely retroperitoneal)	Has the appearances of mature fat	MDM2–, CDK4–, no *MDM2* amplification, *HMGA2* fusions
Angiolipoma	Superficial painful lump(s) of forearm of young adult	Lobulated fat and admixed capillary proliferation, fibrin thrombi	
Spindle cell lipoma	Superficial lesion of shoulder girdle, neck of middle-aged adults, M > F	Uniform spindle cells, fat, wiry collagen, mast cells	CD34+, S100 protein+ in fat, abnormalities of 13q and 16q

Myxoid/round cell liposarcoma	Deep soft tissues of extremities of young adults. Often metastasizes to other soft tissue sites as well as to lungs	Monotonous small uniform rounded cells with abundant (myxoid) or minimal (round cell) myxoid matrix. Rich network of delicate vessels becomes inconspicuous in round cell liposarcoma. Lipoblasts	S100 protein+ in some cases, *CHOP-FUS* or *CHOP-EWS* rearrangements
Pleomorphic lipoma	Superficial lesion of shoulder girdle, neck of middle-aged adults, M > F	Same features as spindle cell lipoma with the addition of enlarged atypical multinucleated cells ("floret" cells) and lipoblasts	CD34+, S100 protein+ in fat, abnormalities of 13q and 16q, MDM2–, CDK4–, no *MDM2* amplification
Chondroid lipoma	Multiple anatomic sites, adults	Lobulated lesion with fat, "bubbly" cells, chondroid matrix, lipoblasts, hypovascular	S100 protein+, balanced translocation t (11, 16) (q13;p12–13)
Myolipoma (lipoleiomyoma)	Deep soft tissues and pelvis/retroperitoneum. Some associated with female genital tract. F > M	Mixture of bland smooth muscle with fat	Desmin+, actin+, caldesmon+, calponin+ in myoid component, S100 protein+ in fat. Typically hormone receptor (ER, PR)+
Myelolipoma	Usually in the adrenal gland of adults, F > M, association with obesity, hypertension, and diabetes	Mixture of fat and trilinear hematopoiesis without erythroid hyperplasia	
Hibernoma	Adults usually younger than 40 y (younger than patients with ordinary lipomas), thigh	Lobulated lesion with prominent capillaries, varying amounts of mature fat cells, cells with fine vacuoles, and cells with granular eosinophilic cytoplasm.	Abnormalities of chromosome 11q13

(Continued)

TABLE 15.1 Differential Diagnosis of Benign Tumors of Adipose Tissue

	Typical clinical features	Microscopic features	Ancillary investigations
Lipoblastoma	Proximal extremities of infants, benign	Lobulated with mature fat and areas with lipoblasts and numerous capillaries (that can be indistinguishable from myxoid liposarcoma)	Variable S100 protein+, amplification of *PLAG1*, rearrangements of *HAS2* or *COL1A2*
Lipofibromatosis	Hands and feet of infants and young children, M > F	Infiltrative admixture of fat and fibrous tissue with lipoblast-like cells in areas where fat and fibrous tissue meet	Variable focal CD34+, Bcl2+, S100 protein+
Fibrous hamartoma of infancy	Infants and small children, anterior or posterior axillary fold, M >> F	Slightly infiltrative borders, fat, fibrous tissue similar to fibromatosis, and small rounded cells	Actin+ in fibromatosis-like areas, can be CD34+
Hemosiderotic fibrohistiocytic lipomatous lesion (possible relationship to pleomorphic hyalinizing angeictatic tumor)	Feet and ankles of middle-aged females, prone to recurrences but no metastases reported	Fat and fibrous areas with hemosiderin and scattered hyperchromatic pleomorphic nuclei	CD34+ in spindle cells, S100+ in fat, t(1;10) and amplification of 3p11–12, which it shares with myxoinflammatory fibroblastic sarcoma
Fibrolipomatous hamartoma of nerve (lipomatosis of nerve)	Distal upper extremities of adults, involving mostly the median and ulnar nerves, benign	Damaged nerve infiltrated by abundant fat forming a mass	
Lipomatous hemangiopericytoma (fat-rich solitary fibrous tumor)	Multiple sites, deep, adults	Spindle cell neoplasm with hemangiopericytoma vascular pattern, angulated nuclei, "patternless pattern"	CD34+, Bcl2+, CD99+

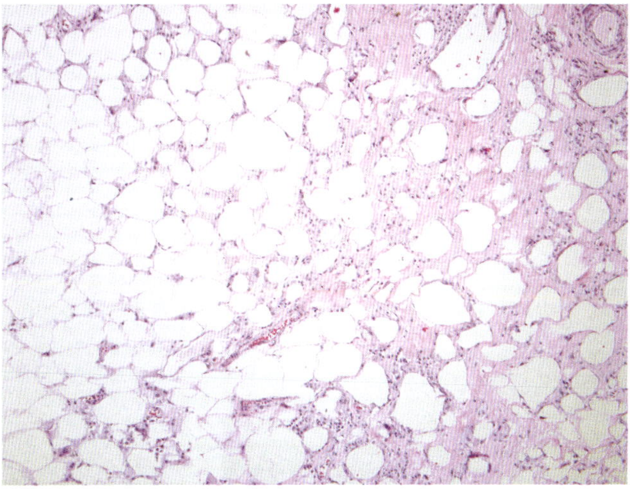

FIGURE 15.1 **Fat Necrosis.** This field shows fat, sclerosis, and sheets of foamy macrophages. Such cases are readily recognizable.

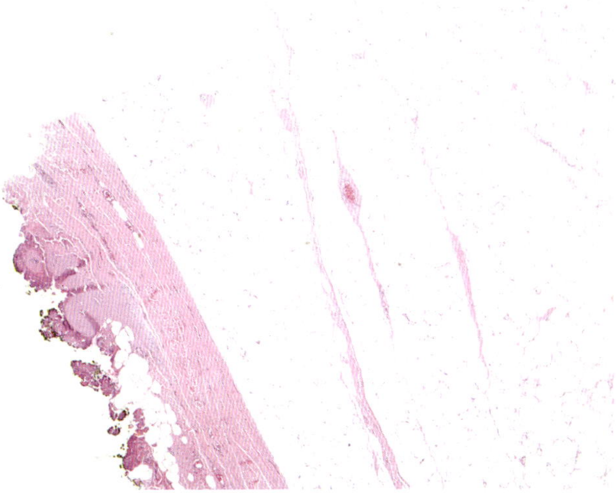

FIGURE 15.2 **Lipoma with Fat Necrosis.** This is how such foci appear at low magnification. Compare this image, original magnification 4×, to Fig. 15.3, which is of a well-differentiated liposarcoma, also prepared at 4×.

Ancillary Investigations

In general, fat necrosis is readily recognizable as such but occasionally CD68 staining can be helpful in recognizing histiocytes.

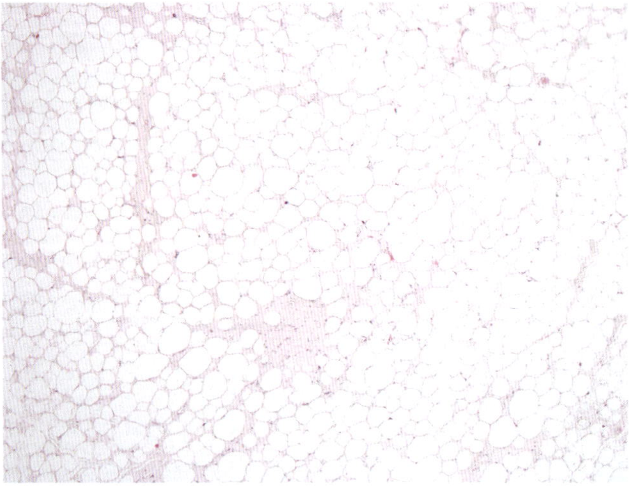

FIGURE 15.3 **Well-Differentiated Liposarcoma.** The original magnification is 4× and the findings can be compared to those in Fig. 15.2. This field shows scattered enlarged hyperchromatic nuclei that are readily apparent.

FAT ATROPHY

Clinical Features

Fat atrophy can be found in diverse settings including starvation, malnutrition (including malnutrition associated with chemotherapy), and local trauma. Patients who lose large amounts of weight by dieting also have fat atrophy. It is often encountered as an incidental finding in specimens removed for any number of reasons and is mostly relevant because it can be confused with myxoid liposarcoma.

Pathologic Features

Atrophy results in adipocyte shrinkage, which causes the adipocytes to assume an epithelioid appearance and lipoblast-like cells. Additionally, capillaries appear more prominent because they move closer together as the intervening fat shrinks (Fig. 15.4, e-Fig. 15.4). However, the overall arrangement remains lobulated as per normal fat.

SILICONE GRANULOMA

Clinical Features

Silicones are chemically inert, synthesized compounds with a wide variety of forms and uses. They are heat resistant, nonstick, and elastic. They are used in cookware, various medical applications, sealants, adhesives, lubricants, and insulation. Their classic medical use has been in breast implants although, in the past, direct injections of gel were used in various

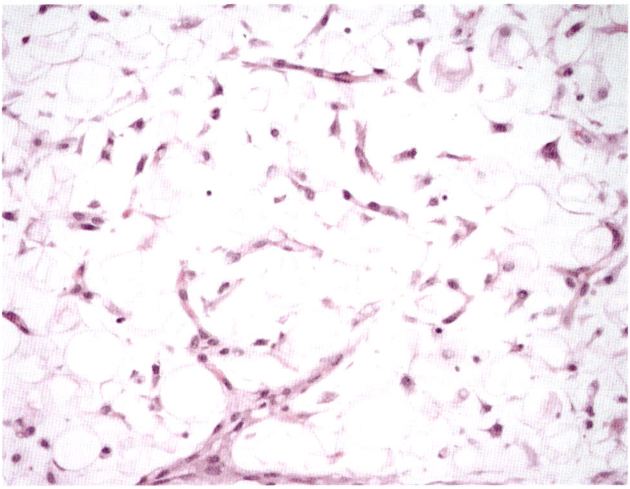

FIGURE 15.4 **Fat Atrophy.** The cytoplasm of individual adipocytesis shrunken with more prominent eosinophilia. The capillaries become less separated and scattered histiocytes are seen closer together than in fat or in a lipoma. This appearance can suggest a liposarcoma.

anatomic sites.[1] In general, silicone gel in mammary implants remains within the capsules of the implants, but these can sometimes rupture with seepage of silicone gel into the surrounding tissue and a histiocytic response. Silica compounds have also been injected in extramammary sites with exuberant histiocytic responses that mimic fibrohistiocytic neoplasms.[2]

Pathologic Features

The scenario most likely to be encountered by the pathologist is finding an unusual liposarcoma-like lesion in the breast (Figs. 15.5 and 15.6, e-Figs. 15.5 and 15.6). At scanning magnification, histiocytes containing crisply demarcated contents are reminiscent of lipoblasts. The silica gel does not consistently polarize, adding to the potential for a misdiagnosis.

The nuclei of the engulfing histiocytes differ dramatically from those of well-differentiated liposarcomas in being small, uniform, and pale rather than large and hyperchromatic. Additionally, liposarcomas seldom involve the breast, whereas leaky implants often do. In the past, a similar diagnostic problem existed with injections of Polyvinylpyrrolidone (a plasma expander no longer used) in which the unusual granulomas resembled chordomas (e-Fig. 15.7)[3] (see Chapter 12).

Ancillary Investigations

CD68 staining can be performed in any doubtful case.

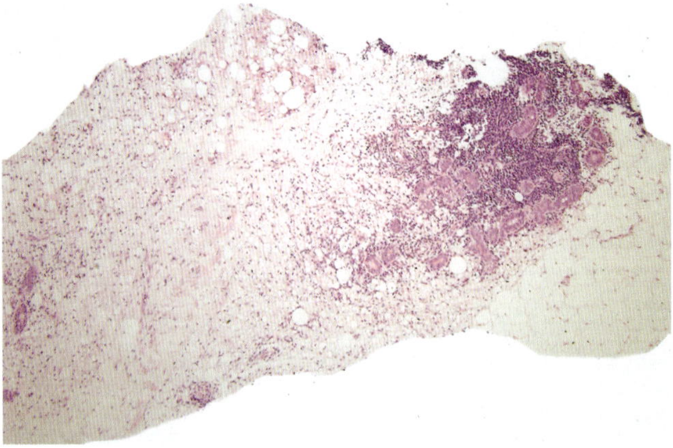

FIGURE 15.5 **Silicone Granuloma.** This image is from a needle core biopsy from a breast mass. There is an infiltrative process that had been interpreted as a liposarcoma. It would be unusual for a well-differentiated liposarcoma to have an infiltrative appearance rather than a pushing mass.

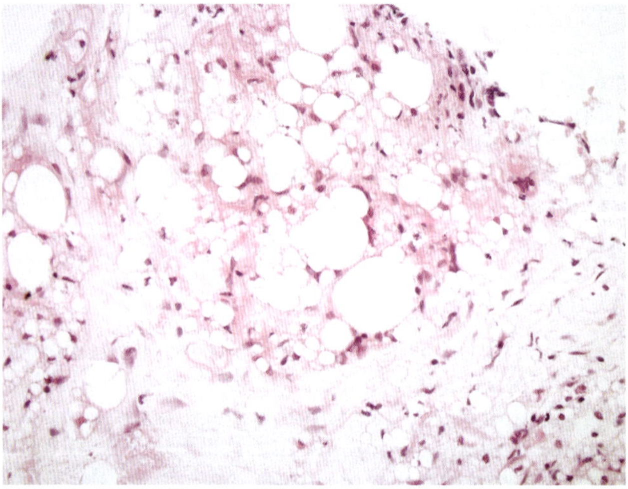

FIGURE 15.6 **Silicone Granuloma.** At high magnification, some of the cells perfectly mimic lipoblasts, but the nuclei are uniform and small. The lesion lacks the cytologic atypia of a well-differentiated liposarcoma and the vascularity of a myxoid liposarcoma (which would also feature small uniform nuclei).

TUMEFACTIVE EXTRAMEDULLARY HEMATOPOIESIS

Clinical Features

Patients with chronic myeloproliferative disorders (especially myelofibrosis) occasionally develop tumor-like deposits of extramedullary hematopoiesis, which some have termed sclerosing extramedullary hematopoietic tumor (SEMHT).[4] They tend to arise in the urinary tract (perirenal area) or mesentery where, because they contain fat, they are easily mistaken for sclerosing liposarcomas, especially when the history of a bone marrow disorder is unknown.

Pathologic Features

At low magnification, these tumors appear similar to well-differentiated liposarcomas in displaying large hyperchromatic nuclei (megakaryocytes) and fibrous bands (e-Fig. 15.8). However, at higher magnification, islands of erythropoiesis and myelopoiesis become readily apparent (Fig. 15.7, e-Fig. 15.9).

Ancillary Investigations

When small crushed needle biopsies from SEMHT are encountered, recognizing megakaryocytes as such can be difficult. Factor VIII–related antigen immunohistochemistry can be helpful in confirming megakaryocytic cells.

LIPOMA

Clinical Features

Lipomas, benign tumors composed of cells resembling mature adipocytes, are the most common soft tissue tumors of adulthood. Most arise in patients between the ages of 40 and 60 years. They are more common in obese individuals. The tumors may arise in the subcutaneous tissue (superficial lipoma) or within deep soft tissues (deep lipoma) or even from the surfaces of bone (parosteal lipoma). Occasionally, lipomas can have areas of bone formation (osteolipoma), nodules of cartilage (chondrolipoma), abundant fibrous tissue

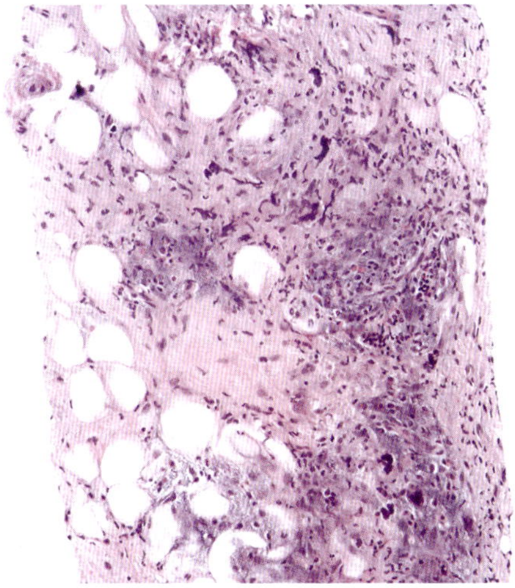

FIGURE 15.7 **Tumefactive Extramedullary Hematopoiesis.** Trilinear hematopoiesis is present within a background of sclerosis.

(fibrolipoma), extensive myxoid change (myxolipoma), or a smooth muscle component (myolipoma).[5] These microscopic subtypes do not have clinical significance. Superficial lipomas present as painless, soft, mobile masses that are generally small at the time of diagnosis (<5.0 cm). They are treated by simple excision. Recurrences are uncommon. Deep lipomas are generally larger at the time of diagnosis (>5.0 cm). They are typically painless but occasionally cause symptoms when they compress peripheral nerves. Deep seated lipomas that arise within, or between skeletal muscles are called intramuscular and intermuscular lipomas, respectively. Intramuscular lipomas affect patients in middle to late adult life. They occur in various locations including the trunk, upper and lower extremities.[6] Intramuscular lipomas may be infiltrative or well circumscribed. This clinicopathologic distinction is important, as the infiltrative type has a tendency to locally recur following incomplete excision. Intermuscular lipoma, as the name implies, arises between muscles. It also affects adults and arises most often in the anterior abdominal wall. These are usually cured by local excision.

Retroperitoneal lipomas are rare.[7] In one small series, there was a slight female predominance, tumors had a medium size of 22 cm, and there were no recurrences.[8]

Pathologic Features

Grossly, most lipomas are well circumscribed, encapsulated, and have a yellow, greasy cut surface. Intramuscular lipomas may appear as ill-defined regions of pallor within skeletal muscles. Typically, they lack a capsule. Microscopically, conventional lipoma is composed of lobules of mature adipocytes (Fig. 15.8, e-Fig. 15.10). In the infiltrative type of intramuscular

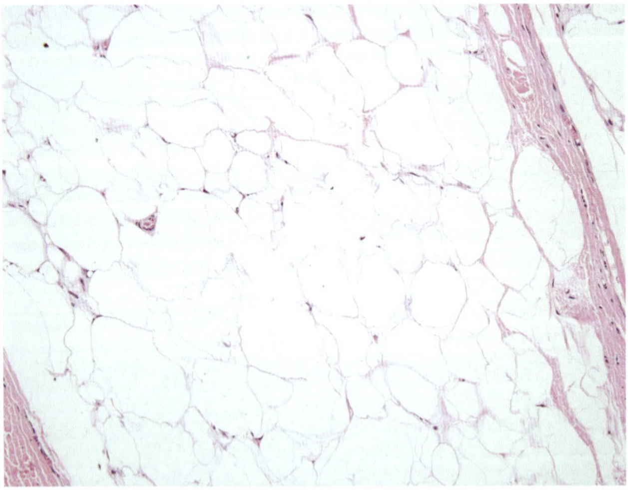

FIGURE 15.8 **Lipoma.** The appearances are similar to those of adipose tissue. Compare the sizes of the lesional nuclei to those of nearby fibroblast and endothelial cell nuclei; they are similar.

lipoma, the mature adipocytes are arranged between skeletal myocytes (Fig. 15.9, e-Fig. 15.11). The most important pathologic differential diagnosis, especially for deep-seated lipomas, is low-grade liposarcoma. Well-differentiated liposarcoma generally has sclerotic bands containing cells with bizarre, hyperchromatic nuclei and occasional lipoblasts, whereas deep lipomas are composed only of mature adipocytes that do not demonstrate hyperchromasia or nuclear enlargement. A common pitfall, especially in evaluating thickly cut sections, in addition to that presented by fat necrosis (see Fig. 15.2, e-Fig. 15.3) is confusion of "lochkern," adipocytic cells with intranuclear lipid invaginations (Fig. 15.10), with the atypical nuclei found in well-differentiated liposarcomas or with lipoblasts (Fig. 15.11). All lipomas and lipoma variants can have foci of myxoid change, which can result in diagnostic problems. This is illustrated in electronic figures in Chapter 20.

Since the majority of adipose tissue tumors in the retroperitoneum are liposarcomas, the pathologist should always be extremely cautious diagnosing lipomas in the retroperitoneum and search for pockets with atypical nuclei. The rare lipomas of the retroperitoneum have no atypical nuclei (e-Figs. 15.12 and 15.13), but confirmation with ancillary testing is often reassuring (e-Fig. 15.13).[8]

Ancillary Investigations

The majority of lipomas demonstrate karyotypic abnormalities involving 12q, and some have gene rearrangements with fusions involving the *HMGA2* gene.[8] Some otherwise typical lipomas have rings/giant marker chromosomes (as do atypical lipomatous tumors) and seem more prone

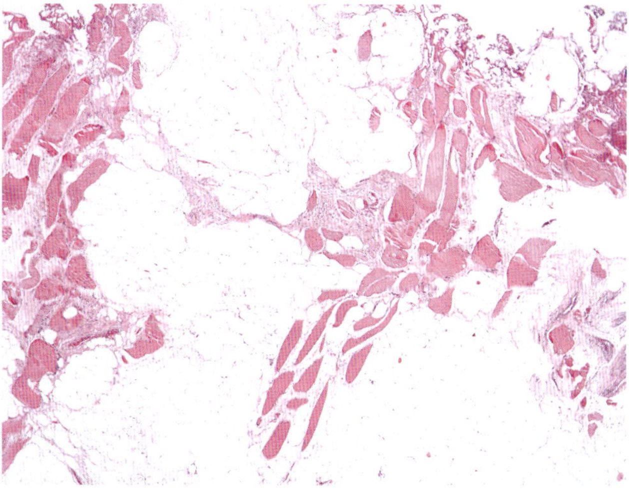

FIGURE 15.9 **Intramuscular Lipoma.** The tumor shows adipose tissue intermingled with skeletal muscle.

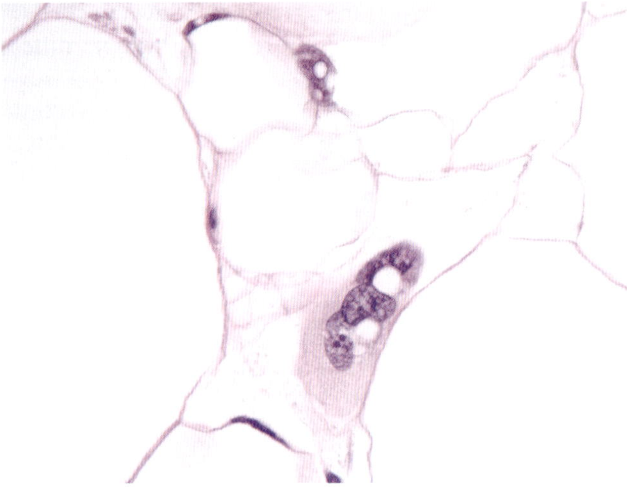

FIGURE 15.10 **Lochkern.** This type of cell from a lipoma contains an intranuclear lipid invagination. The plane of section has captured the nucleus en face such that it is enlarged but not hyperchromatic. Compare it to the nucleus depicted in Fig. 15.12, from a well-differentiated liposarcoma (taken at the same magnification and stained in the same laboratory), which is much more hyperchromatic.

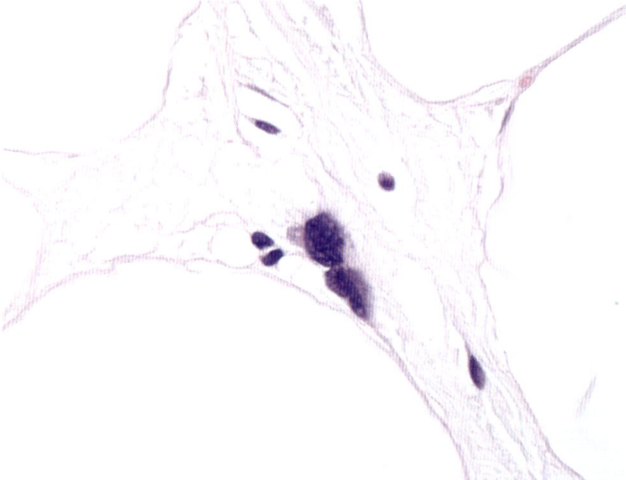

FIGURE 15.11 **Well-Differentiated Liposarcoma.** This image is intended to compare to Fig. 15.11, which depicts a nucleus from a lipoma at the same magnification (100×, oil immersion).

to recurrence than other lipomas, suggesting that these are, in fact, occult atypical lipomatous tumors lacking diagnostic histologic features.[9] Since the usual issue confronting the pathologist is to exclude malignant neoplasms, however, often it is most useful to perform immunohistochemical stains for MDM2 or CDK4, as above (or fluorescence *in-situ* hybridization [*FISH*] for *MDM2* amplification), to exclude well-differentiated liposarcoma. In most instances, however, special studies are not needed.

MULTIPLE LIPOMAS/LIPOMATOSIS

Multiple lipomas are found in about 5% of patients with lipomas. Hundreds of lipomas can be present in these patients. The back, shoulder, and upper arms are the most common location, and men are affected more frequently than women. Familial cases of multiple lipomas have been described that seem to have a dominant inheritance pattern and to be associated with other syndromes. In lipomatosis, there is a diffuse, nonlobular proliferation of fat in the affected tissues. The subcutaneous fat of the back of the neck and shoulder is involved in nearly every individual.[10–13] Lipomatosis is thought to be secondary to a defect in lipid metabolism and patients with diffuse lipomatosis have the clinical appearance of obesity; mediastinal involvement can cause venous obstruction with stasis and airway obstruction.[10–13]

The lipomas in these patients have the same gross and histologic features as conventional lipoma. The adipocytes have a normal appearance, except for slightly smaller size.

ANGIOLIPOMA

Clinical Features

These subcutaneous lesions usually arise in young adults with a small male predominance. The most common site is the forearm followed by the trunk and shoulder girdle area. Most are painful and multiple. The term "angiolipoma" has also been (incorrectly) applied to intramuscular hemangiomas, which tend to be accompanied by abundant fat.[14]

Pathologic Features

Most examples of angiolipoma are easy to diagnose, consisting of subcutaneous well-marginated lobulated adipose tissue lesions punctuated by varying numbers of small vessels, many containing fibrin thrombi. However, some have very cellular areas with numerous capillaries (Fig. 15.12, e-Figs. 15.14–15.17). Such cases are sometimes mistaken for Kaposi sarcoma or angiosarcomas.

Ancillary Investigations

Angiolipomas are interesting in their overall lack of cytogenetic abnormalities on karyotyping.[15] The endothelial cells in the vessels express expected markers, namely CD31 and CD34.

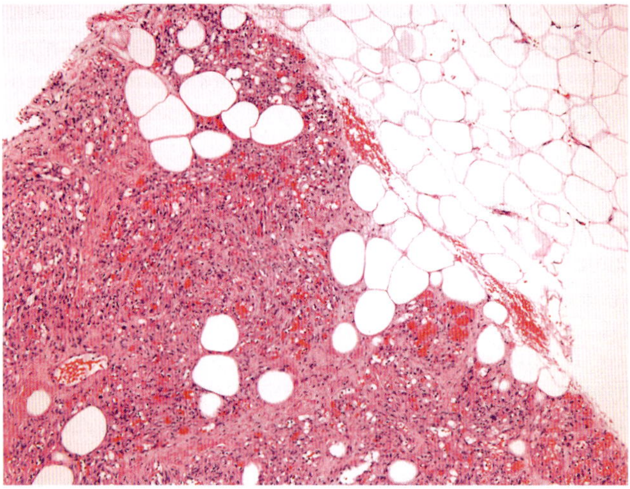

FIGURE 15.12 **Angiolipoma.** This example contains numerous capillaries, some of which contain fibrin thrombi. The capillaries have supporting elements (such as smooth myocytes) surrounding them, an indication that, despite its cellularity, the process is benign.

SPINDLE CELL LIPOMA

Clinical Features

Spindle cell lipoma was first recognized by Enzinger.[16] Although it can arise in various locations, the classic presentation is that of a painless subcutaneous mass involving the shoulder, back, or the posterior neck in a middle-aged to elderly man. Most tumors are solitary, but occasionally they can be multiple. In rare cases, there may be a familial tendency toward multiple lesions.[17] The treatment is excision. Recurrences are rare.

Pathologic Features

Grossly, the tumors are well circumscribed and typically measure between 3 and 5 cm, although occasionally larger examples occur. On sectioning, they have yellow areas, representing the mature fat, and gray-gelatinous areas representing the spindle cell component (e-Fig. 15.18). Microscopically, spindle cell lipoma is usually well circumscribed (Fig. 15.13); however, focal infiltration into surrounding tissue can be seen, especially in those spindle cell lipomas that involve the deeper structures. Spindle cell lipoma is composed of an admixture of mature adipocytes and spindle cells embedded in myxoid matrix that contains collagen fibers. The spindle cell component can be focal or it can involve almost the entire lesion, obscuring its lipomatous nature (e-Figs. 15.19–15.31). It can be palisaded (e-Fig. 15.19), sclerotic (e-Fig. 15.20), or replete with wiry collagen like a neurofibroma, sharing the proclivity to containing prominent mast cells (Fig. 15.14, e-Figs. 15.25–15.27). The mature adipocytes have identical features to those of

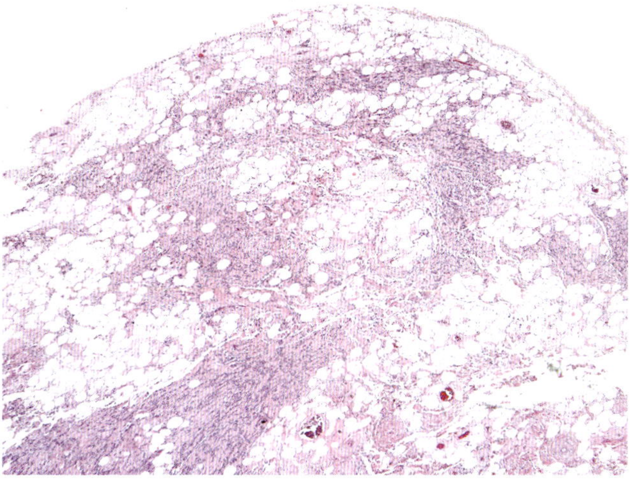

FIGURE 15.13 **Spindle Cell Lipoma.** At low magnification, the tumor contains fat, uniform spindle cells, and cleft-like spaces.

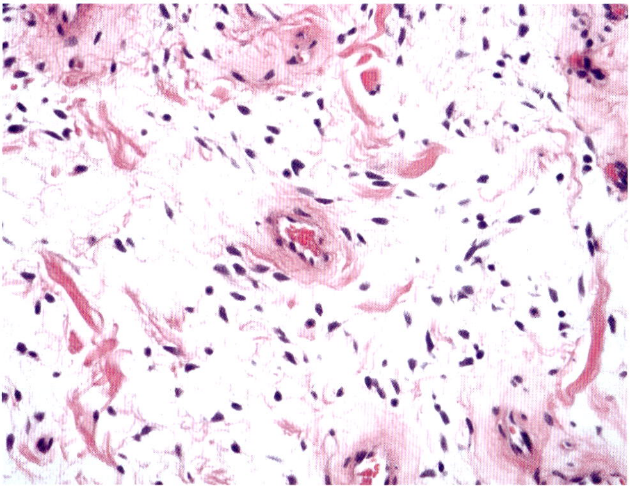

FIGURE 15.14 **Spindle Cell Lipoma.** This example is myxoid, with an admixture of spindle cells, mast cells, and wiry collagen. There is no fat in this field.

conventional lipoma. The spindle cells have oval to elongated uniform dark staining nuclei and bipolar eosinophilic cytoplasm. Mitotic figures are rare. The matrix is variably myxoid, with some examples exclusively so (e-Figs. 15.22–15.24) and characteristically contains bright eosinophilic collagen fibers (e-Fig. 15.20–15.22). The vascular pattern is usually inconspicuous, but occasionally this tumor can have a "pseudoangiomatous" appearance secondary to myxoid degenerative changes, which imparts many cleft-like spaces (e-Figs. 15.28–15.30).

Ancillary Investigations

Immunohistochemically, the mature adipocytes, but not the spindle cells, stain for S-100 protein. The spindle cells stain for CD34[18] (e-Fig. 15.31) and CD10,[19] and some observers believe spindle cell lipoma forms a continuum with extramammary myofibroblastoma.[19] Cytogenetic studies have shown abnormalities involving 13q and 16q.[20]

PLEOMORPHIC LIPOMA

Clinical Features

Pleomorphic lipoma is clinically, morphologically, and cytogenetically related to spindle cell lipoma and can be considered a pleomorphic variant of spindle cell lipoma.[21] Like spindle cell lipoma, pleomorphic lipoma generally occurs in males and involves the posterior neck, shoulder, and back. Patients typically present with a longstanding solitary subcutaneous mass. As is the case with spindle cell lipoma, treatment is excision and recurrences are rare.

Pathologic Features

Grossly, pleomorphic lipomas are well circumscribed with a yellow or grayish-tan cut surface (e-Fig. 15.32). Microscopically, they closely resemble spindle cell lipomas (Fig. 15.15, e-Figs. 15.33–15.40). However, in addition, pleomorphic lipoma contains variable numbers of hyperchromatic multinucleated giant cells that frequently demonstrate a concentric or "floret-like" arrangement of the nuclei (Fig. 15.22, e-Fig. 15.35). These cells have eosinophilic cytoplasm with the nuclei arranged peripherally and circumferentially. The nuclei overlap, have finely dispersed, or less frequently, smudgy chromatin and small eosinophilic nucleoli. These pleomorphic cells are highly variable in number. The extracellular matrix is myxoid and contains thick eosinophilic collagen fibers (e-Fig. 15.37). Lipoblasts are present in about half of cases (e-Figs. 15.36 and 15.38). Pleomorphic lipomas, like other adipose tissue neoplasms, can contain areas of fat necrosis (e-Fig. 15.39).

Ancillary Investigations

On cytogenetic studies, this tumor displays similar chromosomal abnormalities to those found in spindle cell lipoma. Since the differential diagnosis is often with well-differentiated liposarcoma, the absence of evidence of MDM2 or CDK4 alterations in these tumors[22] can be reassuring (e-Figs. 15.40 and 15.41).

CHONDROID LIPOMA

Clinical Features

Chondroid lipoma was first described by Meis[23] although an example of this tumor had been previously reported as "extraskeletal chondroma with lipoblast-like cells."[24] These tumors have a female predominance and usually

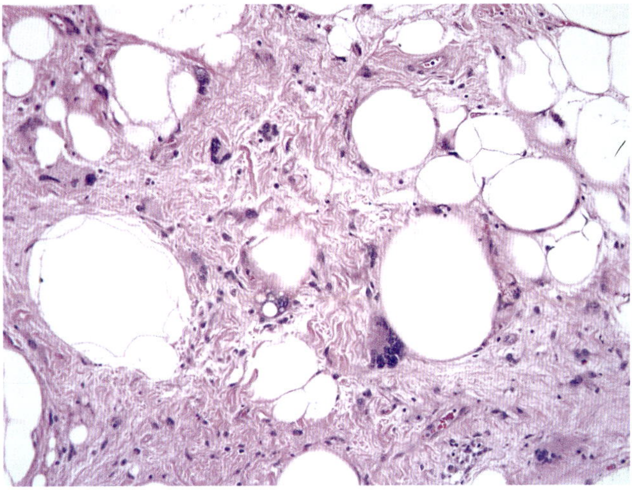

FIGURE 15.15 **Pleomorphic Lipoma.** A characteristic type of cell in these lesions is the multinucleated "floret" cell. Cells with such morphology are characteristic of but not specific for pleomorphic lipoma; virtually identical cells can be encountered in well-differentiated liposarcomas, although the latter usually lack wiry collagen.

affect adults, although rare pediatric cases are known.[25] They usually arise in the extremities but can also involve other sites. All reported examples of chondroid lipoma have behaved in a benign fashion. The treatment is excision.

Pathologic Features

Grossly, chondroid lipoma is well circumscribed and has a yellow cut surface. Microscopically, it is lobulated (Fig. 15.16, e-Figs. 15.42–15.44) with the neoplastic cells growing in sheets, cords, or as single cells, separated by extracellular eosinophilic ("chondroid") matrix (e-Figs. 15.45–15.48). The cells have well-defined cell membranes and small, dark staining nuclei surrounded by granular eosinophilic cytoplasm. Many cells contain clear intracytoplasmic fat vacuoles indenting the nucleus, making them indistinguishable from lipoblasts seen in liposarcomas (e-Figs. 15.47 and 15.48). However, mature adipocytes are present in all of the tumors.

Ancillary Investigations

Immunohistochemically, the chondroid-like cells stain for vimentin and S100 protein in a manner similar to normal adipocytes. Ultrastructural studies have shown a spectrum of differentiation with the cells showing features of prelipoblasts and chondroblasts.[26]

Cytogenetic analysis reveals a balanced translocation t(11, 16)(q13;p12–13) distinct from the known translocation involving 16p11 in myxoid and round-cell liposarcoma. The 11q13 breakpoint was previously noted in hibernomas, raising the possibility of a common genetic deregulation.[27–29]

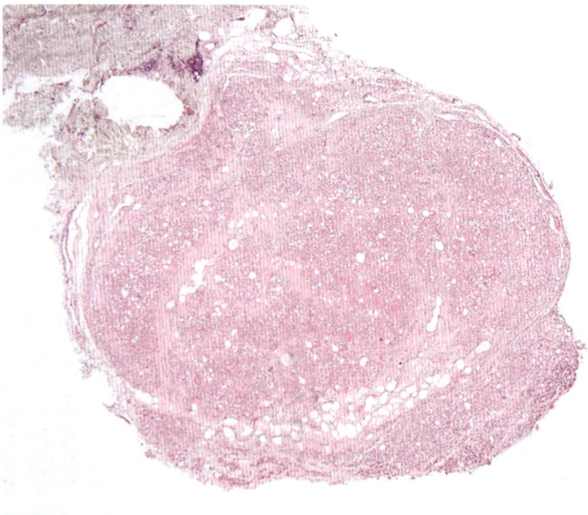

FIGURE 15.16 **Chondroid Lipoma.** This superficial lesion is well circumscribed, lobulated, and small.

MYOLIPOMA (LIPOLEIOMYOMA)

Clinical Features

These lesions have been reported predominantly in the female genital tract (as lipoleiomyoma)[30–34] in adults and occasionally in the pelvis and retroperitoneum (as myolipoma), also in adults. There is a female predominance in myolipomas arising outside the genital tract. In deep sites, these tumors are often large (up to 26 cm).[5] Uterine examples can even present as "benign metastasizing lipoleiomyoma."[31] These tumors are benign.

Pathologic Features

Grossly, myolipoma is well marginated (e-Fig. 15.49) and composed of firm whorled areas punctuated by adipose tissue. As the name implies, myolipoma/lipoleiomyoma is histologically a benign-appearing tumor composed of an admixture of smooth muscle and adipose tissue[5] (Fig. 15.17, e-Figs. 15.50 and 15.51).

Ancillary Investigations

On immunolabeling, the smooth muscle component expresses usual smooth muscle markers (actin, desmin, calponin, caldesmon) and also often expresses hormone receptors[35] (e-Fig. 15.52). The adipose component expresses S100 protein. Occasional cases immunolabel with HMB45[30] although these cases have little morphologic overlap with angiomyolipoma (which has prominent vessels and its smooth muscle component is less differentiated). Dysregulation of *HMGIC* (also called *HMGA2;* high-mobility group AT-hook 2) has been demonstrated in a case.[36]

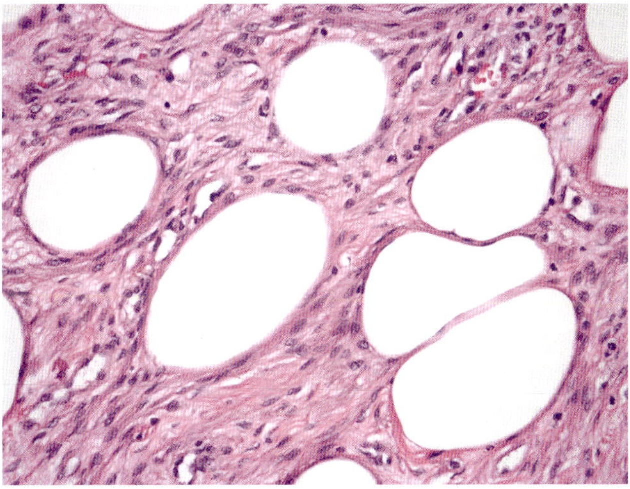

FIGURE 15.17 **Myolipoma.** As their name suggests, myolipomas consist of an admixture of fat and bland-appearing smooth muscle.

MYELOLIPOMA

Clinical Features

These tumors arise in adults. Reported patients have been over 40 years and there is a female predominance as well as an association with obesity, hypertension, and diabetes.[37] By a large margin, the adrenal gland is the most common site, but myelolipomas have been reported in numerous extra-adrenal locations, especially the presacral or retroperitoneal region. These tumors have been reported in individuals with various adrenal-related endocrine disorders, including Conn syndrome and Cushing syndrome.

Pathologic Features

Myelolipomas, as suggested by the name, consist of an admixture of adipose tissue and hematopoietic elements (Fig. 15.18, e-Fig. 15.53), with scattered lymphoid aggregates. They have overlapping features with extramedullary hematopoietic tumors (Fig. 15.7 and e-Figs. 15.8 and 15.9), but differ by having more abundant adipose tissue in general, lacking sclerosis and erythroid hyperplasia, and displaying lymphoid aggregates. Of course, extramedullary hematopoietic tumors arise in individuals with bone marrow disorders, whereas myelolipomas do not.

Ancillary Investigations

There are no studies of genetic alterations in these benign tumors. No immunohistochemistry is required for diagnosis.

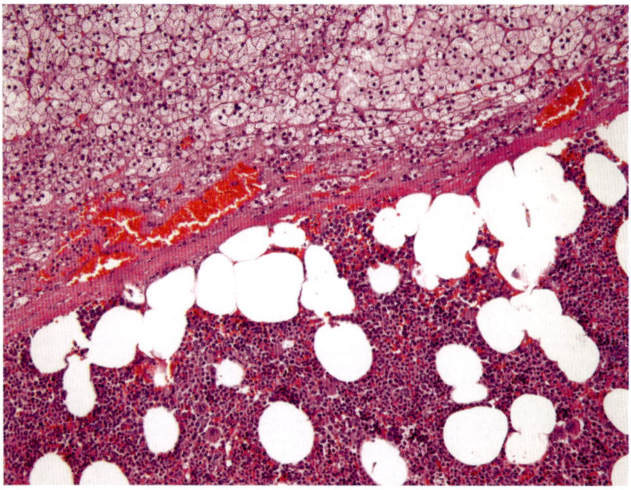

FIGURE 15.18 **Adrenal Myelolipoma.** Note the adrenal tissue at the top of the field. The neoplasm is composed of fat and trilinear hematopoietic tissue.

HIBERNOMA

Clinical Features

Hibernomas generally arise in locations where brown fat is found in fetuses and infants, such as the interscapular region, neck, mediastinum, axilla, posterior abdominal wall, and retroperitoneum adjacent to the kidney and adrenal gland. In the largest reported series,[38] there was a slight male predominance and tumors arose most commonly in adults, with a mean age of about 38.0 years, which is younger than that expected for usual lipomas, with occasional pediatric examples. The most common anatomic locations include the thigh, shoulder, back, neck, chest, and arm, and but some lesions arise in the abdominal cavity/retroperitoneum. Most attain a size of about 9 to 10 cm. Hibernoma presents as a painless slow-growing mass. Hibernomas are benign and treated by local excision.

Pathologic Features

Grossly, hibernomas are tan or red-brown, usually measuring between 5 and 10 cm; tumors >20 cm occasionally occur. Microscopically hibernoma demonstrates a lobular architecture and is composed of large polygonal cells supported by small branching capillaries (Fig. 15.19, e-Figs. 15.54–15.57). Three cell types can be identified; those with abundant mitochondria have a granular eosinophilic cytoplasm. Other cells have granular eosinophilic cytoplasm and numerous lipid vacuoles that typically indent the centrally located nucleus. The third type resembles a mature univacuolar adipocyte.

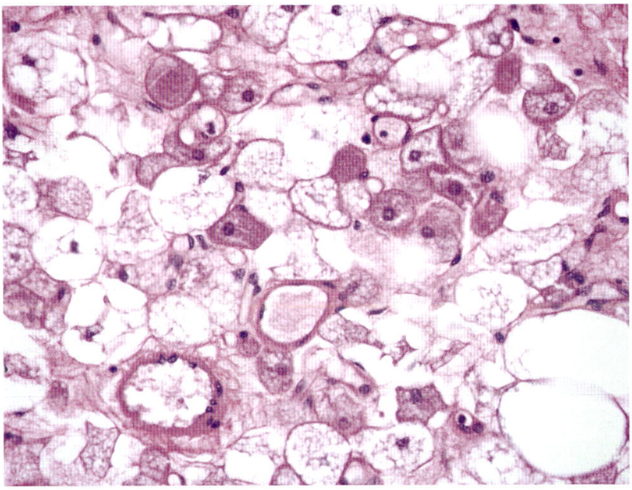

FIGURE 15.19 **Hibernoma.** These tumors recapitulate brown fat in displaying numerous lipid vacuoles and rich vascularity. This example shows all three cell types: those with granular eosinophilic cytoplasm, those with both granular eosinophilic cytoplasm and numerous lipid vacuoles, and a few that look like normal adipocytes.

Ancillary Investigations

Cytogenetically, hibernomas demonstrate aberrations of chromosome 11q13.[39]

LIPOBLASTOMA/LIPOBLASTOMATOSIS

Clinical Features

Lipoblastoma is a benign tumor almost exclusively arising in infants, typically during the first 3 years of life.[40,41] The term lipoblastomatosis is used to describe poorly circumscribed masses of similar immature-appearing adipose tissue. Patients with lipoblastoma tend to be slightly older than those with lipoblastomatosis. Lipoblastoma is more common in boys. It most frequently involves the extremities and presents as a slow-growing painless mass. Other locations include the neck, trunk, retroperitoneum, groin, axilla, back, labia, flank, lung, and mediastinum. Lipoblastoma generally involves the subcutaneous tissue but can also involve deeper tissue especially the diffuse (lipoblastomatosis) form. Lipoblastoma and lipoblastomatosis are treated by local resection. Local recurrence has been reported in about 10% to 20% of patients; recurrences are more common in patients with the diffuse (lipoblastomatosis) form. These lesions do not metastasize.

Pathologic Features

Grossly, lipoblastomas have a lobulated, myxoid, or pale cut surface. Some examples have cystic areas filled with mucoid material. They are typically well circumscribed. Lipoblastomatosis, however, is poorly circumscribed, infiltrates the subcutaneous tissue, and occasionally also underlying skeletal muscle. Most tumors are <5.0 cm in diameter but larger tumors, measuring over 20 cm, rarely occur. Microscopically, lipoblastoma is lobular, with the individual lobules separated by fibrous connective tissue septa (Fig. 15.20, e-Fig. 15.58 and 15.59). It is composed of primitive stellate and spindle-shaped cells, multivacuolated adipocytes, and univacuolated "signet ring" cell adipocytes (lipoblasts; Fig. 15.21, e-Figs. 20.27–20.30). Mitotic figures are rare and always normal in appearance. The supporting extracellular stroma is myxoid and commonly demonstrates a plexiform vascular pattern very much like the vascular pattern in myxoid liposarcoma (Fig. 15.33). Sometimes, these tumors mature to conventional lipomas.

Ancillary Investigations

These tumors have alterations (rearrangements) of the long arm or chromosome 8[42] and often have amplification of *PLAG1* (Pleomorphic adenoma gene 1) and rearrangements with hyaluronic acid synthase 2 (*HAS2*) or collagen 1 alpha 2 (*COL1A2*).[43–46] These alterations differ from those in myxoid liposarcoma, with which lipoblastoma is readily confused. Some observers have used *FISH* as a diagnostic aid for lipoblastoma[47] although most cases can be resolved with attention to the age of the patient and the morphologic features.

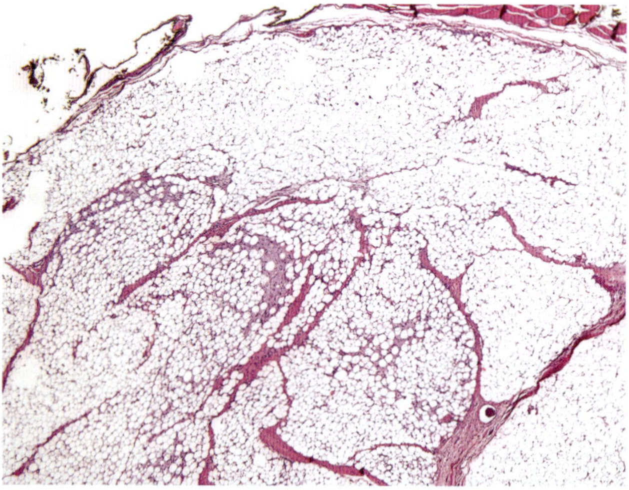

FIGURE 15.20 **Lipoblastoma.** The tumor is lobulated and has myxoid areas.

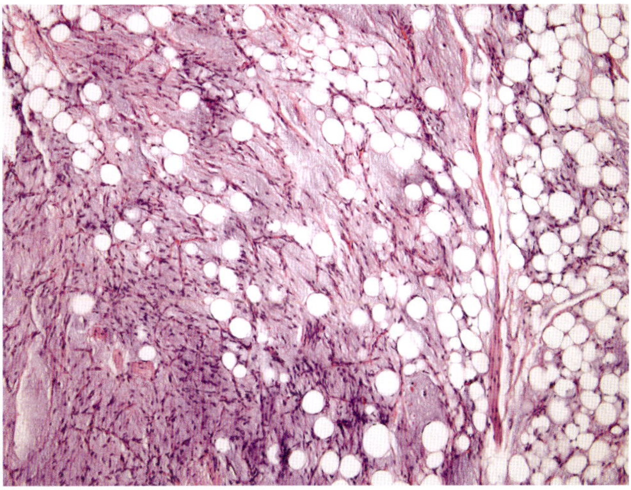

FIGURE 15.21 **Lipoblastoma.** Some lipoblastomas have zones that are indistinguishable from myxoid liposarcomas, with uniform cells, abundant vessels, and lipoblasts. In some cases, molecular testing is required to exclude myxoid liposarcoma.

LIPOFIBROMATOSIS

Lipofibromatosis (e-Figs. 15.60–15.62), covered in Chapter 2, is a pediatric lesion with a characteristic appearance with features of both lipomatosis and fibromatosis.

HEMOSIDEROTIC FIBROHISTIOCYTIC LIPOMATOUS LESION

Clinical Features

These lesions were initially described in the foot/ankle region of primarily middle-aged females with a history of local trauma, usually attaining a size of about 5 cm.[48] They can also be encountered in other sites,[48,49] and some observers believe that they are related to pleomorphic hyalinizing angiectatic tumor.[49] Others have associated these tumors with venous stasis.[50] About half of these lesions recur locally, presumably because they can have an infiltrative growth pattern and are difficult to excise, but no metastases have been reported.

Pathologic Features

The lesions consist of adipose tissue punctuated by short fascicles of hemosiderin-stippled spindled cells that infiltrated fat (Fig. 15.22, e-Figs. 15.63–15.65) and surrounded congeries of small, "Infiltrate" fat vessels. The spindle cells have vesicular nuclei in general, but scattered enlarged hyperchromatic cells can be found in most cases (Fig. 15.36).

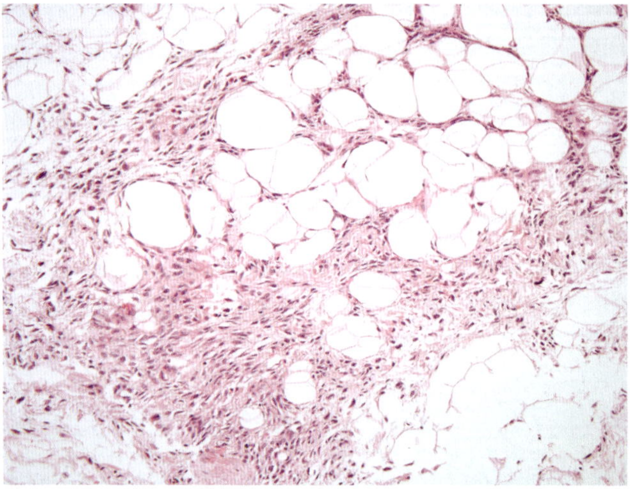

FIGURE 15.22 **Hemosiderotic Fibrohistiocytic Lipomatous Lesion.** These tumors consist of hemosiderin-rich spindle cells within a fatty lesion. There are scattered atypical enlarged hyperchromatic cells.

Ancillary Investigations

Iron is accentuated in most cases by a Prussian blue stain (e-Fig. 15.65). On immunostaining, the spindled component expresses vimentin, calponin, CD34 (e-Fig. 15.66), and occasionally KP1 or lysozyme and negative for caldesmon, S100, and desmin. Interestingly, hemosiderotic fibrohistiocytic lipomatous lesion shares molecular features with myxoinflammatory fibroblastic sarcoma (inflammatory myxohyaline tumor), namely, t(1;10) and amplification of 3p11–12.[51]

FIBROLIPOMATOUS HAMARTOMA OF NERVE

Clinical Features

These tumors were described in a series in 1985,[52] but the subsequent literature consists of isolated case reports. The majority involve the hand, wrist, palm, or finger of adults, with occasional involvement of the foot. About a third of patients have macrodactyly. Most commonly involved nerves are the median and ulnar nerves. About a third of lesions are associated with neurologic symptoms. Most patients had been aware of a mass for several years. These lesions are benign.

Pathologic Features

These are lobulated fatty lesions that the surgeon usually notes to be associated with a peripheral nerve at the time of operation. Microscopically, the tumor is characterized by fibrofatty enlargement of the nerve with marked

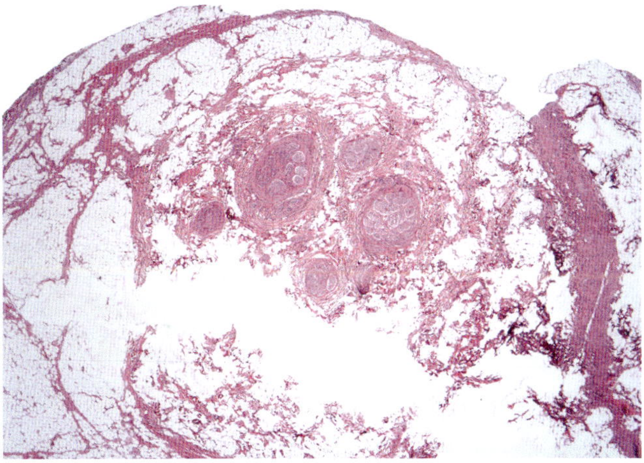

FIGURE 15.23 **Fibrolipomatous Hamartoma of Nerve.** This type of tumor results in a macrodactyly in about a third of cases and histologically consists of fat intermixed with a large peripheral nerve (often of the digits).

epineural and perineural fibrosis. The amount of fat versus fibrous tissue varies between cases (Fig. 15.23, e-Figs. 15.67–15.70); some examples have zones of ossification.

OTHER LESIONS WITH A COMPONENT OF FAT

Fat can be a component of several types of neoplasm. For example, this is a relatively common feature in genital stromal tumors such as angiomyofibroblastoma[53,54] (Fig. 8.6, e-Figs. 8.7–8.9). Solitary fibrous tumors can also contain fat[55,56] (so-called lipomatous hemangiopericytoma)[57–59] (e-Figs. 15.71 and 15.72).

REFERENCES

1. Travis WD, Balogh K, Abraham JL. Silicone granulomas: report of three cases and review of the literature. *Hum Pathol.* 1985;16:19–27.
2. Weiss SW, Enzinger FM, Johnson FB. Silica reaction simulating fibrous histiocytoma. *Cancer.* 1978;42:2738–2743.
3. Hizawa K, Inaba H, Nakanishi S, et al. Subcutaneous pseudosarcomatous polyvinylpyrrolidone granuloma. *Am J Surg Pathol.* 1984;8:393–398.
4. Remstein ED, Kurtin PJ, Nascimento AG. Sclerosing extramedullary hematopoietic tumor in chronic myeloproliferative disorders. *Am J Surg Pathol.* 2000;24:51–55.
5. Meis JM, Enzinger FM. Myolipoma of soft tissue. *Am J Surg Pathol.* 1991;15:121–125.
6. Kindblom LG, Angervall L, Stener B, et al. Intermuscular and intramuscular lipomas and hibernomas. A clinical, roentgenologic, histologic, and prognostic study of 46 cases. *Cancer.* 1974;33;754–762.

7. Ida CM, Wang X, Erickson-Johnson MR, et al. Primary retroperitoneal lipoma: a soft tissue pathology heresy?: report of a case with classic histologic, cytogenetics, and molecular genetic features. *Am J Surg Pathol.* 2008;32:951–954.
8. Marcarenco R, Erickson-Johnson M, Wang X, et al. Retroperitoneal lipomas: A clinicopathologic and molecular study of 16 cases [Abstract 69]. *Mod Pathol.* 2009;22;18A.
9. Bartuma H, Hallor KH, Panagopoulos I, et al. Assessment of the clinical and molecular impact of different cytogenetic subgroups in a series of 272 lipomas with abnormal karyotype. *Genes Chromosomes Cancer.* 2007;46:594–606.
10. Gamez J, Playan A, Andreu AL, et al. Familial multiple symmetric lipomatosis associated with the A8344G mutation of mitochondrial DNA. *Neurology.* 1998;51:258–260.
11. Ronan SJ, Broderick T. Minimally invasive approach to familial multiple lipomatosis. *Plast Reconstr Surg.* 2000;106:878–880.
12. Tsao H, Sober AJ. Multiple lipomatosis in a patient with familial atypical mole syndrome. *Br J Dermatol.* 1998;139:1118–1119.
13. Stoll C, Alembik Y, Truttmann M. Multiple familial lipomatosis with polyneuropathy, an inherited dominant condition. *Ann Genet.* 1996;39:193–196.
14. Austin RM, Mack GR, Townsend CM, et al. Infiltrating (intramuscular) lipomas and angiolipomas. A clinicopathologic study of six cases. *Arch Surg.* 1980;115:281–284.
15. Sciot R, Akerman M, Dal Cin P, et al. Cytogenetic analysis of subcutaneous angiolipoma: further evidence supporting its difference from ordinary pure lipomas: a report of the CHAMP Study Group. *Am J Surg Pathol.* 1997;21:441–444.
16. Enzinger FM, Harvey DA. Spindle cell lipoma. *Cancer.* 1975;36:1852–1859.
17. Fanburg-Smith JC, Devaney KO, Miettinen M, et al. Multiple spindle cell lipomas: a report of 7 familial and 11 nonfamilial cases. *Am J Surg Pathol.* 1998;22:40–48.
18. Templeton SF, Solomon AR Jr. Spindle cell lipoma is strongly CD34 positive. An immunohistochemical study. *J Cutan Pathol.* 1996;23:546–550.
19. Magro G, Caltabiano R, Di Cataldo A, et al. CD10 is expressed by mammary myofibroblastoma and spindle cell lipoma of soft tissue: an additional evidence of their histogenetic linking. *Virchows Arch.* 2007;450:727–728.
20. Maggiani F, Debiec-Rychter M, Verbeeck G, et al. Extramammary myofibroblastoma is genetically related to spindle cell lipoma. *Virchows Arch.* 2006;449:244–247.
21. Shmookler BM, Enzinger FM. Pleomorphic lipoma: a benign tumor simulating liposarcoma. A clinicopathologic analysis of 48 cases. *Cancer.* 1981;47;126–133.
22. Weaver J, Downs-Kelly E, Goldblum JR, et al. Fluorescence in situ hybridization for MDM2 gene amplification as a diagnostic tool in lipomatous neoplasms. *Mod Pathol.* 2008;21:943–949.
23. Meis JM, Enzinger FM. Chondroid lipoma. A unique tumor simulating liposarcoma and myxoid chondrosarcoma. *Am J Surg Pathol.* 1993;17:1103–1112.
24. Chan JK, Lee KC, Saw D. Extraskeletal chondroma with lipoblast-like cells. *Hum Pathol.* 1986;17:1285–1287.
25. Patne SC, Aryya NC, Gangopadhyay AN. Chondroid lipoma in a child. *Indian J Pathol Microbiol.* 2008;51:541–542.
26. Zamecnik M, Michal M, Fakan F. Ultrastructural study of so called chondroid lipoma. *Hum Pathol.* 1998;29:98–100.
27. Gisselsson D, Domanski HA, Hoglund M, et al. Unique cytological features and chromosome aberrations in chondroid lipoma: a case report based on fine-needle aspiration cytology, histopathology, electron microscopy, chromosome banding, and molecular cytogenetics. *Am J Surg Pathol.* 1999;23:1300–1304.
28. Thomson TA, Horsman D, Bainbridge TC. Cytogenetic and cytologic features of chondroid lipoma of soft tissue. *Mod Pathol.* 1999;12:88–91.

29. Thomson TA, Bainbridge TC, Horsman D. Unique cytologic and chromosome aberrations in chondroid lipoma. *Am J Surg Pathol.* 2000;24:1035.
30. Aung T, Goto M, Nomoto M, et al. Uterine lipoleiomyoma: a histopathological review of 17 cases. *Pathol Int.* 2004;54:751–758.
31. Fukunaga M. Benign "metastasizing" lipoleiomyoma of the uterus. *Int J Gynecol Pathol.* 2003;22:202–204.
32. Brannstrom M, Jones I, Lew W, et al. Ovarian lipoleiomyoma–a rare benign ovarian tumor with pre- and intra-operative features suggestive of malignancy. *Acta Obstet Gynecol Scand.* 2001;80:866–868.
33. Bajaj P, Kumar G, Agarwal K. Lipoleiomyoma of broad ligament: a case report. *Indian J Pathol Microbiol.* 2000;43:457–458.
34. Oh MH, Cho IC, Kang YI, et al. A case of retroperitoneal lipoleiomyoma. *J Korean Med Sci* 2001;16:250–252.
35. Akpolat I, Sertcelik A, Comert S, et al. ERRP-29 and ER staining in uterine lipoma and lipoleiomyoma. *Acta Oncol.* 1996;35:108.
36. Pedeutour F, Quade BJ, Sornberger K, et al. Dysregulation of HMGIC in a uterine lipoleiomyoma with a complex rearrangement including chromosomes 7, 12, and 14. Genes Chromosomes *Cancer.* 2000;27:209–215.
37. Fowler MR, Williams RB, Alba JM, et al. Extra-adrenal myelolipomas compared with extramedullary hematopoietic tumors: a case of presacral myelolipoma. *Am J Surg Pathol.* 1982;6:363–374.
38. Furlong MA, Fanburg-Smith JC, Miettinen M. The morphologic spectrum of hibernoma: a clinicopathologic study of 170 cases. *Am J Surg Pathol.* 2001;25:809–814.
39. Gisselsson D, Hoglund M, Mertens F, et al. Hibernomas are characterized by homozygous deletions in the multiple endocrine neoplasia type I region. Metaphase fluorescence in situ hybridization reveals complex rearrangements not detected by conventional cytogenetics. *Am J Pathol.* 1999;155:61–66.
40. Hicks J, Dilley A, Patel D, et al. Lipoblastoma and lipoblastomatosis in infancy and childhood: histopathologic, ultrastructural, and cytogenetic features. *Ultrastruct Pathol.* 2001;25:321–333.
41. Chung EB, Enzinger FM. Benign lipoblastomatosis. An analysis of 35 cases. *Cancer.* 1973;32:482–492.
42. Dal Cin P, Sciot R, De Wever I, et al. New discriminative chromosomal marker in adipose tissue tumors. The chromosome 8q11-q13 region in lipoblastoma. *Cancer Genet Cytogenet.* 1994;78:232–235.
43. Gisselsson D, Hibbard MK, Dal Cin P, et al. PLAG1 alterations in lipoblastoma: involvement in varied mesenchymal cell types and evidence for alternative oncogenic mechanisms. *Am J Pathol.* 2001;159:955–962.
44. Hibbard MK, Kozakewich HP, Dal Cin P, et al. PLAG1 fusion oncogenes in lipoblastoma. *Cancer Res.* 2000;60:4869–4872.
45. Morerio C, Rapella A, Rosanda C, et al. PLAG1-HAS2 fusion in lipoblastoma with masked 8q intrachromosomal rearrangement. *Cancer Genet Cytogenet.* 2005;156:183–184.
46. Ropke A, Kalinski T, Kluba U, et al. PLAG1 activation in lipoblastoma coinciding with low-level amplification of a derivative chromosome 8 with a deletion del(8)(q13q21.2). *Cytogenet Genome Res.* 2007;119:33–38.
47. Bartuma H, Domanski HA, Von Steyern FV, et al. Cytogenetic and molecular cytogenetic findings in lipoblastoma. *Cancer Genet Cytogenet.* 2008;183:60–63.
48. Marshall-Taylor C, Fanburg-Smith JC. Hemosiderotic fibrohistiocytic lipomatous lesion: ten cases of a previously undescribed fatty lesion of the foot/ankle. *Mod Pathol.* 2000;13:1192–1199.

49. Folpe AL, Weiss SW. Pleomorphic hyalinizing angiectatic tumor: analysis of 41 cases supporting evolution from a distinctive precursor lesion. *Am J Surg Pathol.* 2004;28:1417–1425.
50. Kazakov DV, Sima R, Michal M. Hemosiderotic fibrohistiocytic lipomatous lesion: clinical correlation with venous stasis. *Virchows Arch.* 2005;447:103–106.
51. Hallor KH, Sciot R, Staaf J, et al. Two genetic pathways, t(1;10) and amplification of 3p11–12, in myxoinflammatory fibroblastic sarcoma, haemosiderotic fibrolipomatous tumour, and morphologically similar lesions. *J Pathol.* 2009;217;716–727.
52. Silverman TA, Enzinger FM. Fibrolipomatous hamartoma of nerve. A clinicopathologic analysis of 26 cases. *Am J Surg Pathol.* 1985;9:7–14.
53. Laskin WB, Fetsch JF, Tavassoli FA. Angiomyofibroblastoma of the female genital tract: analysis of 17 cases including a lipomatous variant. *Hum Pathol.* 1997;28:1046–1055.
54. Cao D, Srodon M, Montgomery EA, et al. Lipomatous variant of angiomyofibroblastoma: report of two cases and review of the literature. *Int J Gynecol Pathol.* 2005;24:196–200.
55. Guillou L, Gebhard S, Coindre JM. Lipomatous hemangiopericytoma: a fat-containing variant of solitary fibrous tumor? Clinicopathologic, immunohistochemical, and ultrastructural analysis of a series in favor of a unifying concept. *Hum Pathol.* 2000;31:1108–1115.
56. Gengler C, Guillou L. Solitary fibrous tumour and haemangiopericytoma: evolution of a concept. *Histopathology.* 2006;48:63–74.
57. Folpe AL, Devaney K, Weiss SW. Lipomatous hemangiopericytoma: a rare variant of hemangiopericytoma that may be confused with liposarcoma. *Am J Surg Pathol.* 1999;23:1201–1207.
58. Nielsen GP, Dickersin GR, Provenzal JM, et al. Lipomatous hemangiopericytoma. A histologic, ultrastructural and immunohistochemical study of a unique variant of hemangiopericytoma. *Am J Surg Pathol.* 1995;19:748–756.
59. Ceballos KM, Munk PL, Masri BA, et al. Lipomatous hemangiopericytoma: a morphologically distinct soft tissue tumor. *Arch Pathol Lab Med.* 1999;123:941–945.

16

LIPOSARCOMA

INTRODUCTION

This chapter considers malignant tumors with adipocytic differentiation. The differential diagnosis is presented in Table 16.1.

WELL-DIFFERENTIATED LIPOSARCOMA

Clinical Features

Well-differentiated liposarcoma is the commonest subtype of liposarcoma. These tumors virtually always arise in adults with no gender predilection.[1–7] They involve the deep soft tissues of the proximal extremities and the retroperitoneum. Occasionally, retroperitoneal liposarcomas present as groin masses by virtue of extension into the scrotal sac.[8]

Most patients with well-differentiated liposarcomas present with painless slow-growing soft tissue masses. Intra-abdominal tumors typically are larger than extremity tumors and patients with abdominal tumors may present with altered abdominal girth or gastrointestinal obstruction. Primary groin tumors commonly simulate inguinal or femoral herniae.[9] CT and MRI imaging effectively demonstrates these neoplasms, highlighting their relationship to muscle, bone, and neurovascular structures. Using both these modalities, most well-differentiated liposarcomas exhibit similar signal qualities to normal fat and can be presumptively diagnosed on imaging studies with biopsy confirmation. In the absence of dedifferentiation, well-differentiated liposarcomas do not metastasize. Extremity tumors often recur many years after the original surgical procedure. Well-differentiated liposarcoma is managed by wide local excision, if technically possible, avoiding functional compromise. Retroperitoneal tumors are treated by debulking that virtually always results in residual gross or microscopic tumor. Treated in this way, well-differentiated liposarcoma of the extremity demonstrates a recurrence rate of approximately 40% to 50%, whereas the groin and retroperitoneal tumors nearly always recur (80% to 90%). The extremity tumors do not result in patient deaths, but the retroperitoneal and groin tumors have a poor long-term prognosis due to uncontrolled local growth within the abdominal cavity.[1,3,4,10]

When these lesions arise in superficial sites, they have been classified as "atypical lipomas" or "atypical lipomatous tumors" (e-Figs. 16.1–16.3).[1,4,10,11] Some observers have applied these terms to extremity lesions

TABLE 16.1 Differential Diagnosis of Liposarcoma (Continued)

	Typical clinical features	Microscopic features	Ancillary investigations
Fat necrosis	No typical features; can be encountered in normal fat and in neoplasms with fat	Fat with necrosis and many foamy macrophages, some multinucleated	CD68+ in macrophages
Fat atrophy	Cachexia either from dieting, malignancy, or treatment for malignancy	Lobulated fat with adipocyte shrinkage, capillaries appear more prominent	
Tumefactive extramedullary hematopoiesis	Mass in patient with a myeloproliferative disorder, benign	Trilinear hematopoiesis with erythroid hyperplasia and fat	
Lipoma with fat necrosis	Usually superficial well-circumscribed masses in adults (some intramuscular, rarely retroperitoneal)	Has the appearance of mature fat. No hyperchromatic enlarged cells. Multinucleated histiocytes.	MDM2–, CDK4–, no *MDM2* amplification, *HMGA2* fusions
Well-differentiated liposarcoma/ Atypical lipomatous tumor	Deep tumors of adults >50 y	Adipose tissue with scattered enlarged hyperchromatic nuclei, often found in fibrous septa	MDM2+, CDK4±, *MDM2* amplification
Lymphedema in the morbidly obese	Large subcutaneous-based mass in obese individuals, often with overlying skin changes	Dilated lymphatic channels, edema, mildly atypical fibroblasts	MDM2–, CDK4–, no *MDM2* amplification

Myxoid/round cell liposarcoma	Deep soft tissues of extremities of young adults. Often metastasizes to other soft tissue sites as well as to lungs	Monotonous small uniform spindle or rounded cells with abundant (myxoid) or minimal (round cell) myxoid matrix. Rich network of delicate vessels becomes inconspicuous in round cell liposarcoma. Lipoblasts	S100 protein+ in some cases, t(12;16)(q13;p11) or t(12;22)(q13;q12) with *FUS-DDIT3 or EWSR1-DDIT3* fusion genes
Pleomorphic lipoma	Superficial lesion of shoulder girdle, neck of middle-aged adults, M > F	Same features as spindle cell lipoma with the addition of enlarged atypical multinucleated cells ("fleurette" cells) and lipoblasts	CD34+, S100 protein+ in fat, abnormalities of 13q and 16q, MDM2–, CDK4–, no *MDM2* amplification
Chondroid lipoma	Multiple anatomic sites, adults	Lobulated lesion with fat, "bubbly" cells, chondroid matrix, lipoblasts, hypovascular	S100 protein+, balanced translocation t(11, 16)(q13;p12–13)
Silicone granuloma	Often in breast associated with ruptured implant	Infiltrates between lobules and ducts, macrophages	CD68+
Myelolipoma	Usually in the adrenal gland of adults, F > M, association with obesity, hypertension, and diabetes	Mixture of fat and trilinear hematopoiesis without erythroid hyperplasia	

(Continued)

TABLE 16.1 Differential Diagnosis of Liposarcoma

	Typical clinical features	Microscopic features	Ancillary investigations
Hibernoma	Adults usually younger than 40 y (younger than patients with ordinary lipomas), thigh	Lobulated lesion with prominent capillaries, varying amounts of mature fat cells, cells with fine vacuoles and cells with granular eosinophilic cytoplasm.	Abnormalities of chromosome 11q13
Lipoblastoma	Proximal extremities of infants, benign	Lobulated with mature fat and areas with lipoblasts and numerous capillaries (that can be indistinguishable from myxoid liposarcoma)	Variable S100 protein+, amplification of *PLAG1*, rearrangements of *HAS2* or *COL1A2*
Myxofibrosarcoma	Superficial lesions in elderly adults	Richly vascular myxoid lesion with pleomorphic cells	None useful in differential diagnosis. Often CD34+, actin+
Extrakeletal myxoid chondrosarcoma	Deep soft tissues of extremities, slight male predominance	Uniform rounded cells with eosinophilic cytoplasm in hypovascular myxoid background	S100 protein+, synaptophysin+, *EWS-NR4A3* rearrangement
Pleomorphic liposarcoma	Deep soft tissue lesions in adults >50 y	Pleomorphic lipoblasts in background that is either undifferentiated, epithelioid, or myxoid	Can be CD34+, actin+, desmin+, focal S100 protein+. MDM2–, CDK4–Complex karyotypes

Dedifferentiated liposarcoma	Deep tumors of adults >50 y, typically retroperitoneal	Areas of well-differentiated liposarcoma and juxtaposed zones of pleomorphic undifferentiated sarcoma	MDM2+, CDK4±, *MDM2* amplification with additional changes
Pleomorphic rhabdomyosarcoma	Deep neoplasms in adults >50 y, usually proximal thigh	Pleomorphic spindle cell neoplasm with cells with markedly eosinophilic cytoplasm	Desmin+, myogenin+ (nuclear), MyoD1+ (nuclear)
Pleomorphic undifferentiated sarcoma (malignant fibrous histiocytoma)	Deep neoplasms in adults >50 y, usually proximal thigh	Pleomorphic spindle cell neoplasm, often with storiform pattern	Variable actin, desmin, MyoD1–, MDM2–, CDK4–
Pleomorphic leiomyosarcoma	Adults > 50 y, deep extremities	Defined as pleomorphic zones comprising two thirds of the tumor, typical leiomyosarcoma in the remainder with fascicles of brightly eosinophilic cells with blunt-ended nuclei and paranuclear vacuoles	Actin+, desmin+, calponin+, caldesmon+, myogenin–, MyoD1–, focal keratin in some cases

and others restrict them to lesions of the subcutis.[1,4,11] Although atypical lipomatous tumors are histologically and cytogenetically identical to their deep counterparts, the natural history of the superficial tumors is sufficiently different that they may be considered as a separate group. However, they still occasionally undergo dedifferentiation to a high-grade sarcoma (see below).[5,12] On a practical note, using the term "atypical lipomatous tumor" for neoplasms in accessible sites (extremities) is sometimes advantageous as it avoids labeling patients as "sarcoma patients" when their likelihood of dying from their neoplasm is negligible and the risk of dedifferentiation of their tumors is about 5%.[3–5,11] In contrast, the risk of dedifferentiation for retroperitoneal lesions is about 28%.[3–5,11]

Pathologic Features

Well-differentiated liposarcomas are usually large. Tumors in excess of 20 cm are common. They typically demonstrate a multinodular growth pattern. The tumors are soft and pale yellow on cut section. The cut surface often is a paler yellow than adjacent normal fat due to the presence of excessive interstitial collagen within the tumor in comparison to the normal fat. There are three main microscopic variants of well-differentiated liposarcoma, but it is not important to separate them when reporting; they are simply a construct for recognizing well-differentiated liposarcomas. Needle biopsies are usually diagnostic, but occasionally sampling error can be a factor.

The most common pattern is the lipoma-like variant. This subtype is composed predominantly of cells that resemble mature adipocytes. In contrast to lipoma, there is a greater variability in adipocyte size and a diagnosis can be suspected scanning the slide at 4× and identifying enlarged hyperchromatic cells. Additionally, there is usually an increase in interstitial collagen within the tumor, both within thickened fibrous bands that traverse the tumor and diffusely within the extracellular space. The diagnostic hallmark of lipoma-like liposarcoma is atypical hyperchromatic nuclei within the cells showing adipose differentiation in addition to nonspecific spindled cells embedded within the collagenous bands and interstitial matrix (Figs. 16.1 and 16.2, e-Fig. 16.4). These latter nuclei are enlarged and characterized by intense hyperchromasia, coarsely clumped chromatin, and convoluted nuclear membranes (e-Fig. 16.5; see also Figs. 15.3 and 15.11). Lipoblasts are often present in lipoma-like liposarcoma, particularly adjacent to the collagenous septa, but their identification is not required for diagnosis. Mitotic figures are sparse in pure well-differentiated liposarcoma. Focal regions of fat necrosis with cystic change and a histiocytic inflammatory reaction are commonly present. Other microscopic findings that may be present include atypical stromal cells within the muscular walls of veins in the tumor (e-Fig. 16.6), stromal myxoid change (e-Figs. 16.7–16.13), and focal myoid areas.[13–15] The latter finding is more common in dedifferentiated tumors.

The second most common histologic pattern is the so-called sclerosing type (e-Fig. 16.14). When exclusively sclerosing, the radiographic and gross appearance of the neoplasm suggests a nonfatty tumor since

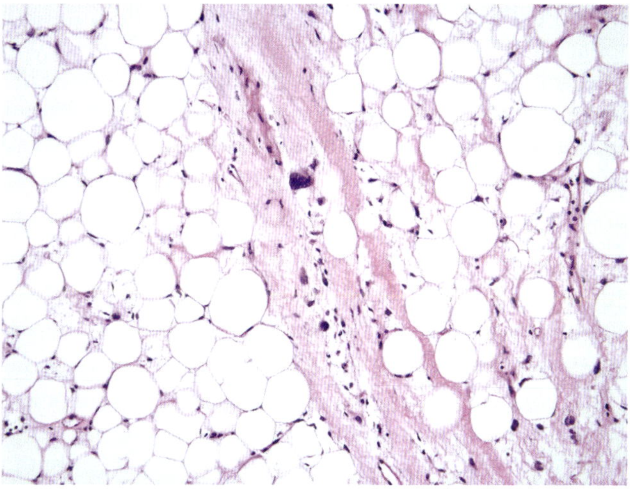

FIGURE 16.1 **Well-Differentiated Liposarcoma.** An enlarged pleomorphic hyperchromatic nucleus is present within a fibrous tissue septum and surrounded by lobules of the adipose tissue neoplasm. Compare the size of this nucleus to that of those in the endothelial cells in a capillary at the right side of the field.

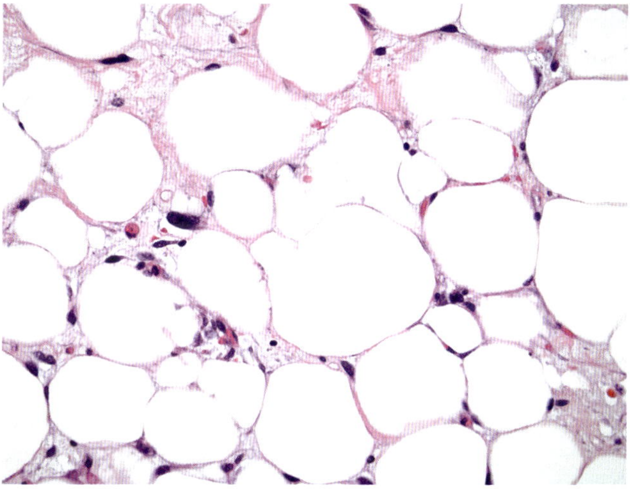

FIGURE 16.2 **Well-Differentiated Liposarcoma.** In this field, there are enlarged hyperchromatic nuclei scattered among the other normal-appearing adipocytic nuclei. Endothelial cells within capillaries can be used to compare nuclear sizes.

adipocytic differentiation may be scant, which may cause some difficulty on needle biopsies, although this can often be resolved using ancillary studies. However, there are usually transitions between lipoma-like and sclerosing regions within a single neoplasm. In sclerosing regions, the tumor is dominated by interstitial collagen that separates tumor cells. Only a minority of the embedded cells exhibit recognizable adipocytic differentiation. The majority appear as nonspecific spindled cells or markedly atypical stromal cells similar to the type present within the lipoma-like variant. The extracellular collagen that separates the lesional cells varies from fibrillary to hyalinized, but the cellularity remains low. Hypercellularity with fascicular growth suggests dedifferentiation (see below). As with the more common lipoma-like variant, mitotic figures are infrequent.

The least common histologic subtype of well-differentiated liposarcoma is the inflammatory type (e-Figs. 16.15 and 16.16).[16] Both lipoma-like and sclerosing well-differentiated liposarcoma may contain focal regions of tumor with extensive lymphoid infiltration. These regions may exhibit follicle formation with germinal centers, sheets and clusters of plasma cells, and even admixed neutrophils and eosinophils. The atypical stromal cells that characterize all types of well-differentiated liposarcoma are found admixed with these inflammatory cells which may cause confusion with malignant lymphoma.

Well-differentiated liposarcomas can also contain areas of heterologous differentiation, especially smooth muscle foci,[14] and areas of ossification.

None of the histologic variants of low-grade liposarcoma are clinically or prognostically relevant.

Ancillary Investigations

Well-differentiated liposarcomas demonstrate ring chromosomes and long marker chromosomes derived from the q13–15 region of chromosome 12. These findings are present regardless of anatomic location, including in tumors that arise in the superficial soft tissue.[17,18] Well-differentiated liposarcomas also have *MDM2* amplification (which correlates with nuclear MDM2 immunoreactivity–see e-Figs. 16.12 and 16.13) and express nuclear CDK4 immunohistochemically,[19–25] a feature they share with dedifferentiated liposarcoma.

DEDIFFERENTIATED LIPOSARCOMA

These tumors are also discussed and illustrated in Chapter 5, since they are usually intra-abdominal, and Chapter 13.

Clinical Features

The term dedifferentiated liposarcoma describes a spindle cell nonlipogenic sarcoma occurring in association with a well-differentiated low-grade liposarcoma (Figs. 16.3 and 16.4, e-Figs. 16.17–16.20).[4,5,10,12,26,27] Dedifferentiated liposarcoma affects the same patient population as well-differentiated liposarcoma. There is no sex predilection. In the past, it was suggested that dedifferentiation only occurred in the setting of retroperitoneal low-grade liposarcoma and that this phenomenon was site dependent, but more recent experience has shown that well-differentiated liposarcomas in all locations may undergo dedifferentiation. The concept that dedifferentiation is "time dependent" rather than "site dependent" has been proposed.[26]

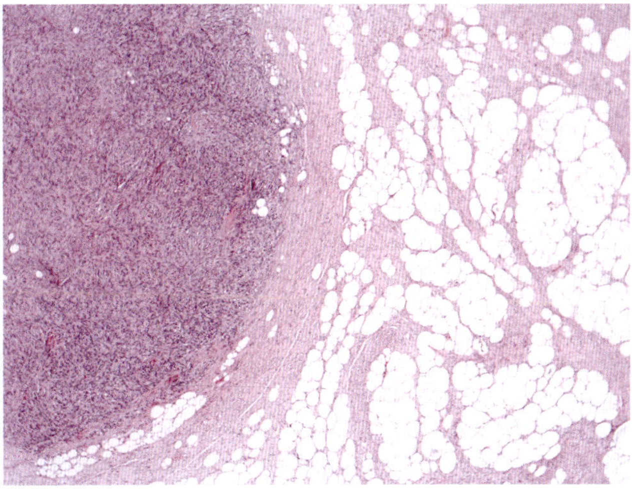

FIGURE 16.3 **Dedifferentiated Liposarcoma.** The residual well-differentiated liposarcoma component is on the right side of the field. On the left side, there is a pleomorphic high-grade sarcoma component. To identify such foci, it is important to sample both solid and fatty components at the time of gross evaluation of these tumors.

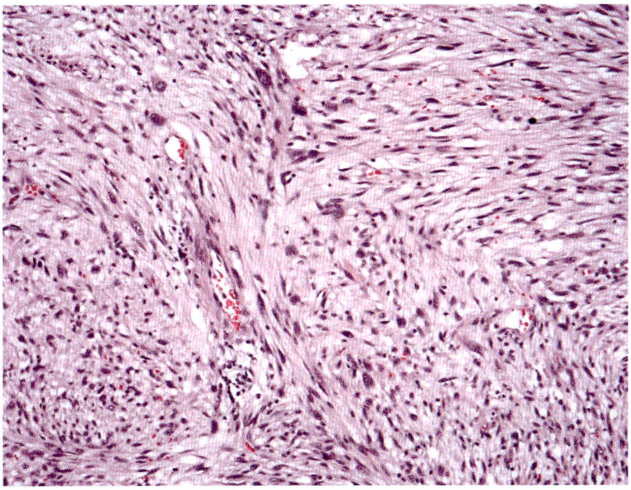

FIGURE 16.4 **Dedifferentiated Liposarcoma.** The high-grade component can display a storiform pleomorphic pattern.

The clinical significance of dedifferentiation is that once it occurs in a well-differentiated liposarcoma the tumor acquires the capacity for distant metastases and hence should be considered biologically high grade. The metastatic rate for dedifferentiated liposarcoma ranges between 15% and 30%. Dedifferentiation also typically portends more aggressive local growth, an increased risk of local recurrence, and higher tumor-related mortality.

Dedifferentiated liposarcoma is treated by radical surgical excision, if feasible. Adjuvant radiation therapy and/or chemotherapy may also be considered as for other high-grade soft tissue sarcomas. Use of antagonists against MDM2 is being explored.[28]

Pathologic Features

In the majority of cases, the spindle cell sarcoma and low-grade liposarcoma regions are found in the same tumor at the time of diagnosis ("primary dedifferentiated liposarcoma").[26] In a minority of cases, the spindle cell sarcoma is identified at the time of a local recurrence of a previously resected low-grade liposarcoma ("secondary dedifferentiated liposarcoma").[26] In the latter situation, the dedifferentiated tumor may contain a mixture of well-differentiated liposarcoma and spindle cell sarcoma or be composed only of the nonlipogenic component. Like well-differentiated liposarcomas, dedifferentiated tumors are typically large (>10 cm) and demonstrate multinodular growth. There is no minimum amount of nonlipogenic spindle cell sarcoma that must be present for a tumor to be classified as dedifferentiated. Approximately, 90% of these tumors are primary dedifferentiated liposarcomas, and these often show admixtures of pale soft yellow fat representing the well-differentiated liposarcoma component and firmer tan tissue representing the nonlipogenic spindle cell sarcoma. At the time of gross evaluation, both solid and fatty components should be sampled for histology. Secondary dedifferentiated tumors may consist only of nonlipogenic sarcoma at the time of recurrence or contain an admixture of both adipose and nonadipose components. The adipose components of the dedifferentiated tumors are histologically identical to usual well-differentiated liposarcoma (e-Figs. 16.17 and 16.18). In the majority of instances, the spindle cell sarcoma component is undifferentiated and histologically high grade, resembling malignant fibrous histiocytoma/high-grade undifferentiated pleomorphic sarcoma (Figs. 16.3 and 16.4, e-Figs. 16.19 and 16.20). These two components may show abrupt interfaces, gradual transitions, or a more diffuse admixture. The first of these is the most typical with the last the least common. The dedifferentiated component of the tumor characteristically demonstrates marked hypercellularity, nuclear pleomorphism, and a high mitotic rate. A number of morphological variations of the dedifferentiated foci of the tumor have been described. It is now clear that in a minority of cases the dedifferentiated regions may appear histologically low grade, resembling fibromatosis or low-grade fibrosarcoma (e-Figs. 16.21–16.23).[26] Some examples have myoid areas (e-Figs. 16.24–16.26) and some dedifferentiated liposarcomas have a striking inflammatory pattern (e-Figs. 16.27–16.32); in the past these were often diagnosed as inflammatory malignant fibrous histiocytoma, but we now recognize that the majority of such lesions are dedifferentiated liposarcomas.[29] Occasionally, the dedifferentiated regions may exhibit a microscopic nodularity resembling meningothelial whorls (e-Figs. 16.33–16.35).[30,31] Finally, heterologous differentiation toward leiomyosarcoma, rhabdomyosarcoma, and/or osteosarcoma (e-Figs. 16.36–16.38) rarely occurs.[13] These histologic variants of dedifferentiation do not appear to be prognostically relevant. "Low-grade" dedifferentiated is believed by some to reflect an earlier step toward high-grade dedifferentiation and is also associated with metastases,[26] although this remains a subject of debate.[32]

Ancillary Investigations

Dedifferentiated liposarcoma is cytogenetically related to well-differentiated liposarcoma. Although these tumors may demonstrate complex karyotypes similar to those found in undifferentiated sarcomas such as malignant fibrous histiocytoma, the majority of dedifferentiated liposarcomas exhibit the ring chromosomes characteristic of well-differentiated liposarcoma. Like well-differentiated liposarcomas, dedifferentiated liposarcomas have *MDM2* amplification, which correlates with nuclear MDM2 immunolabeling, and they express nuclear CDK4 on immunolabeling. They also variably express actin, desmin, and CD34.

MYXOID AND ROUND CELL LIPOSARCOMA

Introduction

These tumors are also discussed in Chapter 21 in light of their myxoid appearances. Myxoid and round cell liposarcoma are the low- and high-grade variants of the same neoplasm.[33-39] Those that have purely myxoid liposarcoma morphology are associated with a better prognosis than those with round cell features.[4,35,38] Pure round cell morphology is rare.

Clinical Features

These tumors typically affect younger adults than do well-differentiated liposarcomas (median–fifth decade) with a slight male predominance. They are occasionally encountered in children. Tumors most commonly arise in the deep soft tissue of the thigh but may also be encountered in the arms, trunk, and retroperitoneum. Most are deep to the fascia as demonstrated in the imaging study in e-Figure 21.1 from Chapter 21. Most patients present with a painless soft tissue mass. Myxoid/ round cell liposarcoma is treated by wide surgical excision with or without radiation therapy.[40] Approximately 30% of patients develop distant metastases. As for most other sarcomas, metastases often involve the lungs, but myxoid/round cell liposarcoma also tends to spread to the retroperitoneum, soft tissue, and skeleton.[37] Histologic grading appears to be of value in predicting those patients at risk for metastases; increasing cellularity increases risk of metastasis.

Pathologic Features

Grossly myxoid/round cell liposarcomas are usually large neoplasms (>10 cm). They are typically lobulated and may appear encapsulated (e-Fig. 16.39). The cut surface of the tumor varies from gelatinous and tan to opaque and yellow with focal hemorrhage. Myxoid liposarcoma is composed of lobules of low to moderately cellular uniform small spindled and oval tumor cells a richly myxoid ground substance (Fig. 16.5, e-Figs. 16.40–16.45; see also Figs. 21.6 and 21.7, e-Figs. 21.8 and 21.9). The tumor cells are arranged as cords and clusters with numerous delicate capillaries within the ground substance. The neoplastic cells are monotonous appearing with scant cytoplasm and uniform dark staining nuclei. Scattered to numerous lipoblasts can be identified (Fig. 16.6). Nucleoli and mitotic figures are inconspicuous. Myxoid liposarcoma is a translocation associated sarcoma and thus displays uniform cells with essentially no nuclear pleomorphism and no abnormal mitoses.[41] Tumor cells often aggregate closer to each other at the periphery of individual tumor lobules and adjacent to blood vessels. Univacuolar and multivacuolar lipoblasts are scattered throughout the tumor. Many tumors have foci of mature-appearing fat (e-Fig. 16.43), a feature that can be seen de novo, as well as associated with treatment.[40] In round cell liposarcoma, the myxoid matrix is overrun by closely packed tumor cells with obscuring of the vascular pattern and enhanced mitotic activity (Fig. 16.7, e-Fig. 16.46). Usually, foci of conventional myxoid liposarcoma are present, allowing for a diagnosis. The "cut-off" as to when a myxoid liposarcoma becomes a round cell liposarcoma is not well defined. The term "transitional" was coined by Smith et al.[38] to describe areas in these tumors that are more cellular than those of myxoid liposarcoma but with preservation of the vascular pattern and readily apparent myxoid matrix (e-Figs. 16.47 and 16.48). When unassociated with round cell areas, transitional morphology appears not to relate to prognosis. Smith et al.[38] suggest that a prognostic "cutoff" occurs at >5% round cell areas, whereas other authors prefer to rely on a higher figure (25%),[10,35] using death as their endpoint. When reporting such tumors, it is worthwhile to estimate the fraction of round cell component. A subset of myxoid liposarcomas in children has either a spindle cell pattern (e-Figs. 16.49 and 16.50) that can be difficult to diagnose as it often lacks readily identifiable lipoblasts[42] or a component of pleomorphic cells ("pleomorphic myxoid liposarcoma").[42]

Ancillary Investigations

Most myxoid/round cell liposarcomas demonstrate the chromosomal translocations that result in *FUS-CHOP* or *EWSR1-CHOP* rearrangements.[18,34,39,43–49] Molecular diagnostic testing is not typically needed for diagnosis, but it is sometimes useful in separating pediatric myxoid liposarcoma from lipoblastoma. Like normal adipose tissue, myxoid liposarcomas express S100 protein but only in about a third of cases.[50]

PLEOMORPHIC LIPOSARCOMA (SEE ALSO CHAPTER 13)

Clinical Features

Pleomorphic liposarcoma is the rarest subtype of liposarcoma. Few series of this variant of liposarcoma have been reported.[51–54] They typically occur in adults over the age of 50 years (median age: 54–63 years). There is

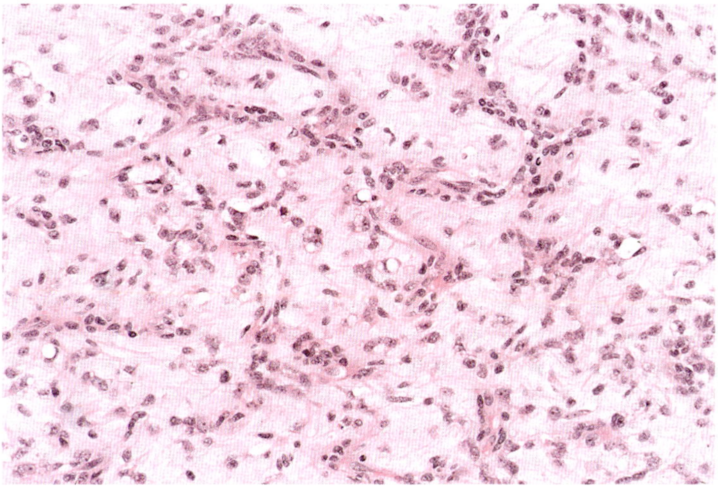

FIGURE 16.5 **Myxoid Liposarcoma.** This tumor show numerous delicate capillaries and is composed of uniform round cells. Several lipoblasts, characterized by lipid droplets that indent the nuclei, are present in this field.

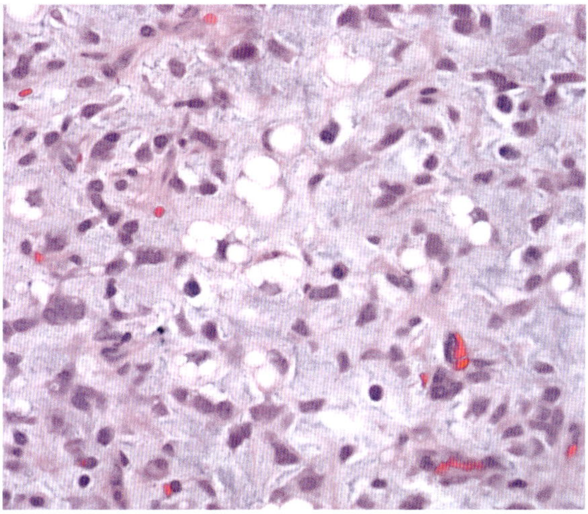

FIGURE 16.6 **Myxoid Liposarcoma.** This field shows prominent myxoid stroma and numerous lipoblasts.

a slight male predominance. Pleomorphic liposarcoma in childhood is extremely uncommon. Most tumors arise in the deep soft tissues of the thigh, trunk, or retroperitoneum where they produce symptoms related to a mass. A subset (about 20%) is superficial (usually subcutaneous, rarely dermal). These tumors are often large and typically exceed 10 cm. Pleomorphic liposarcomas are treated by wide surgical excision with or without adjuvant radiation therapy. The role of chemotherapy remains

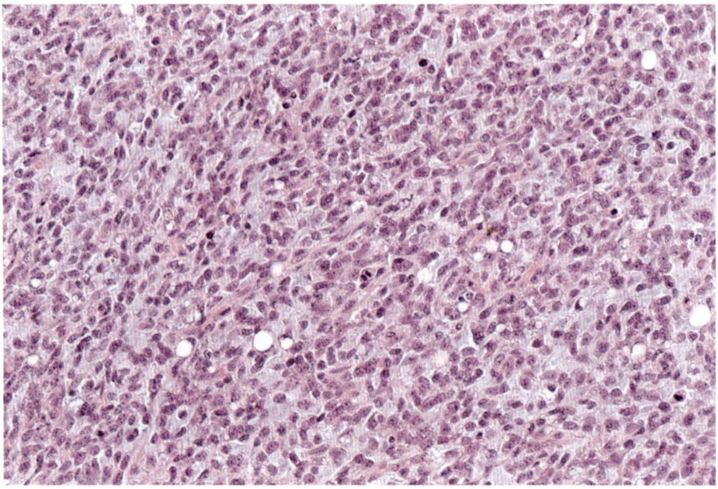

FIGURE 16.7 **Round Cell Liposarcoma.** The neoplasm is composed of the same uniform rounded cells that are featured in myxoid liposarcomas, but it is highly cellular, obscuring the vascular pattern. In this example, lipoblasts are identifiable, but in some cases molecular analysis can be required for diagnosis.

unclear. Pleomorphic liposarcomas have a very high incidence of metastases and tumor-related mortality; the 5-year survival ranges from 50% to 63%. Adverse prognostic factors include central location, origin in deep soft tissue, and large size.

Pathologic Features

Pleomorphic liposarcomas are large multinodular tumors that typically are yellow to tan on their cut surface. Grossly recognizable fat is usually absent. Regions of hemorrhage and/or necrosis are common. There are three microscopic subtypes of pleomorphic liposarcoma. They are unified by the presence of markedly pleomorphic multivacuolated lipoblasts (Fig. 16.8, e-Fig. 16.51), which can be sparse and found only on careful search in some cases. Many tumors consist of predominantly pleomorphic undifferentiated sarcoma (malignant fibrous histiocytoma-like areas) with only scattered diagnostic pleomorphic lipoblasts (e-Fig. 16.52 and 16.53). A second subset is epithelioid with pleomorphic lipoblasts (e-Figs. 16.54 and 16.55), and the last type has prominent myxoid areas and appears similar to myxofibrosarcoma (myxoid malignant fibrous histiocytoma). Pleomorphic liposarcomas often contain markedly bizarre enormous nuclei that are eye catching at low magnification. Mitotic figures, including atypical forms, are readily found. Lipoblasts with excess of 20 separate cytoplasmic vacuoles arranged around a central atypical nucleus are not uncommon. In the more common variant of pleomorphic liposarcoma, these cells comprise the majority of the tumor. In the other histologic variant, clusters of these bizarre lipoblasts are embedded in a background of otherwise

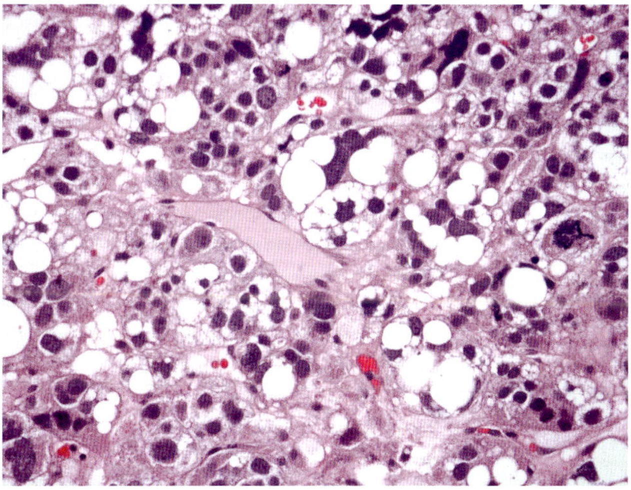

FIGURE 16.8 **Pleomorphic Liposarcoma.** Note the sheets of pleomorphic lipoblasts.

undifferentiated pleomorphic spindle cell sarcoma. There is usually an abrupt transition between these two microscopically distinct regions. All variants of pleomorphic liposarcoma may exhibit a well-developed capillary vascular pattern which may appear somewhat "plexiform."

Ancillary Investigations

There is variable S100 protein expression in lipogenic areas (about 50%) and the spindled areas may show focal immunostaining with antibodies against desmin, actin, CD34, CD68, epithelial membrane antigen, keratin, and S100 protein (in other words, a nonspecific profile). Staining with MDM2 and CDK4 has been negative in these tumors,[22] which should be helpful in separating them from dedifferentiated liposarcomas, but experience with large numbers of cases is lacking. Epithelioid areas can show positivity for cytokeratins and even melan-A. There are no consistent or specific cytogenetic abnormalities within this subgroup of liposarcoma and they display complex karyotypes.[55]

REFERENCES

1. Evans HL, Soule EH, Winkelmann RK. Atypical lipoma, atypical intramuscular lipoma, and well differentiated retroperitoneal liposarcoma: a reappraisal of 30 cases formerly classified as well differentiated liposarcoma. *Cancer.* 1979;43:574–584.
2. Elgar F, Goldblum JR. Well-differentiated liposarcoma of the retroperitoneum: a clinicopathologic analysis of 20 cases, with particular attention to the extent of low-grade dedifferentiation. *Mod Pathol.* 1997;10:113–120.
3. Lucas DR, Nascimento AG, Sanjay BK, et al. Well-differentiated liposarcoma. The Mayo Clinic experience with 58 cases. *Am J Clin Pathol.* 1994;102:677–683.

4. Evans HL. Liposarcoma: a study of 55 cases with a reassessment of its classification. *Am J Surg Pathol.* 1979;3:507–523.
5. Weiss SW, Rao VK. Well-differentiated liposarcoma (atypical lipoma) of deep soft tissue of the extremities, retroperitoneum, and miscellaneous sites. A follow- up study of 92 cases with analysis of the incidence of "dedifferentiation". *Am J Surg Pathol.* 1992;16:1051–1058.
6. Enzinger F, Winslow D. Liposarcoma: a study of 103 cases. *Virchows Arch A Pathol Anat Histopathol.* 1962;335:367–388.
7. Shmookler BM, Enzinger FM. Liposarcoma occurring in children. An analysis of 17 cases and review of the literature. *Cancer.* 1983;52:567–574.
8. Montgomery E, Fisher C. Paratesticular liposarcoma; a clinicopathologic study. *Am J Surg Pathol.* 2003;27:40–47.
9. Montgomery E, Fisher C. Paratesticular liposarcoma: a clinicopathologic study. *Am J Surg Pathol.* 2003;27:40–47.
10. Evans H. Liposarcomas and atypical lipomatous tumors: a study of 66 cases followed for a minimum of 10 years. *Surg Pathol.* 1988;1:41–54.
11. Azumi N, Curtis J, Kempson RL, et al. Atypical and malignant neoplasms showing lipomatous differentiation. A study of 111 cases. *Am J Surg Pathol.* 1987;11:161–183.
12. Yoshikawa H, Ueda T, Mori S, et al. Dedifferentiated liposarcoma of the subcutis. *Am J Surg Pathol.* 1996;20:1525–1530.
13. Evans HL, Khurana KK, Kemp BL, et al. Heterologous elements in the dedifferentiated component of dedifferentiated liposarcoma. *Am J Surg Pathol.* 1994;18:1150–1157.
14. Evans HL. Smooth muscle in atypical lipomatous tumors. A report of three cases. *Am J Surg Pathol.* 1990;14:714–718.
15. Vartanian R, O'Connell J, Holden J, et al. Primary jejunal well-differentiated liposarcoma (atypical lipomatous tumor) with leiomyosarcomatous differentiation. *Int J Surg Pathol.* 1996;4:29–36.
16. Argani P, Facchetti F, Inghirami G, et al. Lymphocyte-rich well-differentiated liposarcoma: report of nine cases. *Am J Surg Pathol.* 1997;21:884–895.
17. Fletcher CD, Akerman M, Dal Cin P, et al. Correlation between clinicopathological features and karyotype in lipomatous tumors. A report of 178 cases from the Chromosomes and Morphology (CHAMP) Collaborative Study Group. *Am J Pathol.* 1996;148:623–630.
18. Rosai J, Akerman M, Dal Cin P, et al. Combined morphologic and karyotypic study of 59 atypical lipomatous tumors. Evaluation of their relationship and differential diagnosis with other adipose tissue tumors (a report of the CHAMP Study Group). *Am J Surg Pathol.* 1996;20:1182–1189.
19. Italiano A, Bianchini L, Keslair F, et al. HMGA2 is the partner of MDM2 in well-differentiated and dedifferentiated liposarcomas whereas CDK4 belongs to a distinct inconsistent amplicon. *Int J Cancer.* 2008.
20. Sirvent N, Coindre JM, Maire G, et al. Detection of MDM2-CDK4 amplification by fluorescence in situ hybridization in 200 paraffin-embedded tumor samples: utility in diagnosing adipocytic lesions and comparison with immunohistochemistry and real-time PCR. *Am J Surg Pathol.* 2007;31:1476–1489.
21. Binh MB, Garau XS, Guillou L, et al. Reproducibility of MDM2 and CDK4 staining in soft tissue tumors. *Am J Clin Pathol.* 2006;125:693–697.
22. Binh MB, Sastre-Garau X, Guillou L, et al. MDM2 and CDK4 immunostainings are useful adjuncts in diagnosing well-differentiated and dedifferentiated liposarcoma subtypes: a comparative analysis of 559 soft tissue neoplasms with genetic data. *Am J Surg Pathol.* 2005;29:1340–1347.

23. Hostein I, Pelmus M, Aurias A, et al. Evaluation of MDM2 and CDK4 amplification by real-time PCR on paraffin wax-embedded material: a potential tool for the diagnosis of atypical lipomatous tumours/well-differentiated liposarcomas. *J Pathol.* 2004;202:95–102.
24. Weaver J, Goldblum JR, Turner S, et al. Detection of MDM2 gene amplification or protein expression distinguishes sclerosing mesenteritis and retroperitoneal fibrosis from inflammatory well-differentiated liposarcoma. *Mod Pathol.* 2009;22:66–70.
25. Weaver J, Downs-Kelly E, Goldblum JR, et al. Fluorescence in situ hybridization for MDM2 gene amplification as a diagnostic tool in lipomatous neoplasms. *Mod Pathol.* 2008;21:943–949.
26. Henricks WH, Chu YC, Goldblum JR, et al. Dedifferentiated liposarcoma: a clinicopathological analysis of 155 cases with a proposal for an expanded definition of dedifferentiation. *Am J Surg Pathol.* 1997;21:271–281.
27. McCormick D, Mentzel T, Beham A, et al. Dedifferentiated liposarcoma. Clinicopathologic analysis of 32 cases suggesting a better prognostic subgroup among pleomorphic sarcomas [see comments]. *Am J Surg Pathol.* 1994;18:1213–1223.
28. Singer S, Socci ND, Ambrosini G, et al. Gene expression profiling of liposarcoma identifies distinct biological types/subtypes and potential therapeutic targets in well-differentiated and dedifferentiated liposarcoma. *Cancer Res.* 2007;67:6626–6636.
29. Coindre JM, Hostein I, Maire G, et al. Inflammatory malignant fibrous histiocytomas and dedifferentiated liposarcomas: histological review, genomic profile, and MDM2 and CDK4 status favour a single entity. *J Pathol.* 2004;203:822–830.
30. Nascimento AG, Kurtin PJ, Guillou L, et al. Dedifferentiated liposarcoma: a report of nine cases with a peculiar neurallike whorling pattern associated with metaplastic bone formation. *Am J Surg Pathol.* 1998;22:945–955.
31. Fanburg-Smith JC, Miettinen M. Liposarcoma with meningothelial-like whorls: a study of 17 cases of a distinctive histological pattern associated with dedifferentiated liposarcoma. *Histopathology.* 1998;33:414–424.
32. Evans HL. Atypical lipomatous tumor, its variants, and its combined forms: a study of 61 cases, with a minimum follow-up of 10 years. *Am J Surg Pathol.* 2007;31:1–14.
33. Antonescu CR, Tschernyavsky SJ, Decuseara R, et al. Prognostic impact of P53 status, TLS-CHOP fusion transcript structure, and histological grade in myxoid liposarcoma: a molecular and clinicopathologic study of 82 cases. *Clin Cancer Res.* 2001;7:3977–3987.
34. Antonescu CR, Elahi A, Healey JH, et al. Monoclonality of multifocal myxoid liposarcoma: confirmation by analysis of TLS-CHOP or EWS-CHOP rearrangements. *Clin Cancer Res.* 2000;6:2788–2793.
35. Kilpatrick SE, Doyon J, Choong PF, et al. The clinicopathologic spectrum of myxoid and round cell liposarcoma. A study of 95 cases. *Cancer.* 1996;77:1450–1458.
36. Oliveira AM, Nascimento AG, Okuno SH, et al. p27(kip1) protein expression correlates with survival in myxoid and round-cell liposarcoma. *J Clin Oncol.* 2000;18:2888–2893.
37. Spillane AJ, Fisher C, Thomas JM. Myxoid liposarcoma–the frequency and the natural history of nonpulmonary soft tissue metastases. *Ann Surg Oncol.* 1999;6:389–394.
38. Smith TA, Easley KA, Goldblum JR. Myxoid/round cell liposarcoma of the extremities. A clinicopathologic study of 29 cases with particular attention to extent of round cell liposarcoma. *Am J Surg Pathol.* 1996;20:171–180.
39. Tallini G, Akerman M, Dal Cin P, et al. Combined morphologic and karyotypic study of 28 myxoid liposarcomas. Implications for a revised morphologic typing, (a report from the CHAMP Group). *Am J Surg Pathol.* 1996;20:1047–1055.
40. Engstrom K, Bergh P, Cederlund CG, et al. Irradiation of myxoid/round cell liposarcoma induces volume reduction and lipoma-like morphology. *Acta Oncol.* 2007;46:838–845.

41. Montgomery E, Wilentz RE, Argani P, et al. Analysis of anaphase figures in routine histologic sections distinguishes chromosomally unstable from chromosomally stable malignancies. *Cancer Biol Ther*. 2003;2:248–252.
42. Alaggio R, Coffin CM, Weiss SW, et al. Liposarcomas in young patients: a study of 82 cases occurring in patients younger than 22 years of age. *Am J Surg Pathol*. 2009;33:645–658.
43. Sreekantaiah C, Karakousis CP, Leong SP, et al. Cytogenetic findings in liposarcoma correlate with histopathologic subtypes. *Cancer*. 1992;69:2484–2495.
44. Sreekantaiah C, Karakousis CP, Leong SP, et al. Trisomy 8 as a nonrandom secondary change in myxoid liposarcoma. *Cancer Genet Cytogenet*. 1991;51:195–205.
45. Paulien S, Turc-Carel C, Dal Cin P, et al. Myxoid liposarcoma with t(12;16) (q13;p11) contains site-specific differences in methylation patterns surrounding a zinc-finger gene mapped to the breakpoint region on chromosome 12. *Cancer Res*. 1990;50:7902–7907.
46. Meis-Kindblom JM, Sjogren H, Kindblom LG, et al. Cytogenetic and molecular genetic analyses of liposarcoma and its soft tissue simulators: recognition of new variants and differential diagnosis. *Virchows Arch*. 2001;439:141–151.
47. Downs-Kelly E, Goldblum JR, Patel RM, et al. The utility of fluorescence in situ hybridization (FISH) in the diagnosis of myxoid soft tissue neoplasms. *Am J Surg Pathol*. 2008;32:8–13.
48. Bridge JA, Shaffer B, Neff JR, et al. A complex translocation involving chromosomes 12 and 16 in a metastatic myxoid liposarcoma. *Cancer Genet Cytogenet*. 1988;34:119–120.
49. Panagopoulos I, Hoglund M, Mertens F, et al. Fusion of the EWS and CHOP genes in myxoid liposarcoma. *Oncogene*. 1996;12:489–494.
50. Hashimoto H, Daimaru Y, Enjoji M. S-100 protein distribution in liposarcoma. An immunoperoxidase study with special reference to the distinction of liposarcoma from myxoid malignant fibrous histiocytoma. *Virchows Arch A Pathol Anat Histopathol*. 1984;405:1–10.
51. Downes KA, Goldblum JR, Montgomery EA, et al. Pleomorphic liposarcoma: a clinicopathologic analysis of 19 cases. *Mod Pathol*. 2001;14:179–184.
52. Miettinen M, Enzinger FM. Epithelioid variant of pleomorphic liposarcoma: a study of 12 cases of a distinctive variant of high-grade liposarcoma. *Mod Pathol*. 1999;12:722–728.
53. Hornick JL, Bosenberg MW, Mentzel T, et al. Pleomorphic liposarcoma: clinicopathologic analysis of 57 cases. *Am J Surg Pathol*. 2004;28:1257–1267.
54. Gebhard S, Coindre JM, Michels JJ, et al. Pleomorphic liposarcoma: clinicopathologic, immunohistochemical, and follow-up analysis of 63 cases: a study from the French Federation of Cancer Centers Sarcoma Group. *Am J Surg Pathol*. 2002;26:601–616.
55. Mertens F, Fletcher CD, Dal Cin P, et al. Cytogenetic analysis of 46 pleomorphic soft tissue sarcomas and correlation with morphologic and clinical features: a report of the CHAMP Study Group. Chromosomes and morphology. *Genes Chromosomes Cancer*. 1998;22:16–25.

17

SUPERFICIAL VASCULAR LESIONS AND MIMICS

INTRODUCTION

This chapter includes reactive and neoplastic lesions arising in the superficial soft tissues in adults and children. The differential diagnosis is presented in Table 17.1.

Benign pediatric vascular lesions can be divided into the two broad categories of tumors (hemangiomas) and vascular malformations. Hemangiomas are characterized by rapid growth during infancy followed by gradual involution, whereas malformations are present at birth (although not necessarily clinically apparent), growing proportionally with the child and persisting without regression. Vascular malformations have subsequently been further subdivided according to the predominant type of vascular channel (capillary, venous, arterial, lymphatic or a combination) and their hemodynamic features (low or high blood flow).

REACTIVE LESIONS

This group includes vascular proliferations that result from infectious processes, immunologic disturbances, or host response to a variety of other etiologies, including trauma. Angiolymphoid hyperplasia with eosinophilia (ALHE; epithelioid hemangioma) is included in this section, in part, to highlight its contrasting features with Kimura disease, with which it has been confused in the past, and in part, as a reflection of the belief that some examples have features consistent with a reactive process although some examples may be neoplasms (epithelioid hemangioma).

BACILLARY ANGIOMATOSIS

Clinical Features

Bacillary (epithelioid) angiomatosis (BA) is a pseudoneoplastic vascular proliferation, first described in HIV-infected individuals.[1] The disease has a predilection for, but is not restricted to, immunocompromised patients. The predominant pathogen is *Bartonella* (*Rochalimaea) henselae*, which

TABLE 17.1 Differential Diagnosis of Superficial Vascular Lesions

	Typical clinical features	Microscopic features	Ancillary investigations
BA	Immunocompromised patients with cutaneous lesions	Lobulated proliferation of capillary-sized vessels, aggregates of neutrophils, leukocytoclastic debris	Warthin Starry stain (pH 4.0) shows clumps of small curved rods of *B. henselae*
Verruga peruana (Oroya fever)	Skin lesions in persons in endemic areas (Peru)	Cutaneous vascular proliferation with plump endothelial cells and inflammation	Weak staining of *B. bacilliformis* organisms with Giemsa
PEH	Within thrombi anywhere in the body, often distal extremities and in hemorrhoids; essentially a variant of organizing thrombus	Fibrin cores coated by monolayers of endothelial cells, typically all within a vessel	Typically not required
Intravascular fasciitis	Distal extremity nodules in young adults	Intravascular myofibroblastic proliferation accompanied by lymphocytes and osteoclast-like giant cells	SMA+, calponin+, caldesmon–, desmin–, vascular markers (CD34, CD31) negative
Intravascular leiomyomatosis	In women with uterine leiomyomas that extend into veins	Essentially a leiomyoma in a vessel; perpendicularly orientated fascicles of brightly eosinophilic cells with blunt-ended nuclei without mitotic activity	SMA+, calponin+, caldesmon+, desmin+, vascular markers (CD34, CD31) negative

ALHE (epithelioid hemangioma)	Adults (20–40 y), head-neck region, single or multiple smooth papules or plaques (superficial)	Lobular vascular proliferation surrounded by lymphoid cuff, often associated with damaged artery. Vessels lined by epithelioid endothelial cells, background eosinophils–benign	Typically not required
Epithelioid hemangioendothelioma	Deep soft tissues, organs (lungs, liver)	Infiltrative lesion composed of single (not forming capillaries) epithelioid endothelial cells in chondroid background, sometimes associated with a vessel–looks similar to lobular breast carcinoma in some cases–malignant	CD34+, CD31+, variable keratin expression
Kimura disease	Asians, head and neck region associated lymphadenopathy and peripheral blood eosinophilia, elevation in the serum IgE, sometimes nephrotic syndrome	Fibroinflammatory lesion with numerous eosinophils, sometimes eosinophilic microabscesses, vessels inconspicuous	Typically not required
Capillary hemangioma (infantile hemangioendothelioma, juvenile hemangioma, strawberry nevus)	Newborns and babies, female predominance, head and neck, grow rapidly and then usually regress	Cellular capillary proliferation with commensurate proliferation of supporting cells (smooth muscle, pericytes)	GLUT1+
Pyogenic granuloma/lobular capillary hemangioma	Head and neck of adults, some associated with pregnancy, do not regress	Lobular capillary proliferation of capillaries, overlying epidermal collarette common	GLUT1–

(Continued)

TABLE 17.1 Differential Diagnosis of Superficial Vascular Lesions (Continued)

	Typical clinical features	Microscopic features	Ancillary investigations
Cavernous hemangioma	Any age, usually upper half of body, do not regress	Gaping blood-filled spaces	GLUT1–
Superficial arteriovenous tumor/malformation	Perioral region and extremities of adults, small red or purple papules, do not regress	Well-circumscribed masses of thick- and thin-walled vessels, in dermis (skin) or submucosa (lip). Some vessels have a "transitional" appearance between arteries and veins	Typically not required
Microvenular hemangioma	Small solitary nodule or plaque involving the extremities of young adults	Permeative proliferation of small irregularly branching vessels that are well formed but often have collapsed, somewhat inconspicuous lumina; vessels are thicker than	Typically not required
Glomeruloid hemangioma	Found in patients with POEMS syndrome–**P**olyneuropathy, **O**rganomegaly (hepatosplenomegaly and lymphadenopathy), **E**ndocrinopathy (amenorrhea, gynecomastia, hypothyroidism, adrenal insufficiency, and glucose intolerance), **M**onoclonal protein (marrow plasmacytosis, paraproteinemia), and **S**kin lesions	Ectatic vessels with intraluminal capillary conglomerates, architecturally resembling renal glomeruli	Typically not required

Angioblastoma (acquired tufted angioma, progressive capillary hemangioma, angioblastoma of Nakagawa)	Children and young adults, upper half of body, some painful, do not regress	Tightly packed clusters of capillaries with a rounded or ovoid ("cannonball") appearance in a plexiform pattern	GLUT1–
Hobnail hemangioma (targetoid hemosiderotic hemangioma)	Solitary lesion, trunk or extremities of young adults. Early examples with central purple, violaceous, or brown-black papule, bordered by an inner pale zone and a more peripherally situated ecchymotic ring ("targetoid").	Ectatic thin-walled vascular channels situated in the superficial dermis and lined by plump, sometimes epithelioid, endothelium. Deeper vessels, located in the reticular dermis, have an angulated, irregular and slit-like appearance.	Typically not required – endothelial cells CD34+, CD31+, podoplanin (D2-40)–
Progressive lymphangioma (benign lymphangioendothelioma)	Head and neck of adults	Anastomosing vascular channels with a "collagen dissection" pattern	CD34+, CD31+, podoplanin (D2-40)+
Angiokeratoma	Some sporadic; systemic type (angiokeratoma corpus diffusum) is associated with Fabry disease, fucosidosis, and deficiency of beta-galactosidase	Dilated vessels that are primarily restricted to the uppermost dermis and are bordered or enclosed by elongate rete ridges	Typically not required
Verrucous hemangioma	Reflects superficial extension (into epidermis) of an underlying deep hemangioma or vascular malformation	Dilated vessels in uppermost dermis enclosed by elongate rete ridges associated with underlying vascular lesion	Typically not required

(Continued)

TABLE 17.1 Differential Diagnosis of Superficial Vascular Lesions (Continued)

	Typical clinical features	Microscopic features	Ancillary investigations
Angioma serpiginosum	Lower extremities of young women	Superficial vascular ectasia	Typically not required
Cutaneous epithelioid angiomatous nodule	Blue papules, usually on the trunk of adults	Circumscribed, unilobular, mainly solid proliferations of large polygonal epithelioid endothelial cells with vesicular nuclei and conspicuous nucleoli and at least focal vasoformation	Variable staining with CD34, CD31, and FVIII-related antigen
Massive localized lymphedema in the morbidly obese	Large soft tissue lesions (usually of thigh) with superficial component of longstanding duration in morbidly obese adults	Dermal fibrosis, expansion of the fibrous septa between fat lobules with increased numbers of stromal fibroblasts, lymphatic proliferation and lymphangiectasia	Typically not required. MDM2, CDK4 both negative if performed to exclude liposarcoma
Well-differentiated liposarcoma	Deep adipose tissue mass of thighs or retroperitoneum, only rarely involves the subcutaneous fat, no skin changes	Mature-appearing fat punctuated by enlarged hyperchromatic nuclei, occasionally lipoblasts	MDM2, CDK4+, nuclear labeling. MDM2 amplification on *FISH*
Spindle cell hemangioma	Slow-growing, often multifocal small painless mass involving the dermis and/or subcutis, usually of hands and feet in young adults. Association with Milroy disease, Maffucci disease, Klippel-Trenaunay syndrome	Cavernous vascular spaces and a spindle cell proliferation vaguely reminiscent of KS	Typically not required; CD34+ and CD31+ in the endothelial cells of the dilated vessels and IL8+ and VEGFR+ in the spindle cells

Malignant endovascular papillary angioendothelioma, papillary intralymphatic angioendothelioma, Dabska tumor	Extremely rare, possibly more common in children but all ages, no favored site	Intercommunicating vascular channels, epithelioid to columnar endothelium, sometimes arranged in papillary (primitive glomeruloid) tufts with a central avascular hyaline core, intravascular lymphocytes may be prominent	CD34+, CD31+, podoplanin (D2-40)+ and VEGFR-3+
Kaposiform hemangioendothelioma	Superficial or deep lesion of children (often) and adults (occasional). In some infants, large retroperitoneal mass associated with a consumptive coagulopathy (Kasabach-Merritt syndrome), aggressive local behavior, and association with lymphangiomatosis.	Infiltrative yet lobular growth of well-formed capillaries admixed with short fascicles of spindle cells with slit-like vascular lumina	Podoplanin D2-40+ in the KS-like proliferative capillaries but not in the surrounding dilated vessels. Endothelial cells in nodules are CD31+, CD34+, VEGFR-3+, FLI1+, but GLUT1−
Atypical vascular lesion	In (usually mammary) skin following radiation. A single or several small papules of patches in the irradiated site. Most benign, but a subset progresses to angiosarcoma, often after several recurrences	Small (<1 cm) resembling benign lymphangiomas lymphangioendothelioma, or a lobular capillary proliferation	CD34+, CD31+, podoplanin (D2-40)+ for lesions that are lymphangioma-like OR CD34+, CD31+, podoplanin (D2-40)− for capillary-like lesions

(Continued)

TABLE 17.1 Differential Diagnosis of Superficial Vascular Lesions (Continued)

	Typical clinical features	Microscopic features	Ancillary investigations
Retiform hemangioendothelioma	Rare neoplasms of young adults without gender preference involving skin and subcutaneous tissue, usually of lower extremities. Occasionally metastases to regional lymph nodes but not distant sites	Narrow arborizing vascular channels lined by plump hobnail endothelial cells with pattern reminiscent of rete testis, often with a striking lymphoid background	CD31+, CD34+, factor VIII-related antigen+, podoplanin (D2-40)–, VEGFR-3–
Composite hemangioendothelioma	Longstanding dermal and subcutaneous nodules and plaques, usually in the extremities of young adults	Admixture of benign-appearing well-formed vessels, areas that resemble spindle cell hemangioma, areas similar to retiform hemangioendothelioma and areas similar to epithelioid hemangioendothelioma	CD34+, CD31+, factor VIII-related antigen +, podoplanin (D2-40)–
Kaposi sarcoma	Lesions of immunosuppressed patients or in endemic areas. Tumors can involve skin or viscera	Spindle cells in fascicles and sheets, extravasated erythrocytes, siderophages, hyaline globules, lymphoplasmacytic infiltrate. Early lesions with more subtle features	CD34+, CD31+, HHV-8+, podoplanin (D2-40)+, VEGFR-3+
Superficial angiosarcoma	Variable tumors: e.g., bruise-like lesions of face and scalp of elderly, associated with lymphedema, postirradiation	Wide range from hemangioma-like with collagen-dissection to overtly malignant epithelioid neoplasms	Variable staining with CD34, CD31, podoplanin (D2-40), Fli-1, keratins, HHV-8–

Angiomatoid fibrous histiocytoma	Small lesions usually of proximal limb girdle, trunk, head and neck arising in first 2 decades, slight female predominance. About 15% recurrences, rare metastases to nodes, rarer systemic metastases	Multinodular sheets of ovoid cells Some cases with focal nuclear pleomorphism and multinucleated giant cells, variable hemorrhage, some cases with large cysts lined by tumor cells, not endothelium, variable fibrous and lymphoid cuff	Desmin+, about 60%, variable calponin+, caldesmon+, SMA−, myogenin−. *EWSR1-CREB1*; *EWSR1-ATF1*, *FUS-ATF1*
Aneurysmal fibrous histiocytoma	Trunk and extremities of adults, cutaneous	Overlying epidermal hyperplasia, dermal short spindle cells with focal storiform pattern, peripheral thickened collagen bundles and minimal extension into subcutis, variably sized cystic spaces filled with blood but lacking endothelial lining cells, abundant hemosiderin, multinucleated giant cells.	CD34, CD31, HHV-8, S100 protein, desmin all negative, factor XIIIa+
Multinucleate cell angiohistiocytoma	Violaceous erythematous papules of acral regions in middle-aged to elderly women	Capillaries and small venules of subpapillary plexus and the mid-dermis, in association with angulated multinucleate cells	Vessels: CD34+, CD31+, podoplanin (D2-40)−. Multinucleate cells: variable CD68 and FXIIIa.

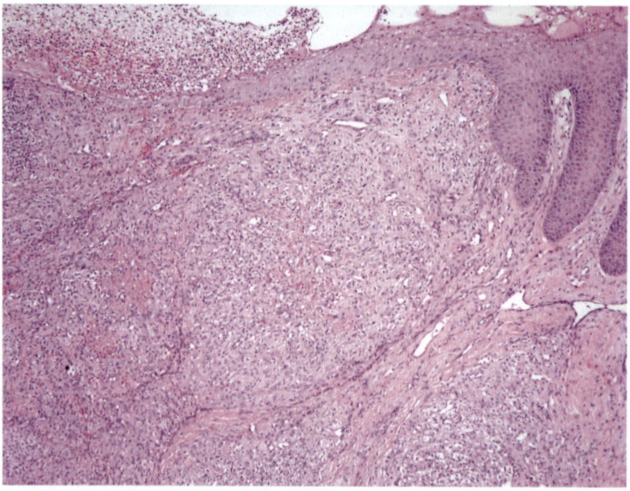

FIGURE 17.1 **Bacillary Angiomatosis.** This lesion arose in the knee area a patient who had had a renal transplant. Beneath the ulcerated skin is a lobular but solid endothelial proliferation. The centers of the lobules contain eosinophilic necrotic material.

is also the etiologic agent of cat scratch disease. The organism is commonly harbored by domestic cats (which have a seroprevalence of about 5% to over 60% depending on geographic area[2]) and transmitted to their owners. These organisms are susceptible to antibiotics, but the disease can prove fatal if untreated. Although cutaneous lesions are the most frequently recognized manifestation of BA (e-Fig. 17.1), a systemic infection typically ensues in the immunosuppressed host. In immunocompetent individuals, lesions are believed to remain localized to the inoculation site.

Pathologic Features

The lesions of BA consist of a lobulated proliferation of capillary-sized vessels, which are often well formed (Fig. 17.1, e-Figs. 17.2–17.4). The endothelium lining the vessels may be plump with an "activated" or mildly atypical appearance. Aggregates of neutrophils, leukocytoclastic debris, and granular flocculent material are present both within the vascular lobules and the adjacent soft tissue (e-Figs. 17.5 and 17.6). The infectious agent is harbored within these foci and appears, with aid of the Warthin Starry stain (pH 4.0), as clumps of small curved rods approximately 0.5 to 1.0 μm in length (Fig. 17.2, e-Figs. 17.7 and 17.8).

Ancillary Investigations

Classically, organisms are recognized on Warthin Starry staining but can also be detected by PCR.

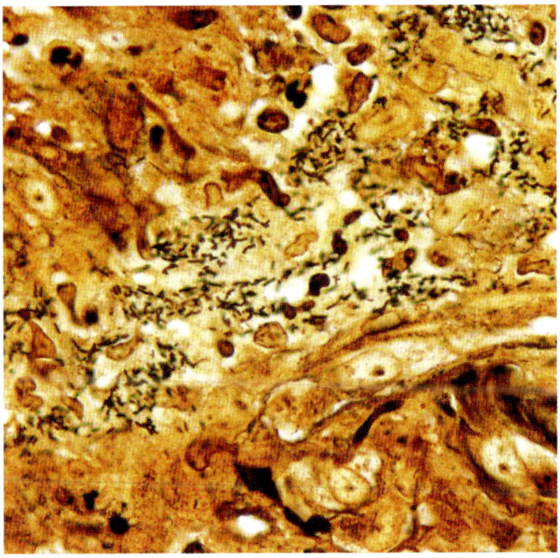

FIGURE 17.2 **Bacillary Angiomatosis, Warthin-Starry Stain.** Numerous *B. henselae* organisms are apparent.

VERRUGA PERUANA (OROYA FEVER, CARRION DISEASE)

Clinical Features

The etiologic agent is *Bartonella bacilliformis*, a hemotropic, mobile, pleomorphic, Gram-negative bacterium that has been shown to elaborate an angiogenesis factor *in vitro*.[3,4] The disease is transmitted by *Lutzomyia (Phlebotomus) verrucarum*, a nocturnal sandfly. Humans are the only known reservoir. After an incubation period of approximately 3 weeks, individuals without tolerance develop a fever and an acute, severe, hemolytic anemia, the result of virtually 100% parasitization of circulating erythrocytes by the microorganism. Infiltration of the reticuloendothelial system results in hepatosplenomegaly and lymphadenopathy. In the preantibiotic era, the mortality at this stage was approximately 40%; the current figure is around 8%. A tissue phase, which signals improvement in the patient's condition, appears approximately 2 months after the hematic phase and is characterized by the development of verruga peruana nodules (e-Fig. 17.9), which primarily involve the face and extremities.

Pathologic Features

The lesions can be subclassified histologically as miliary, when small and confined to the papillary dermis; nodular, when small to medium sized and present in the reticular dermis or subcutis; or mular, when large and involving both skin and subcutaneous tissue.[5] All contain vasoformation elements, commonly admixed with inflammatory cells, and typically arranged in a multinodular or lobulated pattern (Fig. 17.3, e-Figs. 17.10–17.13). Superficial

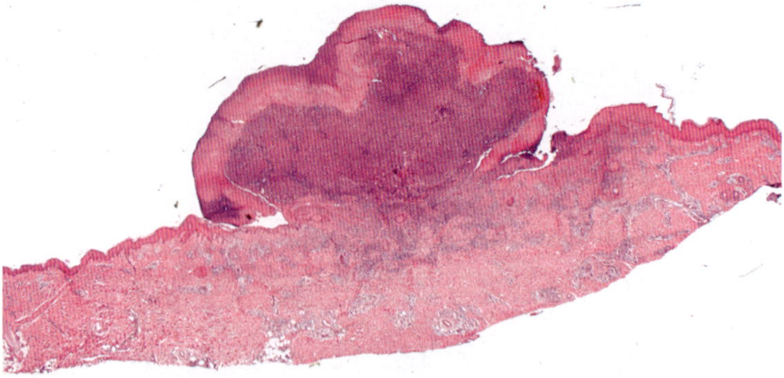

FIGURE 17.3 **Verruga Peruana.** This lesion appears similar to those associated with BA (image courtesy of Dr. Javier Arias-Stella); diagnosis requires correlation with the clinical history.

examples may be polypoid and, when accompanied by well-formed vessels with patent lumina, may be suggestive of a pyogenic granuloma or BA. Lesions that arise in less distensible tissues may exhibit more solid "angioblastic" growth suggestive of a neoplastic process.[5] All examples are unified by the presence of plump atypical appearing endothelial (verruga) cells. Depending on the stage of the lesions, lymphocytes and plasma cells or polymorphonuclear leukocytes with microabscess formation may be the predominant inflammatory constituents. Fibrin deposition, cellular necrosis, and fibrosclerosis may also be evident. The identification of Rocha-Lima inclusions, which may be fleeting, assists in confirming the diagnosis. These granular structures are best seen when tissues are fixed in buffered neutral formalin, embedded in glycol methacrylate, and stained with Giemsa.[6] They also stain lightly, though less convincingly, with the Warthin-Starry and PAS/D stains.

PAPILLARY ENDOTHELIAL HYPERPLASIA

This benign reactive process, which is an exuberant form of organizing vascular thrombus, was first described in 1923 by Pierre Masson as "vegetant intravascular hemangioendothelioma," reflecting his belief that it was neoplastic.

Clinical Features

Papillary endothelial hyperplasia (PEH) occurs at any age and involves virtually any vessel, including those of neoplastic processes and vascular malformations. However, in its "pure" form, it presents as a solitary,

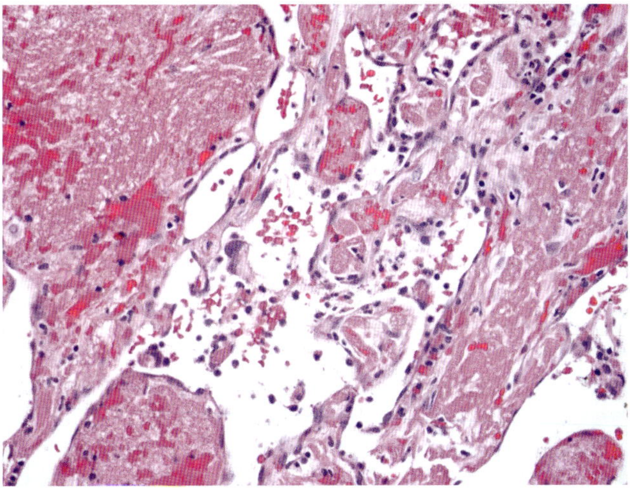

FIGURE 17.4 **Papillary Endothelial Hyperplasia.** This is an exaggerated form of organisation of vascular thrombi. Note the fibrin cores coated by a monolayer of endothelial cells.

superficial, firm, bluish, or erythematous mass, involving the fingers, head and neck, or anorectal region. Physical examination reveals limited mobility of the process about its longitudinal axis. Astute gross examination by the surgeon or the pathologist may reveal confinement of the process to the lumen of a dilated vessel, usually a vein.

Pathologic Features

There is a proliferation of endothelial cells within vessels (hemorrhoidal; e-Figs. 17.14 and 17.15) forming papillary fronds associated with thrombus. The fronds contain a core of fibrin or hyalinized collagen, depending upon the stage of the lesion, and are lined by a single layer of endothelial cells, which may be plump or swollen but lack significant atypia and mitotic activity (Fig. 17.4, e-Figs. 17.16 and 17.17).[7] Occasionally, due to the plane of sectioning or an actual event, the fronds appear to be "free-floating" within the vessel lumen. Extravascular extension may occasionally be seen, although it is usually not extensive. However, large, predominantly extravascular examples arising in hematomas have also been reported.

ANGIOLYMPHOID HYPERPLASIA WITH EOSINOPHILIA (EPITHELIOID HEMANGIOMA)

Clinical Features

These are lesions of adults (20–40 years) without gender predominance and unaccompanied by systemic symptoms.[8] They are most common in the head-neck region and are characterized by single or multiple smooth papules or plaques of varying color.[9] Most are unilateral. Local recurrence has been noted in up to one third of patients. Whether this is the result of a persisting underlying vascular anomaly (i.e., arteriovenous shunt) or an indication of inherent neoplastic potential is unresolved. Occasional multicentric lesions have been reported. There are no reported deaths due to this process. Optimal management is complete local excision.

Pathologic Features

Subcutaneous examples of ALHE are characterized by a prominent proliferation of capillary-sized vessels that, although well formed, often have an "immature," uncanalized appearance. Many are lined by plump epithelioid (histiocytoid[10]) endothelial cells (Fig. 17.5, e-Figs. 17.18–17.23). Mild cytologic atypia may be noted but generally the nuclei have small nucleoli, an abundance of euchromatin, and little heterochromatin clumping along the nuclear membranes. Lobulation and folds in the nucleus may occasionally be observed. The vascular proliferation is frequently centered about, and emanates radially from, a medium-sized artery or vein which shows histologic evidence of damage.[8] The process is commonly well marginated and bordered peripherally by lymphoid follicles (e-Figs. 17.20 and 17.21). Eosinophils (e-Fig. 17.18) without eosinophilic microabscesses and lymphocytes are usually present.

Dermal examples of ALHE[9] are similar to subcutaneous lesions but less well marginated. They more frequently have a mature, canalized appearance, and are not generally associated with a medium-sized artery or vein. Lymphoid follicles are also less commonly observed in this superficial location.

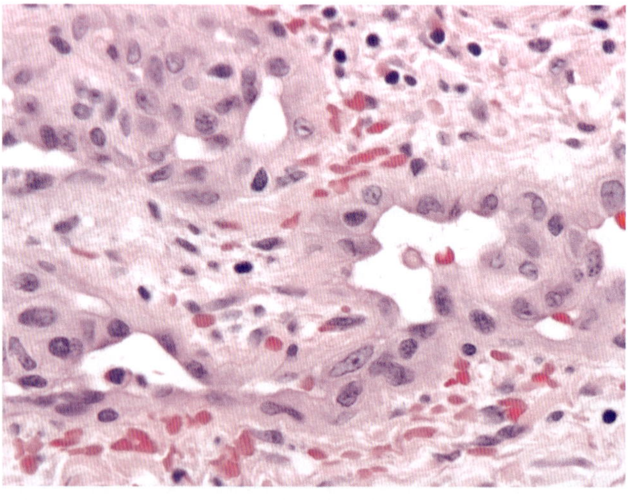

FIGURE 17.5 **Angiolymphoid Hyperplasia with Eosinophilia/Epithelioid Hemangioma.** This lesion shows well-formed vessels lined by plump epithelioid endothelial cells.

Ancillary Investigations

The endothelial cells are reactive for CD31 and CD34 but not GLUT1[11]; the latter feature confirms that they differ from juvenile-type hemangiomas (see below).

KIMURA DISEASE

This is not actually a vascular lesion but has been confused with epithelioid hemangioma/ALHE in the past and is thus listed here.

Clinical Features

Kimura disease appears almost exclusively in the Orient where it presents as a mass lesion, primarily in the head and neck region. Other reported sites of involvement include the groin, upper limb, axilla, and chest wall.[12] The masses may be multifocal or bilateral. Regional lymphadenopathy and peripheral blood eosinophilia are commonly noted, and serum IgG can be elevated. Some cases have been associated with renal disease.

Pathologic Features

The condition is characterized by a poorly marginated fibroinflammatory mass (Fig. 17.6) predominantly involving the subcutaneous tissue but also occasionally extending into the dermis, underlying musculature, or adjacent structures such as the salivary glands. Although the microscopic features vary somewhat with the duration of the lesion, all stages feature fibrosis, a reactive vascular proliferation, and an inflammatory infiltrate dominated

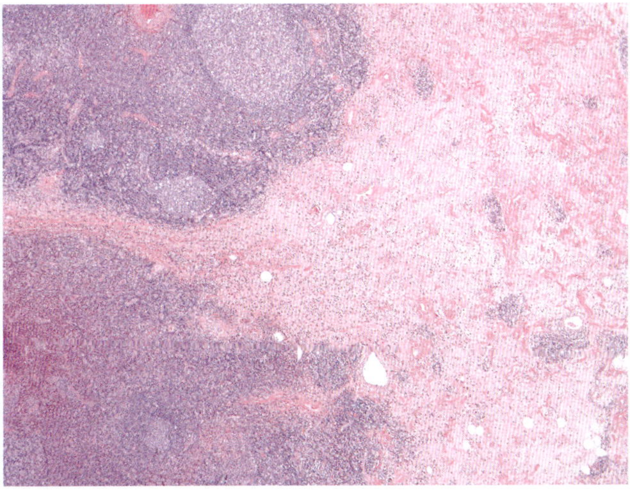

FIGURE 17.6 **Kimura Disease.** Kimura disease is not a vascular lesion but, rather, a fibroinflammatory process. It is included here based on confusion between it and ALHE/epithelioid hemangioma in the past.

by eosinophils and lymphocytes (e-Figs. 17.24–17.26). Earlier examples typically exhibit a more pronounced inflammatory reaction, while later stages are more fibrotic. Lymphoid follicles are a universal finding and are generally distributed through the process. Eosinophilic microabscesses are sometimes present (Fig. 17.7). In contrast to ALHE (epithelioid hemangioma), the vessels in Kimura disease are typically well canalized, lack epithelioid morphology, and, for the most part, tend to be a relatively minor or inconspicuous component of the process.

Ancillary Investigations

HHV-8 and EBV are negative.

HEMANGIOMAS

In general, the following morphologic features in a vascular tumor support a benign diagnosis: (a) zonated/lobular growth, (b) bland morphology with minimal mitotic activity, (c) arrangement of the endothelium in a monolayer, and (d) the presence of a "mature" vascular pattern with appropriate supporting elements or evidence of intralesional maturation. However, as is commonly the case in surgical pathology in general, no single feature can be relied upon with absolute certainty. For example, angiosarcomas may contain deceptively bland foci closely reminiscent of hemangioma, and pediatric vascular tumors (infantile or juvenile hemangiomas) are often cellular with prominent mitotic activity.

Hemangiomas of all types often contain additional supporting elements that include pericytes, smooth muscle, and interstitial fibroblast-like cells.

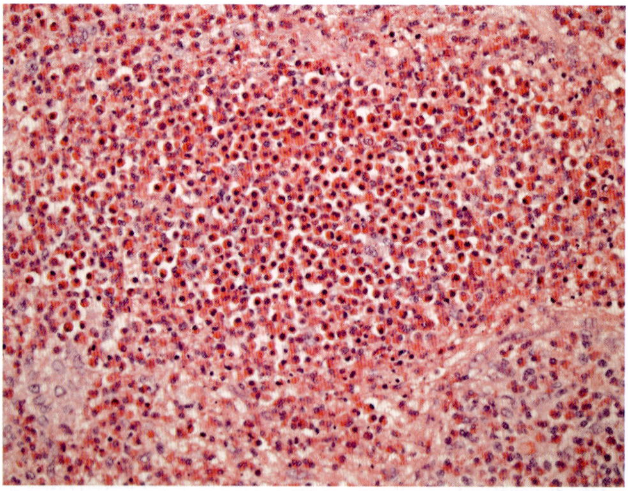

FIGURE 17.7 **Kimura Disease.** Eosinophilic microabscesses are a feature of Kimura disease but not of ALHE/epithelioid hemangioma.

These components are frequently more pronounced in pediatric tumors and can be highlighted with special histochemical stains (i.e., reticulin, Movat, pentachrome, etc.), as well as by immunohistochemical techniques.

CAPILLARY HEMANGIOMA

Clinical Features

Capillary hemangiomas are the most common tumor of infancy, seen in about 10% of term and 20% of preterm babies.[13] There is a female preponderance with an F:M ratio up to 3:1. In children, capillary hemangiomas are typically cellular and have thus been referred to as infantile hemangioendothelioma, juvenile hemangioma, strawberry nevus, and, perhaps most appropriately, cellular capillary hemangioma.

They may, on rare occasion, be associated with right-sided aortic arch coarctation, sternal clefting, midline abdominal raphe, and sacral and genitourinary tract defects[14] or with anomalies of the brain, cerebral vasculature, eyes, aorta, and chest wall in the neurocutaneous disorder called PHACE syndrome.[15] The PHACE acronym refers to posterior fossa anomalies, hemangioma, arterial lesions, cardiac abnormalities/aortic coarctation, and abnormalities of the eye, although the vascular lesions in these syndromes may in fact be malformations.

Sporadic capillary hemangiomas most frequently involve the skin or subcutis of the head and neck region, although a wide variety of other sites may also be involved. Rarely, they may grow to sufficient size to damage adjacent structures and even less frequently, they may have life-threatening or fatal consequences. The vast capillary surface area associated with large lesions can cause platelet trapping, thrombocytopenia, and a consumptive coagulopathy (Kasabach–Merritt syndrome), which can also occur in a variety of large vascular lesions of diverse histologic type.

Capillary hemangiomas typically proliferate in the first few months of life, then regress and, in many instances, completely involute. Approximately half of untreated patients with superficial lesions are left with normal skin by 5 years of life and from 70% to 90% of patients are "cured" by 7 years of age.[16] These results do not appear to be influenced by gender, duration of the proliferative phase, size or site of the lesions. The rare examples with life-threatening or severely disfiguring consequences due to massive size or strategic location have been managed by embolization, laser, corticosteroid therapy, interferon alpha-2A or 2B, or vincristine.[17]

Superficial capillary hemangioma (strawberry nevus or hemangioma) needs to be differentiated from vascular stains. The term nevus flammeus has been used in the past to encompass a wide variety of congenital macular stains, including both small, transient lesions (e.g., nevus simplex) and the larger, persistent, port-wine stains. Common sites of involvement include the glabella, eyelids, and the nape of the neck. Those located in the center of the face commonly disappear by 1 year of life, whereas nape lesions fade more slowly and often incompletely with faint vestiges persisting into adulthood. Port-wine stains (nevus venosus), on the other hand, occur far less frequently. They consist of larger macules with irregular borders that tend to enlarge in proportion to the growth of the child and generally do not fade. They are typically flat in infancy and childhood but may become elevated and nodular later in life.

Lateral facial port-wine stains in the distribution of the trigeminal nerve with abrupt termination at the midline are a component of the Sturge-Weber (leptomeningeal nevus flammeus or encephalotrigeminal angiomatosis) syndrome. Port-wine stains are also associated with the Klippel-Trenaunay (osteohypertrophic nevus flammeus) and Parkes Weber syndromes, which are further discussed in Chapter 18.

Pathologic Features

During the proliferative phase, capillary hemangiomas are characterized histologically by a mixture of endothelial cells, pericytes, and fibroblast-like cells (e-Fig. 17.27). The endothelial cell nuclei can have prominent nucleoli and mitotic activity may be pronounced. Many of the vessels may lack apparent lumina, although tubular or cord-like angiogenic growth can be highlighted with a reticulin stain. On low-power examination, the lesions often have a marginated or circumscribed appearance and the proliferating vessels are typically arranged in a lobular pattern (Fig. 17.8). Maturation is first noted at the periphery of these lobules and is characterized by the presence of flattened, or less active appearing endothelium lining vessels with patent lumina. Over time, a greater

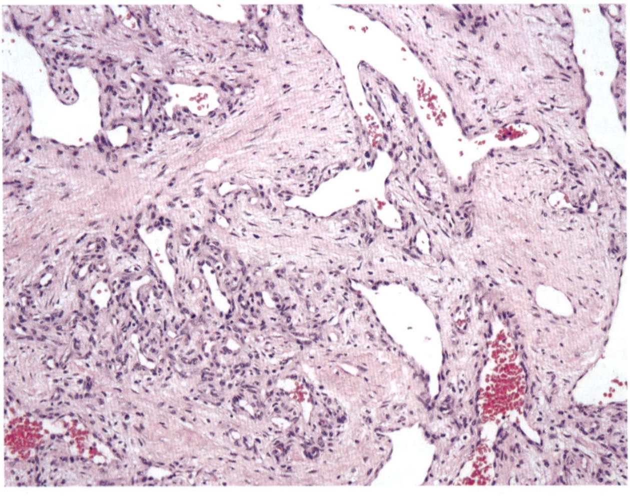

FIGURE 17.8 **Capillary Hemangioma.** This lesion from a small child has a lobular growth pattern, showing larger capillaries branching into smaller ones. The smallest are supported by cells other than endothelial cells (such as myoid cells and pericytes).

percentage of the capillaries assume this morphology. The vascular lobules also become more accentuated due to an ingrowth of fibrous and adipose connective tissue.

Unlike capillary hemangiomas, congenital macular stains lack endothelial proliferation. In fact, when biopsied early in life, they typically reveal minimal or no apparent histologic abnormality. Persistent, laterally located lesions of the port-wine stain type, however, eventually develop pronounced capillary ectasia. Macular stains are regarded as telangiectasias rather than true hemangiomas (and do not regress).

Ancillary Investigations

GLUT1 is usually strongly and diffusely expressed in the lesional endothelial cells of most infantile hemangiomas (which are likely to regress) during all stages of their natural history but usually not in other vascular tumors or malformations (which will not regress).[18–20] GLUT1 also labels a variety of nonvascular neoplasms.[21] The endothelial cells in capillary hemangiomas express CD34 and CD31 but not podoplanin (D2-40).[22]

PYOGENIC GRANULOMA/LOBULAR CAPILLARY HEMANGIOMA

The term pyogenic granuloma is a misnomer that has been retained over time. An infectious etiology has long been disproved and current observers favor a lobular variant of capillary hemangioma, but there are some important distinctions from classic (pediatric) capillary hemangioma.

Clinical Features

The lesions may involve mucosal, cutaneous, subcutaneous, or even intravascular sites. Patients under the age of 18 are predominantly males, whereas those between 19 and 40 are mostly females, with equal sex incidence over 40. About a third have a history of trauma. Local recurrence develops in about 10% of cases treated by simple excision. The most common sites are gingiva and fingers, followed by lips, face, and tongue. Tumors of the oral and nasal mucosa (but not other sites) show a marked predilection for women in their reproductive years.[23]

Approximately 1% of pregnant women develop pyogenic granulomas in the oral mucosa, especially the interdental regions of the gingiva. These typically appear in the first trimester and regress post partum. Similar lesions may develop with oral contraceptive use. These associations suggests hormonal sensitivity although ER and PgR are negative.[24]

Pyogenic granulomas are solitary or rarely multiple. Disseminated lesions can occur spontaneously or be associated with an underlying malignancy. Superficial pyogenic granulomata, involving the mucous membranes or skin, may be sessile, polypoid, or pedunculated. They frequently have a rapid onset but stabilize at a maximum size of several millimeters to a few centimeters after several weeks or months. The lesions range in color from bluish-purple to bright red. Their epithelial surface may be attenuated or ulcerated.

Some pyogenic granulomas are intravascular (e-Figs. 17.28–17.30).[25] These lesions present in the third decade over a period of 2 to 8 weeks and have a predilection for small to medium-sized veins of the neck and upper extremities. They have polypoid intraluminal architecture. Apart from the intravascular location, their histology is typical of pyogenic granuloma.

Pathologic Features

On histological examination, pyogenic granuloma is characterized by a relatively well-marginated proliferation of small capillary-sized vessels arranged in a multilobular pattern (Fig. 17.9, e-Figs. 17.31 and 17.32). Larger feeder vessels may be seen in association with the vascular lobules. The process is set in a fibromyxoid stroma that, in the absence of surface ulceration, has minimal inflammation. Both endothelial and stromal elements are mitotically active. Polypoid or pedunculated lesions often have a collarette of hyperplastic epithelium (Fig. 17.9). Deep-seated have less edema and vascular dilatation.

Ancillary Investigations

The endothelial cells express CD34 and CD31 but not GLUT1

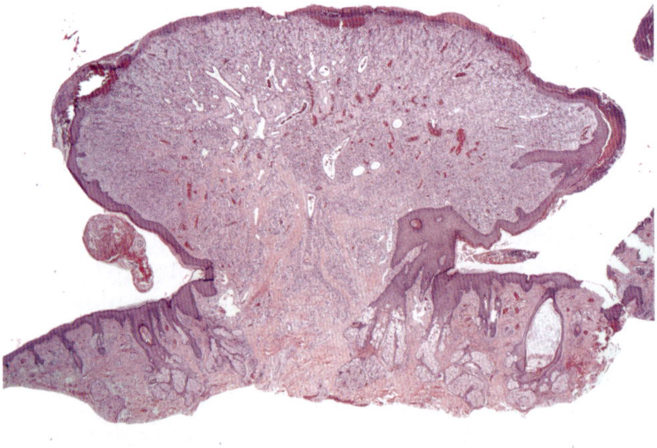

FIGURE 17.9 **Pyogenic Granuloma (Lobular Capillary Hemangioma).** The histologic appearances of these lesions are similar to those of capillary hemangiomas found in infants and small children but, in contrast to those of infants, these are not as likely to regress. Note again the lobular configurations of the proliferating vessels. This example has a collarette of hyperplastic skin.

CAVERNOUS HEMANGIOMA

Clinical Features

Cavernous hemangiomas are common in both children and adults and predilect for the upper half of the body. Roughly equal numbers of males and females are affected. Unlike capillary hemangiomas, cavernous hemangiomas do not regress. Examples occurring in deep soft tissue and organs (liver, bone, intestines, and lung) are also well known. Rarely, large deep-seated examples may be associated with the Kasabach-Merritt consumptive coagulopathy syndrome.

Cutaneous cavernous hemangiomas are soft, elevated, dark blue or purplish masses that compress easily and blanch with pressure. Deep-seated examples may be inapparent clinically and, on occasion, are incidental radiologic findings. Cavernous hemangiomas have been listed as a component of a number of dysmorphic and genetic syndromes including blue-rubber bleb nevus, Maffucci, Klippel-Trenaunay, and Parkes Weber syndromes.[26] Maffucci syndrome (dyschondroplasia and hemangiomas) is a congenital (nonhereditary) syndrome in which multiple vascular lesions occur shortly after birth or prior to puberty. During skeletal growth, there is enchondromatosis complicated by chondrosarcomas in about 15% of patients. While the vascular lesions in some reports seem to be cavernous hemangiomas, many instead appear to be examples of spindle cell hemangioma,[27] discussed below.

Patients with blue rubber bleb syndrome, which is an autosomal dominant,[28] present with multiple small dome-shaped vascular lesions involving the skin and internal organs. Profound iron deficiency is common and attributable to numerous lesions lining the gastrointestinal tract, especially the small bowel.

Pathologic Features

The histology of cavernous hemangiomas is characterized by either a lobulated or a poorly marginated collection of engorged thin-walled vascular channels lined by flattened endothelium (Fig. 17.10). Supporting elements (pericytes, smooth muscle cells, and fibroblastic cells) are less pronounced than in capillary hemangiomas. Sometimes, especially in the superficial portion of cutaneous tumors, a coexisting small vessel component may be evident. One variant, termed "sinusoidal hemangioma" (e-Figs. 17.33 and 17.34), occurs in adults and consists of clustered markedly dilated interconnecting (sinusoidal) vascular spaces.[29]

Biopsied cutaneous lesions of blue rubber bleb syndrome demonstrate relatively well-demarcated collections of dilated thin-walled vessels in the upper and midreticular dermis and lined by attenuated endothelium. The overlying skin is flattened and hyperkeratotic. Gastrointestinal tract lesions have similar vessels, which may be located in any layer of the bowel wall, but frequently protrude into the mucosa where they are prone to ulceration. The presence of prominent strands of organized smooth muscle

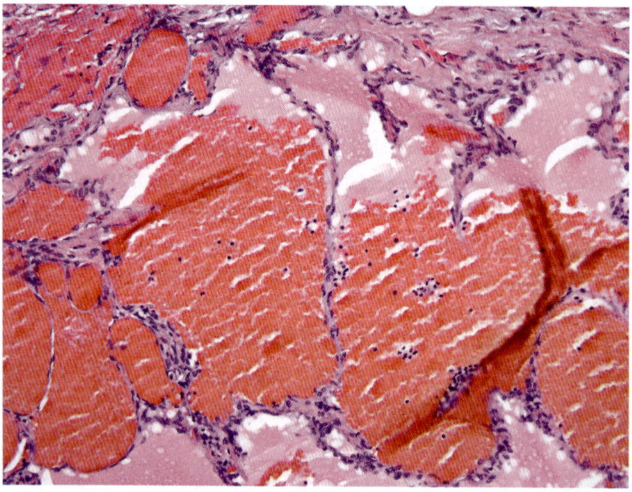

FIGURE 17.10 **Cavernous Hemangioma.** This lesion features ectatic engorged thin-walled vessels.

and wisps of elastic lamina in some vessel walls suggests that these lesions are multiple vascular malformations of venous type rather than cavernous hemangiomas. PEH can be encountered within these anomalous vessels.

OTHER HEMANGIOMA (AND LYMPHANGIOMA) VARIANTS

Superficial Arteriovenous Tumor/Malformation

Cutaneous arteriovenous hemangiomas (acral arteriovenous tumors) have a predilection for the perioral region and the extremities of adults.[30] Clinically, they are small (<1 cm) red or purple papules with little tendency for spontaneous regression. Some examples may resemble basal cell carcinoma or a nevus. Local excision is usually curative.

On microscopic examination, the tumors consist of relatively well-circumscribed masses of thick- and thin-walled vessels, located primarily in the dermis of the skin or submucosa of the lip. Many of the vessels have a "transitional" appearance between arteries and veins, and in some cases, a direct communication between the latter may be noted. The endothelial cells may be plump but are not cytologically atypical.

Microvenular Hemangioma

This lesion generally presents as a small solitary nodule or plaque involving the extremities of young adults.[31] The ten patients reported by Hunt et al. ranged in age from 9 to 39 years (median age = 29.5 years). The clinical features are in keeping with hemangioma although the acquired nature of the lesion, evidence of lesional growth, and an origin within an extremity indicate inclusion of the patch stage of Kaposi sarcoma (KS) in the differential diagnosis. One lesion has been described as HHV-8 reactive,[32] although it was reported in a patient with POEMS syndrome (see below), and may not have been a typical microvenular hemangioma.

Microvenular hemangioma is characterized microscopically by a permeative proliferation of small irregularly branching vessels that are well formed but often have collapsed, somewhat inconspicuous lumina (e-Figs. 17.35–17.37). The vessel walls are said to be thicker than those of capillary hemangiomas. The endothelium lacks cytologic atypia and inflammation is only rarely noted. Hemosiderin deposits may be present. In contrast to KS, microvenular hemangioma lacks the promontory sign (i.e., an irregular proliferation of small vessels, adjacent to and protruding into a more ectatic vessel), a spindle cell element, apoptotic endothelium, intracytoplasmic hyaline globules, and an inflammatory infiltrate rich in plasma cells.

Glomeruloid Hemangioma

Glomeruloid hemangioma occurs as a component of the POEMS syndrome.[33] This syndrome, also known as Takatsuki syndrome, Crow-Fukase syndrome, and plasma cell dyscrasia with polyneuropathy and endocrine disorder, is characterized by **P**olyneuropathy, **O**rganomegaly (hepatosplenomegaly and lymphadenopathy), **E**ndocrinopathy (amenorrhea, gynecomastia, hypothyroidism, adrenal insufficiency, and glucose intolerance), **M**onoclonal protein (marrow plasmacytosis, paraproteinemia), and **S**kin lesions. The latter include glomeruloid and cherry angiomas, acanthosis, hyperpigmentation, and hypertrichosis. The syndrome differs from ordinary myeloma in that bone lesions tend to be sclerotic, plasma cells are frequently only mildly increased in the marrow, the paraprotein titer commonly is lower, and the patients are typically younger. Enlarged lymph nodes in POEMS patients frequently show features of Castleman disease.[33] While some patients with Castleman disease are reported to have HHV-8 in lesional cells,[34] this has not been reported in glomeruloid hemangiomas.

Glomeruloid hemangiomas are commonly multifocal. The majority of examples involved the skin of the trunk or proximal extremities where they appear as pin-sized to pea-sized papules. However, internal structures may also be affected. Histologic examination reveals dilated, ectatic vessels with intraluminal capillary conglomerates, architecturally resembling renal glomeruli. The vessels are lined by flattened or slightly plump endothelium with bland nuclear features (e-Figs. 17.38–17.42). Interposed between the capillary loops are plump "stromal" cells with clear cytoplasm. These latter cells occasionally contain PAS-positive, diastase-resistant globules that are believed to represent phagocytosed immunoglobulin.

As noted earlier, cherry hemangiomas have also been described in POEMS syndrome and a few lesions having hybrid features with glomeruloid hemangioma have been identified. Thus, it has been suggested that, in this setting, the two hemangioma types may represent either a different stage in the evolution of a single process or a variation in the degree of the vascular response to the angiogenic stimuli.

Angioblastoma (Acquired Tufted Angioma, Progressive Capillary Hemangioma, Angioblastoma of Nakagawa)

Almost 60% of cases have an onset in the first year of life and over 70% are evident before the age of ten. The lesions are frequently painful. They typically develop insidiously, with slow growth for several years before stabilizing. Occasionally, however, more rapid growth is noted. Spontaneous regression or involution is rare (and these lesions lack GLUT1 staining). Metastases have not been reported.

The most frequent sites of involvement are the neck, upper chest, and shoulders. There is considerable variability in size and appearance although commonly they are macular or plaque-like, with slight granularity or nodularity due to a superimposed papular component.

At low magnification, there are tightly packed clusters of capillaries with a rounded or ovoid ("cannonball") appearance (e-Figs. 17.43–17.45). The process is usually concentrated in the mid and deep dermis, although involvement of the papillary dermis and superficial subcutis may also be evident. The intervening dermal collagen has a normal appearance with minimal, if any, inflammation. Coalescence of the capillary aggregates occasionally results in the presence of larger, more geographic, vascular expanses. The vascular tufts contain plump or spindled endothelium, pericytes, and occasional smooth muscle cells, all with bland morphology (e-Fig. 17.45). The constituents are frequently arranged in a whorled or concentric pattern such that individual capillary lumina are compressed and slit-like. Dilated vascular channels may be evident at the periphery of the capillary aggregates. Mitotic activity is usually scant. Mast cells may be abundant in and about the tumor.

Since the morbidity associated with angioblastoma appears to be primarily cosmetic, aggressive intervention is not required. Local recurrence may occur following incomplete excision.

Hobnail Hemangioma (Targetoid Hemosiderotic Hemangioma)

These tumors typically occur as a solitary lesion on the trunk or extremities of young adults. Early examples have a central purple or brown-black papule, bordered by an inner pale zone, and a more peripherally situated ecchymotic ring and have been termed "targetoid hemosiderotic hemangioma."[35] The outer ring fades with maturation, leaving behind a small papule which can clinically resemble a fibrous histiocytoma. These lesions are not always targetoid but do feature hobnail endothelium, so the term "hobnail hemangioma" has prevailed.[36]

The histology of hobnail hemangioma varies with the duration of the lesion. First, there are ectatic thin-walled vascular channels and lined by plump, sometimes epithelioid, endothelium (e-Figs. 17.46–17.51), in the superficial dermis. Intraluminal papillary endothelial projections and fibrin thrombi may be present. Deeper vessels infiltrate reticular dermis and have an angulated, irregular, and slit-like appearance. They exhibit a permeative, collagen "dissecting," growth pattern and are lined by attenuated, relatively inconspicuous endothelium. Extension into the superficial subcutis may also be noted. Hemorrhage, hemosiderin deposition, edema, and a mild lymphocytic infiltrate are commonly present. In later stages, the superficial ectatic vascular channels are lost and collapsed; anastomosing, small vessels predominate.

Progressive Lymphangioma (Benign Lymphangioendothelioma)

Acquired progressive lymphangioma (benign lymphangioendothelioma)[37] differs clinically from targetoid hemosiderotic hemangioma in being a more extensive, slowly progressive process, often having the appearance of a large bruise-like macule. Most examples arise in adults but pediatric cases have been reported. The head and neck is a favored site followed by the rest of the upper part of the body. Histologically, both hobnail hemangioma and acquired progressive lymphangioma feature numerous anastomosing vascular channels with a "collagen dissection" pattern (e-Fig. 17.52–17.58). However, acquired progressive lymphangioma typically lacks hemosiderin deposition and hobnail endothelium, and its vascular channels are generally bloodless. On immunolabeling, the lesional cells express podoplanin (D2-40) but not HHV-8.

Angiokeratoma

There are several clinical forms of angiokeratoma. The generalized systemic type (angiokeratoma corpus diffusum) is associated with Fabry disease, fucosidosis, and a deficiency of beta-galactosidase. The lesions are characterized histologically by the presence of dilated vessels that are primarily restricted to the uppermost dermis and are bordered or enclosed by elongate rete ridges (e-Fig. 17.59–17.61). With time, the overlying epidermis often becomes hyperkeratotic and, sometimes, papillomatous. The process is commonly regarded as a form of telangiectasia rather than true neoplasm.

Verrucous Hemangioma

Verrucous hemangioma shares many similarities with angiokeratoma, the key distinction being the added presence of an underlying hemangioma/vascular malformation within the deep dermis or subcutis (e-Figs. 17.62–17.64). This entity has a high local recurrence rate attributable to incomplete resection of the anomalous vascular proliferation.

Angioma Serpiginosum

Angioma serpiginosum is a benign vascular ectasia with a distinct gyrate or serpiginous clinical appearance. It typically appears in females in the first 2 decades of life and favors the lower extremities. Although there may be periods of relative stability, this process has a tendency for slow progression.

CUTANEOUS EPITHELIOID ANGIOMATOUS NODULE

Clinical Features

These lesions present as erythematous to blue papules, usually on the trunk of adults.[38,39] Most are single, but the lesions sometimes occur in an eruptive fashion.[38,39] These lesions are benign.

Pathologic Features

The lesions are centered superficially in the dermis and are circumscribed, unilobular, mainly solid proliferations of large polygonal epithelioid endothelial cells with vesicular nuclei and conspicuous nucleoli and at least focal vasoformation (Fig. 17.11, e-Figs. 17.65 and 17.66). The endothelial cells contain abundant and cytoplasm and frequent intracytoplasmic vacuoles. Nuclear atypia is absent. Mitotic figures can be abundant. Many cases are associated with adjacent dilated dermal vessels, hemosiderin deposition, and mild fibrosis. Like epithelioid hemangioma described above, these lesions are accompanied by a chronic inflammatory infiltrate with a lymphoplasmacytic component, most pronounced at the periphery of the lesion, usually contain eosinophils.

Ancillary Investigations

Variable staining with CD34, CD31, and FVII-related antigen has been reported.

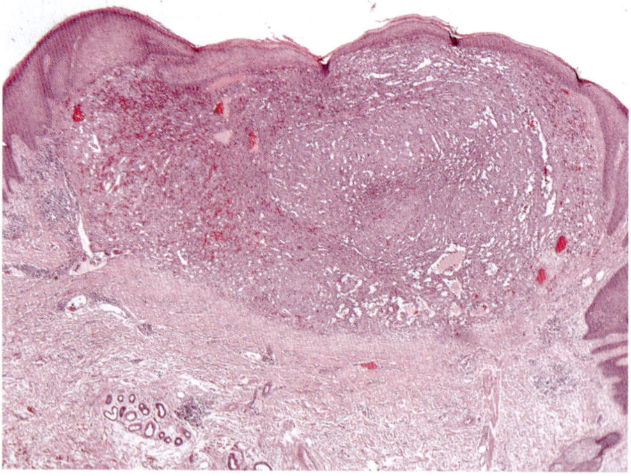

FIGURE 17.11 **Cutaneous Epithelioid Angiomatous Nodule.** Small vessels are accompanied by sheets of mitotically active spindle cells without a well-formed lobular configuration. Like pyogenic granulomas, these lesions also feature a hyperplastic epidermal collarette.

MASSIVE LOCALIZED LYMPHEDEMA IN THE MORBIDLY OBESE

Clinical Features

These lesions present as unilateral, large soft tissue masses of longstanding in morbidly obese adults (mean patient weight: 409 and 372 lb in two series[40,41]). Most involve the thigh, but they can also arise in the calf and lower leg (e-Fig. 17.67). Clinically, they resemble pedunculated lipoma, lymphocele, or recurrent cellulitis, although soft tissue sarcoma is occasionally suspected. These lesions are benign.

Pathologic Features

Grossly, these are large lesions with a superficial component. The overlying skin is markedly thickened with a "cobblestone" appearance. The lesions are ill-defined, unencapsulated, lobulated, and very large (mean size: 31 cm, range: 15–61.5 cm, mean weight: 3,386 g, range: 1,133–10,800 g in one series[41]). Histologically, there is striking dermal fibrosis, expansion of the fibrous septa between fat lobules with increased numbers of stromal fibroblasts (Fig. 17.12, e-Figs. 17.68–17.73), lymphatic proliferation, and lymphangiectasia (Fig. 17.13). Some cases have multinucleated fibroblastic cells (Fig. 17.12, e-Fig. 17.73), marked vascular proliferation, moderate stromal cellularity, and fascicular growth (Fig. 17.12).

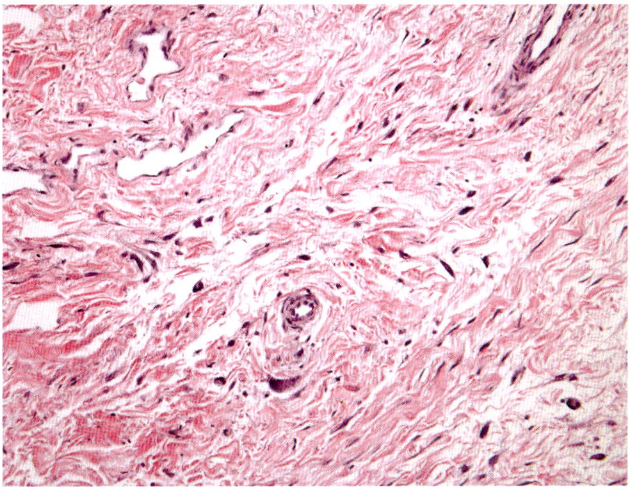

FIGURE 17.12 **Lymphedema in the Morbidly Obese.** This area features fascicular growth of spindle cells, some multinucleated.

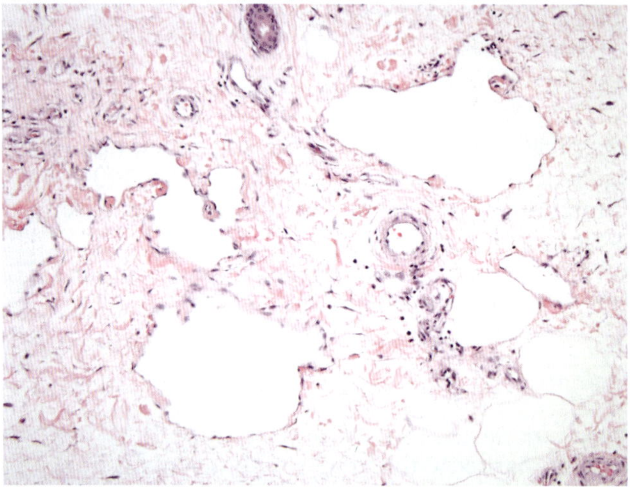

FIGURE 17.13 **Lymphedema in the Morbidly Obese.** This field shows ecstatic lymphatic spaces near the skin surface. Part of a skin adnexal structure is present at the top of the field.

SPINDLE CELL HEMANGIOMA

This was originally called "spindle cell hemangioendothelioma."[42] However, the lesion probably arises in response to abnormal blood flow, perhaps in a preexisting vascular malformations and is currently classified as spindle cell hemangioma.[43]

Clinical Features

Spindle cell hemangioma typically presents as a superficial slow-growing painless mass involving the dermis and/or subcutis. Most lesions are 2 cm or less and develop in the third and fourth decades. Over half involve the hands or feet with the remainder occurring elsewhere in the extremities or on the trunk. Multifocality is common. Some cases have been associated with other disease processes including Milroy disease, Maffucci disease, Klippel-Trenaunay syndrome, and an early-onset of varicose veins.[44]

Pathologic Findings

The process is typically well marginated. There are cavernous vascular spaces, similar to those seen in a cavernous hemangioma, sometimes containing phleboliths and a spindle cell proliferation vaguely reminiscent of KS (Fig. 17.14, e-Figs. 17.74–17.76). Smooth muscle may be evident around or within the lesion, in association with the cavernous spaces or the more solid spindled areas. Epithelioid endothelial cells, sometimes with intracytoplasmic lumina, are an additional feature of these lesions. Lesions are often partially or completely intravascular. The vein containing the tumor often has an irregularly attenuated wall with small intimal herniations and intimal papillae traversing the lumen.

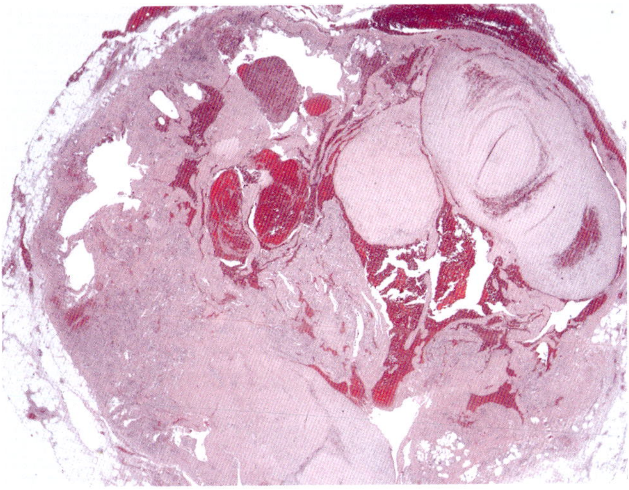

FIGURE 17.14 **Spindle Cell Hemangioma.** At low magnification, the lesion is characterized by cavernous hemangioma-like areas, thrombi, and spindle cell areas.

Ancillary Investigations

CD34 and CD31 are positive in the endothelial cells but not in the spindle cells that display SMA, IL8, and VEGFR.[45]

MALIGNANT ENDOVASCULAR PAPILLARY ANGIOENDOTHELIOMA, PAPILLARY INTRALYMPHATIC ANGIOENDOTHELIOMA, DABSKA TUMOR

The majority of these tumors appear to occur in infants and children, but they can also arise in adults.[46] They primarily involve the skin and subcutis, but if left untreated, they can extend into muscle and bone and have rarely been reported as isolated muscle or bone lesions. No anatomic site appears to be favored. These tumors are considered "intermediate" (rare metastases)

Pathologic Findings

Histologic examination shows a tumor composed of intercommunicating vascular channels of varying caliber, some large and irregular, with a cavernous appearance, others smaller and capillary-like (e-Figs. 17.77–17.84). The vessels contain endothelium with diverse morphology, ranging from a normal flattened appearance to plump and epithelioid to distinctly columnar. The latter endothelial variants may exhibit cytologic atypia and are sometimes arranged in papillary (primitive glomeruloid) tufts with a central avascular hyaline core (Fig. 17.15). This feature is the true *sine qua non* of the process. Endothelial cells lining the papillae have nuclei that are eccentrically located along the luminal aspect of the tuft, a feature that Dabska likened to the appearance of match heads (Fig. 17.16).[47]

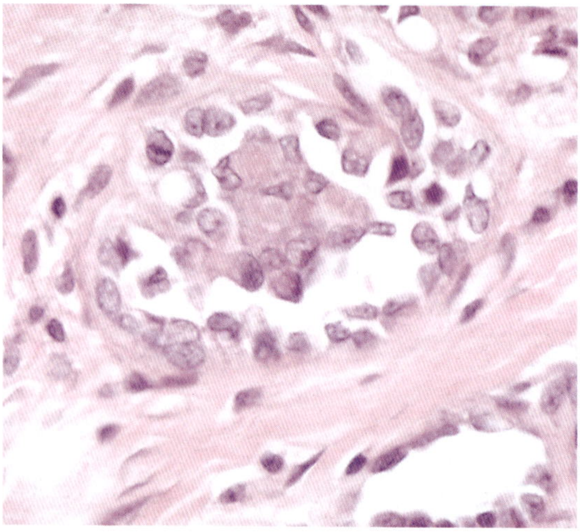

FIGURE 17.15 **Dabska Tumor (Malignant Endovascular Papillary Angioendothelioma, Papillary Intralymphatic Angioendothelioma).** This vascular space is lined by hobnail endothelium and contains a papilla with a central acellular core.

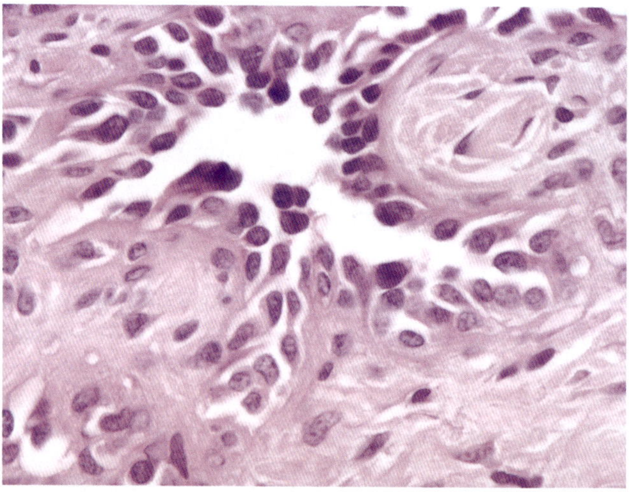

FIGURE 17.16 **Dabska Tumor (Malignant Endovascular Papillary Angioendothelioma, Papillary Intralymphatic Angioendothelioma).** The apical nuclei of the tall endothelial cells in this lesion reminded Dr. Dabska of match heads.

Intravascular lymphocytes may be prominent and are sometimes intimately associated with the endothelium. The surrounding soft tissue can have a relatively normal appearance or it may be fibrotic. Occasionally, lymphoid aggregates, foci of hemorrhage, and degenerative elements (i.e., cholesterol clefts, siderophages, etc.) are noted.

This tumor has many overlapping features with retiform hemangioendothelioma with which it may form a spectrum representing an adult variant,[48] although they have slightly different immunolabeling patterns.

Ancillary Investigations

These lesions express CD34, CD31, podoplanin (D2-40), and vascular endothelial growth factor receptor-3 (VEGFR-3). Retiform hemangioendothelioma is usually negative for podoplanin and VEGRF-3.[49]

KAPOSIFORM HEMANGIOENDOTHELIOMA

Clinical Features

This lesion was initially reported as kaposiform infantile hemangioendothelioma as a rare but distinctive vascular tumor that primarily arose as retroperitoneal lesions in infants and children.[50] These tumors were later recognized in adults[51] and in superficial sites.[52] Overall, superficial lesions outnumber deep ones. In infants, the tumor may manifest as a large retroperitoneal mass that is frequently associated with a consumptive coagulopathy (Kasabach-Merritt syndrome) and is sometimes complicated by intestinal obstruction, jaundice, and hemoperitoneum.[19,50] Although the tumor has proven lethal for many patients with intra-abdominal disease, due to aggressive local behavior, distant metastases have not been reported. Local spread to lymphoid tissue is documented.[19] Some are associated with lymphangiomatosis.[50]

A consensus approach to management of intra-abdominal examples has not been developed; treatment has ranged from supportive care to attempts at surgical resection. With varying degrees of success, prednisone, radiation, and chemotherapy have also been used in an attempt to reduce tumor burden. Optimal management for peripherally situated examples is believed to be wide local excision.[52]

Pathologic Features

The tumors are characterized histologically by infiltrative but yet lobular growth with intervening fibrous septa (Fig. 17.17). Well-formed capillaries, sometimes containing fibrin thrombi, are admixed with short fascicles of spindle cells with slit-like vascular lumina (e-Figs. 17.85 and 17.86). The latter component results in a pattern reminiscent of KS and serves as a distinguishing feature from other pediatric vascular tumors such as cellular capillary hemangioma (juvenile or infantile hemangioendothelioma). The lobulated growth pattern, lack of a prominent interanastomosing vascular pattern, and paucity of significant cytologic atypia aid in distinguishing this tumor from angiosarcoma.

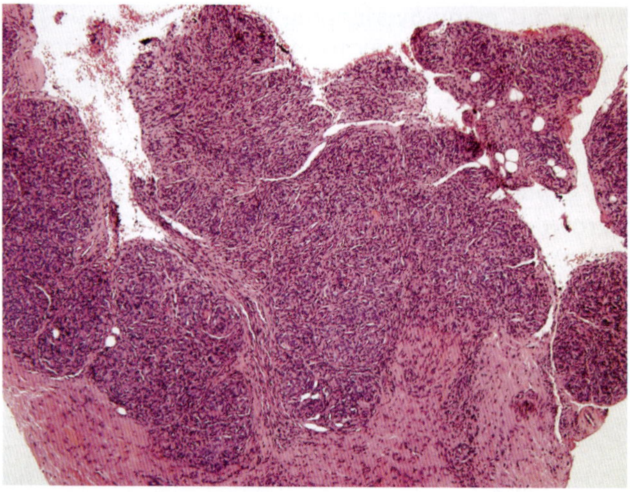

FIGURE 17.17 **Kaposiform Hemangioendothelioma.** This highly cellular lesion has a lobular configuration.

Ancillary Investigations

Kaposiform hemangioendothelioma shows marked D2-40 expression in the KS-like proliferative capillaries but not in the surrounding dilated vessels.[53] Endothelial cells in nodules are CD31, CD34, VEGFR-3, and FLI1 positive but negative for GLUT1. The lesions lack HHV-8.[19]

ATYPICAL VASCULAR LESION

Clinical Features

These lesions are classically encountered in mammary skin following radiation for mammary carcinoma. They appear as a single or several small papules of patches in the irradiated site. Most such lesions behave in a benign fashion, but a subset progresses to angiosarcoma, often after several recurrences so that complete excision has been suggested.[54] These lesions are difficult to separate from highly differentiated angiosarcomas, both clinically and histologically. However, most atypical vascular lesions are small (<1 cm), whereas angiosarcomas have a median size of about 7 cm.[55]

Pathologic Features

These lesions can have several patterns. Some resemble benign lymphangiomas (Fig. 17.18, e-Fig. 17.87), consisting of a well-marginated proliferation of thin-walled vascular channels. These channels have an interanastomosing pattern and bland flat or hobnail endothelium and lack erythrocytes. Others appear more like lymphangioendothelioma,[37] displaying a more infiltrative pattern but featuring bland appearing endothelium.[54]

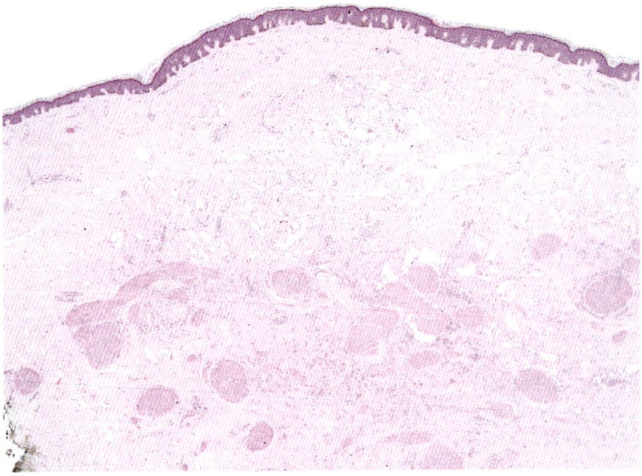

FIGURE 17.18 **Atypical Vascular Lesion.** This example arose in irradiated breast skin and shows features reminiscent of a lymphangioma. The lesion was <1 cm and did not extend deeper than the arrector pili muscles.

However, a subset can have endothelium that appears as a lobular capillary proliferation. These cases may be more likely to progress to angiosarcoma (e-Figs. 17.88–17.90), although the lymphatic types can progress as well.[56]

Ancillary Investigations

The endothelial cells in these lesions express CD34 and CD31 and those with lymphatic differentiation express podoplanin (D2-40).[56]

RETIFORM HEMANGIOENDOTHELIOMA

Clinical Features

These are extremely rare neoplasms typically affecting young adults without gender preference.[49,57] These lesions involve the skin and subcutaneous tissues and usually arise on the lower extremities. The lesions grow slowly, forming plaques and nodules that measure about 3 cm. Rarely lesions are multiple[58] or arise in previously radiated sites or areas of lymphedema.[57] This tumor occasionally metastasizes to regional lymph nodes but not distant sites, and tumor-associated deaths have not been reported.

Histologic Features

The lesions consist of elongated narrow arborizing vascular channels (Fig. 17.19, e-Figs. 17.91–17.94). The channels are lined by plump endothelial cells that are reminiscent of epithelium at low magnification, and hence the overall appearance suggests rete testis. The endothelial cells themselves are monomorphic and hyperchromatic with a hobnail appearance (Fig. 17.20).

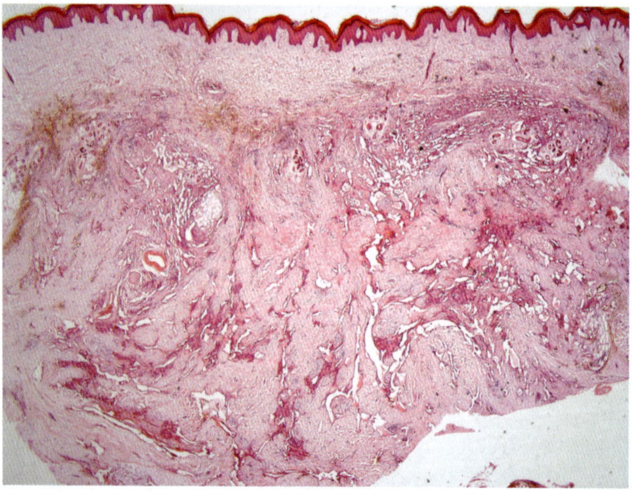

FIGURE 17.19 **Retiform Hemangioendothelioma.** The configuration of the vessels is reminiscent of the pattern of rete testis. This was an extensive lesion. Note the hemosiderin deposition at the superficial portion of the tumor.

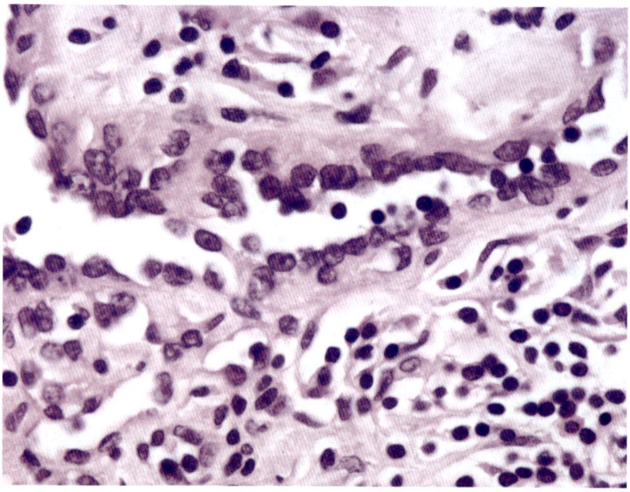

FIGURE 17.20 **Retiform Hemangioendothelioma.** The endothelial cells are reminiscent of those in Dabska tumors. This example has numerous associated lymphocytes.

Mitotic activity is negligible. There is often a striking lymphoid background with numerous lymphocytes both between the vessels and admixed with the endothelium (Fig. 17.20, e-Figs. 17.91 and 17.92). Some of the lesions display intravascular papillae with hyaline cores resembling those in the Dabska tumor.

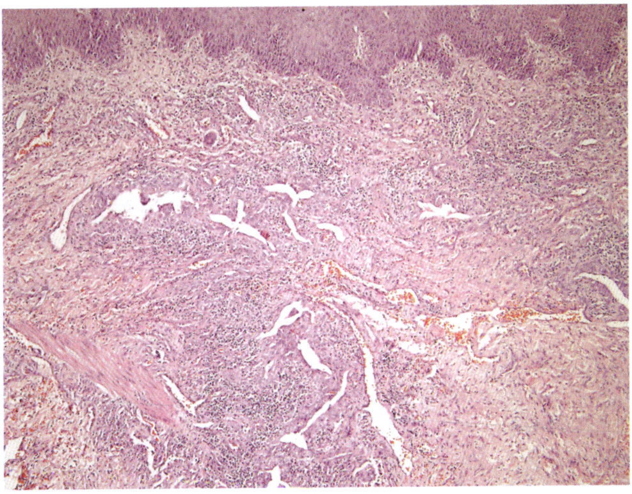

FIGURE 17.21 **Composite Hemangioendothelioma.** This example features epithelioid endothelial cells but a growth pattern similar to that of retiform hemangioendothelioma with many intralesional lymphocytes.

Ancillary Investigations

The endothelial cells in retiform hemangioendothelioma react with vascular endothelial markers CD31, CD34, and factor VIII–related antigen but usually do not express podoplanin or VEGFR-3 (D2-40).[49] There is an isolated report of detection of HHV-8 viral transcripts,[59] but presumably this reflected a PCR contaminant as similar lesions lack HHV-8.[19]

COMPOSITE HEMANGIOENDOTHELIOMA

These extremely rare neoplasms show elements of with histologic features of both epithelioid hemangioendothelioma and retiform hemangioendothelioma.[60,61]

Clinical Features

These lesions present as longstanding dermal and subcutaneous nodules and plaques, usually in the extremities of young adults.[60,61] Other lesions have arisen in the tongue and oral cavity.[60,61] A few of these lesions are congenital and the lesions are associated with Mafucci syndrome (multiple enchondromas and vascular tumors).[61] Recurrences are common. Metastases have been reported to regional lymph nodes, but no systemic metastases are recorded.

Pathologic Features

These lesions are found in the subcutaneous tissue and dermis (or mucosa) and are highly infiltrative (Fig. 17.21, e-Figs. 17.95 and 17.96). They consist of a complex admixture of benign-appearing well-formed vessels, areas that resemble spindle cell hemangioma, areas that appear similar to retiform hemangioendothelioma with long vessels and prominent lymphocytes, and areas with epithelioid endothelial cells in a chondroid background (similar to epithelioid hemangioendothelioma). Some display zones of vacuolated cells. Mitotic activity is sparse in these neoplasms.

Ancillary Investigations

The endothelial cells in these lesions express CD34, CD31, and factor VIII–related antigen but not podoplanin (D2-40).[61]

KAPOSI SARCOMA

Clinical Features

Epidemiologic Subtypes of KS. In the "classic" or European form of the disease, KS typically affects male patients of Mediterranean descent or Ashkenazi Jewish extraction between the ages of 50 and 80. Patients typically survive an average of 10 to 15 years following their initial diagnosis and commonly die of an unrelated cause. Secondary malignancies have been reported in over a third of the patients[62] with approximately half of these tumors being of hematopoietic/lymphoreticular derivation (i.e., leukemia, lymphoma, and multiple myeloma). Cutaneous lesions usually appear in the distal lower extremities and evolve in stages, consisting initially of purple patches, followed by plaques and nodules. Over time, the lesions extend proximally, gradually coalesce, and may ulcerate. Some foci may regress while others progress. Upper extremity and internal involvement may develop although the latter is often clinically silent.

The African or "endemic" form of KS occurs in adults or children. In adults, the median age at presentation is in the fourth decade. Over ninety percent are in males. The majority have a clinically benign, nodular form of the disease although both florid and aggressive variants also occur. Affected children have a male to female ratio of 3:1 and a mean age at presentation of three. They typically exhibit lymph node involvement without cutaneous manifestations and the disease is fulminant and fatal within 2 or 3 years. Some patients who are uninfected with the HIV virus seem to have an endemic form of KS; this presumably relates to HHV-8 serotypes in various endemic areas.[63]

A third epidemiologic subgroup at risk for KS is composed of individuals (primarily transplant patients) receiving potent, high-dose, or long-term immunosuppressive therapy. The overall risk to these patients is relatively low. KS is estimated to account about 5% of all malignancies in the transplant population.[64] The mean interval to onset after transplantation is 16.5 months.[65] Many of these individuals are also of Jewish or Mediterranean descent. However, females comprise a higher percentage of those affected; the male to female ratio ranges from 2 to 3:1.[64] Although KS may assume a chronic or aggressive course in these patients, regression frequently follows discontinuation of the immunosuppressive treatment. Patients receiving immunosuppressive agents for various other collagen vascular and skin disorders are also included in this category.

"Epidemic" or AIDS-related KS occurs in HIV-positive individuals. The clinical definition for AIDS-KS is lymphadenopathic and/or oral, genital, gastrointestinal, pulmonary, or disseminated cutaneous KS. These criteria distinguish "endemic" and "epidemic" (i.e., HIV seropositive) KS with 91% and 95% sensitivity and specificity, respectively.[66] The presence of oral KS (e-Fig. 17.97) is particularly helpful, having a sensitivity of 73% and a predictive value of 99% for HIV seropositivity.[66] In this group, KS frequently assumes an aggressive course. Areas prone to KS in the adult AIDS population include the oral cavity, especially the hard palate, the tip of the nose, behind the ears, and the trunk, penis, legs, and feet. Lesions more often involve the upper half of the body than in classic KS. Postmortem studies have demonstrated a high incidence of concurrent disease in lymph nodes, the gastrointestinal tract, and lungs. Pediatric cases of AIDS-KS have a proclivity for lymphadenopathic disease. HHV-8 has been found in all forms of KS previously mentioned as well as in primary effusion lymphomas, in multicentric Castleman disease (MCD), and in a plasmablastic lymphoma variant associated with MCD, sometimes all in the same person.[67] Various chemotherapeutic agents and targeted therapies have been offered for the subset (AIDS-related lesions) that is more aggressive.

Histologic Features

There are no well-defined morphologic or immunohistochemical differences between the clinical forms of KS. In the early, patch stage of KS (e-Fig. 17.98), changes predominate in the upper half of the reticular dermis, consisting of a proliferation of capillaries around preexisting dermal vessels and adnexa. These newly formed vessels often have a collapsed, jagged, or angulated appearance, but on occasion, they may be somewhat ectatic. The endothelial lining is flattened or slightly plump. Some endothelial cells may contain apoptotic nuclei. The protrusion of small proliferating capillary channels into the vascular lumen of a larger, pre,-existing dermal vessel, the "promontory" sign (e-Fig. 17.99), also has diagnostic importance. Bland-appearing spindled cells may be associated with the neovasculature, although at this stage, they tend to be a minor component. A variable inflammatory infiltrate, dominated by lymphocytes, with or without plasma cells, is frequently present. Extravasated erythrocytes, hemosiderin deposition, and intracytoplasmic PAS-positive, diastase-resistant, hyaline globules may or may not be noted. As the process progresses to involve the full thickness of the dermis, it becomes palpable and is clinically recognized as a plaque.

In the plaque stage (e-Figs. 17.100 and 17.101), the spindled component of KS becomes more prominent. These cells are dispersed among the dermal collagen bundles and are also noted in and around the network of new vessels. They form slit-like spaces, which frequently contain red blood cells. Plasma cells and hemosiderin deposits are also usually apparent. Eosinophilic hyaline globules (e-Fig. 17.102), 1 to 7 μm in size, are commonly present and form grape-like agglomerations that are predominantly intracellular. They are various stages of erythrophagolysosomes.

Nodular Kaposi lesions represent further development and organization beyond the plaque stage (Fig. 17.22, e-Figs. 17.103 and 17.104). On gross examination, cutaneous lesions have a well-circumscribed, violaceous, dome-shaped, or polypoid appearance. The spindle cell population often dominates, forming fascicles and sheets. Extravasated erythrocytes, siderophages, hyaline globules, and a peripheral lymphoplasmacytic infiltrate are typically present. Single cell necrosis is also seen.

Lymphangioma-like KS has also been described (e-Fig. 17.105). Its clinical presentation does not appear to vary substantially from more typical cases. However, its histology differs by featuring a predominance of ectatic lymphatic-like channels that permeate the dermis. Associated inflammation is minimal but hemosiderin deposition is seen. A minor, ill-defined, spindle cell component may be present, but it is not usually intermingled with the vascular clefts as in more typical Kaposi lesions.

KS may involve lymph nodes (e-Fig. 17.106), either as an initial, sometimes isolated, manifestation, or as a later component of disseminated disease. Like cutaneous examples, it is readily recognized when the disease is fully established but is difficult to characterize in its initial stages. Early changes include subcapsular sinus ectasia and intrasinusoidal vascular proliferation.

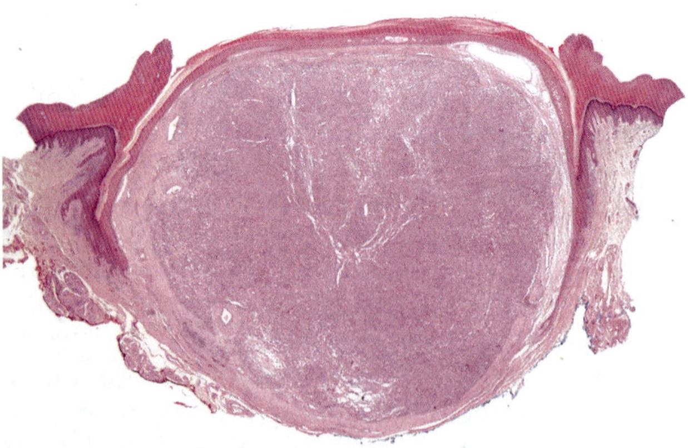

FIGURE 17.22 **Nodular Kaposi Sarcoma.** This spindle cell lesion is arranged in a lobular configuration like a pyogenic granuloma, even displaying an epidermal collarette.

Ancillary Investigations

KS can be regarded as a lesion of lymphatic endothelial cells, since it expresses CD34, CD31, Fli-1, VEGFR-3, and podoplanin (D2-40). Virtually all examples show nuclear labeling with HHV-8 antibodies (Fig. 17.23, e-Fig. 17.107).

SUPERFICIAL ANGIOSARCOMA (SEE ALSO CHAPTER 18; DEEP VASCULAR TUMORS)

In this book, angiosarcoma is used in a generic sense to encompass fully malignant neoplasms of endothelial derivation whether originating from lymphatics (lymphangiosarcoma) or blood vessels (hemangiosarcoma). This seem justifiable for the following reasons: (a) it can be difficult or impossible to make a definitive statement with regard to the precise origin of a malignant endothelial tumor; (b) the morphologic, immunohistochemical, and ultrastructural features of tumors previously classified as lymphangiosarcoma or hemangiosarcoma overlap; and (c) there appears to be little if any therapeutic or prognostic relevance to the distinction.

Angiosarcoma is a rare tumor, comprising <1% of all sarcomas. It can develop in practically any site, but there is a particularly strong predilection for the skin and subcutis. In this superficial location, angiosarcoma occurs in three distinct clinical settings: (a) the face and scalp of the elderly, (b) the extremities of patients with chronic lymphedema, and (c) at sites previously subjected to radiation therapy. Other key primary sites for angiosarcoma are the breast parenchyma, liver, deep soft tissue, skeleton,

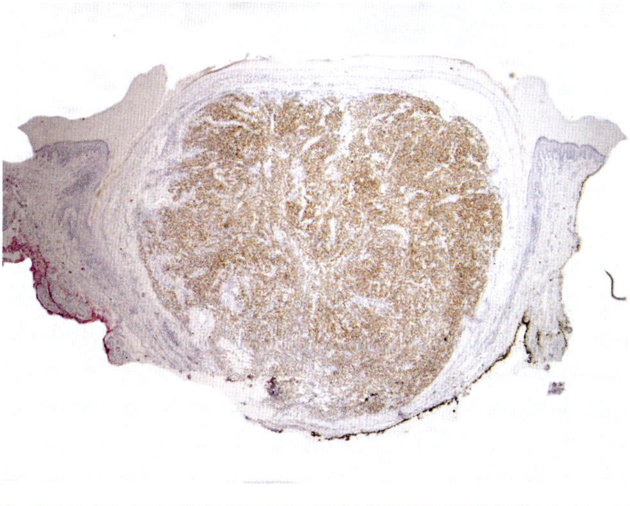

FIGURE 17.23 **Nodular Kaposi Sarcoma, HHV-8 Immunolabeling.** Regardless of the stage of the lesion or its epidemiologic characteristics, KS essentially always shows nuclear expression of HHV-8 on immunohistochemistry.

heart, and spleen. There are reports of this tumor developing in association with foreign bodies, and defunctionalized arteriovenous fistulae in transplant recipients, and an increased frequency has been reported in neurofibromatosis[68] where the tumor may occur either as an independent finding or in association with benign or malignant peripheral nerve sheath tumors. Angiosarcomas may also arise in association with various skin diseases.[69]

Arsenical compounds (i.e., Fowler solution, arsenical insecticides), vinyl chloride, and thorium dioxide (Thorotrast) exposure have been implicated in the development of approximately one fourth of angiosarcomas arising in the liver but not usually in other sites.

Clinical Features, Angiosarcoma of the Face and Scalp

The most common location for angiosarcoma is the scalp and midfacial region (e-Fig. 17.108). The vast majority of affected individuals are Caucasian and in their seventh or eighth decade of life. The disease is uncommon under the age of 50. The neoplasms may be well marginated or ill-defined, solitary or multifocal and flat, elevated, nodular, or cystic. Consistency varies from firm and solid to soft and fluctuant or spongy. The majority of tumors are red or bluish-purplish. However, a few edematous examples may retain normal skin coloration. The early stage of superficial angiosarcomas can be misinterpreted as a bruise (e-Fig. 17.109). Large or longstanding lesions frequently ulcerate and may become secondarily infected.

In one large series, the 5-year survival rate was 12%, with half of the patients dying within 15 months of presentation,[70] but in a more recent series, the 5-year survival was about 50% for head and neck angiosarcomas.[71] Tumors <5 cm in diameter tend to recur and metastasize less frequently than larger ones, and a prominent lymphoid reaction may also be associated with a better prognosis. Age >70 years, tumor necrosis, and epithelioid features have also been associated with an adverse outcome in head and neck lesions. Cervical lymph nodes and lungs are the most frequent metastatic sites, followed in frequency by the liver, spleen, skeleton, kidneys, and heart. The best chance for cure seems to entail radical surgical removal of the primary tumor, supplemented with wide-field electron beam radiotherapy and, in selected instances, regional lymph node clearance.

Clinical Features, Lymphedema-associated Angiosarcoma

Patients treated for breast carcinoma by radical mastectomy with or without supplemental irradiation can develop (lymph) angiosarcoma in the ipsilateral extremity following chronic postoperative edema (Stewart-Treves syndrome). This is rare, occurring in < 1% of postmastectomy patients surviving at least 5 years, and its incidence is decreasing, given the current, more conservative surgical approach to breast carcinoma. Chronic lymphedema is considered the predominant factor in the development of these tumors.

The average interval from the onset of postmastectomy lymphedema to the appearance of angiosarcoma is approximately 9 years. Gross examination typically reveals pitting, indurated, or "pachydermatous" skin with red or bluish-purple macular, papular, polypoid, or fungating lesions. The tumors may be either solitary or multicentric. Sometimes, a dominant mass with multiple satellite lesions is noted.

Similar neoplasms are reported following persistent lymphedema associated with other postoperative settings. Angiosarcoma may also develop in association with chronic congenital, posttraumatic, idiopathic, postirradiation, and filariasis-associated lymphedema. Examples arising in the setting of chronic congenital, and idiopathic, and filariasis lymphedema often have a later onset (>20 years), and the affected individuals appear to have a somewhat longer mean survival than patients with postmastectomy lymphedema-associated tumors.

Optimal management is generally considered to be early, radical, and ablative surgery in the form of limb, forequarter, or hindquarter amputation.

Clinical Features, Postirradiation Angiosarcoma

Postirradiation angiosarcomas have a predilection for the skin and subcutis, although they occasionally arise in more deep-seated sites. The usual antecedent malignancies are breast or gynecologic carcinomas, but 29% arise following radiotherapy for a benign disorder (i.e., eczema, sinusitis, hemangiomas, or lymphangiomas).[72] The mean interval to angiosarcoma is 11 years (range, 2.5–25 years) following treatment for a malignancy, contrasted with 22 years (range, 4–52 years) for benign antecedent conditions (which usually received less irradiation).

Clinical Features, Angiosarcoma of the Breast Parenchyma

Primary, noniatrogenic angiosarcomas of the breast parenchyma occur in a wide age range and commonly present as a painless, soft mass with bluish-red, or black discoloration of the overlying skin (e-Fig. 17.110). The outcome is poor with a mean interval to death of 22 months and a 3-year disease-free survival rate of <15%. However, small well-differentiated tumors fare better.

Optimal management is generally considered to be complete surgical excision with a wide resection margin as tumors of this type typically invade well beyond their grossly apparent margin.

Pathologic Features

Angiosarcoma has a broad morphologic spectrum (Figs. 17.24, e-Figs. 17.88–17.90, 17.111–17.113, Fig. 18.8, e-Figs. 18.46–18.61). At one extreme, the tumor may consist entirely of well-developed hemangioma or lymphangioma-like vascular spaces (angiomatous or collagen dissection pattern), in which the only clues of malignancy are the interanastomosing and infiltrative nature of the process, the presence of mild nuclear hyperchromasia and occasional crowding or piling up of the endothelium, sometimes forming small papillations. The opposite end of the spectrum includes both a spindle cell pattern reminiscent of fibrosarcoma or KS and an "undifferentiated"

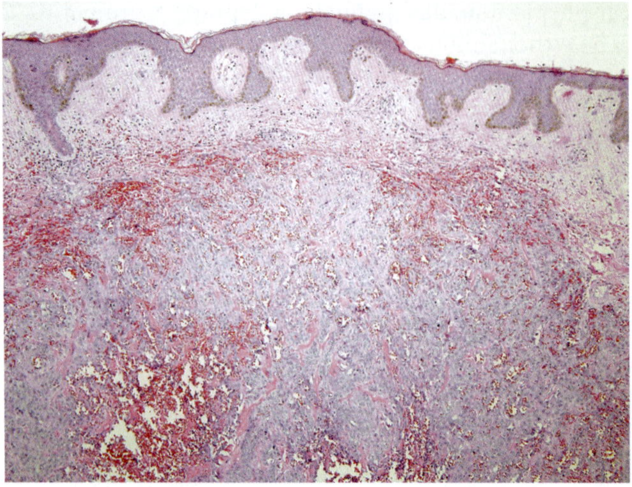

FIGURE 17.24 **Angiosarcoma.** This high-grade angiosarcoma features epithelioid endothelial cells; such cases often require immunolabeling to confirm the impression of endothelial differentiation.

pattern that consists of plump epithelioid neoplastic cells with prominent nucleoli and diffuse sheet-like growth, suggestive of carcinoma or melanoma. A high index of suspicion, knowledge of the clinical findings, and thorough tumor sampling are essential to establish the correct diagnosis at these morphologic extremes. Since angiosarcomas have variable morphology, adequate sampling is needed to find vasoformative architecture and cytologically malignant features. Where the histologic grade has been shown to have prognostic significance, as in the breast, sampling is also critical for appropriate management. When well-developed vessels are not apparent, the presence of cytoplasmic vacuolization consistent with early lumen development and a red blood cell or hemosiderin-rich milieu may serve as important clues to endothelial differentiation.

Ancillary Investigations

Angiosarcomas react with markers of endothelial differentiation such as FVIII-related antigen, CD31, UEA-1, FKBP12, podoplanin (D2-40), and Fli-1. CD31 is a sensitive marker of endothelial differentiation but not a wholly specific one; it is important to recognize that histiocytes, as well as plasma cells, can express CD31, to avoid overdiagnosis of angiosarcoma. Cytokeratins can also be expressed, especially in epithelioid angiosarcoma, notably CK8 and CK18 (~50%), and less commonly showed CK7 and CK19; they are negative for CK14 and with the antibody 34betaE12. Nonepithelioid angiosarcomas less commonly show keratin expression with CK7, CK8, and CK18 being positive in 20% of cases, and CK14 and CK19 in none.[73] Epithelial membrane antigen (EMA) is reported in 25% of epithelioid angiosarcomas and 35% of nonepithelioid angiosarcomas.[73] Over half of angiosarcomas express CD117 (c-kit) but lack *C-KIT* mutations.[74]

NONENDOTHELIAL LESIONS THAT CAN MIMIC VASCULAR TUMORS

A number of non-endothelial neoplasms, can be misdiagnosed as vascular tumors principally because of hemorrhage.

ANGIOMATOID FIBROUS HISTIOCYTOMA

This tumor was originally described as angiomatoid malignant fibrous histiocytoma (MFH) and considered to be part of the MFH family.[75,76] The term "malignant" was removed from its name in the 2002 WHO Classification, and the entity was recategorized as an intermediate (rarely metastasizing) tumor of uncertain differentiation.[43] It has a distinctive morphology and immunophenotype that is unrelated to histiocytic differentiation, and is now known to be characterized by specific chromosomal translocations.[77]

Clinical Features

Angiomatoid fibrous histiocytoma (AFH) occurs at any age from infancy to over 70 years, but is most common in the first 2 decades, and is slightly more frequent in females. The favored sites are the deep dermis/subcutis (or rarely skeletal muscle) of proximal limb girdle (especially upper limb), trunk, and head and neck, including sites of normal lymphoid tissue such as axilla, antecubital fossa, and groin. Some cases are associated with systemic clinical manifestations including fever and anemia. Most are <4 cm in maximum dimension, though examples have been reported exceeding 12 cm. Up to 15% recur, and wide local excision is appropriate management. Fewer than 3% have been reported to metastasize, usually to regional lymph nodes and exceptionally to lung and brain.[75,78] Deep location, origin in head and neck region, and infiltrating histologic margins are risk factors for recurrence.[75]

Pathologic Features

This tumor is circumscribed (or rarely infiltrative) and the cut surface can be solid or show blood-filled cystic spaces. It is composed of multinodular sheets of ovoid cells with mostly uniform vesicular nuclei, scanty cytoplasm, and low mitotic index (e-Figs. 17.114–17.116). Some cases show focal nuclear pleomorphism and multinucleated giant cells are occasionally seen. The amount of hemorrhage is variable and absent from some examples; others have extensive interstitial hemorrhage with large cysts that are lined by tumor cells, not endothelium. The tumor is characteristically surrounded by a variable fibrous and lymphoid cuff (Fig. 17.25), which can manifest germinal centre formation and adjacent plasmacytic proliferation and be misinterpreted as a lymph node with metastatic tumor.

Ancillary Investigations

About 60% of AFH express desmin, either focally or diffusely (e-Fig. 17.116), and sometimes calponin and h-caldesmon but SMA and myogenin are negative. Other positive markers include EMA, CD99, and CD68. The lymphoid

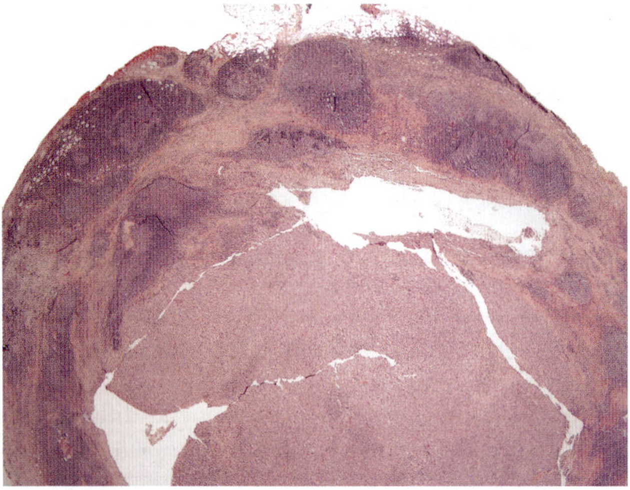

FIGURE 17.25 **Angiomatoid (Malignant) Fibrous Histiocytoma.** This example has a prominent lymphoid cuff and is composed of uniform cells. This is not a vascular tumor, but these lesions often have blood-filled cystic spaces (that lack an endothelial lining).

cuff comprises a mixture of B and T cells, and the plasma cells are polyclonal. Electron microscopy has not revealed specific differentiation in the lesional cells, with features suggestive of endothelial, epithelial, and myoid differentiation being variously described. Genetically, AFH is characterized by several chromosomal rearrangements. The most common is t(2;22)(q33;q12), associated with *EWSR1-CREB1*; t(12;22)(q13;q12), resulting in *EWSR1-ATF1* (which can have four chimeric forms), and t(12;16)(q13;p11) leading to *FUS-ATF1* fusion gene, have also been described. The first two translocations are of special interest because they are also found in clear cell sarcoma of GI tract and soft tissues, respectively. The reasons for the different phenotypes in tumors with the same genotype are not known. High transcript levels for TFE3 have also been found in AFH.

ANEURYSMAL FIBROUS HISTIOCYTOMA

This is an uncommon variant of cutaneous fibrous histiocytoma characterized by intralesional hemorrhage. This arises on the extremities or trunk, usually in adults, and can grow rapidly raising the clinical suspicion of malignancy.[79]

Pathologic Features

This has the usual features of fibrous histiocytoma with epidermal hyperplasia (Fig. 17.26), a dermal aggregate of short spindle cells with focal storiform pattern, peripheral thickened collagen bundles, and minimal extension into subcutis (e-Figs. 17.117–17.121). In addition, there are variably sized cystic spaces filled with blood but lacking endothelial lining cells, abundant hemosiderin often in macrophages, and multinucleated giant cells. A focal

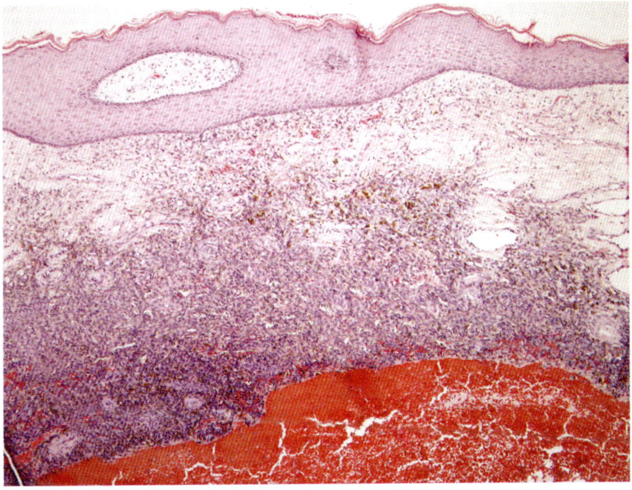

FIGURE 17.26 **Aneurysmal Fibrous Histiocytoma.** This is not a vascular tumor but simply a fibrous histiocytoma (dermatofibroma) with hemorrhage. There is overlying epidermal hyperplasia and collagen trapping at the interface of the lesion with the dermis.

hemangiopericytomatous pattern and areas of cellular fibrous histiocytoma are sometimes seen. Angiosarcoma, Kaposi sarcoma, and melanoma, which this lesion can clinically simulate, are readily excluded with immunohistochemistry should there be morphologic doubt. Partly because of the terminology, aneurysmal fibrous histiocytoma can be confused with AFH, which also has cystic intralesional hemorrhage. The latter, however, is located in subcutis, has a fibrous and inflammatory cuff or pseudocapsule, often displays immunoreactivity for desmin, and has specific translocations.

Ancillary Investigations

The lesions cells lack CD34, CD31, HHV-8, S100 protein, and desmin. A Perls stain demonstrates abundant hemosiderin pigment.

MULTINUCLEATE CELL ANGIOHISTIOCYTOMA

Clinical Features

Multinucleate cell angiohistiocytoma is an infrequent disorder seen predominantly in acral regions in middle-aged to elderly women, although rare head and neck lesions and lesions in men have been reported.[80] It presents clinically as asymptomatic discrete grouped violaceous erythematous papules, sometimes clinically mimicking KS, with a tendency to confluence. Local excision has been used to treat this benign process.

Pathologic Features

The lesions consist of a proliferation of capillaries and small venules at the level of the subpapillary plexus and the mid-dermis, in association with angulated multinucleate cells (e-Figs. 17.122 and 17.123).

Ancillary Investigations

The vessels in these lesions express CD34 and CD31 but not podoplanin (D2-40). The multinucleate cells variably express CD68 and FXIIIa.

REFERENCES

1. Stoler MH, Bonfiglio TA, Steigbigel RT, et al. An atypical subcutaneous infection associated with acquired immune deficiency syndrome. *Am J Clin Pathol.* 1983;80:714–718.
2. Nutter FB, Dubey JP, Levine JF, et al. Seroprevalences of antibodies against *Bartonella henselae* and *Toxoplasma gondii* and fecal shedding of Cryptosporidium spp, Giardia spp, and Toxocara cati in feral and pet domestic cats. *J Am Vet Med Assoc.* 2004;225:1394–1398.
3. Garcia FU, Wojta J, Broadley KN, et al. *Bartonella bacilliformis* stimulates endothelial cells in vitro and is angiogenic in vivo. *Am J Pathol.* 1990;136:1125–1135.
4. O'Connor SP, Dorsch M, Steigerwalt AG, et al. 16S rRNA sequences of *Bartonella bacilliformis* and cat scratch disease bacillus reveal phylogenetic relationships with the alpha-2 subgroup of the class Proteobacteria. *J Clin Microbiol.* 1991;29:2144–2150.
5. Arias-Stella J, Lieberman PH, Erlandson RA, et al. Histology, immunohistochemistry, and ultrastructure of the verruga in Carrion's disease. *Am J Surg Pathol.* 1986;10:595–610.
6. Arias-Stella J, Lieberman PH, Garcia-Caceres U, et al. Verruga peruana mimicking malignant neoplasms. *Am J Dermatopathol.* 1987;9:279–291.
7. Hashimoto H, Daimaru Y, Enjoji M. Intravascular papillary endothelial hyperplasia. A clinicopathologic study of 91 cases. *Am J Dermatopathol.* 1983;5:539–546.
8. Fetsch JF, Weiss SW. Observations concerning the pathogenesis of epithelioid hemangioma (angiolymphoid hyperplasia). *Mod Pathol.* 1991;4:449–455.
9. Olsen TG, Helwig EB. Angiolymphoid hyperplasia with eosinophilia. A clinicopathologic study of 116 patients. *J Am Acad Dermatol.* 1985;12:781–796.
10. Rosai J. Angiolymphoid hyperplasia with eosinophilia of the skin. Its nosological position in the spectrum of histiocytoid hemangioma. *Am J Dermatopathol.* 1982;4:175–184.
11. Dyduch G, Okon K, Mierzynski W. Benign vascular proliferations–an immunohistochemical and comparative study. *Pol J Pathol.* 2004;55:59–64.
12. Chan JK, Hui PK, Ng CS, et al. Epithelioid haemangioma (angiolymphoid hyperplasia with eosinophilia) and Kimura's disease in Chinese. *Histopathology.* 1989;15:557–574.
13. Amir J, Metzker A, Krikler R, et al. Strawberry hemangioma in preterm infants. *Pediatr Dermatol.* 1986;3:331–332.
14. Burns AJ, Kaplan LC, Mulliken JB. Is there an association between hemangioma and syndromes with dysmorphic features? *Pediatrics.* 1991;88:1257–1267.
15. Metry D, Heyer G, Hess C, et al. Consensus statement on diagnostic criteria for PHACE syndrome. *Pediatrics.* 2009;124:1447–1456.
16. Sachatello CR, McSwain B. Regression of cutaneous capillary hemangioma. *Am J Surg.* 1968;116:113–114.
17. Marler JJ, Mulliken JB. Current management of hemangiomas and vascular malformations. *Clin Plast Surg.* 2005;32:99–116, ix.
18. Leon-Villapalos J, Wolfe K, Kangesu L. GLUT-1: an extra diagnostic tool to differentiate between haemangiomas and vascular malformations. *Br J Plast Surg.* 2005;58:348–352.
19. Lyons LL, North PE, Mac-Moune Lai F, et al. Kaposiform hemangioendothelioma: a study of 33 cases emphasizing its pathologic, immunophenotypic, and biologic uniqueness from juvenile hemangioma. *Am J Surg Pathol.* 2004;28:559–568.
20. North PE, Waner M, Mizeracki A, et al. GLUT1: a newly discovered immunohistochemical marker for juvenile hemangiomas. *Hum Pathol.* 2000;31:11–22.

21. Ahrens WA, Ridenour RV, III, Caron BL, et al. GLUT-1 expression in mesenchymal tumors: an immunohistochemical study of 247 soft tissue and bone neoplasms. *Hum Pathol.* 2008;39:1519–1526.
22. Kahn HJ, Bailey D, Marks A. Monoclonal antibody D2-40, a new marker of lymphatic endothelium, reacts with Kaposi's sarcoma and a subset of angiosarcomas. *Mod Pathol.* 2002;15:434–440.
23. Mills SE, Cooper PH, Fechner RE. Lobular capillary hemangioma: the underlying lesion of pyogenic granuloma. A study of 73 cases from the oral and nasal mucous membranes. *Am J Surg Pathol.* 1980;4:470–479.
24. Nichols GE, Gaffey MJ, Mills SE, et al. Lobular capillary hemangioma. An immunohistochemical study including steroid hormone receptor status. *Am J Clin Pathol.* 1992;97:770–775.
25. Cooper PH, McAllister HA, Helwig EB. Intravenous pyogenic granuloma. A study of 18 cases. *Am J Surg Pathol.* 1979;3:221–228.
26. Esterly NB. Cutaneous hemangiomas, vascular stains and associated syndromes. *Curr Probl Pediatr.* 1987;17:1–69.
27. Fanburg JC, Meis-Kindblom JM, Rosenberg AE. Multiple enchondromas associated with spindle-cell hemangioendotheliomas. An overlooked variant of Maffucci's syndrome. *Am J Surg Pathol.* 1995;19:1029–1038.
28. Fine RM, Derbes VJ, Clark WH Jr. Blue rubber bleb nevus. *Arch Dermatol.* 1961;84:802–805.
29. Calonje E, Fletcher CD. Sinusoidal hemangioma. A distinctive benign vascular neoplasm within the group of cavernous hemangiomas. *Am J Surg Pathol.* 1991;15:1130–1135.
30. Connelly MG, Winkelmann RK. Acral arteriovenous tumor. A clinicopathologic review. *Am J Surg Pathol.* 1985;9:15–21.
31. Hunt SJ, Santa Cruz DJ, Barr RJ. Microvenular hemangioma. *J Cutan Pathol.* 1991;18:235–240.
32. Hudnall SD, Chen T, Brown K, et al. Human herpesvirus-8-positive microvenular hemangioma in POEMS syndrome. *Arch Pathol Lab Med.* 2003;127:1034–1036.
33. Chan JK, Fletcher CD, Hicklin GA, et al. Glomeruloid hemangioma. A distinctive cutaneous lesion of multicentric Castleman's disease associated with POEMS syndrome. *Am J Surg Pathol.* 1990;14:1036–1046.
34. Tohda S, Murakami N, Nara N. Human herpesvirus 8 DNA in HIV-negative Japanese patients with multicentric Castleman's disease and related diseases. *Int J Mol Med.* 2001;8:549–551.
35. Santa Cruz DJ, Aronberg J. Targetoid hemosiderotic hemangioma. *J Am Acad Dermatol.* 1988;19:550–558.
36. Mentzel T, Partanen TA, Kutzner H. Hobnail hemangioma ("targetoid hemosiderotic hemangioma"): clinicopathologic and immunohistochemical analysis of 62 cases. *J Cutan Pathol.* 1999;26:279–286.
37. Guillou L, Fletcher CD. Benign lymphangioendothelioma (acquired progressive lymphangioma): a lesion not to be confused with well-differentiated angiosarcoma and patch stage Kaposi's sarcoma: clinicopathologic analysis of a series. *Am J Surg Pathol.* 2000;24:1047–1057.
38. Sangueza OP, Walsh SN, Sheehan DJ, et al. Cutaneous epithelioid angiomatous nodule: a case series and proposed classification. *Am J Dermatopathol.* 2008;30:16–20.
39. Brenn T, Fletcher CD. Cutaneous epithelioid angiomatous nodule: a distinct lesion in the morphologic spectrum of epithelioid vascular tumors. *Am J Dermatopathol.* 2004;26:14–21.
40. Farshid G, Weiss SW. Massive localized lymphedema in the morbidly obese: a histologically distinct reactive lesion simulating liposarcoma. *Am J Surg Pathol.* 1998;22:1277–1283.

41. Manduch M, Oliveira AM, Nascimento AG, et al. Massive localised lymphoedema: a clinicopathological study of 22 cases and review of the literature. *J Clin Pathol.* 2009;62:808–811.

42. Weiss SW, Enzinger FM. Spindle cell hemangioendothelioma. A low-grade angiosarcoma resembling a cavernous hemangioma and Kaposi's sarcoma. *Am J Surg Pathol.* 1986;10:521–530.

43. Fletcher C, Unni K, Mertens FE. *World Health Organization Classification of Tumours. Pathology and Genetics of Tumours of Soft Tissue and Bone.* Lyon: IACR Press, 2002.

44. Fletcher CD. The non-neoplastic nature of spindle cell hemangioendothelioma. *Am J Clin Pathol.* 1992;98:545–546.

45. Sato H, Takahashi T, Fujisawa Y, et al. Interleukin-8 and CXCR2 expression in spindle cell haemangioendothelioma. *J Eur Acad Dermatol Venereol.* 2008;22:638–640.

46. Fanburg-Smith JC, Michal M, Partanen TA, et al. Papillary intralymphatic angioendothelioma (PILA): a report of twelve cases of a distinctive vascular tumor with phenotypic features of lymphatic vessels. *Am J Surg Pathol.* 1999;23:1004–1010.

47. Dabska M. Malignant endovascular papillary angioendothelioma of the skin in childhood. Clinicopathologic study of 6 cases. *Cancer.* 1969;24:503–510.

48. Argani P, Athanasian E. Malignant endovascular papillary angioendothelioma (Dabska tumor) arising within a deep intramuscular hemangioma. *Arch Pathol Lab Med.* 1997;121:992–995.

49. Parsons A, Sheehan DJ, Sangueza OP. Retiform hemangioendotheliomas usually do not express D2-40 and VEGFR-3. *Am J Dermatopathol.* 2008;30:31–33.

50. Zukerberg LR, Nickoloff BJ, Weiss SW. Kaposiform hemangioendothelioma of infancy and childhood. An aggressive neoplasm associated with Kasabach-Merritt syndrome and lymphangiomatosis. *Am J Surg Pathol.* 1993;17:321–328.

51. Mentzel T, Mazzoleni G, Dei Tos AP, et al. Kaposiform hemangioendothelioma in adults. Clinicopathologic and immunohistochemical analysis of three cases. *Am J Clin Pathol.* 1997;108:450–455.

52. Mac-Moune Lai F, To KF, Choi PC, et al. Kaposiform hemangioendothelioma: five patients with cutaneous lesion and long follow-up. *Mod Pathol.* 2001;14:1087–1092.

53. Arai E, Kuramochi A, Tsuchida T, et al. Usefulness of D2-40 immunohistochemistry for differentiation between kaposiform hemangioendothelioma and tufted angioma. *J Cutan Pathol.* 2006;33:492–497.

54. Gengler C, Coindre JM, Leroux A, et al. Vascular proliferations of the skin after radiation therapy for breast cancer: clinicopathologic analysis of a series in favor of a benign process: a study from the French Sarcoma Group. *Cancer.* 2007;109:1584–1598.

55. Brenn T, Fletcher CD. Radiation-associated cutaneous atypical vascular lesions and angiosarcoma: clinicopathologic analysis of 42 cases. *Am J Surg Pathol.* 2005;29:983–996.

56. Patton KT, Deyrup AT, Weiss SW. Atypical vascular lesions after surgery and radiation of the breast: a clinicopathologic study of 32 cases analyzing histologic heterogeneity and association with angiosarcoma. *Am J Surg Pathol.* 2008;32:943–950.

57. Calonje E, Fletcher CD, Wilson-Jones E, et al. Retiform hemangioendothelioma. A distinctive form of low-grade angiosarcoma delineated in a series of 15 cases. *Am J Surg Pathol.* 1994;18:115–125.

58. Duke D, Dvorak A, Harris TJ, et al. Multiple retiform hemangioendotheliomas. A low-grade angiosarcoma. *Am J Dermatopathol.* 1996;18:606–610.

59. Schommer M, Herbst RA, Brodersen JP, et al. Retiform hemangioendothelioma: another tumor associated with human herpesvirus type 8? *J Am Acad Dermatol.* 2000;42:290–292.

60. Nayler SJ, Rubin BP, Calonje E, et al. Composite hemangioendothelioma: a complex, low-grade vascular lesion mimicking angiosarcoma. *Am J Surg Pathol.* 2000;24:352–361.

61. Fukunaga M, Suzuki K, Saegusa N, et al. Composite hemangioendothelioma: report of 5 cases including one with associated Maffucci syndrome. *Am J Surg Pathol.* 2007;31:1567–1572.
62. Safai B, Mike V, Giraldo G, et al. Association of Kaposi's sarcoma with second primary malignancies: possible etiopathogenic implications. *Cancer.* 1980;45:1472–1479.
63. Mosam A, Aboobaker J, Shaik F. Kaposi's sarcoma in sub-Saharan Africa: a current perspective. *Curr Opin Infect Dis.* 2009;23:119–123.
64. Penn I. Kaposi's sarcoma in transplant recipients. *Transplantation.* 1997;64:669–673.
65. Penn I. Kaposi's sarcoma in immunosuppressed patients. *J Clin Lab Immunol.* 1983;12:1–10.
66. Desmond-Hellmann SD, Mbidde EK, Kizito A, et al. The value of a clinical definition for epidemic KS in predicting HIV seropositivity in Africa. *J Acquir Immune Defic Syndr.* 1991;4:647–651.
67. Horenstein MG, Moontasri NJ, Cesarman E. The pathobiology of Kaposi's sarcoma: advances since the onset of the AIDS epidemic. *J Cutan Pathol.* 2008;35(suppl 2): 40–44.
68. Mentzel T, Katenkamp D. Intraneural angiosarcoma and angiosarcoma arising in benign and malignant peripheral nerve sheath tumours: clinicopathological and immunohistochemical analysis of four cases. *Histopathology.* 1999;35:114–120.
69. Hudson CP, Hanno R, Callen JP. Cutaneous angiosarcoma in a site of healed herpes zoster. *Int J Dermatol.* 1984;23:404–407.
70. Holden CA, Spittle MF, Jones EW. Angiosarcoma of the face and scalp, prognosis and treatment. *Cancer.* 1987;59:1046–1057.
71. Deyrup AT, McKenney JK, Tighiouart M, et al. Sporadic cutaneous angiosarcomas: a proposal for risk stratification based on 69 cases. *Am J Surg Pathol.* 2008;32:72–77.
72. Edeiken S, Russo DP, Knecht J, et al. Angiosarcoma after tylectomy and radiation therapy for carcinoma of the breast. *Cancer.* 1992;70:644–647.
73. Miettinen M, Fetsch JF. Distribution of keratins in normal endothelial cells and a spectrum of vascular tumors: implications in tumor diagnosis. *Hum Pathol.* 2000;31:1062–1067.
74. Miettinen M, Sarlomo-Rikala M, Lasota J. KIT expression in angiosarcomas and fetal endothelial cells: lack of mutations of exon 11 and exon 17 of C-kit. *Mod Pathol.* 2000;13:536–541.
75. Costa MJ, Weiss SW. Angiomatoid malignant fibrous histiocytoma. A follow-up study of 108 cases with evaluation of possible histologic predictors of outcome. *Am J Surg Pathol.* 1990;14:1126–1132.
76. Enzinger FM. Angiomatoid malignant fibrous histiocytoma: a distinct fibrohistiocytic tumor of children and young adults simulating a vascular neoplasm. *Cancer.* 1979;44:2147–2157.
77. Thway K. Angiomatoid fibrous histiocytoma: a review with recent genetic findings. *Arch Pathol Lab Med.* 2008;132:273–277.
78. Fanburg-Smith JC, Miettinen M. Angiomatoid "malignant" fibrous histiocytoma: a clinicopathologic study of 158 cases and further exploration of the myoid phenotype. *Hum Pathol.* 1999;30:1336–1343.
79. Calonje E, Fletcher CD. Aneurysmal benign fibrous histiocytoma: clinicopathological analysis of 40 cases of a tumour frequently misdiagnosed as a vascular neoplasm. *Histopathology.* 1995;26:323–331.
80. Perez LP, Zulaica A, Rodriguez L, et al. Multinucleate cell angiohistiocytoma. Report of five cases. *J Cutan Pathol.* 2006;33:349–352.

18

DEEP VASCULAR TUMORS

INTRODUCTION

Benign deep vascular lesions comprise a disease spectrum with considerable clinicopathologic overlap. All share the capacity to be infiltrative and therefore may be difficult to cure with local surgical excision. The predominant vessel pattern and anatomic location seem to have little influence on the recurrence rate; it has thus been proposed that the intramuscular tumors be grouped under the generic designation of "angiomas."[1] However, lesions that conform to the definition of angiomatosis, as used elsewhere in this section,[2] warrant separate distinction since they are more likely to recur than tumors confined to one soft tissue site. Extensive arteriovenous malformations may also warrant separation, especially if shunting is sufficient to produce clinical symptoms. However, there is considerable overlap between all these deep lesions. In fact, radiologists simply view deep vascular lesions based on their blood flow characteristics.[3] The differential diagnosis is presented in Table 18.1.

ARTERIOVENOUS MALFORMATIONS

Clinical Features

Vascular malformations can be classified on imaging into high-flow arteriovenous malformations and low-flow venous or lymphatic malformations.[3] All of these have the ability to cross multiple tissue boundaries.

Lesions featuring arteriovenous anastomoses may be either acquired or congenital. The former are usually solitary and traumatic in origin. Congenital arteriovenous connections are often multiple, involving a significant portion of an extremity or the head and neck region.[4–6] Arteriovenous malformations that have a prominent superficial component, associated with substantial shunting, present as pulsating collections of tortuous vessels and are sometimes referred to as cirsoid aneurysms, racemose aneurysms, aneurysms by anastomosis, or pulsating angiomas. Examples that contain large dilated vessels have been designated arteriovenous aneurysms.

The most common presenting complaint is swelling of the extremity, followed by cosmetic disfigurement and visible pulsations. Pain is less common. Superficial varicosities, increased warmth, and thrills or bruits are often present over the affected site. Systemic hemodynamic effects, such

TABLE 18.1 Differential Diagnosis of Deep Vascular Tumors

	Typical clinical features	Microscopic features	Ancillary investigations
Vascular malformations	Presents early in life, often with an enlarged extremity. Diagnosis is typically by imaging studies–considerable overlap with intramuscular hemangioma and angiomatosis. Does not regress.	Ectatic vascular spaces, often accompanied by fat. Arterialized veins (with irregular elastic tissue)	Typically not required; imaging appearance is important
Intramuscular hemangioma/angioma	Intramuscular mass in young patients, often congenital–considerable overlap with vascular malformation and angiomatosis. Does not regress.	Intramuscular vascular proliferation can be composed of capillaries of cavernous spaces, often accompanied by fat.	Typically not required; imaging appearance is important
Intramuscular lipoma	Adults in sixth decade or older, intramuscular fatty mass	Mature-appearing fat infiltrating skeletal muscle. Vessels not a prominent feature	MDM2–, CDK4– no *MDM2* amplification
Venous hemangioma	Often involves organs (e.g., kidney) of adults	Blood-filled, endothelial-lined channels with prominent muscular walls	Typically not required; imaging appearance is important
Angiomatosis/ lymphangiomatosis	Extensive lesion, usually in babies and children, growing contiguously in multiple tissue planes or extensively in tissues of the same type (e.g., apposed muscles). Considerable overlap with intramuscular angioma and vascular malformation. Does not regress.	Ectatic irregular vessels, often accompanied by fat. Irregular small vessels proliferate within walls of larger vessels	Typically not required; imaging appearance is important

(Continued)

TABLE 18.1 Differential Diagnosis of Deep Vascular Tumors (Continued)

	Typical clinical features	Microscopic features	Ancillary investigations
Angiomyolipoma	Usually adults involving the kidney and retroperitoneum	Myoid spindle cells, fat, and prominent vessels	Spindle cells: Actin+, CD34–, CD31–, HMB-45+
Synovial hemangioma	Painful masses of (usually) knee joint arising in childhood	Synovial vascular proliferation, can be composed of capillaries of cavernous spaces, often accompanied by fat.	Typically not required; imaging appearance is important
Hemangioma of bone	Usually incidental radiographic findings of skull, vertebrae of adults	Skeletal tumor that can be composed of capillaries of cavernous spaces, often accompanied by fat.	Typically not required; imaging appearance is important
Epithelioid hemangioma of bone	Young adults, usually involving long tubular bones, no gender predilection	Lobular architecture, epithelioid endothelial cells that form vascular lumina or grow in solid sheets. No hyalinized or solid appearing extracellular myxoid or chondromyxoid matrix	Typically not required; CD34+, CD31+
Littoral cell hemangioma of the spleen	Predominantly lesions of adults (occasional children) with no gender predilection	Cavernous-like hemangioma lined by unique endothelial cells similar to those of splenic sinuses	CD34+, CD68 +, CD8–

Anastomosing hemangioma of genitourinary tract (kidney)	Adult tumors, often renal with solid appearance on imaging	Sinusoidal vessels with hobnail endothelium. Thrombi and extramedullary hematopoiesis common	CD34+, CD31+, HHV8–
Epithelioid hemangioendothelioma	Deep lesions of soft tissues, lungs, and liver of adults	Epithelioid cells in a chondromyxoid background. The cells infiltrate singly, in cords or small nests, and do not form vascular channels, but individual cells can have intracytoplasmic lumina	CD34+, CD31+, Fli-1+ keratins variably +, VEGFR-3–, nuclear INI1+
Epithelioid sarcoma-like hemangioendothelioma	Rare tumors of extremities of young adults	Sheets, ill-defined nodules, fascicles of deeply eosinophilic cells in desmoplastic stroma but no overt vascular channel formation. Occasional cells with vacuoles suggest intracytoplasmic vascular lumen formation.	Keratin+, CD31+, Fli-1+, CD34–, nuclear INI1+
Epithelioid sarcoma	Superficial lesions of distal extremities, often of young adults	Epithelioid cells arranged in granuloma-like configurations with central necrosis	Pan-keratin+, CK5/6–, CD34+, CD31–, loss of nuclear INI1

(Continued)

TABLE 18.1 Differential Diagnosis of Deep Vascular Tumors (Continued)

	Typical clinical features	Microscopic features	Ancillary investigations
Kaposi sarcoma	Lesions of immunosuppressed patients or in endemic areas. Tumors can involve skin or viscera	Spindle cells in fascicles and sheets, extravasated erythrocytes, siderophages, hyaline globules, lymphoplasmacytic infiltrate. Early lesions with more subtle features	CD34+, CD31+, HHV8+, D2-40+, VEGFR-3+
Deep angiosarcoma	Rare tumor of extremities and body cavities, no age predominates	Often epithelioid, overtly malignant neoplasms. Finding vasoformation often requires extensive sampling	Variable staining with CD34, CD31, D2-40, Fli-1, keratins. HHV8–, S100 protein–, can be CD117+ but *C-KIT* mutations absent
Metastatic carcinoma	Any site, usually adults	When sarcomatoid, can resemble deep angiosarcoma	Usually keratin +, CD34–, CD31–, PAX8 can be used to identify sarcomatoid renal cell carcinoma
Metastatic melanoma	Any site, usually adults	When epithelioid, can resemble EHE or epithelioid angiosarcoma	S100 protein+, CD34–, HMB-45+, Melan-A+, MITF1+

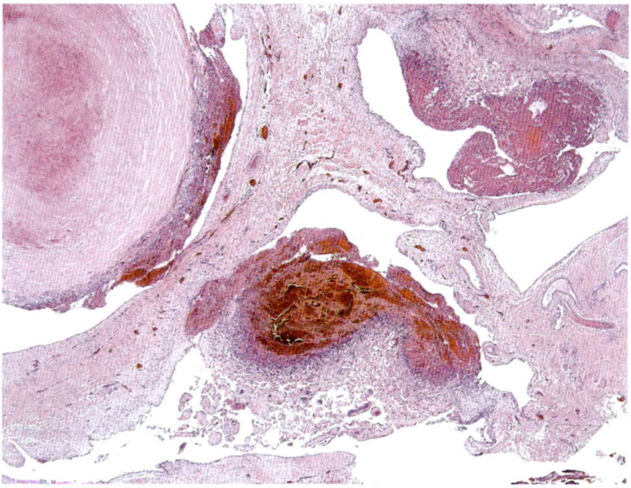

FIGURE 18.1 **Vascular Malformation.** By imaging studies, this was a high-flow lesion (in keeping with an arteriovenous malformation). The lesion consists of irregular malformed vessels. This lesion has areas of thrombi and is complicated by papillary endothelial hyperplasia (best seen at the bottom of the field).

as cardiac enlargement, high output cardiac failure, and Branham sign (bradycardia elicited by digital pressure on the afferent arterial supply), are identified only rarely in congenital arteriovenous malformations. Traumatic fistulas, however, are more likely to be associated with these findings.

In 1900, Klippel and Trenaunay[4] summarized a group of patients with the following triad: (a) a lower extremity port wine stain, (b) varicose veins, and (c) skeletal and soft tissue hypertrophy of the affected site with lengthening of the limb. Later, Parkes Weber[6] described a similar group of cases but included two individuals who also had extensive arteriovenous malformations. The Parkes Weber or Klippel-Trenaunay-Weber syndrome is diagnosed in patients with all four of the aforementioned features.

The diagnosis of arteriovenous malformation is made with greater accuracy on the basis of clinical and radiographic findings than by histological examination. Arteriography can be used to confirm the presence of arteriovenous anastomoses but also to identify cases where superficial varicosities are attributable to deep venous obstruction or the congenital absence of deep veins rather than an arteriovenous malformation; excision of superficial veins in the latter cases is contraindicated.[5] Magnetic resonance imaging (MRI) can also be used to characterize vascular malformations.[3]

Histologic Features

The histology of arteriovenous malformations may vary considerably; foci identical to capillary or cavernous hemangiomas may be present (Fig. 18.1, e-Figs. 18.1–18.4). The identification of direct arteriovenous anastomoses may require extensive tissue sampling. When these are not seen, the presence of juxtaposed medium-sized or larger arteries and veins and the identification of arterialized veins, characterized by prominent fibrointimal hyperplasia and medial muscular hypertrophy aid in this diagnosis.

Ancillary Investigations

Elastic stains may be useful in searching for arterialized veins. Vascular malformations do not express GLUT1.[7]

INTRAMUSCULAR HEMANGIOMAS

Intramuscular hemangiomas/angiomas are relatively uncommon, accounting for 0.8% to 4.4% of all vascular tumors in two large series.[1,8] There does not appear to be a distinct gender predilection. The majority of cases are identified in the first 3 decades of life.[1,8,9] The lower extremity, in particular the quadriceps femoris, is the most frequent site. However, any muscle may be involved. Soft tissue swelling and pain are the most frequent sign and symptom, respectively.

Recurrences are common and attributable to incomplete excision.

Pathologic Features

The gross appearance varies widely, depending on the type and size of vessels that predominate and the extent to which supporting elements such as adipose and fibrous connective tissue are represented. Tumors composed predominantly of small capillary-sized vessels tend to be poorly marginated and vary from whitish-tan to reddish-brown. Tumors dominated by large vessels (i.e., cavernous spaces) are much more likely to be recognized grossly as vascular anomalies. When intramuscular hemangiomas are accompanied by abundant adipose tissue, an incorrect diagnosis of lipoma or liposarcoma may be entertained both clinically and histologically. (Lesions with this appearance have, in the past, been referred to as "infiltrating angiolipomas."[10]) Occasionally, foci of ossification may be seen; this seems to occur most frequently in lesions with an arteriovenous component.[1]

As suggested above, intramuscular vascular tumors can be histologically categorized according to vessel size or type (Fig. 18.2, e-Figs. 18.5–18.7). Some authors have suggested that all of these lesions, including capillary, cavernous, arteriovenous, lymphangiomatous, and complex malformation-types be regarded as intramuscular "angiomas"[1] since most examples have mixed features, despite a frequently dominant vessel pattern, and there is no correlation between the predominant vessel type and the clinical outcome. There is, however, some correlation between vessel pattern and anatomic site; intramuscular capillary hemangiomas and lymphangiomas favor the upper half of the body. All types of vessels can be accompanied by abundant fat. Atrophic skeletal muscle is seen intermixed with the lesion.

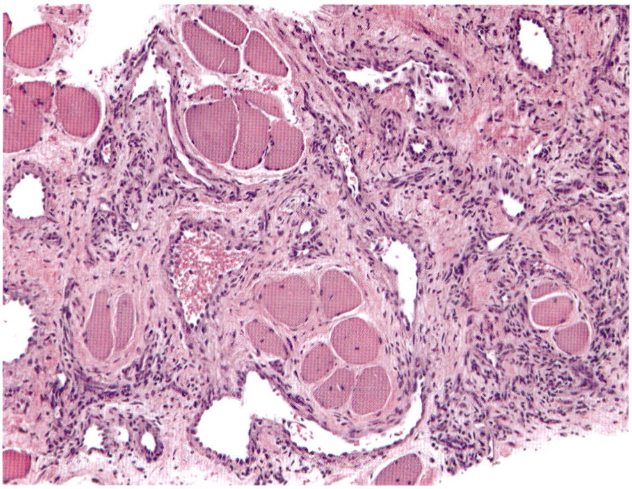

FIGURE 18.2 **Intramuscular Hemangioma.** This lesion has capillary hemangioma features.

VENOUS HEMANGIOMAS/MALFORMATIONS

Clinical Features

Venous hemangiomas are rare tumors that often involve deep structures and solid organs (liver, spleen, kidney). Adults are reported to be affected more frequently than children. Sites that may be involved include the skeletal muscle, bones, mediastinum, joint spaces, mucosa-lined hollow organs, and the spinal cord. Due to sluggish blood flow and thrombosis of feeding vessels, these lesions are often not visualized by arteriography but have been characterized on MRI.[3]

Pathologic Features

On microscopic examination, one sees blood-filled, endothelial-lined channels with prominent muscular walls (e-Figs. 18.8 and 18.9). These walls frequently have disorganized smooth muscle bundles.[11] It is the thickened muscular walls that distinguish venous from cavernous hemangiomas.

Ancillary Investigations

Elastic stains can demonstrate the absence or paucity of elastic tissue in the lesional vessels.[11]

ANGIOMATOSIS

Angiomatosis is a term that over the years has been applied to a variety of processes, including papillary endothelial hyperplasia, encephalofacial vascular malformations in Sturge-Weber syndrome, and extensive multifocal benign vascular proliferations in children.[12] For the purposes of this discussion, angiomatosis is used to described a histologically benign vascular proliferation growing contiguously in multiple tissue planes or extensively in tissues of the same type (e.g., apposed muscles).[2,13] The lesions tend to be based in the deep subcutaneous tissue and muscles, but more superficial tissues or underlying bone may also be involved.

Although the true incidence of these lesions is unknown, they appear to be relatively rare. For example, in a review by Watson and McCarthy[8]of 1,056 patients with benign vascular lesions, only seven individuals, briefly mentioned under the heading "diffuse systemic hemangiomata," seem to fulfill criteria for a diagnosis of angiomatosis.

Clinical Features

Most patients present within childhood and frequently in the first year of life.[2] The most common symptoms are persistent diffuse swelling, pain, and tenderness. Limb hypertrophy is present only infrequently. Vascular lesions are usually not suspected clinically since superficial discoloration is frequently absent and arteriovenous shunting is unapparent. The lower extremity, including the buttock, is the most frequently affected site, followed by the trunk and the upper extremity. Less commonly, the head and neck, back, pelvis, and retroperitoneum may be involved. When excised these lesions typical recur based on their extensive growth.

Pathologic Features

Angiomatosis is characterized histologically by an admixture of large irregular venous segments with disorganized muscular walls, cavernous vessels and capillary channels, scattered diffusely throughout tissue planes and often associated with large amounts of adipose tissue (e-Fig. 18.10). Arteries and lymphatic channels may also be noted but are typically not seen in direct communication with the former. A characteristic features is the presence of capillary-sized vessels proliferating adjacent to, and within the walls of, the disorganized venous segments (Fig. 18.3). Similar extensive lesions composed of lymphatic vessels can be referred to as "lymphangiomatosis" or "lymphatic malformation" (e-Figs. 18.11–18.18).

OTHER BENIGN DEEP ANGIOMATOUS LESIONS

Synovial (e-Figs. 18.19 and 18.20) and tendinous, neural, and intraosseous hemangiomas (e-Figs. 18.21 and 18.22)[14] are all well documented in the literature. Synovial hemangiomas most frequently affect the knee joint. They produce signs and symptoms that often begin during childhood, including pain, swelling, and recurrent joint effusions. Hemangiomas arising within peripheral nerves are rare, and there is no established age predilection or favored site of involvement. Signs and symptoms may include pain, hypoesthesia, and muscle wasting of the innervated region. Both synovial and neural hemangiomas are often of the cavernous type.

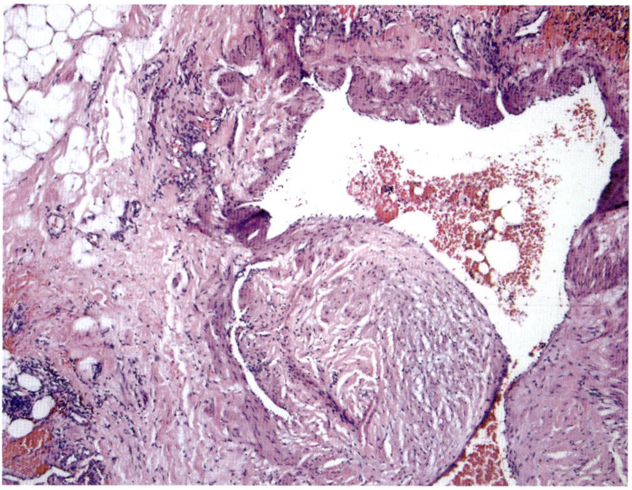

FIGURE 18.3 **Angiomatosis.** This extensive lesion involved the lower extremity of a young patient. There was extensive overgrowth of adipose tissue (upper left) and some of the irregular ecstatic vessels had smaller vessels within their muscular walls.

Hemangiomas of bone most frequently affect the skull and vertebrae. They are usually first noted in adulthood and are more frequently solitary than multifocal. The majority of these lesions are asymptomatic, incidental radiographic findings. However, they may be associated with local pain, swelling and, infrequently, a pathologic fracture. The vasculature may have cavernous, capillary, or, rarely, venous or arteriovenous features. Synovial hemangiomas are also known.

Diffuse skeletal hemangiomatosis (diffuse cystic angiomatosis) refers to extensive, multicentric angiomatous lesions of bone.[15,16] This disorder is often associated with visceral and soft tissue hemangiomas.

Some hemangiomas of organs assume somewhat organ-specific appearances. For example, littoral cell hemangioma of the spleen is reminiscent of the normal sinuses of the spleen (e-Figs. 18.23–18.25).[17] In contrast to normal sinus endothelia, which express only endothelial markers and CD8 but not histiocytic markers, neoplastic cells express both endothelial and histiocytic (CD68, lysozyme) antigens but lack CD8. Angiosarcomas of the spleen showing similar features have also been reported.[18]

In the kidney, a peculiar hemangioma variant has been termed "anastomosing hemangioma" (e-Figs. 18.26–18.28).[19] These lesions consist of anastomosing sinusoidal capillary-sized vessels with scattered hobnail endothelial cells within a framework of nonendothelial supporting cells. Vascular thrombi are typical and the lesions show zones of central sclerosis with focal necrosis. Some tumors feature prominent extramedullary hematopoiesis or hyaline globules reminiscent of those seen in Kaposi sarcoma.

EPITHELIOID HEMANGIOENDOTHELIOMA

Clinical Features

Epithelioid hemangioendothelioma (EHE) is a malignant vascular tumor that generally pursues a less aggressive course than angiosarcoma. It can occur at any age although it is rare in childhood. The predominant sites of involvement are the soft tissue (e-Fig. 18.29), lungs, liver, and bones (e-Figs. 18.30 and 18.31).

Soft tissue examples have no gender predilection.[20–23] The median age at presentation is in the fifth decade. The tumors are typically solitary and have a predilection for the extremities. Either the subcutis or deeper soft tissue sites may be involved. About half of cases are associated with a medium-sized or larger vessel, usually a vein. Involvement of the jugular, femoral, and iliac veins has been documented. Metastases and tumor related deaths were reported in 31% and 13% of patients, respectively, in the 1980s[20]–figures that have changed little over time. In a 2008 study, 22% of patients experiences metastases and 18% died of disease.[23]

Intravascular bronchioloalveolar tumor, sclerosing endothelial tumor, sclerosing interstitial vascular sarcoma, primary chondrosarcoma of the lung, and pulmonary deciduosis is a partial list of designations previously used to describe examples of EHE of the lungs.[24] Approximately, 80% of patients are women. The median age at presentation is forty. Multiple and bilateral nodules are typically noted at presentation. Over half of patients die of disease, often after a protracted course.[24] Although both the pattern and the extent of disease in pulmonary EHE suggest a metastatic process, this has generally been viewed as a primary, possibly multicentric, neoplasm since past experience has indicated that an extrapulmonary primary does not become apparent clinically although metastatic spread can sometimes be documented.[25] However, imaging studies and autopsy examinations are commonly limited to the torso and, as such, some extremity tumors may have escaped detection in early studies.

Before the vascular nature of EHE was recognized, hepatic examples were interpreted as sclerosing hepatic carcinomas, cholangiocarcinomas, or calcifying mixed malignant tumors.[26] Hepatic involvement is commonly multifocal and bilobar. There is a slight female predominance. The mean age at presentation is approximately forty.[27] As with pulmonary examples, identification of hepatic EHE should prompt a clinical investigation to exclude the possibility of metastases from other potential primary sites. The most common management has been liver transplantation, followed by no treatment, chemotherapy or radiotherapy, and liver resection. The reported 1- and 5-year patient survival rates are 96% and 54.5%, respectively, after liver transplant; 39.3% and 4.5%, respectively, after no treatment; 73.3% and 30%, respectively, after chemotherapy or radiotherapy; and 100% and 75%, respectively, after liver resection (performed in patients deemed resectable and thus with less extensive disease).[27]

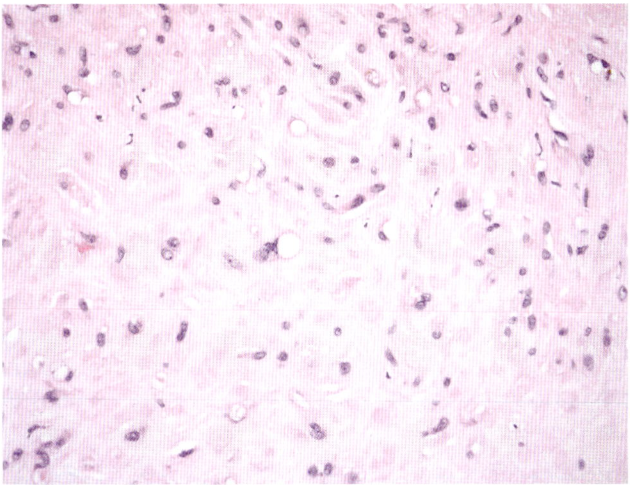

FIGURE 18.4 **Epithelioid Hemangioendothelioma.** There are single epithelioid cells (they do not form organized lumina—compare this to Figure 17.5, an epithelioid hemangioma) in a chondromyxoid background. Some of the cells contain intracytoplasmic vacuoles/lumina.

Skeletal EHEs typically may involve any bone and have been recognized in the femur, tibia, fibula, small bones of the hands and feet, humerus, radius, ulna, ribs, vertebral bodies, pelvis, and scapula. Affected patients have a slight male predominance and a wide age distribution extending from the second through the eighth decade of life.[28] EHE of bone is multifocal in approximately half of cases, and it is unclear whether the separate lesions reflect multicentric or metastatic disease. The indolent clinical course supports the concept that they are independent primary tumors.

Pathologic Features

The gross and microscopic features of EHE are similar in all sites. The tumor nodules have a white-tan, well-marginated appearance and a firm, rubbery or "cartilaginous" consistency. Calcifications may occasionally be present. Microscopic examination reveals a tumor composed of epithelioid (histiocytoid) and, occasionally, spindle or dendritic cells, embedded singly, in cord-like arrangements, or clusters within a matrix variably described as "myxohyaline" or "chondromyxoid" (Fig. 18.4, c-Figs. 18.32 18.37). The matrix frequently has a hyalinized or collagenized appearance centrally and a more myxoid quality peripherally. Scattered neoplastic cells have prominent cytoplasmic vacuoles. Occasionally, the vacuoles may contain intraluminal erythrocytes, a sign of "early" or "primitive" vasoformative differentiation. Features of soft tissue EHEs that may correlate with more aggressive behavior include finding >3 mitotic figures per 50 hpf and size >3.0 cm.[23]

EHE generally features mildly to moderately atypical cytology, although, on rare occasions, foci with significant pleomorphism may be noted. Tumors with the latter appearance can sometimes be difficult to distinguish from epithelioid angiosarcoma, a finding that suggests the possibility of a histologic (diagnostic) continuum.

Ancillary Investigations

On immunolabeling, EHEs variably express CD31, CD34 (e-Fig. 18.35), and Fli-1[29]and may also express (usually focally) keratins.[30] They lack VEGFR-3, which argues against lymphatic endothelial differentiation.[31] A chromosomal translocation involving chromosomes 1 and 3 [t(1;3)(p36.3;q25)] has been detected in a limited number of cases[32] and a separate translocation (t(10;14)(p13;q24),+r) has been detected in another case.[33]

EPITHELIOID SARCOMA-LIKE HEMANGIOENDOTHELIOMA

This rare lesion has been reported as a small series and case reports.[34–36] In the original series,[34] the patients (four male; three female) ranged in age from 17 to 54 years (median: 23 years). Their tumors were small (1–3.5 cm), and involved the extremities ($n = 5$), scalp ($n = 1$), and chest wall ($n = 1$), both in deep ($n = 3$) and superficial ($n = 3$) soft tissue, or both ($n = 1$). In the original series, local (but not systemic) metastases were reported but not tumor-associated deaths.[34]

Pathologic Features

Epithelioid sarcoma-like hemangioendothelioma is characterized by sheets, ill-defined nodules, or fascicles of deeply eosinophilic cells set within a desmoplastic stroma (Fig. 18.5, e-Figs. 18.38–18.41). Overt vascular channel formation and/or hemorrhage are absent. Some cases display cells with vacuolization suggestive of intracytoplasmic vascular lumen formation (e-Fig. 18.41). The lesional cells are large and rounded to spindled. Mitotic activity is low, nuclear pleomorphism is mild to moderate, and necrosis is absent.

Ancillary Investigations

Epithelioid sarcoma-like hemangioendothelioma expresses cytokeratin, vimentin, CD31, and Fli-1, but not CD34[34] (e-Figs. 18.42–18.44).

KAPOSI SARCOMA

Kaposi sarcoma can arise in the deep soft tissues and viscera (e-Figs. 18.45 and 18.46). It is discussed in Chapters 10 and 17.

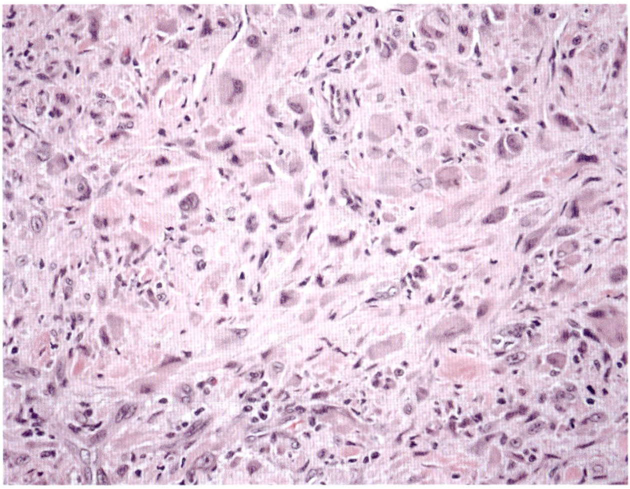

FIGURE 18.5 **Epithelioid Sarcoma-Like Hemangioendothelioma.** This lesion arose in the foot of a teenage boy. Epithelioid cells without overt vasoformation are seen in sclerotic stroma. On immunolabeling, this lesion expressed CD31 and keratin but not CD34.

ANGIOSARCOMA OF DEEP SOFT TISSUE

Clinical Features

The true incidence of angiosarcoma arising in deep soft tissue is unknown. This assumption is supported by the rarity of published series.[37,38] Deep soft tissue angiosarcomas occur throughout life, without predilection for one age group and pediatric examples are known.[39] The extremities and abdominal cavity are favored sites.

Pathologic Features

In general, deep soft tissue angiosarcomas seem to have a propensity for high-grade histology (e-Figs. 18.46–18.61). Epithelioid morphology is well documented in this group.[38]and may lead to an erroneous diagnosis of carcinoma or melanoma (Fig. 18.6). Some deep-seated examples appear to originate from medium or large-sized vessels. Deep angiosarcomas are frequently hemorrhagic and multinodular. There is a wide morphologic spectrum within and between cases, including areas similar to cavernous and capillary hemangioma, Dabska tumor, spindle cell and EHE, various spindle cell sarcomas, or carcinoma. In epithelioid angiosarcomas, epithelioid cells are arranged in nests, clusters, papillae, and gaping vascular channels. Hemorrhage can obscure the diagnosis and be accompanied by papillary endothelial hyperplasia-like areas.

Ancillary Investigations

Deep angiosarcomas display variable expression of endothelial markers (CD34, CD31, Fli-1; e-Figs. 18.47, 18.56, and 18.57.) and some

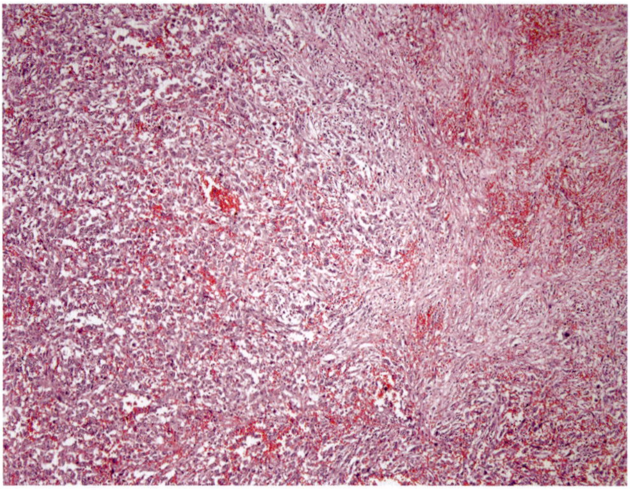

FIGURE 18.6 **Epithelioid Angiosarcoma.** This lesion arose in the retroperitoneum. The malignant cells have large nuclei with prominent nucleoli and abundant eosinophilic cytoplasm. Such cases often require immunolabeling for diagnosis and often express cytokeratins.

display lymphatic endothelial markers podoplanin (D2-40, VEGFR-3).[38–41] Epithelioid examples frequently express keratins[30] (e-Fig. 18.48) and CD117 labels a subset but is unassociated with *C-KIT* mutations.[42] Human herpesvirus type 8 (HHV8) transcripts are not detected.[43]

FOREIGN BODY-ASSOCIATED ANGIOSARCOMA

Infrequently, angiosarcoma has developed in association with foreign body material (i.e., Dacron vascular graft, shrapnel, bullet, surgical sponge, metallic orthopedic appliances).[44–47] As with other angiosarcomas, the tumors are typically aggressive and lethal.

REFERENCES

1. Beham A, Fletcher CD. Intramuscular angioma: a clinicopathological analysis of 74 cases. *Histopathology.* 1991;18:53–59.
2. Rao VK, Weiss SW. Angiomatosis of soft tissue. An analysis of the histologic features and clinical outcome in 51 cases. *Am J Surg Pathol.* 1992;16:764–771.
3. Fayad LM, Hazirolan T, Bluemke D, et al. Vascular malformations in the extremities: emphasis on MR imaging features that guide treatment options. *Skeletal Radiol.* 2006;35:127–137.
4. Klippel M, Trenaunay P. Du naevus variqueux osteo-hypertrophique. *Arch Gen Med (Paris).* 1900;185:641–672.
5. Lindenauer SM. Congenital arteriovenous fistula and the Klippel-Trenaunay syndrome. *Ann Surg.* 1971;174:248–263.
6. Parkes Weber F. Angioma formation in connection with hypertrophy of limbs and hemihypertrophy. *Br J Dermatol.* 1907;19:231–235.

7. Leon-Villapalos J, Wolfe K, Kangesu L. GLUT-1: an extra diagnostic tool to differentiate between haemangiomas and vascular malformations. *Br J Plast Surg*. 2005;58:348–352.
8. Watson W, McCarthy W. Blood and blood vessel tumors: 1056 cases. *Surg Gynecol Obstet*. 1940;71:569–588.
9. Allen PW, Enzinger FM. Hemangioma of skeletal muscle. An analysis of 89 cases. *Cancer*. 1972;29:8–22.
10. Austin RM, Mack GR, Townsend CM, et al. Infiltrating (intramuscular) lipomas and angiolipomas. A clinicopathologic study of six cases. *Arch Surg*. 1980;115:281–284.
11. Ichikawa MM, Ishida-Yamamoto A, Hashimoto Y, et al. Venous hemangioma. An immunohistochemical and ultrastructural study. *Acta Derm Venereol*. 1997;77:382–384.
12. Holden KR, Alexander F. Diffuse neonatal hemangiomatosis. *Pediatrics*. 1970;46:411–421.
13. Howat AJ, Campbell PE. Angiomatosis: a vascular malformation of infancy and childhood. Report of 17 cases. *Pathology*. 1987;19:377–382.
14. Unni KK, Ivins JC, Beabout JW, et al. Hemangioma, hemangiopericytoma, and hemangioendothelioma (angiosarcoma) of bone. *Cancer*. 1971;27:1403–1414.
15. Pulido-Zamudio T, Orr W, Lertzman M. Cystic angiomatosis of the bone appearing as intrathoracic lung masses. *Can Respir J*. 2001;8:187–190.
16. Boyle WJ. Cystic angiomatosis of bone. A report of three cases and review of the literature. *J Bone Joint Surg Br*. 1972;54:626–636.
17. Falk S, Stutte HJ, Frizzera G. Littoral cell angioma. A novel splenic vascular lesion demonstrating histiocytic differentiation. *Am J Surg Pathol*. 1991;15:1023–1033.
18. Rosso R, Paulli M, Gianelli U, et al. Littoral cell angiosarcoma of the spleen. Case report with immunohistochemical and ultrastructural analysis. *Am J Surg Pathol*. 1995;19:1203–1208.
19. Montgomery E, Epstein JI. Anastomosing hemangioma of the genitourinary tract: a lesion mimicking angiosarcoma. *Am J Surg Pathol*. 2009;33:1364–1369.
20. Weiss SW, Ishak KG, Dail DH, et al. Epithelioid hemangioendothelioma and related lesions. *Semin Diagn Pathol*. 1986;3:259–287.
21. Weiss SW, Enzinger FM. Epithelioid hemangioendothelioma: a vascular tumor often mistaken for a carcinoma. *Cancer*. 1982;50:970–981.
22. Mentzel T, Beham A, Calonje E, et al. Epithelioid hemangioendothelioma of skin and soft tissues: clinicopathologic and immunohistochemical study of 30 cases. *Am J Surg Pathol*. 1997;21:363–374.
23. Deyrup AT, Tighiouart M, Montag AG, et al. Epithelioid hemangioendothelioma of soft tissue: a proposal for risk stratification based on 49 cases. *Am J Surg Pathol*. 2008;32:924–927.
24. Dail DH, Liebow AA, Gmelich JT, et al. Intravascular, bronchiolar, and alveolar tumor of the lung (IVBAT). An analysis of twenty cases of a peculiar sclerosing endothelial tumor. *Cancer*. 1983;51:452–464.
25. Verbeken E, Beyls J, Moerman P, et al. Lung metastasis of malignant epithelioid hemangioendothelioma mimicking a primary intravascular bronchioalveolar tumor. A histologic, ultrastructural, and immunohistochemical study. *Cancer*. 1985;55:1741–1746.
26. Ishak KG, Sesterhenn IA, Goodman ZD, et al. Epithelioid hemangioendothelioma of the liver: a clinicopathologic and follow-up study of 32 cases. *Hum Pathol*. 1984;15:839–852.
27. Mehrabi A, Kashfi A, Fonouni H, et al. Primary malignant hepatic epithelioid hemangioendothelioma: a comprehensive review of the literature with emphasis on the surgical therapy. *Cancer*. 2006;107:2108–2121.
28. O'Connell JX, Nielsen GP, Rosenberg AE. Epithelioid vascular tumors of bone: a review and proposal of a classification scheme. *Adv Anat Pathol*. 2001;8:74–82.

29. Folpe AL, Chand EM, Goldblum JR, et al. Expression of Fli-1, a nuclear transcription factor, distinguishes vascular neoplasms from potential mimics. *Am J Surg Pathol.* 2001;25:1061–1066.
30. Miettinen M, Fetsch JF. Distribution of keratins in normal endothelial cells and a spectrum of vascular tumors: implications in tumor diagnosis. *Hum Pathol.* 2000;31:1062–1067.
31. Folpe AL, Veikkola T, Valtola R, et al. Vascular endothelial growth factor receptor-3 (VEGFR-3): a marker of vascular tumors with presumed lymphatic differentiation, including Kaposi's sarcoma, kaposiform and Dabska-type hemangioendotheliomas, and a subset of angiosarcomas. *Mod Pathol.* 2000;13:180–185.
32. Mendlick MR, Nelson M, Pickering D, et al. Translocation t(1;3)(p36.3;q25) is a nonrandom aberration in epithelioid hemangioendothelioma. *Am J Surg Pathol.* 2001;25:684–687.
33. He M, Das K, Blacksin M, et al. A translocation involving the placental growth factor gene is identified in an epithelioid hemangioendothelioma. *Cancer Genet Cytogenet.* 2006;168:150–154.
34. Billings SD, Folpe AL, Weiss SW. Epithelioid sarcoma-like hemangioendothelioma. *Am J Surg Pathol.* 2003;27:48–57.
35. Watabe A, Okuyama R, Hashimoto A, et al. Epithelioid sarcoma-like haemangioendothelioma: a case report. *Acta Derm Venereol.* 2009;89:208–209.
36. Tokyol C, Uzum N, Kuru I, et al. Epithelioid sarcoma-like hemangioendothelioma: a case report. *Tumori.* 2005;91:436–439.
37. Fletcher CD, Beham A, Bekir S, et al. Epithelioid angiosarcoma of deep soft tissue: a distinctive tumor readily mistaken for an epithelial neoplasm. *Am J Surg Pathol.* 1991;15:915–924.
38. Meis-Kindblom JM, Kindblom LG. Angiosarcoma of soft tissue: a study of 80 cases. *Am J Surg Pathol.* 1998;22:683–697.
39. Deyrup AT, Miettinen M, North PE, et al. Angiosarcomas arising in the viscera and soft tissue of children and young adults: a clinicopathologic study of 15 cases. *Am J Surg Pathol.* 2009;33:264–269.
40. Kahn HJ, Bailey D, Marks A. Monoclonal antibody D2-40, a new marker of lymphatic endothelium, reacts with Kaposi's sarcoma and a subset of angiosarcomas. *Mod Pathol.* 2002;15:434–440.
41. Fukunaga M. Expression of D2-40 in lymphatic endothelium of normal tissues and in vascular tumours. *Histopathology.* 2005;46:396–402.
42. Miettinen M, Sarlomo-Rikala M, Lasota J. KIT expression in angiosarcomas and fetal endothelial cells: lack of mutations of exon 11 and exon 17 of C-kit. *Mod Pathol.* 2000;13:536–541.
43. Martinez-Escribano JA, del Pino Gil-Mateo M, Miquel J, et al. Human herpesvirus 8 is not detectable by polymerase chain reaction in angiosarcoma. *Br J Dermatol.* 1998;138:546–547.
44. Ben-Izhak O, Vlodavsky E, Ofer A, et al. Epithelioid angiosarcoma associated with a Dacron vascular graft. *Am J Surg Pathol.* 1999;23:1418–1422.
45. Ben-Izhak O, Kerner H, Brenner B, et al. Angiosarcoma of the colon developing in a capsule of a foreign body. Report of a case with associated hemorrhagic diathesis. *Am J Clin Pathol.* 1992;97:416–420.
46. Jennings TA, Peterson L, Axiotis CA, et al. Angiosarcoma associated with foreign body material. A report of three cases. *Cancer.* 1988;62:2436–2444.
47. Hayman J, Huygens H. Angiosarcoma developing around a foreign body. *J Clin Pathol.* 1983;36:515–518.

19

OSTEOCHONDROID LESIONS OF SOFT TISSUE

INTRODUCTION

Bone or cartilage formation occurs in a wide variety of soft tissue lesions. Benign osseous, chondroid, or osteochondroid metaplasia is an occasional feature in many benign and malignant tumors, examples of which include calcifying aponeurotic fibroma (Chapter 2), lipoma (Chapter 15), fibromatosis (Chapter 2), ossifying fasciitis (Chapter 3), synovial sarcoma (Chapter 10), sclerosing epithelioid fibrosarcoma (Chapter 10), and liposarcoma (Chapter 16). Divergent differentiation to osteosarcoma or chondrosarcoma can occur in malignant peripheral nerve sheath tumors (MPNSTs) (Chapter 10), dedifferentiated liposarcoma (Chapters 5 and 16), mesothelioma (Chapter 5), and sarcomatoid carcinomas. This chapter discusses those lesions in which such changes are the principal or sole form of differentiation. Extraskeletal myxoid chondrosarcoma is a translocation sarcoma without cartilaginous differentiation and is considered in Chapter 21. The differential diagnosis is summarized in Table 19.1.

TUMORS FORMING BONE

These include reactive and neoplastic conditions, and their diagnosis often requires clinical and radiologic information in addition to careful histologic assessment.

FIBRO-OSSEOUS PSEUDOTUMOR OF THE DIGITS

Clinical Features

Fibro-osseous pseudotumor is a benign, reactive zonal lesion, similar to myositis ossificans (MO), which occurs in the digits, often with a history of repetitive manual activity or trauma. Unlike MO, it chiefly involves the dermis or subcutaneous tissue and adjacent fibrous structures,[1] has a slight predilection for women,[2,3] and involves a slightly older age group.[2,4] The lesion usually occurs in the fingers, most commonly the proximal phalanx of the index or middle fingers, and small numbers occur in the toes. It may rarely occur in nondigital sites such as the wrist. The usual presenting feature is a localized, often painful and erythematous mass in soft tissue that is not

TABLE 19.1 Differential Diagnosis of Osteochondroid Lesions

	Typical Clinical Features	Microscopic Features	Ancillary Investigations
Myositis ossificans	Young adults, proximal extremities or trunk. Usually intramuscular and often history of trauma	Zonal pattern. Highest cellularity in early stage. Spindle and stellate fibroblasts resembling nodular fasciitis centrally. Vascular or myxoid stroma with inflammation and extravasated erythrocytes. Transition zone of active bone formation. Peripheral layer of well-formed bone	Fibroblastic cells SMA+, occasionally desmin+
Fibro-osseous pseudotumor	Adults, digits; infrequently nondigital sites such as wrist. Dermis or subcutis. May have history of trauma	Variably cellular fascicles of spindle cells in myxoid stroma, similar to nodular fasciitis. Focal irregular bony trabeculae with osteoid and osteoblastic rimming. May display zoning pattern, but less organized than in MO	Variably SMA and calponin+
Ossifying fibromyxoid tumor	Subcutaneous circumscribed nodule	Cords of small rounded glomus like cells in fibromyxoid stroma. About 80% have partial or complete rim of mature bone in capsule, extending long septa. Atypical variants can have intratumoral osteoid and rarely spindle cells.	S100 protein+, GFAP+, desmin±, SMA±, CK+ rarely

Extraskeletal osteosarcoma	Older adults. May occur at sites of previous irradiation. Deep soft tissue of extremities, retroperitoneum	Atypical osteoblasts producing malignant osteoid and bone. Surrounding tumor varies in morphology, but most resemble pleomorphic sarcoma. Atypical mitoses. Calcification, mature bone, and atypical cartilage can be present	Similar immunoprofile to skeletal counterpart, e.g., osteocalcin and osteonectin+. Can show divergent differentiation with variable muscle marker, S100 protein and CK+
Ossifying synovial sarcoma	Young adults, often ankle or foot, slowly growing	Irregular distribution of mature bone spicules within tumor. Can be biphasic or monophasic, but are often the latter that can be only sparsely cellular. Frequent mast cells. Metaplastic bone can also be seen within fibrous septa	CK+, EMA+, bcl-2+, CD909+, S100 protein+, TLE1+
Lipoma with metaplastic bone	Usually superficial well-circumscribed masses in adults (some intramuscular, rarely retroperitoneal)	Resembles mature fat with variation in adipocyte size. Mature-type bone	MDM2–, CDK4–, no *MDM2* amplification, *HMGA2* fusions
Schwannoma with metaplastic bone	Adults, superficial or deep, head and neck, limbs, retroperitoneum, posterior mediastinum	Circumscribed, fibrous capsule. Spindle cells with wavy nuclei in palisades or patternless patterns. Inflammatory cells, hyalinization. Mature-type bone	S100 protein+ (diffuse). Peripheral rim of EMA+ perineurial cells

(Continued)

TABLE 19.1 **Differential Diagnosis of Osteochondroid Lesions (Continued)**

	Typical Clinical Features	Microscopic Features	Ancillary Investigations
Soft tissue chondroma	Adults, extraosseous and extra-articular sites, hands and feet	Lobules of mature hyaline cartilage, with clusters of chondrocytes. Atypia and normal mitoses can be present, but more mature and sparsely cellular areas elsewhere identify lesion as benign	S100 protein+ in chondroid areas
Synovial chondromatosis	Adults. Synovium of joints, bursae, and tendon sheaths. Most common in large joints, e.g., knee and hip. Rarely in soft tissue adjacent to, but without communication with the joint. Has potential for malignant transformation to chondrosarcoma	Variably cellular nodules and islands of hyaline cartilage, present within the synovial membrane. Atypia, mitoses, and ossification can be present	S100 protein+ in chondroid areas
Extraskeletal mesenchymal chondrosarcoma	Young adults. Head and neck, extremities. Exclude metastasis from extraosseous site	Biphasic morphology. Hypercellular sheets of primitive small cells with round, ovoid, or spindled nuclei. Discrete or intermingled islands of variably differentiated hyaline cartilage. Hemangiopericytic vascular pattern	Small cell component CD99+. Cartilaginous component S100 protein+
Lipoma with metaplastic cartilage	Usually superficial well-circumscribed masses in adults (some intramuscular, rarely retroperitoneal)	Resembles mature fat with variation in adipocyte size. Well-differentiated cartilage	MDM2–, CDK4–, no *MDM2* amplification, *HMGA2* fusions

Atypical lipomatous tumor with metaplastic osteochondroid differentiation	Deep tumors of adults >50 y	Adipose tissue with scattered enlarged hyperchromatic nuclei, often found in fibrous septa. Mature-type bone	MDM2+, CDK4±, *MDM2* amplification
Myxoid liposarcoma with metaplastic osteochondroid differentiation	Deep soft tissues of extremities of young adults. Often metastasizes to other soft tissue sites as well as to lungs	Monotonous small uniform spindle or round cells with abundant (myxoid) or minimal (round cell) myxoid matrix. Rich network of delicate vessels becomes inconspicuous in round cell liposarcoma. Lipoblasts.	S100 protein+ in some cases t(12;16)(q13;p11) or t(12;22)(q13;q12) with *FUS-DDIT3 or EWSR1-DDIT3* fusion
MPNST with divergent osteochondroid differentiation	M > F. In NF1 or sporadic, axial or in limbs. Origin in nerve or neurofibroma	Elongated spindle cells, wavy or buckled nuclei. Variably cellular and myxoid, fascicular pattern. Nuclei wavy, buckled, or lanceolate. Palisading, neuroid whorls, vascular wall involvement, collagenous "rosettes"	S100 protein+ focally, occasional GFAP+
Dedifferentiated liposarcoma with divergent osteochondroid differentiation	Older adults, large retroperitoneal tumor, recurrences frequent M > F	Low-grade dedifferentiation: cellular fascicles with mild pleomorphism	MDM2+, CDK4+, both amplified on FISH. P16+
		High-grade dedifferentiation: pleomorphic undifferentiated sarcoma, or myofibrosarcoma-like. Malignant osteochondroid or rhabdomyosarcomatous elements. WD liposarcomatous component present or absent	Variable desmin, SMA, CD34

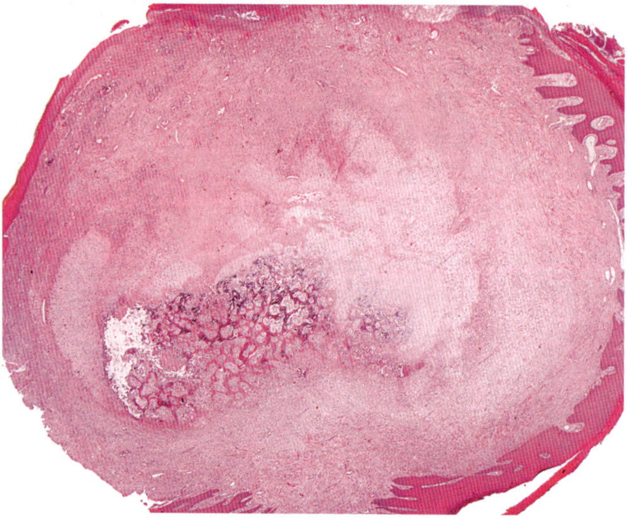

FIGURE 19.1 **Fibro-osseous Pseudotumor.** This is an ill-defined lesion in the dermis and subcutis with a cellular spindle cell background and focal bone formation.

connected to the adjacent bone. Radiologically, there is randomly distributed lesional calcification. Complete local excision is usually curative.

Pathologic Features

Fibro-osseous pseudotumor is macroscopically fairly well circumscribed, although the surface can be ulcerated. It can display a "zonal" pattern of immature spindled areas admixed with more mature areas showing osteoid metaplasia. The features are similar to those of MO but tend to be less well organized, and generally the bone is more randomly distributed (Fig. 19.1, e-Fig. 19.1). There is an irregular multinodular growth pattern with variably cellular fascicles of spindle cells with minimal to mild atypia within myxoid stroma (Fig. 19.2, e-Figs. 19.1 and 19.2) reminiscent of nodular fasciitis. Mitotic figures can be abundant. All cases show at least focal irregular bony trabeculae with osteoid formation and osteoblastic rimming,[3] with occasional osteoclast-like giant cells (e-Fig. 19.3), and a component of cartilage is sometimes seen (e-Fig. 19.4). Importantly, there is no significant atypia, which helps to exclude osteosarcoma.

Ancillary investigations. The spindle cells show variable positivity for smooth muscle actin and calponin and are negative for S100 protein, desmin, and h-caldesmon.

MYOSITIS OSSIFICANS

Clinical Features

MO is a rare lesion that can occur at any age, although chiefly affects young adults, with a predilection for males. It is a localized, reactive,

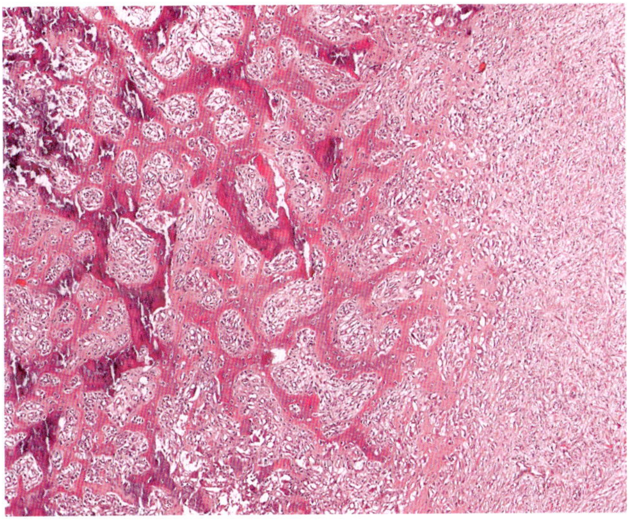

FIGURE 19.2 **Fibro-osseous Pseudotumor.** Irregular trabeculae of bone are formed within plump fasciitis-like spindle cell stroma.

self-limiting lesion that generally matures over several weeks to form a peripheral bony rim. It is a reactive process but its clinical features of rapid growth and histological features of hypercellularity, mitotic activity, and sometimes focal atypia can mimic malignancy, particularly osteosarcoma. Patients present with a rapidly growing mass at any site, but typically the proximal extremities or trunk. The lesion is separate from bone, and usually within skeletal muscle, but sometimes occurs in or extends into subcutaneous tissue. Patients are typically physically active and often have a history of trauma. The radiological features reflect the stage of development of the lesion. When fully developed, they usually show a circumscribed lesion with peripheral lacy bone deposition, in contrast with extraskeletal osteosarcoma (EO) where the bone formation is more frequently in the center of the tumor. After time the lesion may remain stable or undergo resorption, with some lesions regressing completely. Recurrence is rare if the lesion is completely excised.

Pathologic Features

Grossly lesions are circumscribed and of variable size. There is a spectrum of microscopic features, but characteristically the lesion is composed of fibroblasts and osteoblastic elements that form bone with a "zonal" pattern (Figs. 19.3 and 19.4, e-Figs. 19.5 and 19.6). The appearance varies according to the stage of development. The lesion is most cellular in its earliest stage. The central aspect of the lesion resembles nodular fasciitis, with loosely fascicular or patternless arrays of spindle and stellate fibroblasts and myofibroblasts with vesicular nuclei and small nucleoli (e-Figs. 19.5 and 19.6). There is no significant atypia, unlike in EO. Mitotic figures can be frequent, although atypical ones are not seen. The stroma is

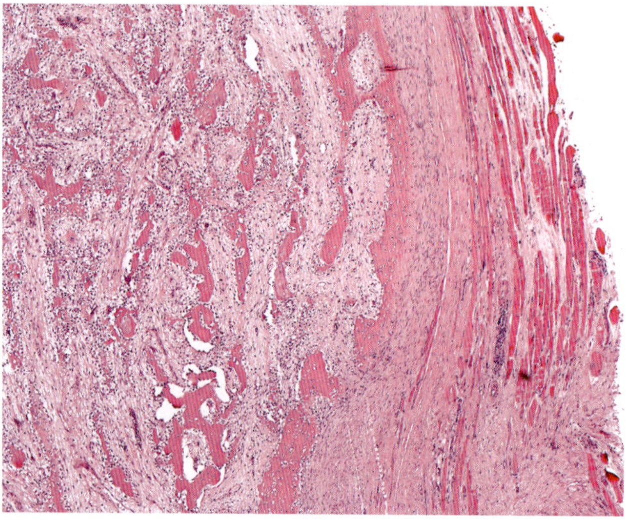

FIGURE 19.3 **Myositis Ossificans.** The tumor typically has a zonal pattern, with a peripheral rim of more mature bone and a central loose spindle to stellate cell element with metaplastic bone formation.

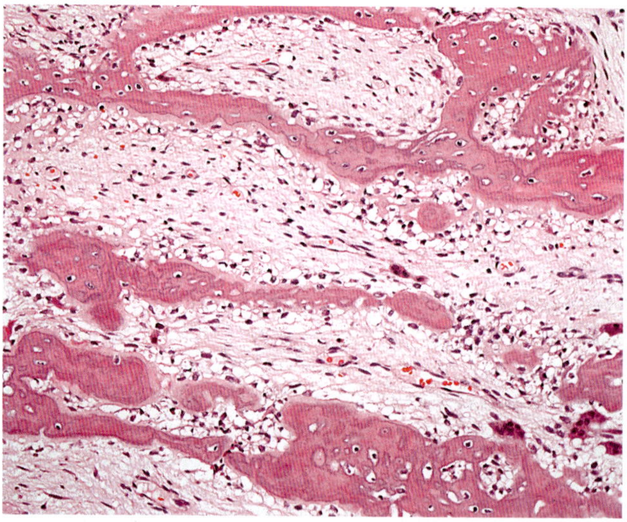

FIGURE 19.4 **Myositis Ossificans.** This is composed of fibroblastic and osteoblastic elements that form bone. The appearances vary according to the stage of development.

myxoid and vascular (Fig. 19.4, e-Figs. 19.6), with variable chronic inflammation, extravasated erythrocytes, and fibrinoid material. Osteoclast-like giant cells can be present (e-Fig. 19.6), as well as damaged muscle fibers. There is a transition zone with active bone formation, with trabeculae of woven bone with osteoblastic rimming, and sometimes admixed areas of

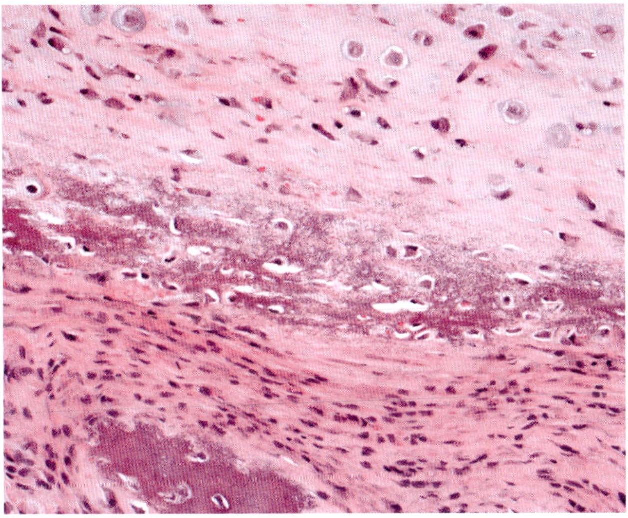

FIGURE 19.5 **Myositis Ossificans.** Foci of cartilage formation can sometimes be a feature.

hyaline cartilage (Fig. 19.5, e-Fig. 19.7). Peripherally, the lesion comprises a layer of well-formed bone (e-Fig. 19.8), initially of woven appearance and later remodeled to lamellar bone. A thin layer of fibrous tissue usually surrounds the lesion. Eventually, the cellular areas within the center become more fibrotic and paucicellular (e-Fig. 19.9) and undergo ossification. In the latest stages, the lesion comprises bone with hematopoietic or fatty marrow.

Ancillary Investigations

The fibroblastic cells show variable expression of smooth muscle actin or less commonly desmin.

Variants

Heterotopic mesenteric ossification is a similar lesion that occurs in the abdomen, often following surgery (see Chapter 5).[5]

Fibrodysplasia ossificans progressive (MO progressive) is a rare genetic disorder due to mutations in the *ACVR1* gene located in chromosome 2q23–24.[6,7] This encodes for bone morphogenetic protein type-1 receptor, which is involved in the normal process of bone ossification. There is also overproduction of bone morphogenetic protein 4. Following injury, skeletal muscle, tendons, and ligaments are gradually replaced by bone. The disease is inherited in an autosomal dominant fashion and presents congenitally or in childhood with a typical clinical feature of deformed toes. Ossification begins in upper back muscles and spreads peripherally to other parts of trunk and to limbs. The diagnosis is best made by clinical and radiologic features, and biopsy should be avoided since it provokes further bone formation. Histologically, there is initially a nodular fasciitis-like proliferation (e-Figs. 19.10–19.12) that can also resemble infantile fibromatosis. This is succeeded by calcification and metaplastic bone and cartilage formation with replacement of muscle.

OSSIFYING FIBROMYXOID TUMOR

This is discussed in Chapter 21. Mature bone is present in about 75% of cases as a partial shell in the fibrous capsule or septa. Cartilage is less commonly seen. In atypical ossifying fibromyxoid tumor, there can be osteoid and bone formation within the tumor, and rarely this can appear malignant, overlapping with EO.

EXTRASKELETAL OSTEOSARCOMA

EO is a malignant tumor of soft tissue characterized by neoplastic bone or osteoid formation. This is a common feature of all EO, but some also demonstrate chondroblastic differentiation. EO is rare, accounting for fewer than 5% of osteosarcomas, and in contrast to osteosarcoma of bone that predominantly occurs during the first 2 decades of life, it occurs most often in older adults.[8]

Clinical Features

EO arises predominantly during mid to late adulthood, affecting both sexes but more often in males. Some tumors arise in an area of prior therapeutic irradiation for other neoplasms. Tumors are subcutaneous or located in deep soft tissue, without skeletal attachment, although underlying bone

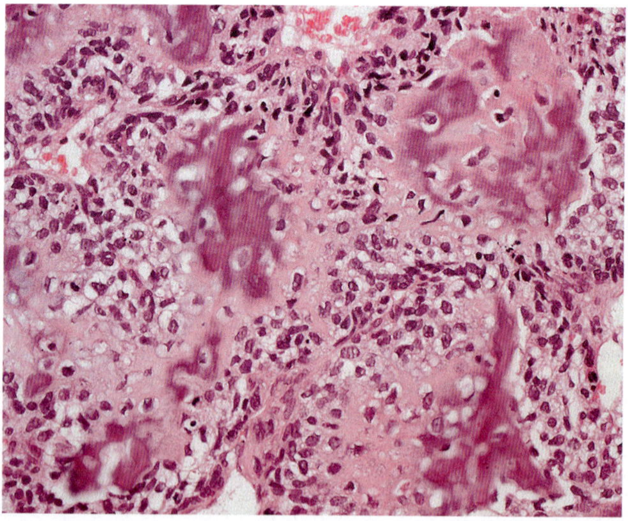

FIGURE 19.6 **Extraskeletal Osteosarcoma.** Pleomorphic tumor cells produce malignant osteoid and bone.

can be secondarily involved. Common sites include the extremities, especially thigh, and retroperitoneum (here often representing dedifferentiated liposarcoma), but other sites can also be affected. Patients usually present with an enlarging, sometimes painful mass. Most tumors are aggressive with 65% metastasizing, mostly to lung, and a 5-year survival rate of 37%.[9]

Pathologic Features

EO is often circumscribed and large, pale or light brown on cut surface with hemorrhage, necrosis, and a firm finely or coarsely gritty consistency. There may be cystic change. By definition, EO contains malignant cells of osteoblastic type, which produce osteoid and bone (Fig. 19.6, e-Fig. 19.13). The amount of the latter components can vary and sometimes involve only a small proportion of the specimen. EO can display any of the histological patterns of its counterpart in bone. These include osteoblastic, chondroblastic, fibroblastic, telangiectatic, well-differentiated,[10] and malignant fibrous histiocytoma (MFH)-like (Fig. 19.7) subtypes, as well as rare examples with aneurysmal bone cyst-like features.[11] The constituent cells vary from spindled to polygonal, and show cytological atypia that is often marked (Fig. 19.7, e-Figs. 19.14 and 19.15) Mitotic figures are prominent, including atypical forms. Most EO resemble pleomorphic undifferentiated sarcoma ("MFH-like") (Fig. 19.7, e-Fig. 19.15), with a varying degree of deposition of tumoral (malignant) osteoid and bone (e-Figs. 19.16 and 19.17). Osteoid deposits comprise trabecular (Fig. 19.8, e-Fig. 19.16) or ramifying (e-Fig. 19.18) areas of eosinophilic material containing anaplastic cells, often in prominent lacunae. Within the osteoid deposits, there is

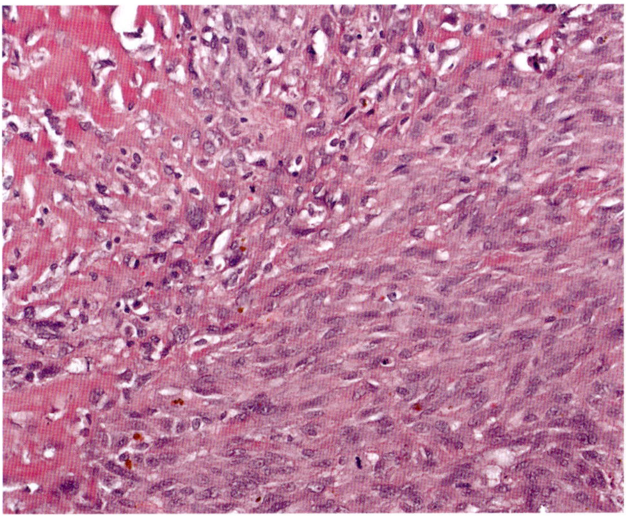

FIGURE 19.7 **Extraskeletal Osteosarcoma.** Tumor cells here show a fibrosarcoma-like fascicular architecture.

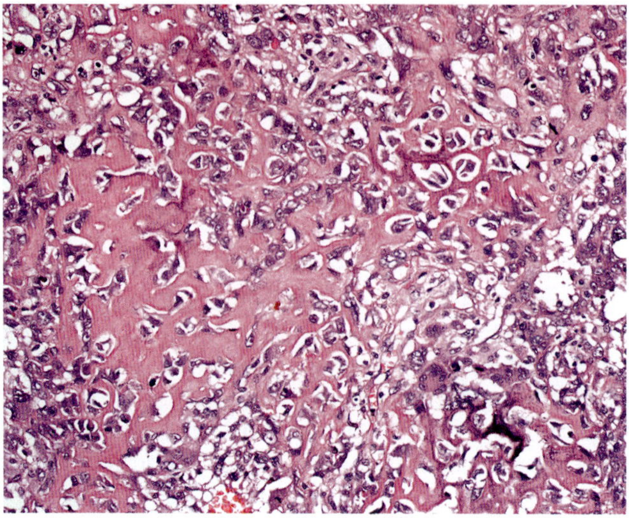

FIGURE 19.8 **Extraskeletal Osteosarcoma.** Tumoral osteoid in broad trabeculae, with lacunae containing atypical polygonal cells.

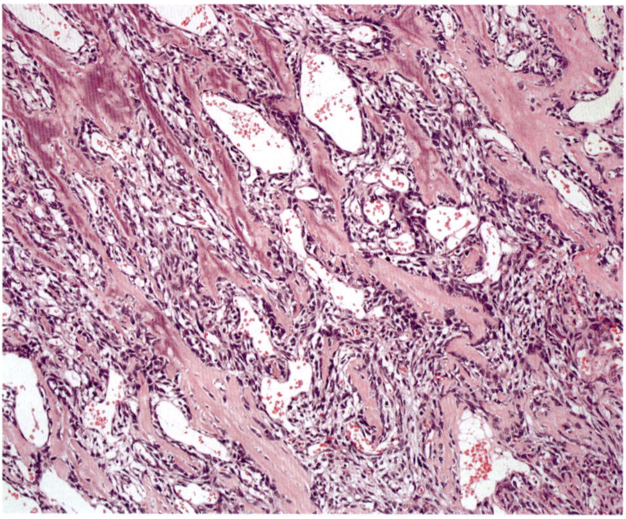

FIGURE 19.9 **Extraskeletal Osteosarcoma.** The bone forms a regular filigree pattern of branching trabeculae.

variable calcification (e-Fig. 19.18) and ossification, with the bone sometimes assuming a filigree pattern (Fig. 19.9). In EO, bone formation is found more centrally, in contrast to MO where bony deposition tends to be at the periphery of the lesion. Malignant cartilage can also be present (e-Fig. 19.19).

When EO is found in a biopsy, especially in tumors of deep soft tissue or retroperitoneum, the possibility of divergent differentiation should be considered and features of associated MPNSTs, dedifferentiated liposarcoma, or sarcomatoid carcinomas should be excluded, by both careful microscopic examination and appropriate immunohistochemistry.

Ancillary Investigations

EO expresses osteocalcin and osteonectin, although immunohistochemical detection of these is only necessary for diagnosis of osteoid in occasional cases. There is also positivity for CD99, and variable focal expression of muscle markers, S100 protein, and cytokeratins.[12] These and other immunohistochemical findings should be evaluated in light of the morphology in case the osteosarcoma represents a divergent component of a different tumor type.

TUMORS FORMING CARTILAGE

Metaplastic mature or immature cartilage formation is seen in a variety of benign and malignant neoplasms including lipoma (Chapter 15), well-differentiated and myxoid liposarcoma (Chapter 16), nerve sheath tumors (Chapter 9), and embryonal rhabdomyosarcoma (Chapter 10). Care must be taken to recognize the underlying tumor and not to misinterpret as chondrosarcoma. Malignant cartilage generally has increased cellularity, variation in cell size, binucleation, nuclear pleomorphism, and (rarely) mitotic activity. The lower grades, however, can sometimes be difficult to diagnose as malignant, and careful attention must be paid to clinical and other morphologic features.

SOFT TISSUE CHONDROMA

Clinical Features

Soft tissue chondromas are benign cartilaginous tumors occurring in extraosseous and extra-articular soft tissue sites, and mostly in the extremities.[13,14] They are most frequent in middle-aged adults,[13] and are most common in the fingers, but also occur on the hands, toes, feet and trunk and rarely in the skin, dura, or fallopian tube. In the lung, chondroma can be associated with epithelioid gastric stromal tumor and extra-adrenal paraganglioma as Carney triad, usually in females (c-Fig. 19.19a).[15] Soft tissue chondroma typically forms a slowly enlarging, usually painless solitary mass, often close to tendons and joint capsules.[16] Tumors can recur locally, but excision is usually curative, and malignant transformation to chondrosarcoma is not reported.

Pathologic Features

Grossly, the lesion is usually <3 cm in diameter, circumscribed, lobulated, and often multinodular. The cut surface is firm and cartilaginous, with

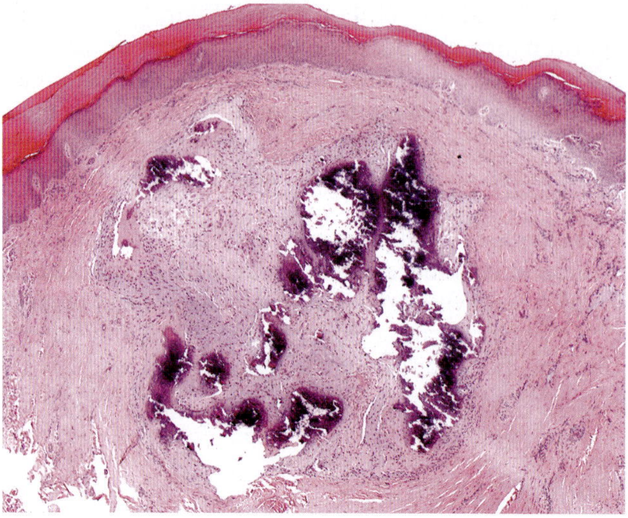

FIGURE 19.10 **Soft Tissue Chondroma.** The lesion is subcutaneous and comprises lobules of mature hyaline cartilage with foci of calcification.

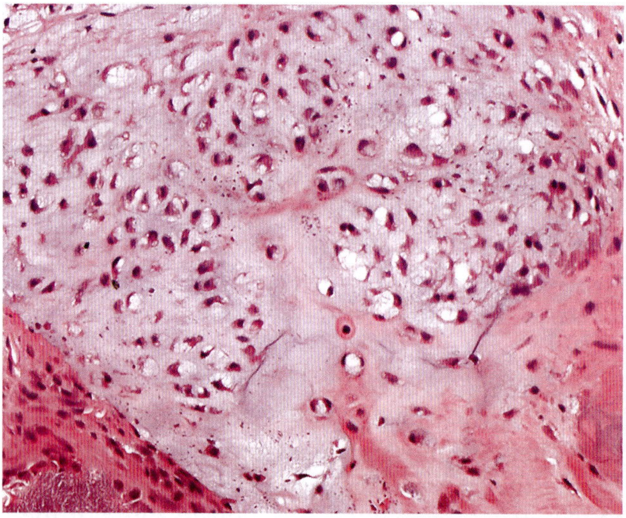

FIGURE 19.11 **Soft Tissue Chondroma.** Lesional cellularity varies. This lesion is moderately cellular.

variable calcification and cystic and myxoid areas. Histologically, the tumor is composed predominantly of lobules of hyaline cartilage, in which chondrocytes are present in nests and clusters (Fig. 19.10, e-Fig. 19.20). Cellularity varies from sparse (e-Fig. 19.21) to moderate (Fig. 19.11), and hypercellular areas may be noted (e-Fig. 19.22). Most chondrocytes are small, but there can be variation in shape and size, with plump, hyperchromatic, more immature-appearing forms (e-Fig. 19.23), and there may

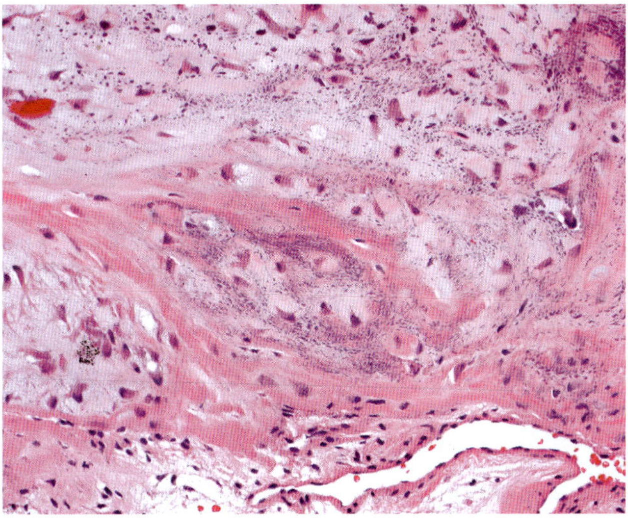

FIGURE 19.12 **Soft Tissue Chondroma.** There are plump, immature chondrocytes and early fine calcification in a pericellular distribution.

be atypia ranging from mild to moderate. Although cells with immature appearances can resemble chondrosarcoma, more mature and sparsely cellular cartilaginous areas in other areas identify the lesion as a chondroma. Small numbers of mitoses can occur, without atypical forms. Some lesions show ossification, focal fibrosis, or marked myxoid stromal change, which is occasionally so abundant that the tumor resembles myxoid chondrosarcoma. Calcification can be present (Fig. 19.12, e-Figs. 19.24–19.27), particularly centrally, and typically, there is a stippled pattern of deposition with a ring-like layer of calcification around the tumor cells (e-Fig. 19.24). The calcification can be widespread (e-Fig. 19.27), and in some cases a careful search is required to identify the lesional cells. Some lesions show a surrounding granuloma-like reaction,[17] with clusters of epithelioid and multinucleated histiocytes surrounding tumor lobules (e-Figs. 19.27–19.29).

Ancillary Investigations

Immunohistochemically, the chondrocytes are positive for S100 protein. Clonal chromosomal abnormalities have been shown in some cases of soft tissue chondroma,[18] including rearrangements of HMGA2 gene at 12q15.[19]

SYNOVIAL CHONDROMATOSIS

This is a rare neoplasm of unknown cause, associated with the formation of cartilaginous or osteocartilaginous nodules in the synovial membranes.[20]

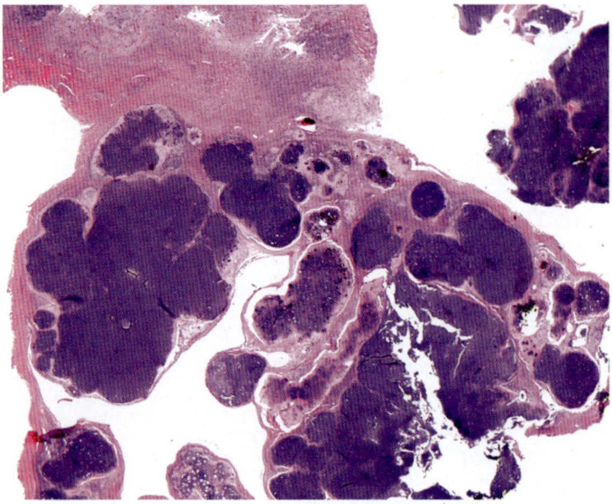

FIGURE 19.13 **Synovial Chondromatosis.** Variably cellular nodules of hyaline cartilage.

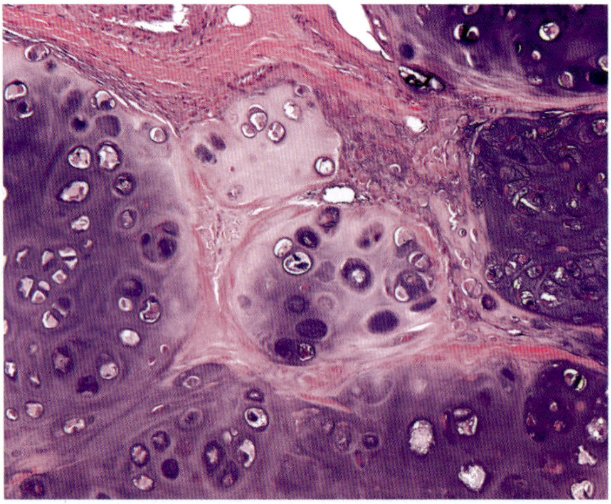

FIGURE 19.14 **Synovial Chondromatosis.** Cells are arranged in clusters and are frequently plump. Binucleate forms are notable.

Clinical Features

Synovial chondromatosis occurs in adults, with a male predilection.[21] The lesion affects the synovium of joints, bursae or tendon sheaths, and most commonly occurs in large joints such as the knee or hip, although other joints, such as those in the ankle, the upper limb, and the temporomandibular joint, can be affected. Rarely, a similar lesion can develop within soft tissue adjacent to but not communicating with the joint.[22,23] Symptoms are nonspecific and include pain and swelling or locking of the joint. The nodules can be confined to the synovium, or become detached and present in the joint cavity as loose bodies.[24] When calcified or ossified, the nodules can be detected by imaging as multiple discrete radio-opaque bodies. Treatment of primary disease is surgical synovectomy with removal of chondroid fragments; recurrence rates range from 3% to 23%.[25] Synovial chondromatosis has the potential for malignant transformation to chondrosarcoma,[21,26,27] with a relative risk of 5% in one large series.[21] Malignant change is suggested in chronic cases with sudden exacerbation of symptoms or by multiple recurrences and marrow invasion.[25]

Pathologic Features

Macroscopically, the lesion comprises multiple irregular, glistening, white nodules within synovial tissue, which vary in size from millimeters to several centimeters. Microscopically, the nodules are variably cellular and consist of islands of hyaline cartilage (Fig. 19.13, e-Fig. 19.30) covered by a thin layer of fibrous tissue (Fig. 19.14), or by synovial lining cells. Histological diagnosis requires the nodules to be present within the synovial membrane, as loose bodies within the joint cavity can also occur in other joint conditions such as osteoarthritis and osteochondritis dissecans. The cells are often plump and arranged in clusters (e-Fig. 19.31). Binucleate forms can be present (Fig. 19.14), as well as mild to moderate atypia (e-Fig. 19.32). These features, as well as areas of hypercellularity, do not indicate malignancy but may cause confusion with chondrosarcoma. Mitotic figures may be present, calcification can be extensive, and ossification sometimes occurs.

Ancillary Investigations

Cytogenetic analyses have shown clonal chromosomal aberrations in a few lesions,[28,29] consistent with neoplastic etiology, including rearrangement of 1p and anomalies of chromosome 6.[30]

Well-differentiated chondrosarcoma is usually found in soft tissue by extension from a tumor of skeletal origin. It is composed of lobules of differentiated, variably cellular hyaline cartilage. In a small biopsy of a soft tissue tumor, the presence of differentiated cartilage with cytologically malignant features should prompt careful examination for other components including osteosarcoma, MPNST, and (especially in the abdomen) dedifferentiated liposarcoma.

EXTRASKELETAL MESENCHYMAL CHONDROSARCOMA

Extraskeletal mesenchymal chondrosarcoma (EMC) is a rare, malignant tumor of bone and soft tissue, composed of islands of variably differentiated cartilage interspersed among sheets of undifferentiated primitive mesenchymal cells resembling other small round cell tumors. The expression in EMC of *Sox-9*, a gene that is a key regulator of chondrogenesis, supports interpretation of this tumor as a variant of chondrosarcoma.

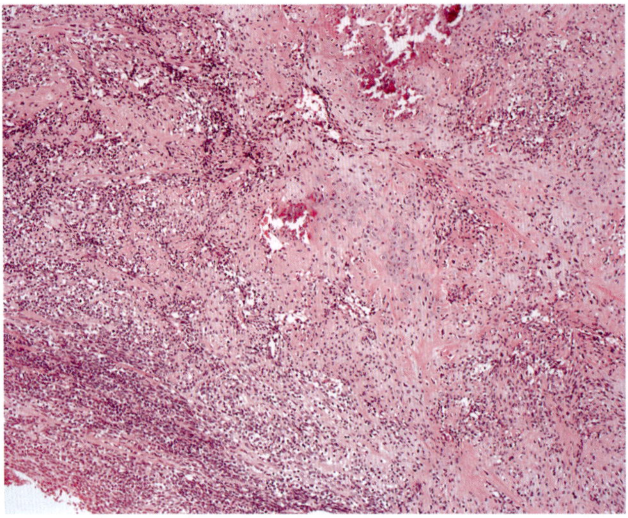

FIGURE 19.15 **Extraskeletal Mesenchymal Chondrosarcoma.** The tumor has a biphasic appearance, with a primitive component of small round cells and a cartilaginous component. The boundary is well demarcated in this lesion.

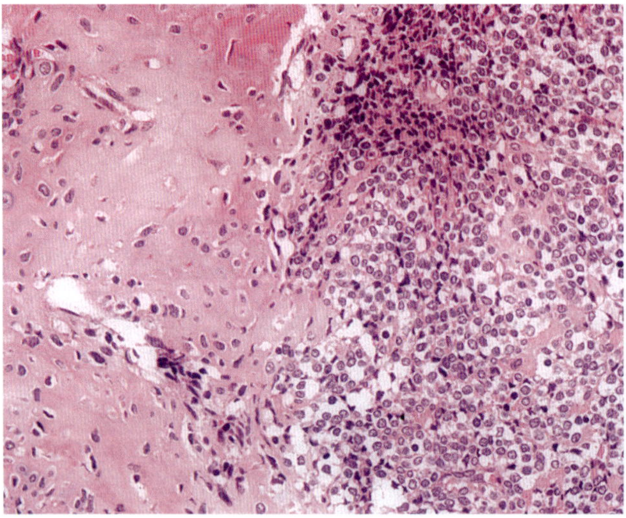

FIGURE 19.16 **Extraskeletal Mesenchymal Chondrosarcoma.** Islands of well-differentiated hyaline cartilage are interspersed.

Clinical Features

EMC predilects for young adults and occurs slightly more frequently in females than males. Although most mesenchymal chondrosarcomas occur in bone, up to a third occur in soft tissues and meninges. Common soft tissue sites are the head and neck, including nose, and the extremities,

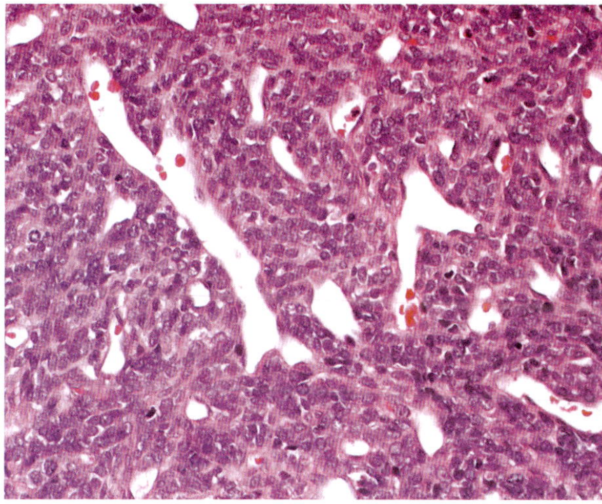

FIGURE 19.17 **Extraskeletal Mesenchymal Chondrosarcoma.** A hemangiopericytic vascular pattern is often prominent, imparting resemblance to synovial sarcoma.

although it is important to exclude metastasis from an intraosseous site. The microscopic features of EMC are similar to those in bone. EMC generally has a poor prognosis, with local recurrence and metastases in a high proportion of cases.

Pathologic Features

Grossly, the tumor is a lobulated circumscribed mass, which can vary in size. The cut surface is gray to tan, with firm areas of cartilage or bone. Hemorrhage and necrosis may be prominent. Microscopically, the tumor has a characteristic biphasic appearance (Fig. 19.15). The primitive or undifferentiated component comprises hypercellular collections of small cells with round, ovoid (e-Figs. 19.33 and 19.34), or sometimes more spindled nuclei (e-Figs. 19.35 and 19.36) and scanty cytoplasm, resembling the cells of Ewing Sarcoma/primitive neuroectodermal tumor (PNET) (e-Fig. 19.37). Interspersed are islands of hyaline cartilage (Fig. 19.15, e-Fig. 19.38) that can show calcification or ossification. Although the cartilage often has a “benign” appearance, it may also have the morphology of well-differentiated chondrosarcoma (e-Fig. 19.39). The boundaries between the two components are usually abrupt (Fig. 19.16), but there can also be a more gradual blending of areas (e-Fig. 19.40). The proportions of the two components can also vary, with either predominating, and cartilage can be absent in many blocks so that extensive sampling is indicated. There is often a prominent hemangiopericytic vascular pattern, with large thin-walled vascular spaces (Fig. 19.17, e-Figs. 19.41 and 19.42), and the tumor can be mistaken for poorly differentiated synovial sarcoma. Necrosis can be present (e-Fig. 19.43), and osteoclast-like giant cells may also be seen.

Ancillary Investigations

In general, the diagnosis is morphological, and immunohistochemistry is of limited use. The small cell component is positive for CD99, similar to the cells in Ewing sarcoma/PNET, but the latter tumor only very exceptionally shows cartilage formation. The tumor does not express cytokeratin, EMA, or muscle markers. S100 protein may be positive in scanty numbers of cells, but is usually absent, whereas the cartilaginous areas show strong expression of S100 protein as in other forms of chondrosarcoma. EMC expresses Sox-9, unlike other small round cell tumors, which can be useful in diagnosis.[31] Also, EMC lacks *EWSR1* or *SS18* gene rearrangements, which assists the distinction from Ewing sarcoma and synovial sarcoma, respectively.

REFERENCES

1. Dupree WB, Enzinger FM. Fibro-osseous pseudotumor of the digits. *Cancer.* 1986;58:2103–2109.
2. Moosavi CA, Al-Nahar LA, Murphey MD, et al. Fibroosseous [corrected] pseudotumor of the digit: a clinicopathologic study of 43 new cases. *Ann Diagn Pathol.* 2008;12:21–28.
3. Chaudhry IH, Kazakov DV, Michal M et al. Fibro-osseous pseudotumor of the digit: a clinicopathological study of 17 cases. *J Cutan Pathol.* 2010;37:323–329.
4. de Silva MV, Reid R. Myositis ossificans and fibroosseous pseudotumor of digits: a clinicopathological review of 64 cases with emphasis on diagnostic pitfalls. *Int J Surg Pathol.* 2003;11:187–195.
5. Patel RM, Weiss SW, Folpe AL. Heterotopic mesenteric ossification: a distinctive pseudosarcoma commonly associated with intestinal obstruction. *Am J Surg Pathol.* 2006;30:119–122.
6. Shore EM, Xu M, Feldman GJ, et al. A recurrent mutation in the BMP type I receptor ACVR1 causes inherited and sporadic fibrodysplasia ossificans progressiva. *Nat Genet.* 2006;38:525–527.
7. Shore EM, Kaplan FS. Insights from a rare genetic disorder of extra-skeletal bone formation, fibrodysplasia ossificans progressiva (FOP). *Bone.* 2008;43:427–433.
8. Chung EB, Enzinger FM. Extraskeletal osteosarcoma. *Cancer.* 1987;60:1132–1142.
9. Lee JS, Fetsch JF, Wasdhal DA, et al. A review of 40 patients with extraskeletal osteosarcoma. *Cancer.* 1995;76:2253–2259.
10. Yi ES, Shmookler BM, Malawer MM, et al. Well-differentiated extraskeletal osteosarcoma. A soft-tissue homologue of parosteal osteosarcoma. *Arch Pathol Lab Med.* 1991;115:906–909.
11. Laforga JB, Jover A, Martinez P. Soft-tissue osteosarcoma with prominent aneurysmatic bone cyst-like features: a case report. *Diagn Cytopathol.* 2001;24:209–214.
12. Lidang Jensen M, Schumacher B, Myhre Jensen O, et al. Extraskeletal osteosarcomas: a clinicopathologic study of 25 cases. *Am J Surg Pathol.* 1998;22:588–594.
13. Chung EB, Enzinger FM. Chondroma of soft parts. *Cancer.* 1978;41:1414–1424.
14. Dahlin DC, Salvador AH. Cartilaginous tumors of the soft tissues of the hands and feet. *Mayo Clin Proc.* 1974;49:721–726.
15. Carney JA. Carney triad: a syndrome featuring paraganglionic, adrenocortical, and possibly other endocrine tumors. *J Clin Endocrinol Metab.* 2009;94:3656–3662.
16. Bansal M, Goldman AB, DiCarlo EF, et al. Soft tissue chondromas: diagnosis and differential diagnosis. *Skeletal Radiol.* 1993;22:309–315.

17. Yamada T, Irisa T, Nakano S, et al. Extraskeletal chondroma with chondroblastic and granuloma-like elements. *Clin Orthop Relat Res.* 1995;257–261.
18. Buddingh EP, Naumann S, Nelson M, et al. Cytogenetic findings in benign cartilaginous neoplasms. *Cancer Genet Cytogenet.* 2003;141:164–168.
19. Dahlen A, Mertens F, Rydholm A, et al. Fusion, disruption, and expression of HMGA2 in bone and soft tissue chondromas. *Mod Pathol.* 2003;16:1132–1140.
20. Baunsgaard P, Nielsen BB. Primary synovial chondrometaplasia. Histologic variations in the structure of metaplastic nodules. *Acta Pathol Microbiol Immunol Scand A.* 1984;92:455–460.
21. Davis RI, Hamilton A, Biggart JD. Primary synovial chondromatosis: a clinicopathologic review and assessment of malignant potential. *Hum Pathol.* 1998;29:683–688.
22. Sim FH, Dahlin DC, Ivins JC. Extra-articular synovial chondromatosis. *J Bone Joint Surg Am.* 1977;59:492–495.
23. Sviland L, Malcolm AJ. Synovial chondromatosis presenting as painless soft tissue mass–a report of 19 cases. *Histopathology.* 1995;27:275–279.
24. Milgram JW. Synovial osteochondromatosis: a histopathological study of thirty cases. *J Bone Joint Surg Am.* 1977;59:792–801.
25. Murphey MD, Vidal JA, Fanburg-Smith JC, et al. Imaging of synovial chondromatosis with radiologic-pathologic correlation. *Radiographics.* 2007;27:1465–1488.
26. Hallam P, Ashwood N, Cobb J, et al. Malignant transformation in synovial chondromatosis of the knee? *Knee.* 2001;8:239–242.
27. Blokx WA, Rasing LA, Veth RP, et al. Late malignant transformation of biopsy proven benign synovial chondromatosis: an unexpected pitfall. *Histopathology.* 2000;36:564–566.
28. Mertens F, Jonsson K, Willen H, et al. Chromosome rearrangements in synovial chondromatous lesions. *Br J Cancer.* 1996;74:251–254.
29. Sciot R, Dal Cin P, Bellemans J, et al. Synovial chondromatosis: clonal chromosome changes provide further evidence for a neoplastic disorder. *Virchows Arch.* 1998;433:189–191.
30. Buddingh EP, Krallman P, Neff JR, et al. Chromosome 6 abnormalities are recurrent in synovial chondromatosis. *Cancer Genet Cytogenet.* 2003;140:18–22.
31. Wehrli BM, Huang W, De Crombrugghe B, et al. Sox9, a master regulator of chondrogenesis, distinguishes mesenchymal chondrosarcoma from other small blue round cell tumors. *Hum Pathol.* 2003;34:263–269.

20

MYXOID TUMORS OF SUPERFICIAL SOFT TISSUE

INTRODUCTION

As a general rule, superficial myxoid lesions are benign, and deep ones are often malignant, with the important exceptions that intramuscular myxoma is deep and myxofibrosarcoma (also called myxoid malignant fibrous histiocytoma) is classically superficial. These latter two lesions are covered in Chapter 21 and are likely to be sampled on needle biopsies, whereas superficial lesions are typically managed by excisional biopsy. The classic myxoid lesions of the genital region (aggressive angiomyxoma and angiomyofibroblastoma) are considered in Chapter 8.

CUTANEOUS MYXOMA AND SUPERFICIAL ANGIOMYXOMA (CUTANEOUS ANGIOMYXOMA)

Myxomas of the dermis and subcutaneous tissue are less well characterized than the more frequently encountered deep intramuscular myxomas and those arising in the jaw bones and heart. In 1985, Carney et al.[1] described a complex of myxomas, including cutaneous myxomas, spotty pigmentation, and endocrine overactivity. In 1988, Allen et al.[2] delineated the clinicopathologic features of histologically similar appearing myxoid lesions of the dermis and subcutaneous tissue that lacked an association with Carney's complex. After a critical review of the literature, Allen et al.[2] concluded that the lesions he described, many previously reported and variously named myxoid lesions of the dermis and subcutis, as well as the "cutaneous myxomas" of Carney's complex, were all closely related. The term, "superficial angiomyxoma" was proposed to encompass both syndromic and sporadic superficial myxomas. Superficial angiomyxomas were unassociated with Carney's complex in a subsequent series.[3]

Clinical Features

Allen et al.[2] described three clinical presentations of superficial myxomas. The most common presentation is that of a solitary lesion unassociated with Carney's complex, followed by multiple lesions unassociated with Carney's complex, and lastly, lesions associated with the fully expressed Carney's complex.

Superficial angiomyxoma/cutaneous myxoma unassociated with Carney's complex presents as a painless, slow-growing, solitary skin nodule with a slight male predominance. Lesions arise primarily on the trunk and lower extremity, followed by the head and neck region and arm. They have also been reported in the female and male genital regions.[4]

Carney's complex[1] includes pigmented skin lesions (lentigines and giant cell blue nevi), endocrine disorders (primary pigmented nodular adrenocortical disease, a variety of stromal tumors of the testis, and growth hormone-producing pituitary adenoma), psammomatous melanocytic schwannoma, and myxomatous tumors (cardiac myxoma, myxoid fibroadenoma of the breast, myxoma of the external ear canal,[5] and cutaneous myxoma). The disorder is familial and transmitted as an autosomal dominant trait. Females are affected slightly more often than males and the initial lesions manifest at an early age (mean age of 18 years). Most patients do not have all of the lesions. However, as the cardiac myxoma and the psammomatous melanocytic schwannoma are the main causes of morbidity and mortality in this disorder,[1,6] it is important to identify patients at risk so that proper evaluation for these potentially lethal tumors can be performed.

Superficial myxomas associated with Carney's complex are usually multiple and vary from small sessile papules to large pedunculated lesions. They most commonly occur on the eyelid.[1]

Cutaneous myxomas are benign, but local recurrence is common, especially with superficial angiomyxomas containing epithelial components.[2]

Pathologic Features

On gross examination, the tumor consists of soft, lobulated nodules, which may appear as polypoid or pedunculated skin lesions. The majority of lesions range between 1 and 5 cm. The cut surface is glistening, mucoid or gelatinous, and gray to white. Incomplete collagenous bands traverse the cut surface, resulting in a nodular configuration.

Microscopically, the process typically involves both the dermis and the subcutaneous fat, but, occasionally, only one location is affected (Fig. 20.1). The tumor consists of multiple, variably demarcated angiomyxoid nodules (Fig. 20.2, e-Fig. 20.1). The nodules are composed of a hypo- to moderately cellular population of bland-appearing, short spindled, stellate-shaped (Fig. 20.3, e-Fig. 20.2), and, occasionally, multinucleated cells scattered haphazardly throughout a highly myxoid stroma. Mitotic activity is negligible.

The stroma contains abundant hyaluronic acid-rich matrix that forms microcysts within the nodules and cleft-like spaces at the interface of the nodule with the surrounding tissue. Thin, wavy collagen fibers course through the stroma. The vascular element consists of small to medium sized, thin-walled, nonarborizing vessels. The vascular density of the nodules varies. Other features observed in superficial angiomyxoma include some perivascular hyalinization, a mixed inflammatory infiltrate (including neutrophils, Fig. 20.4, e-Fig. 20.3, and mast cells), fibrin and hemosiderin deposition, and interstitial hemorrhage.

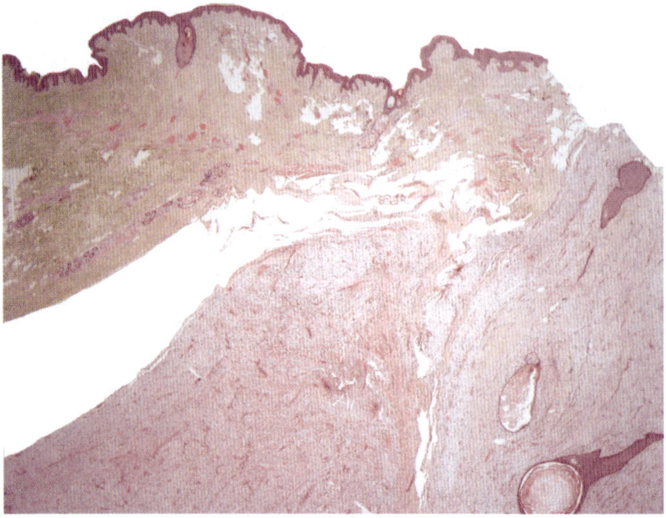

FIGURE 20.1 **Cutaneous Myxoma/Superficial Angiomyxoma.** This lesion is multilobulated and superficial. On the right of the field, the tumor has entrapped skin adnexal structures.

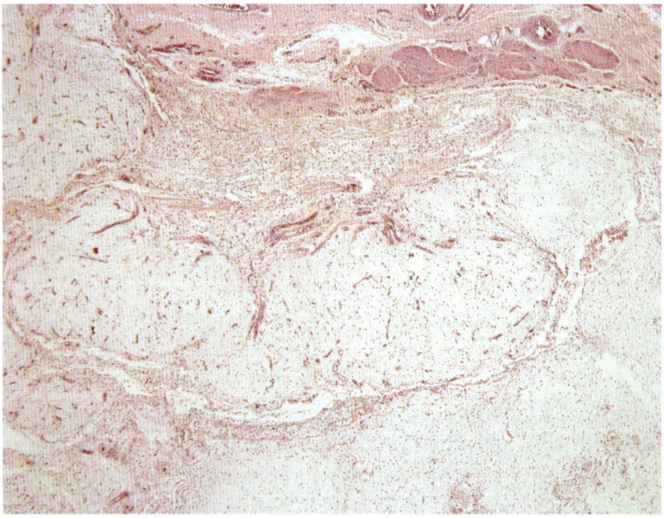

FIGURE 20.2 **Cutaneous Myxoma/Superficial Angiomyxoma.** The tumor lobules have numerous small delicate capillaries.

Epithelial structures within the tumor nodules (Fig. 20.5), including epidermal cysts with keratinous debris and linear strands of squamous cells emanating from the epidermal surface or from a cyst wall, have been identified in about a third of cases and have contributed to the plethora of names given to superficial angiomyxoma in the past.

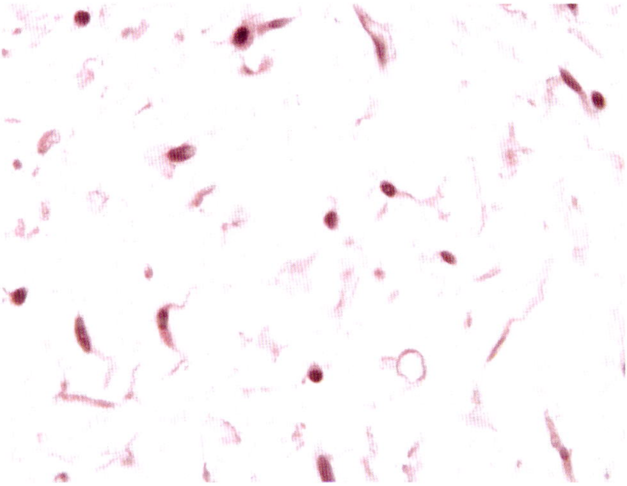

FIGURE 20.3 **Cutaneous Myxoma/Superficial Angiomyxoma.** The proliferating cells are small and bland in this example. Occasional examples are more cellular with larger cells (see also e-Figs. 20.2 and 20.3).

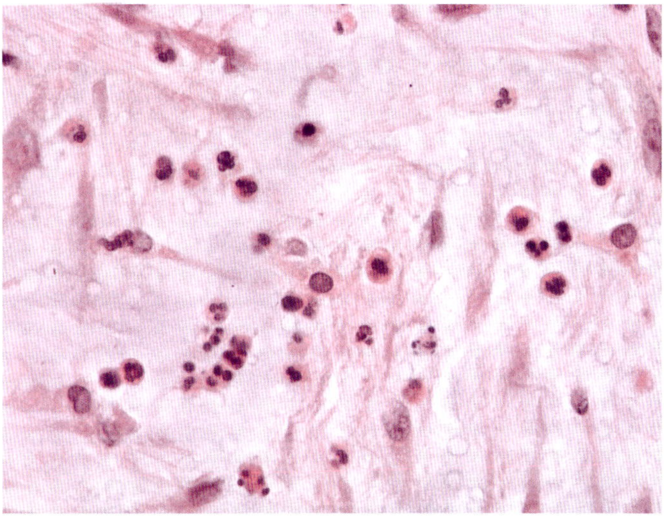

FIGURE 20.4 **Cutaneous Myxoma/Superficial Angiomyxoma.** These tumors often have abundant intralesional neutrophils.

The differential diagnosis is summarized in Table 20.1.

Ancillary Investigations

The reported immunoprofile of myxomas is rather broad with variable immunoreactivity reported for vimentin, CD34, muscle-specific and alpha-smooth muscle actins, and, to a lesser extent, for factor XIIIa and S100 protein.[4]

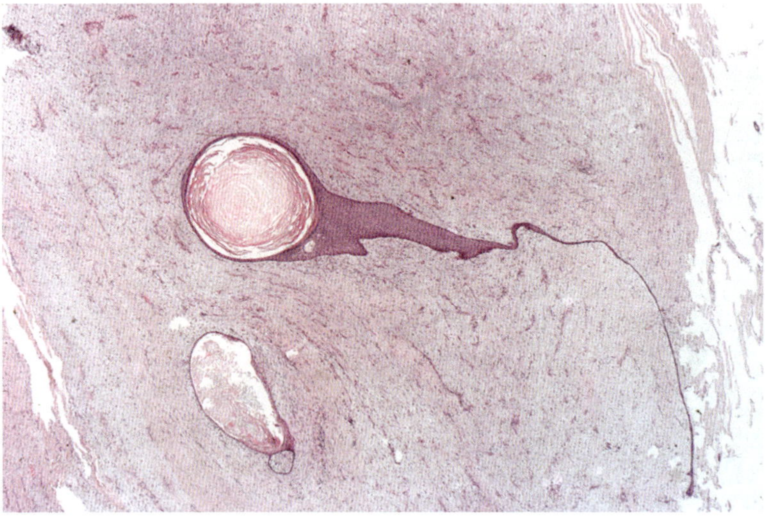

FIGURE 20.5 **Cutaneous Myxoma/Superficial Angiomyxoma.** This example shows entrapped adnexal structures.

TABLE 20.1 Differential Diagnosis of Cutaneous Myxoma/ Angiomyxoma

Lesion	Key features	Distinction from cutaneous myxoma/ angiomyxoma
Cutaneous focal mucinosis	Asymptomatic flesh-colored papule or nodule occurring commonly on face, trunk, or extremities; localized collection of mucin in the dermis with an increased number of fibroblasts	Larger, multilobulated, often involves cutaneous and subcutaneous tissue
Digital mucous cyst	Small and composed of a single mucous cyst of fingers	Smaller, not multilobulated, restricted to digits
Nerve sheath myxoma	Multilobulated myxoid lesion, S100 protein reactive	Multilobulated myxoid lesion, S100 protein–
Neurofibroma	Usually not multilobulated. Contains abundant wiry collagen and mast cells, S100 protein reactive	Multilobulated myxoid lesion, S100 protein–

(Continued)

TABLE 20.1 **Differential Diagnosis of Cutaneous Myxoma/ Angiomyxoma (Continued)**

Lesion	Key features	Distinction from cutaneous myxoma/ angiomyxoma
Lipoma with myxoid stroma	Has fat as an integral part of the lesion	Fat is not an integral part of the lesion
Myxoid dermatofibrosarcoma protuberans (DFSP)	Cellular, large. Usually has areas that show typical nonmyxoid DFSP with repetitive storiform pattern. Consistent CD34+ (e-Figs. 20.4–20.9)	Paucicellular, no storiform pattern, variable CD34+
Low-grade mxyofibrosarcoma	Large lesions composed of scattered overtly hyperchromatic pleomorphic cells, curvilinear vessels	Bland cytology
Embryonal rhabdomyosarcoma	"Cambium layer" under mucosa or epithelium, atypical markedly eosinophilic cells	Desmin+, myogenin+, MyoD1+

SUPERFICIAL ACRAL FIBROMYXOMA

Clinical Features

Fetsch et al.[4] described superficial acral fibromyxoma. They identified 37 cases from 25 men and 12 women ranging in age from 14 to 72 years. The tumors were solitary, involving a toe (20 cases), a finger (13 cases), or the palmar surface of the hand (4 cases), and often (16 cases) involved the nail region. The lesions were slow growing and typically asymptomatic (three were painful). In the original series, about 15% of the lesions recurred, but there were no metastases. In a more recent series that included 32 cases[7] there were 22 males and 10 females with an age range between 23 and 82 years (mean: 51, median: 53). Their lesions had an average size of 2 cm and involved the toes ($n = 15$) and fingers ($n = 13$) with 66.6% of tumors close to or involving the nail bed. Four tumors occurred in the heel. Local recurrences developed in 3 of 14 patients (22%).

Pathologic Features

Tumors range in size from <1 to 5 cm and most are well marginated grossly. Microscopically, these lesions are moderately cellular, consisting

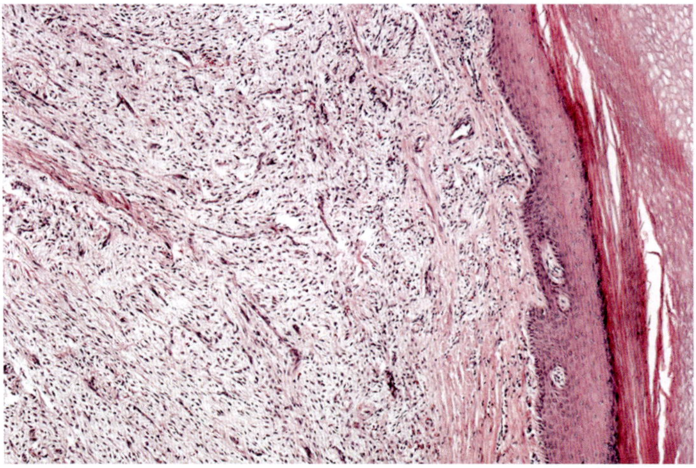

FIGURE 20.6 **Superficial Acral Fibromyxoma.** These tumors often proliferate under the nail bed. They are often richly vascular like this tumor, but some examples are more cellular.

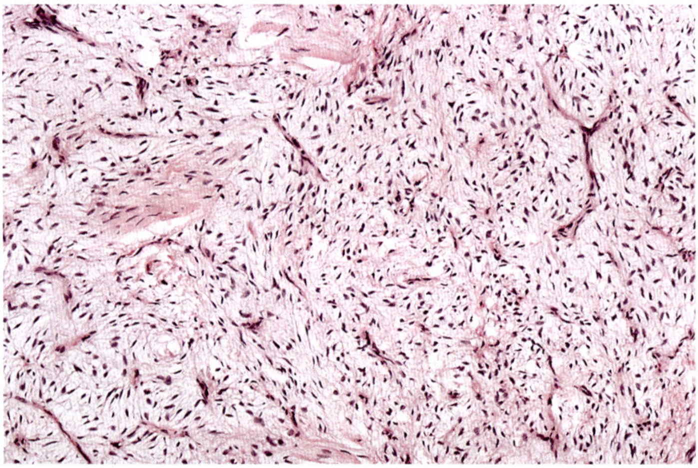

FIGURE 20.7 **Superficial Acral Fibromyxoma.** The tumor is Composed of More Hyperchromatic Cells Than Those Seen in Cutaneous Myxomas. The cells are Stellate to Spindled. Mast cells are usually abundant in these tumors (see e-Figs. 20.12 and 20.13).

of stellate to spindled fibroblastic cells set in myxoid to collagenous stroma with numerous slender vessels (Fig. 20.6, e-Fig. 20.10). Some cases display a focal loose storiform growth similar to fibrous histiocytoma (Fig. 20.7). Scattered multinucleated cells are found in about half of cases (e-Fig. 20.11). Only slight nuclear pleomorphism is detected and mitoses are usually sparse and not atypical. With the exception of mast cells,

TABLE 20.2 Cellular Neurothekeoma and Nerve Sheath Myxoma

Lesion	Clinical features	Histologic features	Ancillary investigations
Cellular neurothekeoma	Common on head, arms, upper limb girdles, recurrences common (about a third)	Multilobulated, large epithelioid cells	S100 protein–, NKI/C3+
"Mixed" cellular neurothekeoma		Multilobulated, mixture of epithelioid cells and myxoid areas with spindle cells.	S100 protein–, NKI/C3+
Myxoid cellular neurothekeoma		Multilobulated, myxoid areas with spindle cells.	S100 protein–, NKI/C3+
Nerve sheath myxoma	Upper extremities, especially hands. Head and neck lesions unusual. Recurrences very common (about half)	Superficial myxoid multinodular masses composed of small spindled cells.	S100 protein+, GFAP+

which are present in most cases (e-Figs. 20.12 and 20.13), there is minimal inflammation.

Ancillary Investigations

Most cases display immunoreactivity for CD34 (e-Fig. 20.14). Epithelial membrane antigen (EMA) and CD99 are detected in some cases but not actins, desmin, glial fibrillary acid protein (GFAP), keratins, HMB-45, and S100 protein.

MYXOID NEURAL AND NEURAL-LIKE LESIONS

Lesions in this general category have been called nerve sheath myxoma, neurothekeoma, cellular neurothekeoma, and myxoid neurothekeoma.[8–11] The literature is confusing on this family of lesions since the terms neurothekeoma and nerve sheath myxoma were used interchangeably in the past when there are actually two entities (Table 20.2), but all are benign and most are superficial. Some, however, are prone to local recurrences based on their infiltrative growth pattern. Remember, however, before considering these more esoteric myxoid lesions, that ordinary neurofibromas are often myxoid (e-Figs. 20.15–20.17).

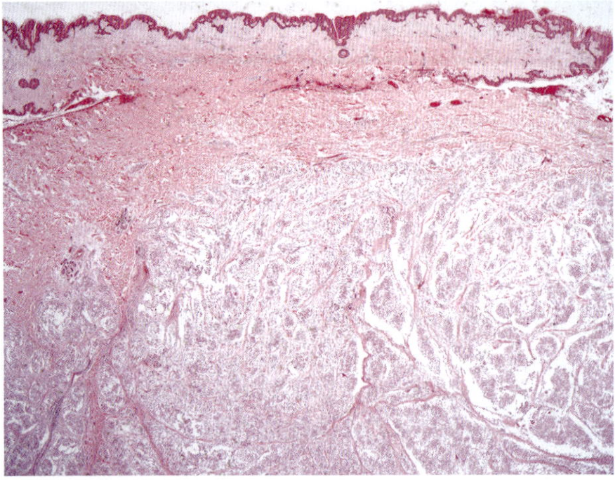

FIGURE 20.8 **Cellular Neurothekeoma.** The tumor consists of Multiple Nodules That Occupy the Deep Dermis and Extend into Subcutaneous Adipose Tissue. The lobules are composed of rounded epithelioid cells.

CELLULAR NEUROTHEKEOMA (See also Chapter 22)

Clinical Features

Cellular neurothekeomas typically present as asymptomatic, solitary, slow-growing, dome-shaped masses that involve the skin and superficial subcutis. Deep involvement of the subcutis is uncommon, and skeletal muscle involvement is rare and largely restricted to the facial region. In a comprehensive series,[8] there was a wide age (i.e., 20 months to 85 years), but most examples presented in the second decade (median age: 17 years). Female patients outnumbered males by a margin of almost 2:1. The tumors had a strong predilection for the head (especially the nose, scalp, orbital regions, cheeks, and chin), arms, and upper limb girdles, with more than 3/4 of cases involving these three sites. The trunk, pelvic girdle, legs, hands, and feet were less commonly affected.

Recurrences are relatively uncommon (up to 10%) and mostly represent incompletely excised lesions. Neurothekeomas are benign neoplasms.

Pathologic Features

Since neurothekeomas are typically biopsied by dermatologists, few data are available concerning their gross appearances. Histologically, the tumors can be segregated into three subgroups, based primarily on the amount of myxoid matrix. Fetsch et al.[4] regarded examples with ≤10% myxoid matrix as cellular neurothekeomas (Figs. 20.8 and 20.9), tumors with >10% but ≤50% myxoid matrix as mixed-type neurothekeomas, and those with >50% myxoid matrix as cellular myxoid neurothekeomas (Figs. 20.10 and 20.11).[8]

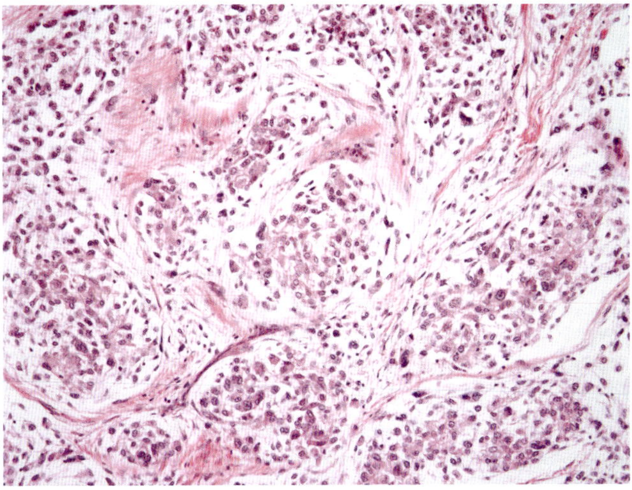

FIGURE 20.9 **Cellular Neurothekeoma.** At high magnification, these tumors can Appear Alarming Since They Display Scattered Enlarged Hyperchromatic Cells. Note the lack of mitotic activity.

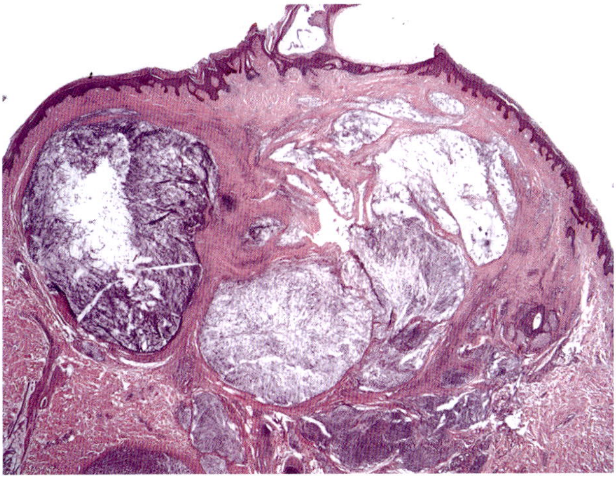

FIGURE 20.10 **Myxoid Neurothekeoma.** Like Cutaneous Myxoma, This tumor is Multilobulated But Differs by Being Less Vascular with More Basophilic Mucinous Matrix.

Despite the differences in matrix, all tumors have certain features, including (a) epithelioid and spindle cells with relatively abundant, somewhat granular-appearing, eosinophilic cytoplasm, (b) a tendency for tumor cells to form multiple small nodules with whorled and sometimes focal fascicular growth, (c) an association with variable amounts of sclerotic collagen, (d) occasional osteoclast-like giant cells, (e-Figs. 20.18–20.22), and (e) a similar immunoprofile (see below). Most have minimal cytologic atypia and

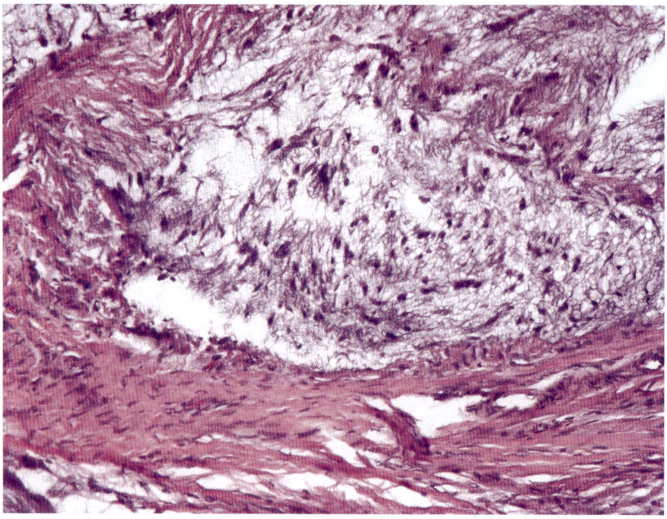

FIGURE 20.11 **Myxoid Neurothekeoma.** These tumors Show Mild Cytologic Atypia.

mitotic activity, but there are some examples displaying atypical nuclei and scattered mitoses.

Ancillary Investigation

On immunohistochemical staining, neurothekeomas nearly invariably express vimentin, NKI/C3, and CD10, and usually MITF, CD99, collagen type IV, NSE, PGP9.5, and CD68. There is variable expression of muscle specific and alpha actin. However, most critically, the consistent lack of S100 protein is the key feature in distinguishing these from true nerve sheath myxomas. Lesions also lack GFAP, melan-A, tyrosinase, NFP, CD34, and desmin.

NERVE SHEATH MYXOMA

Nerve sheath myxomas are far less common than cellular neurothekeomas. In the past, they have been included within the myxoid subgroup of cellular neurothekeoma, but it is now clear, on the basis of the clinical demographics, histomorphology, and immunohistochemical findings, that they are a separate clinicopathologic entity. The distinction is clinically relevant, because nerve sheath myxomas are more likely to recur than cellular neurothekeomas (about half of cases).

Clinical Features

True nerve sheath myxomas have a peak incidence in the fourth decade, occur with approximately equal frequency in males and females, and have a strong predilection for the extremities (especially the hands), and have

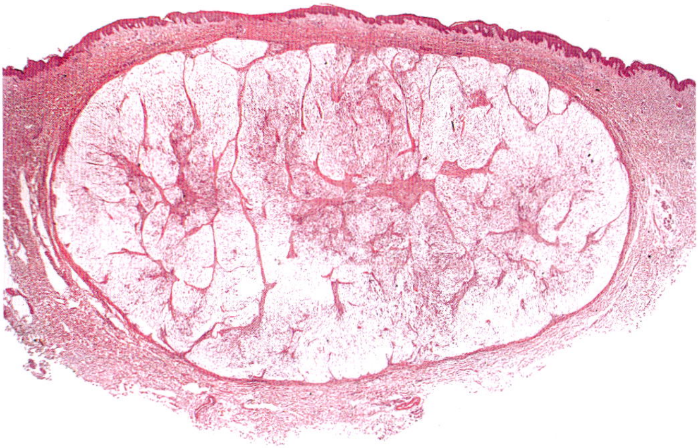

FIGURE 20.12 **Nerve Sheath Myxoma.** Like lesions in the cellular neurothekeoma family, they are lobulated and appear quite similar. Often, the individual lobules are less sharply defined than those of cellular neurothekeoma, as seen in e-Figure 20.23. Immunohistochemistry for S100 protein is positive.

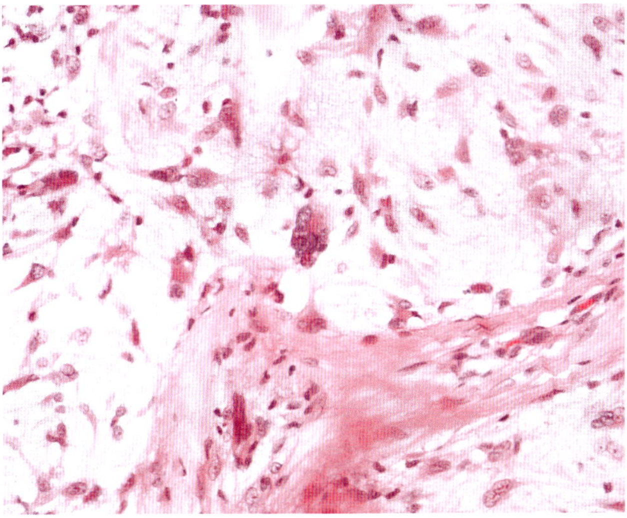

FIGURE 20.13 **Nerve Sheath Myxoma.** Some examples have Scattered Atypical Cells.

a high local recurrence rate when incompletely excised. They only rarely involve the head and neck region.

Pathologic Features

Nerve sheath myxomas characteristically form superficial, highly myxoid, multinodular/multilobular masses with a prominent peripheral fibrous border (Fig. 20.12). They contain spindled (Fig. 20.13, e-Figs. 20.23–20.25),

TABLE 20.3 **Adipose Tissue Lesions That May Be Myxoid**

Lesion	Clinical features	Pathologic features	Ancillary investigations
Lipoblastoma	Found in infants, usually involves extremities, poorly marginated benign lesions.	Lobulated lesions with foci with myxoid stroma, prominent vessels, and lipoblasts (e-Figs. 20.26–20.30).	*PLAG1-HAS2* or *PLAG1-COL1A2* rearrangements
Spindle cell lipoma	Superficial well-marginated benign tumors of neck of middle-aged men	Spindle cell, mast cells, wiry collagen, fat (e-Figs. 20.31–20.40).	CD34+
Chondroid lipoma	Well-marginated superficial benign lesions of extremities of adult females	Epithelioid to chondroid cells, lipoblasts, mature fat (e-Figs. 20.41–20.45).	S100 protein+, t(11, 16)(q13;p12–13)
Myxoid liposarcoma	Deep low- and intermediate-grade malignant lesions of young adults	Myxoid neoplasms with abundant vessels, lipoblasts.	*FUS-CHOP* and *EWS-CHOP* rearrangements
Round cell Liposarcoma	High-grade variant of myxoid liposarcoma. Deep lesions of young adults	Cellular neoplasms with obscured vessels, rare lipoblasts.	*FUS-CHOP* and *EWS-CHOP* rearrangements

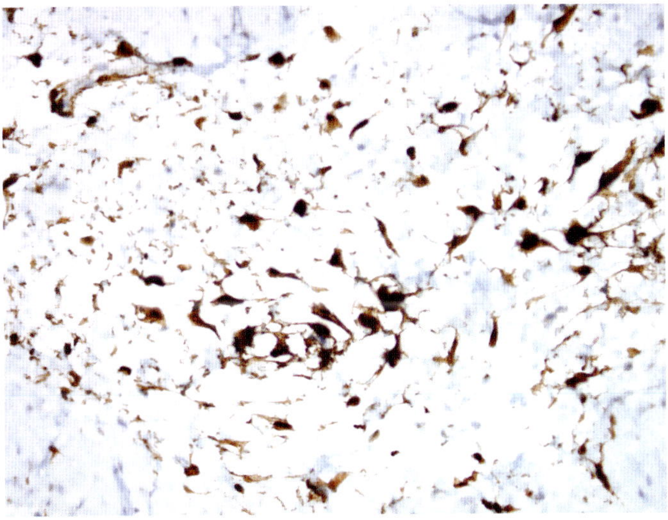

FIGURE 20.14 **Nerve Sheath Myxoma. These neoplasms are S100 Protein Reactive, in Contrast to Neurothekeomas.** Immunoperoxidase.

stellate-shaped, ring-shaped, and epithelioid Schwann cells, and the last are often organized into cords and closely packed syncytial-like aggregates.

Ancillary Investigations

The tumor cells are strongly immunoreactive for S100 protein (Fig. 20.14), GFAP (e-Fig. 20.25), NSE, and CD57; and EMA is sometimes detectable in residual perineurial cells at the tumor periphery.[9]

ADIPOSE TISSUE NEOPLASMS THAT MAY HAVE PROMINENT MYXOID AREAS

This category includes lipoblastoma and lipoblastomatosis,[12-21] spindle cell lipomas,[22-25] chondroid lipoma,[26-35] and, the prototype myxoid lesion with lipid droplets, myxoid liposarcoma (addressed in Chapters 15 and 16). These lesions are listed in Table 20.3 and shown in e-Figs. 20.26–20.45).

REFERENCES

1. Carney JA, Gordon H, Carpenter PC, et al. The complex of myxomas, spotty pigmentation, and endocrine overactivity. *Medicine (Baltimore)*. 1985;64:270–283.
2. Allen PW, Dymock RB, MacCormac LB. Superficial angiomyxomas with and without epithelial components. Report of 30 tumors in 28 patients. *Am J Surg Pathol*. 1988;12:519–530.
3. Calonje E, Guerin D, McCormick D, et al. Superficial angiomyxoma: clinicopathologic analysis of a series of distinctive but poorly recognized cutaneous tumors with tendency for recurrence. *Am J Surg Pathol*. 1999;23:910–917.

4. Fetsch JF, Laskin WB, Tavassoli FA. Superficial angiomyxoma (cutaneous myxoma): a clinicopathologic study of 17 cases arising in the genital region. *Int J Gynecol Pathol.* 1997;16:325–334.
5. Ferreiro JA, Carney JA. Myxomas of the external ear and their significance. *Am J Surg Pathol.* 1994;18:274–280.
6. Carney JA. Psammomatous melanotic schwannoma. A distinctive, heritable tumor with special associations, including cardiac myxoma and the Cushing syndrome. *Am J Surg Pathol.* 1990;14:206–222.
7. Al-Daraji WI, Miettinen M. Superficial acral fibromyxoma: a clinicopathological analysis of 32 tumors including 4 in the heel. *J Cutan Pathol.* 2008;35:1020–1026.
8. Fetsch JF, Laskin WB, Hallman JR, et al. Neurothekeoma: an analysis of 178 tumors with detailed immunohistochemical data and long-term patient follow-up information. *Am J Surg Pathol.* 2007;31:1103–1114.
9. Fetsch JF, Laskin WB, Miettinen M. Nerve sheath myxoma: a clinicopathologic and immunohistochemical analysis of 57 morphologically distinctive, S-100 protein- and GFAP-positive, myxoid peripheral nerve sheath tumors with a predilection for the extremities and a high local recurrence rate. *Am J Surg Pathol.* 2005;29:1615–1624.
10. Hornick JL, Fletcher CD. Cellular neurothekeoma: detailed characterization in a series of 133 cases. *Am J Surg Pathol.* 2007;31:329–340.
11. Laskin WB, Fetsch JF, Miettinen M. The "neurothekeoma": immunohistochemical analysis distinguishes the true nerve sheath myxoma from its mimics. *Hum Pathol.* 2000;31:1230–1241.
12. Hicks J, Dilley A, Patel D, et al. Lipoblastoma and lipoblastomatosis in infancy and childhood: histopathologic, ultrastructural, and cytogenetic features. *Ultrastruct Pathol.* 2001;25:321–333.
13. Mentzel T, Calonje E, Fletcher CD. Lipoblastoma and lipoblastomatosis: a clinicopathological study of 14 cases. *Histopathology.* 1993;23:527–533.
14. Collins MH, Chatten J. Lipoblastoma/lipoblastomatosis: a clinicopathologic study of 25 tumors. *Am J Surg Pathol.* 1997;21:1131–1137.
15. Chung EB, Enzinger FM. Benign lipoblastomatosis. An analysis of 35 cases. *Cancer.* 1973;32:482–492.
16. Dal Cin P, Sciot R, De Wever I, et al. New discriminative chromosomal marker in adipose tissue tumors. The chromosome 8q11-q13 region in lipoblastoma. *Cancer Genet Cytogenet.* 1994;78:232–235.
17. Gisselsson D, Hibbard MK, Dal Cin P, et al. PLAG1 alterations in lipoblastoma: involvement in varied mesenchymal cell types and evidence for alternative oncogenic mechanisms. *Am J Pathol.* 2001;159:955–962.
18. Hibbard MK, Kozakewich HP, Dal Cin P, et al. PLAG1 fusion oncogenes in lipoblastoma. *Cancer Res.* 2000;60:4869–4872.
19. Morerio C, Rapella A, Rosanda C, et al. PLAG1-HAS2 fusion in lipoblastoma with masked 8q intrachromosomal rearrangement. *Cancer Genet Cytogenet.* 2005;156:183–184.
20. Ropke A, Kalinski T, Kluba U, et al. PLAG1 activation in lipoblastoma coinciding with low-level amplification of a derivative chromosome 8 with a deletion del(8)(q13q21.2). *Cytogenet Genome Res.* 2007;119:33–38.
21. Bartuma H, Domanski HA, Von Steyern FV, et al. Cytogenetic and molecular cytogenetic findings in lipoblastoma. *Cancer Genet Cytogenet.* 2008;183;60–63.
22. Enzinger FM, Harvey DA. Spindle cell lipoma. *Cancer.* 1975;36:1852–1859.
23. Fanburg-Smith JC, Devaney KO, Miettinen M, et al. Multiple spindle cell lipomas: a report of 7 familial and 11 nonfamilial cases. *Am J Surg Pathol.* 1998;22:40–48.
24. Dal Cin P, Sciot R, Polito P, et al. Lesions of 13q may occur independently of deletion of 16q in spindle cell/pleomorphic lipomas. *Histopathology.* 1997;31:222–225.

25. Mandahl N, Mertens F, Willen H, et al. A new cytogenetic subgroup in lipomas: loss of chromosome 16 material in spindle cell and pleomorphic lipomas. *J Cancer Res Clin Oncol*. 1994;120:707–711.
26. Meis JM, Enzinger FM. Chondroid lipoma. A unique tumor simulating liposarcoma and myxoid chondrosarcoma. *Am J Surg Pathol*. 1993;17:1103–1112.
27. Chan JK, Lee KC, Saw D. Extraskeletal chondroma with lipoblast-like cells. *Hum Pathol*. 1986;17:1285–1287.
28. Zamecnik M, Michal M, Fakan F. Ultrastructural study of so called chondroid lipoma. *Hum Pathol*. 1998;29:98–100.
29. Nielsen GP, O'Connell JX, Dickersin GR, et al. Chondroid lipoma, a tumor of white fat cells. A brief report of two cases with ultrastructural analysis. *Am J Surg Pathol*. 1995;19:1272–1276.
30. Kindblom LG, Meis-Kindblom JM. Chondroid lipoma: an ultrastructural and immunohistochemical analysis with further observations regarding its differentiation. *Hum Pathol*. 1995;26:706–715.
31. Ballaux F, Debiec-Rychter M, De Wever I, et al. Chondroid lipoma is characterized by t(11;16)(q13;p12–13). *Virchows Arch*. 2004;444:208–210.
32. Gisselsson D, Domanski HA, Hoglund M, et al. Unique cytological features and chromosome aberrations in chondroid lipoma: a case report based on fine-needle aspiration cytology, histopathology, electron microscopy, chromosome banding, and molecular cytogenetics. *Am J Surg Pathol*. 1999;23:1300–1304.
33. Gisselsson D, Domanski HA, Hoglund M, et al. Unique cytological features and chromosome aberrations in chondroid lipoma: a case report based on fine-needle aspiration cytology, histopathology, electron microscopy, chromosome banding, and molecular cytogenetics. *Am J Surg Pathol*. 1999;23:1300–1304.
34. Thomson TA, Horsman D, Bainbridge TC. Cytogenetic and cytologic features of chondroid lipoma of soft tissue. *Mod Pathol*. 1999;12:88–91.
35. Thomson TA, Bainbridge TC, Horsman D. Unique cytologic and chromosome aberrations in chondroid lipoma. *Am J Surg Pathol*. 2000;24:1035.

21

MYXOID TUMORS OF DEEP SOFT TISSUE

INTRODUCTION

Any soft tissue lesion can be myxoid, but the most commonly biopsied ones are those of the deep soft tissue, where the differential diagnosis is limited. Additionally, knowledge of a uniform myxoid appearance on imaging studies (myxoid lesions are bright on T2-weighted magnetic resonance imaging studies [Fig. 21.1, e-Fig. 21.1]) can be helpful. In general, when the pathologist encounters a small biopsy of a myxoid lesion, the top three contenders in the differential diagnosis are intramuscular myxoma (IM), myxoid liposarcoma, and myxofibrosarcoma/myxoid malignant fibrous histiocytoma (MFH). Immunohistochemical stains are typically not required for diagnosis of myxoid lesions, although a few immunohistochemical features will be pointed out for some of the entities. Probably the most important factor to consider when initially assessing a biopsy of a lesion noted to be myxoid is the depth of the lesion, which should guide the differential diagnosis. For example, myxoid liposarcomas are seldom superficial, whereas myxoid dermatofibrosarcoma protuberans virtually always is. Fortunately, most deep myxoid lesions can be diagnosed on a core biopsy, whereas superficial myxoid lesions have considerable overlap but are usually managed with excisional biopsies.

INTRAMUSCULAR MYXOMA

Clinical Features

IM affects individuals over a wide age range but has a peak incidence in middle-aged female adults.[1,2] The tumor develops in deep skeletal muscle. The thigh and pelvic girdle, shoulder, and upper arm are the common sites in decreasing order of frequency. The lesion usually presents as a slow-growing, painless mass with <25% of tumors associated with discomfort or pain. The mass is moveable when the affected muscle relaxes, but becomes fixed when the muscle contracts. The duration of signs and symptoms prior to presentation varies from months to years.

The rare presence of multiple lesions is usually associated with coexistent fibrous dysplasia of bone.[3,4] In such cases, the fibrous dysplasia typically appears first. In most reported cases, the fibrous dysplasia involves

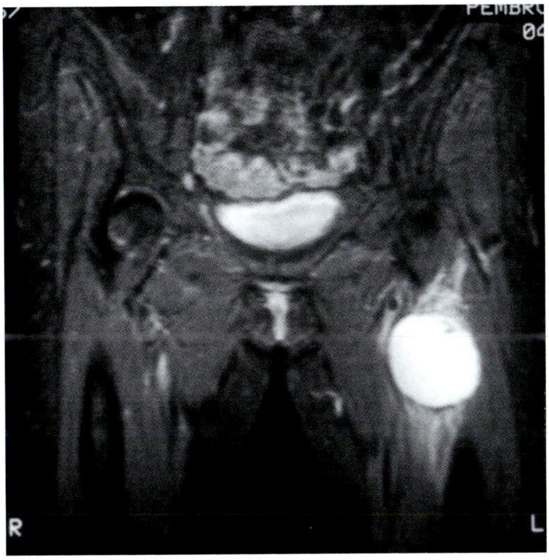

FIGURE 21.1 **Myxoid Neoplasm, T2-weighted MRI Image. On such images, myxoid lesions appear bright as does this intramuscular myxoma.** Compare it to the myxoid lesion depicted in e-Figure 21.1, which is a myxoid liposarcoma. Biopsy is required to distinguish the lesions, but the images tell the pathologist that the tumors are relatively homogeneous.

more than one bone (polyostotic) and, in some instances, can be associated with Albright's syndrome (polyostotic fibrous dysplasia, café au lait spots on the skin, and endocrine abnormalities). The IMs typically arise in the same general vicinity as the affected bone(s). IM is a benign tumor that rarely recurs following local excision.

Pathologic Features

The tumors are located within the skeletal muscle or attached to the muscular fascia. Most range in size between 5 and 10 cm. On gross inspection, the tumor has an oval or lobular shape and appears well circumscribed (Fig. 21.2, e-Fig. 21.2). The cut surface has a soft, mucoid consistency and a gray-white color with thin, traversing fibrous trabeculae and small mucin-filled cysts. On close inspection, the process can be observed infiltrating into surrounding, edematous skeletal muscle.

On microscopic examination, IM is characterized by scattered, bland spindled, and stellate-shaped cells; sparse small vessels; and numerous thin collagen fibers suspended in a richly myxoid stromal matrix (Fig. 21.3). The spindled and stellate-shaped cells have a small nucleus and a meager amount of pale, occasionally vacuolated, eosinophilic cytoplasm. The ill-defined cytoplasmic processes of the lesional cells are often continuous with delicate strands of collagen that run haphazardly throughout the tumor. The mitotic activity is virtually nonexistent. The hyaluronic acid–rich, mucinous stroma often contains small cystic spaces. Occasionally, residual atrophic skeletal muscle fibers, foamy histiocytes and, rarely, mast

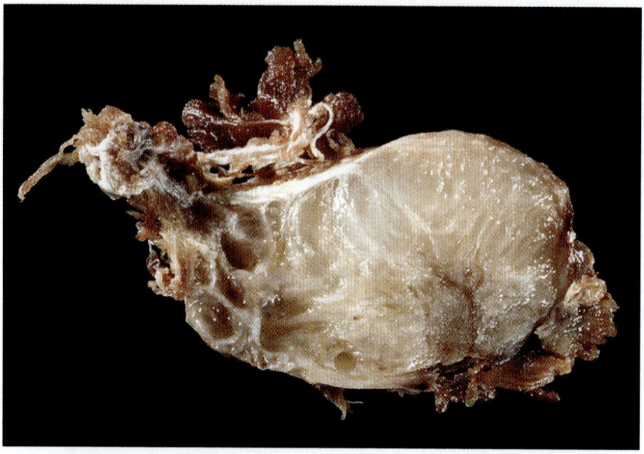

FIGURE 21.2 **IM, Gross Image. The tumor is overall well circumscribed with a glairy cut surface.**

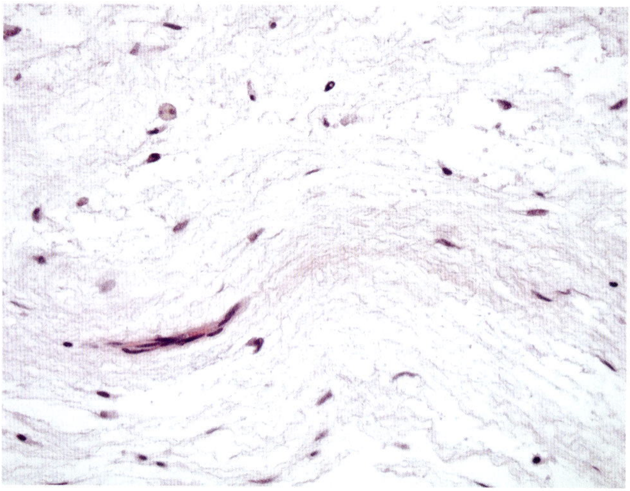

FIGURE 21.3 **Intramuscular Myxoma. Note the hypocellular bland appearance.** The small capillary on the left part of the field serves as an internal size control; the lesional nuclei are small.

cells are identified within the myxoid matrix. Simple, nonarborizing, capillary-sized vessels are scattered throughout the process. At the periphery of the lesion, skeletal muscle fibers adjacent to the tumor are atrophic and separated by edema fluid or infiltrating tumor. Fat cells are commonly interspersed in the skeletal muscle.

Rarely, IM may have areas exhibiting increased cellularity, more abundant collagen, and an increase in the number of vessels (e-Fig. 21.3). These cellular myxomas lack the mitotic activity, cytologic atypia, branching vascular network, and necrosis characteristic of a sarcoma.[2]

Generally, IMs can be readily recognized on needle biopsies, but it is important to correlate with the clinical findings. The imaging should show a relatively uniform myxoid lesion (Fig. 21.1). The pitfall is that small foci in low-grade fibromyxoid sarcomas can be indistinguishable from IMs. Obtaining several cores can forestall this problem as can correlation with imaging by the pathologist. Usually, sarcomas have less monotonous imaging patterns, with the exception of myxoid liposarcoma, which is indistinguishable from IM on imaging (e-Fig. 21.1) but easily distinguished on routine histology.

JUXTA-ARTICULAR MYXOMA

Clinical Features

Juxta-articular myxoma (JAM) arises in association with large joints.[5] As this tumor may exhibit large size, poor circumscription, and focal hypercellularity, recognition of JAM as a distinct benign entity is important.

Although JAM affects patients over a wide age range (16–83 years), almost three fourths of cases occur in men in the third to fifth decades. Most lesions develop around the lateral or medial aspect of the knee. JAM usually presents as a swelling or mass with over 50% of patients giving a history of pain or tenderness. There is often a history of trauma.

Although JAM is a benign tumor with no potential for metastatic spread, it recurs in about a third of patients. Half of these patients experience more than one recurrence.

JAM is centered primarily within the subcutaneous tissue, but can extend into the overlying dermis or the deep fibrous structures of the joint. It may abut the synovium or invade skeletal muscle. When the process involves the knee, the main tumor mass may be associated with smaller, ganglion-like structures within the lateral or medial semilunar cartilage. The tumors range in size from lesions approximating the dimensions of a ganglion to masses over 10 cm in greatest dimension.

Pathologic Features

The lesion appears as a lobulated, unilocular, or multilocular cyst lined by a thin fibrous membrane (Fig. 21.4, e-Figs. 21.4 and 21.5). The tumor has a soft, jelly-like consistency. The cut surface is myxoid, gelatinous, or slimy in appearance and has a white to tan-yellow color.

JAM is chiefly composed of bland-appearing, oval, spindled and stellate-shaped cells embedded in a relatively hypovascular, hyaluronic acid–rich mucinous stroma through which run numerous strands of delicate collagen. Variably sized cystic spaces are identified in the majority of cases (Fig. 21.5, e-Figs. 21.6 and 21.7). JAM is often seen infiltrating and entrapping subcutaneous fat. Focal increased cellularity or fibrosis may be present, especially in recurrent lesions. In the cellular foci, the spindled cells maintain their benign cytologic appearance and lack increased mitotic activity.

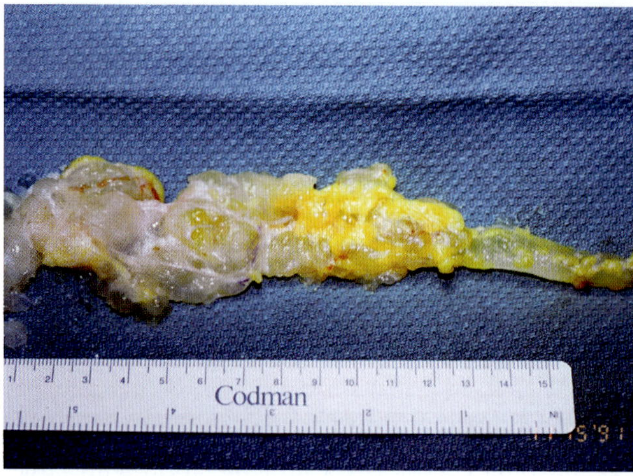

FIGURE 21.4 **JAM, Gross Image. This lesion arose in the wrist of a young woman, an unusual location (most involve the knee joint).**

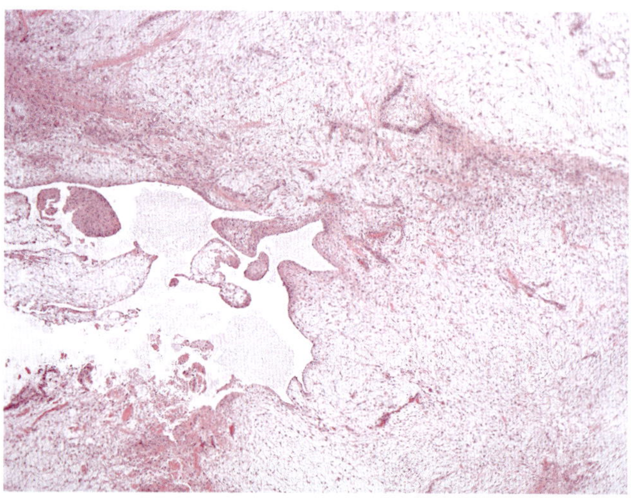

FIGURE 21.5 **Juxta-Articular Myxoma. Cystic spaces are typical.** Note that this tumor is far more cellular than the intramuscular myxoma seen in Fig. 21.3.

Both ganglion and JAM exhibit cystic change and, rarely, a ganglion may show a modest cellular proliferation. However, the former entity occurs more commonly in females, is a smaller lesion, and arises chiefly in the joint capsule or tendinous tissue of the wrist. Ganglion cyst also contains less mucin than does IM or JAM.

MYXOID AND ROUND CELL LIPOSARCOMA

Myxoid/round cell liposarcomas are also discussed in Chapter 16. Although these two lesions were historically considered as separate histologic entities, it is now apparent that these two diagnostic terms describe different histologic and clinical ends of a spectrum that is genetically homogeneous.[6–12] Tumors with pure myxoid liposarcoma morphology are associated with a better prognosis than those with round cell features.[8,11,13] Pure round cell morphology is extremely uncommon, and most tumors classified as round cell liposarcoma are composed of mixtures of myxoid and round cell components.

Clinical Features

These tumors typically affect adults and are most common in the fifth decade. Rare myxoid/round cell liposarcomas occur in children. Males are affected more commonly than females. The deep soft tissue of the thigh is the single most common location for these neoplasms. Primary tumors also arise in the soft tissue of the arms, trunk, and retroperitoneum. The majority are deep to the fascia as demonstrated in the imaging study in e-Figure 21.1. Patients typically complain of a painless soft tissue mass. Myxoid/round cell liposarcoma is treated by wide surgical excision with or without radiation therapy. Approximately 30% of patients develop distant metastases. As for most other sarcomas, metastases often involve the lungs, but myxoid/round cell liposarcoma also has a proclivity for metastases to nonpulmonary sites including the retroperitoneum, soft tissue, and skeleton.[10] Histologic grading appears to be of value in predicting those patients at risk for metastases. Specifically, as the cellularity of the tumor increases and the degree of tumor composed of round cell liposarcoma or so-called cellular myxoid liposarcoma increases, there is an increased risk of metastasis.

Pathologic Features

Grossly myxoid/round cell liposarcomas have a wide size range although most measure >10 cm. They typically demonstrate a lobulated smooth outline and may appear encapsulated. The cut surface of the tumor varies from gelatinous and tan to opaque and yellow. Focal hemorrhage is common; however, necrosis or gross cystic change is unusual. It is usually not possible to grossly distinguish those parts of the tumor that harbor round cell foci. As stated above, virtually all tumors in the myxoid/round cell spectrum contain myxoid regions. Myxoid liposarcoma is composed of aggregated lobules of low to moderately cellular uniform small spindled and oval tumor cells embedded in a richly myxoid ground substance (Figs. 21.6 and 21.7, e-Figs. 21.8 and 21.9). The tumor cells are arranged as cords and clusters although individual cells are usually readily separable from adjacent ones by ground substance. Most characteristically, an acute angle (plexiform) branching capillary vasculature is present within the ground substance. The majority of the tumor cells have scant cytoplasm and

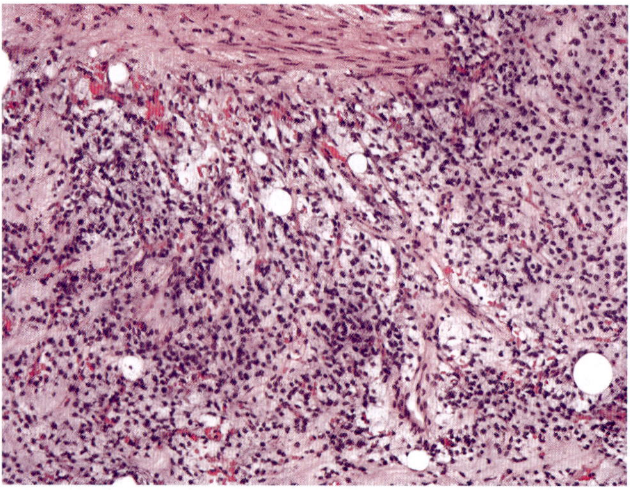

FIGURE 21.6 **Myxoid Liposarcoma.** This tumor features uniform round nuclei, a rich capillary network, and scattered lipoblasts.

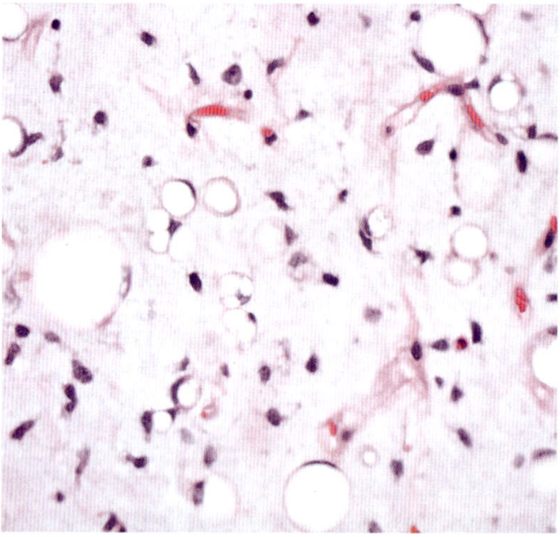

FIGURE 21.7 **Myxoid Liposarcoma.** This classic field shows several lipoblasts—cells with lipid droplets that crisply indent the nucleus. The lipoblasts themselves have uniform small nuclei.

uniform dark staining nuclei. Nucleoli or mitotic figures are typically not prominent. Since myxoid liposarcoma is a translocation associated sarcoma, it tends to have uniform cells with essentially no nuclear pleomorphism and no abnormal mitoses.[14] This feature makes it easy to distinguish from myxofibrosarcoma/myxoid MFH, which has pleomorphic cells (and is also usually more superficial, see Table 21.1). On needle biopsies, the classic features can become obscured either by crush artifact or sampling error and well-formed lipoblasts are inapparent (e-Figs. 21.10–21.13).

TABLE 21.1 Differential Diagnosis of Deep Myxoid Lesions

	Typical clinical features	Microscopic features	Ancillary investigations
Intramuscular myxoma	F > M, thighs	Intramuscular hypocellular myxoid neoplasm with few vessels	Can be CD34+, S100 protein–
Juxta-articular myxoma	Near large joints, especially knee	Similar to IM, but more infiltrative, with cysts and focal cellular areas, scattered mitoses	Can be CD34+, S100 protein–
Myxoid/round cell liposarcoma	Deep soft tissues of extremities of young adults. Often metastasizes to other soft tissue sites as well as to lungs	Monotonous small uniform rounded cells with abundant (myxoid) or minimal (round cell) myxoid matrix. Rich network of delicate vessels becomes inconspicuous in round cell liposarcoma. Lipoblasts	S100 protein+ in some cases, t(12;16)(q13;p11) or t(12;22)(q13;q12) with *FUS-DDIT3 or EWSR1-DDIT3* fusion
Myxofibrosarcoma	Superficial soft tissues of extremities of elderly adults	Pleomorphic cells embedded in myxoid matrix with abundant vessels	Can be CD34+, no characteristic tic genetic feature
Ossifying fibromyxoid tumor	Adults with slight male predominance involving the subcutaneous tissue or skeletal muscle, of proximal extremities	Circumscribed, with pseudocapsule, often with shell of bone, uniform small rounded cells	Often S100 protein+, variable desmin, GFAP, no consistent genetic finding
Extracellular myxoid chondrosarcoma	Deep soft tissues of extremities, slight male predominance	Uniform rounded cells with eosinophilic cytoplasm in hypovascular myxoid background	S100 protein+, synaptophysin+ in some, t(9;22)(q22;q12), t(9;17)(q22;q11) or t(9;15)(q22;q21) with *EWSR1-NR4A3*, *TAF1168-NR4A3*, or *TCF12-NR4A3 fusion*

(Continued)

TABLE 21.1 Differential Diagnosis of Deep Myxoid Lesions (Continued)

	Typical clinical features	Microscopic features	Ancillary investigations
Low-grade fibromyxoid sarcoma	Deep soft tissues of extremities, any age	Hyperchromatic uniform spindle cells in swirled pattern with variable myxoid stroma and variable vascularity	EMA+, Claudin-1+, t(7;16)(q33;p11) with *FUS-CREB3L2* (rarely *FUS-CREB31*) fusion
Myxoinflammatory fibroblastic sarcoma	Distal extremities of adults	Infiltrative masses, pleomorphic cells, myxoid and hyalinized areas, mixed inflammation	Nonspecific
Myxoid dermatofibrosarcoma protuberans	Superficial, usually in shoulder girdle area of adults	Uniform spindle cells with inconspicuous cytoplasm in myxoid stroma	CD34+, t(17;22)(q21;q13) with *COL1A1-PDGFB* fusion
Myxoid solitary fibrous tumor	Multiple anatomic sites, adults	Spindle cells with irregularly shaped nuclei and inconspicuous cytoplasm in myxoid stroma with hemangiopericytoma-like vascular pattern	CD34+, Bcl2+, CD99+
Myxoid leiomyosarcoma	Multiple anatomic sites, adults	Spindle cells with abundant eosinophilic cytoplasm in myxoid stroma	Desmin+, actin+, caldesmon+, calponin+

Myxoid synovial sarcoma	Deep soft tissues of extremities, young adults	Uniform spindle cells with inconspicuous cytoplasm in myxoid stroma	Focal EMA, focal S100 protein, focal keratin, Bcl2+, *SYT-SSX* fusions
Myxoid follicular dendritic cell sarcoma	Multiple anatomic sites, some involving lymph nodes and associated with Castleman's disease, in adults	Spindle cells in a syncytial arrangement embedded with lymphoid cells in a myxoid background	CD21+, CD35+, fascin+, survivin+, podoplanin (D2-40)+
Myxoid melanoma	Multiple anatomic sites, adults	Variable appearances, prominent nucleoli, atypical nuclei, myxoid stroma	S100 protein+, variable HMB45, MART1, Melan-A ("specific" melanoma markers often negative in spindle cell melanomas)

In these cases, attention to the vascularity and uniform cytologic features can be helpful. At times, smears stained with the Diff-Quik preparation can disclose lipoblasts that are otherwise inapparent (e-Fig. 21.14).

As for prognosis, although Smith et al.[11] suggest that a prognostic "cutoff" occurs at >5% cellular areas, other authors prefer to rely on a higher figure (25%[8,15]). When we report such tumors, we attempt to provide an estimate of the fraction of round cell component. Unfortunately, this can be difficult in needle biopsies.

Ancillary Investigations

Most myxoid/round cell liposarcomas demonstrate the chromosomal translocation t(12;16)(q13;p11) that results in the rearrangement of the *CHOP* and *FUS* or a less common alteration that involves the *CHOP* and *EWS* genes.[7,12,16–23] Molecular diagnostic testing is not typically needed for diagnosis, but it is sometimes useful in separating myxoid liposarcoma from lipoblastoma or even for confirming an impression of round cell liposarcoma. Like normal adipose tissue, myxoid liposarcomas express S100 protein (e-Fig. 21.15) but only in about a third of cases.[24]

MYXOFIBROSARCOMA (MYXOID MALIGNANT FIBROUS HISTIOCYTOMA [MFH])

Myxoid MFH as described by Weiss and Enzinger[25] comprised 20% of all MFH, and was defined as having over 50% of myxoid change, with characteristic nodularity, vascular pattern, atypical spindle cells, and a tendency to superficial location. The myxoid nodules merged into areas of pleomorphic MFH. The likelihood of metastasis related to depth from the skin and was inversely proportional to the amount of myxoid change.

Myxofibrosarcoma (the term adopted for the WHO[26]) was described at the same time[27] as a subcutaneous or deep multinodular tumor of older adults composed of thin tapered spindle cells in a myxoid pattern, with a prominent vascular pattern. Four grades were initially recognized depending on degree of cellularity and pleomorphism; higher grades were considered equivalent to myxoid MFH. Comparing grade with outcome in a large series, metastases were found in 0%, 21%, 47%, and 38% of patients with grades I to IV, respectively.[28]

A later series[29] reaffirmed the morphologic findings. On follow-up in this series, in which tumors were graded using a three-tier system, 23% of patients developed metastases, all of whom had intermediate- or high-grade tumors. Over half of the low-grade tumors (6/11) recurred locally. Two of the latter six tumors recurred as higher-grade lesions.

Clinical Features

These are tumors of the elderly, found mainly in patients in the sixth to eighth decades with a slight male predominance. They involve mostly the lower extremities and limb girdles and are uncommon on the trunk. The majority are superficial (dermis and subcutis). They are seldom retroperitoneal and

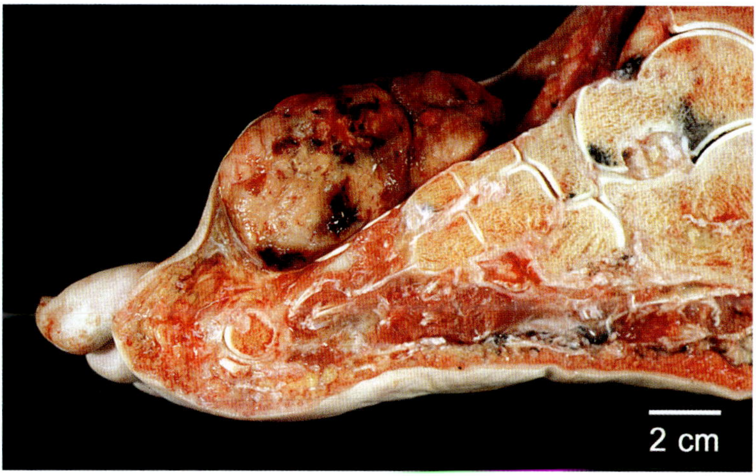

FIGURE 21.8 **Myxofibrosarcoma.** Although the distal presentation of this tumor is unusual (most involve the thigh), the superficial location is typical.

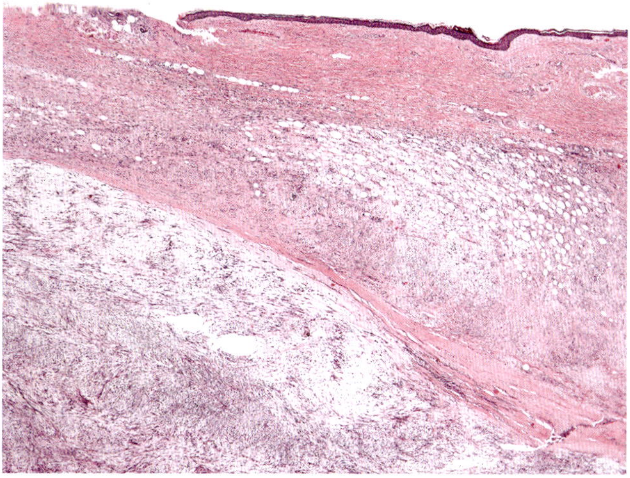

FIGURE 21.9 **Myxofibrosarcoma.** Even at this magnification, the nuclei are pleomorphic, a feature that readily distinguishes this tumor from myxoid liposarcoma. Note that the lesion is close to the overlying skin, which would also be unusual for a myxoid liposarcoma.

most lesions of the retroperitoneum believed to be these are probably simply dedifferentiated liposarcomas. Tumors are usually slow growing and painless.

Pathologic Features

Superficial lesions are typically multilobulated and gelatinous appearing (Figs. 21.8 and 21.9), while deep lesions appear more solid and form a single mass. Although originally lesions were classified as myxoid MFH based on

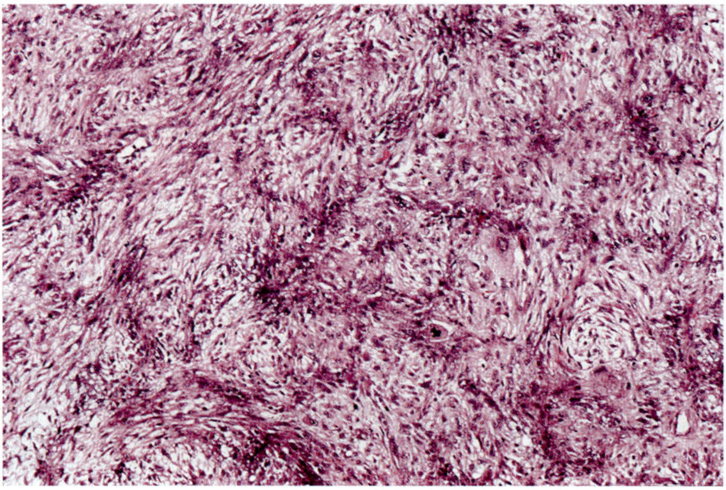

FIGURE 21.10 **Myxofibrosarcoma.** The neoplasm is richly vascular and punctuated by pleomorphic nuclei.

the identification of at least 50% myxoid zones,[25] later authors required only 20%[29] and some authors simply assess for "prominent" myxoid stroma.[30]

There is a broad histologic spectrum depending on tumor grade, but all lesions have spindled to stellate cells with varying degrees of nuclear pleomorphism embedded in abundant mucopolysaccharide matrix (Fig. 21.10, e-Figs. 21.16 and 21.17). At low magnification, most lesions have a multilobular arrangement with incomplete fibrous septa. Vascularity can be rich and similar to that in myxoid liposarcoma (vessels are described as "curvilinear"; Fig. 21.10, e-Figs. 21.18 and 21.19). The individual cells are stellate and some have markedly pleomorphic nuclei. Some of the cells contain abundant cytoplasmic mucin and thus superficially mimic lipoblasts (Fig. 21.11, e-Figs. 21.20–21.23), but this material, unlike lipid, does not crisply indent the nucleus (compare Fig. 21.7 to Fig. 21.11). A subset of cases displays epithelioid morphology[31] (e-Figs. 21.24 and 21.25). In the latter, neoplastic cells were arranged singly and in small clusters in the myxoid areas or formed sheets in the hypercellular areas, where epithelioid cells contain round nuclei, vesicular chromatin, prominent nucleoli, and moderate amounts of eosinophilic cytoplasm. The epithelioid areas are multifocal with admixed areas of conventional myxofibrosarcoma.

Ancillary Investigations

By immunohistochemistry, there is variable expression of actins, CD68, and CD34, but no S100 protein. The epithelioid variant lacks keratins, actins, desmin, and S100 protein.[31] These neoplasms have no characteristic genetic alteration, yielding complex karyotypes in keeping with their nuclear pleomorphism (see http://cgap.nci.nih.gov/Chromosomes/Mitelman).

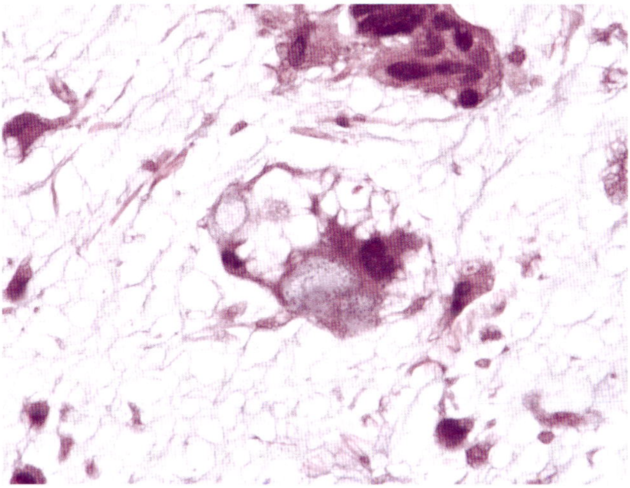

FIGURE 21.11 **Myxofibrosarcoma.** This cell contains mucopolysaccharide matrix rather than a lipid droplet.

OSSIFYING FIBROMYXOID TUMOR

In 1989, Enzinger et al.[32] described the clinicopathologic features of 59 examples of ossifying fibromyxoid tumor of soft parts (OFT).

Clinical Features

OFT occurs over a wide age range with a peak incidence in the fifth decade.[32] Men are affected more often than women. The tumor clinically presents as a slow-growing, asymptomatic nodule or mass within the subcutaneous tissue or, less often, skeletal muscle. Multiple lesions have been documented at presentation[33] and are usually grouped in the same general area. The shoulder, upper arm, buttock, and thigh are the preferentially involved sites. The tumor arises less frequently in the head and neck region and trunk. Duration of preoperative disease varied from <1 year to over 20 years in the initial study.[32]

OFT appears to have low-grade malignant potential. In the original series, the local recurrence rate was 27%, with multiple recurrences documented in three patients. One patient with three recurrences developed a presumed metastasis to the opposite thigh 20 years after initial excision.[32] A subset of "atypical and malignant" OFTs characterized by increased cellularity and mitotic activity has been reported.[34,35] Two of the six patients in the 1995 study of "atypical" lesions developed recurrent disease and one experienced a pulmonary metastasis. Other examples of metastatic lesions have also been documented as case reports.[36,37] In the largest series of patients with follow-up to date,[38] 8 out of 51 patients with OFT had metastases, with metastases tending to occur in atypical lesions. However, in a separate report restricted to more classic cases,[39] there were

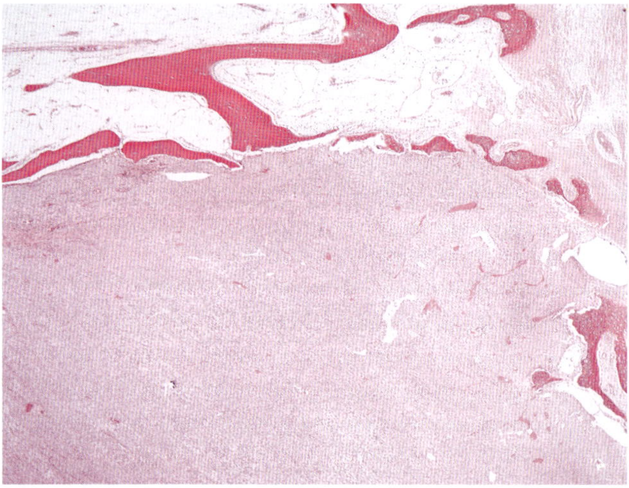

FIGURE 21.12 **Ossifying Fibromyxoid Tumor.** These tumors often have a shell of mature bone. The nuclei in this example are small and uniform.

only recurrences (22%) but no metastases in 41 patients with follow-up. Surgery is presently the mainstay of therapy for OFT.

Pathologic Findings

The tumors vary in size from about 1 cm to as large as 17 cm. OFT appears as either a well-circumscribed, single round to oval nodule, or as a multinodular or lobulated mass. Most lesions have a firm to hard, cartilage-like consistency. The tumor may feel gritty on sectioning due to its variably calcified or ossified pseudocapsule.

Most tumors have calcified lamellar (sometimes with marrow) or woven bone within the pseudocapsule (Fig. 21.12). At low-power magnification, OFT is composed of uniform-appearing, small round to polygonal–shaped cells embedded in a myxohyalin to collagenous stromal matrix (Figs. 21.12 and 21.13). The cells are arranged in lobules that vary in size and cellularity, and are partially separated by fibrous bands. The tumor is surrounded by an incomplete fibrous pseudocapsule composed of dense fibrous and hyalinized connective tissue. Nests of tumor may be seen infiltrating through rents in this fibrous shell. The proliferating cells are small with lightly eosinophilic to clear cytoplasm and a cytologically bland-appearing, round to spindle-shaped nucleus containing a small nucleolus (e-Figs. 21.26–21.28). The occasional presence of a clear space around the cell mimics of appearance of chondrocytic differentiation. In zones with an abundant myxocollagenous stromal matrix, the cells interconnect to form anastomosing, thin cord-like arrangements (e-Fig. 21.28). A vaguely fascicular growth pattern of spindled cells occurs in the more collagenous areas of the tumor. Polygonal-shaped cells with distinct cell borders may aggregate around vessels in a manner reminiscent of a glomus tumor. In

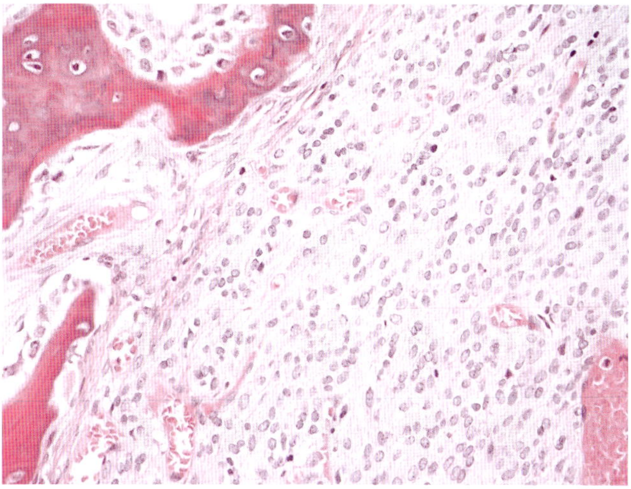

FIGURE 21.13 **Ossifying Fibromyxoid Tumor.** This is a higher magnification image of the lesion depicted in Fig. 21.12.

conventional examples, the mitotic activity is low. In fact, many examples of this tumor lack bone in their capsule (nonossifying variant).[38] The stromal mucin is chiefly composed of hyaluronic acid. Collagen deposition varies from delicate fibers in the myxoid zones to thick bands of hyalinized collagen that occasionally contain spicules of bone or osteoid. Mature cartilage is infrequently identified in OFT. A rich network of thin-walled vessels, often showing perivascular fibrosis, is a consistent finding.

OFTs with aggressive histopathologic features have been described. Tumors reported in the literature as "atypical" or "malignant" OFTs show increased cellularity and are composed of a more pleomorphic cell population exhibiting nuclear hyperchromatism and increased mitotic activity (>2 mitoses per 10 hpf).[34]

Ancillary Investigations

The immunohistochemical profile of conventional OFT includes immunoreactivity for neural and myogenic markers. Along with strong and diffuse expression of vimentin, approximately half to three quarters of tumors tested variably express S100 protein[38] and over one half express CD57 (Leu-7).[33,40,41] In one study,[40] 70% of tumors expressed desmin. Limited expression of neuronal specific enolase, GFAP, alpha-smooth muscle actin, and muscle-specific actin has also been documented.[33,40,41]

The immunoexpression of neural markers, including S100 protein in the majority of these tumors (e-Fig. 21.29), and the presence of discontinuous runs of thick basal lamina and interdigitating cytoplasmic processes on ultrastructural examination support the view that the OFT is closely related to elements of the peripheral nerve sheath.[42]

Cytogenetic and flow-cytometric studies have not yielded consistent findings.[37,43,44]

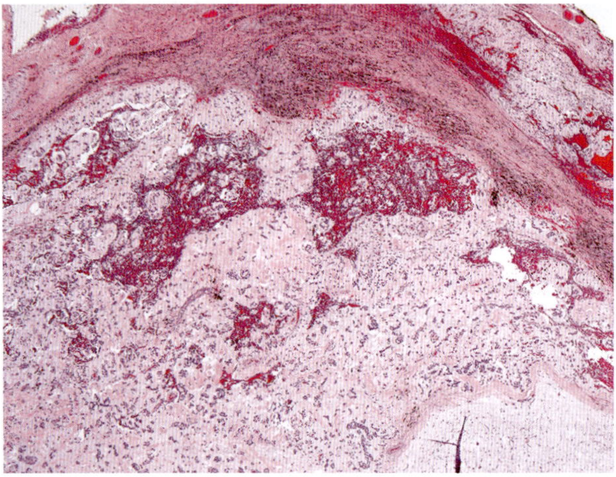

FIGURE 21.14 **Extraskeletal Myxoid Chondrosarcoma.** At low magnification, these tumors are lobulated, consisting of small uniform cells. Hemosiderin deposition in common in these lesions.

EXTRASKELETAL MYXOID CHONDROSARCOMA

Clinical Features

Extraskeletal myxoid chondrosarcomas (EMCs) are rare soft tissue sarcomas that predominantly occur in adulthood.[45–47] There is a slight male predilection. The tumors most commonly occur in the deep soft tissues of the extremities. They usually present as a painless or minimally tender slow-growing mass. Most of the tumors are >5.0 cm. In Enzinger's original series, this tumor was considered relatively low grade with a low incidence of metastasis and an indolent clinical course.[46] More recent experience shows that the estimated 5-, 10-, and 15-year survival rates were 90%, 70%, and 60%, respectively. Older patient age, larger tumor size, and tumor location in the proximal extremity or limb girdle were adverse prognostic factors identified by multivariate analysis. EMC has a unique clinical course, including a high rate of local recurrence, prolonged survival after metastasis in some cases, and eventually a high rate of death due to tumor. These features distinguish EMC from other low-grade sarcomas. Histologic grading is of no prognostic value in EMC because prognosis is dictated primarily by clinical features.[45]

Pathologic Features

EMCs are lobulated myxoid tumors that characteristically demonstrate low cellularity (Figs. 21.14–21.16, e-Figs. 21.30–21.35). The individual tumor cells are small, oval, and have minimal amounts of eosinophilic cytoplasm surrounding the nucleus. The nuclei are central, dark staining, and usually lack visible nucleoli. Tumor cells are arranged in linear arrays that appear as straight lines or curves. Mitotic figures are usually inconspicuous. The tumor cells are embedded within a hypovascular basophilic

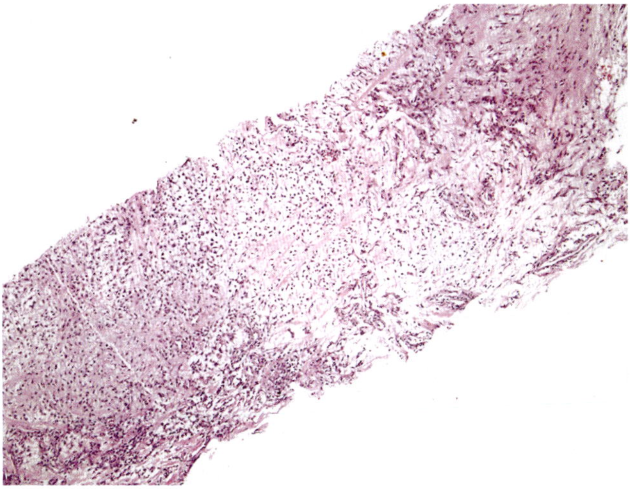

FIGURE 21.15 **Extraskeletal Myxoid Chondrosarcoma.** In this needle biopsy, the appearances are similar to those of myxoid liposarcoma but the rich capillary network is lacking.

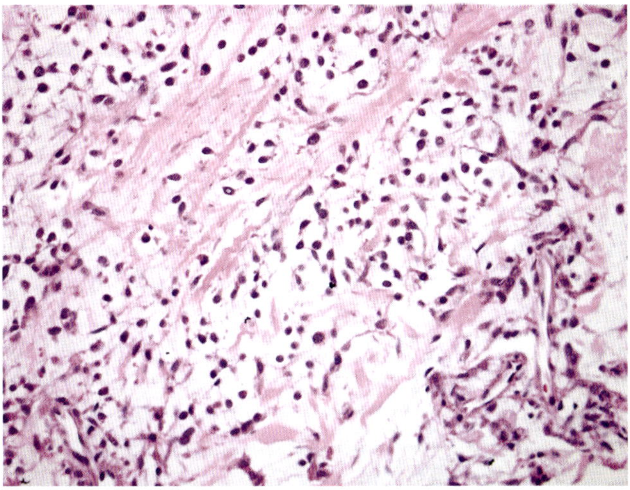

FIGURE 21.16 **Extraskeletal Myxoid Chondrosarcoma.** The tumor consists of small spindled to rounded cells suspended in myxoid matrix. Some examples feature more prominent eosinophilic cytoplasm (see e-Figs. 21.30–21.38).

flocculent matrix. A distinctly nodular/lobular growth is evident. The lobules are separated by strands of eosinophilic collagen. In low-grade tumors, there is low cellularity, and higher-grade tumors typically show greater cellularity with less extracellular matrix. Hyaline cartilage is not found in EMC. Rarely dedifferentiation to a high-grade sarcoma occurs in EMC.[47] Additionally, a subset of cases has zones that are solid, consisting of sheets of small round uniform cells (e-Figs. 21.36 and 21.37).

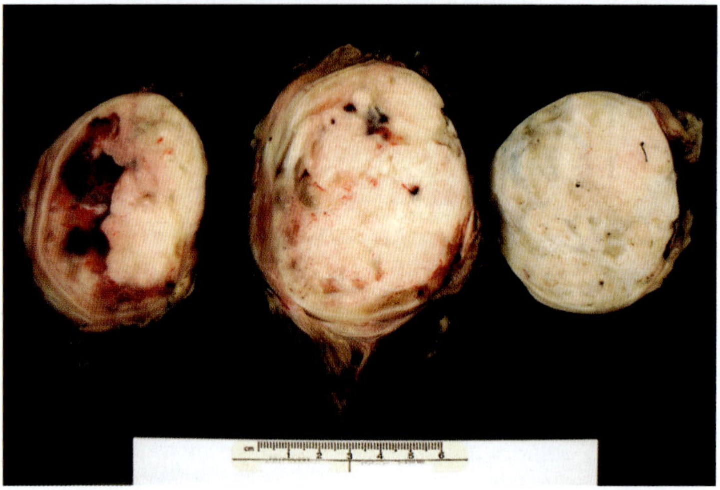

FIGURE 21.17 **Low-Grade Fibromyxoid Sarcoma, Gross Specimen.** The neoplasm has solid areas, myxoid zones, and cystic regions, a heterogeneous appearance compared to that of the intramuscular myxoma seen in Fig. 21.2.

EMC should be distinguished from soft tissue chondroma and from myxoid liposarcoma. It is typically more myxoid than the former and lacks the vascular pattern of the latter.

Ancillary Investigations

Immunohistochemical stains demonstrate vimentin and S100 protein expression (e-Fig. 21.38) in the majority of cases. Interestingly, many tumors express endocrine markers, especially synaptophysin[48–50] as well as neuronspecific enolase and occasionally chromogranin.

Cytogenetic analysis of EMC demonstrates a consistent translocation between chromosomes 9 and 22, t(9;22)(q22–31;q11–12), which serves as a diagnostic marker for this neoplasm since it results in a specific fusion product, *EWSR1-NR4A3*[45] that can be exploited for diagnosis.[21,49]

LOW-GRADE FIBROMYXOID SARCOMA AND HYALINIZING SPINDLE CELL TUMOR WITH GIANT ROSETTES

Additional information on this tumor appears also in Chapter 10–it is predominantly a spindle cell sarcoma but is reiterated here as a myxoid lesion based on its myxoid foci, which can result in a misdiagnosis of myxoma on needle biopsy if sampling error is a factor. However, LGFMS is radiologically heterogeneous whereas myxomas are more uniform. Low-grade fibromyxoid sarcoma is a tumor composed of bland, fibroblast-like cells with a swirling, whorled, vaguely storiform pattern in a fibrous and focally myxoid stroma, occasionally with plexiform vasculature (Figs. 21.17–21.19, e-Figs. 21.39–21.41).

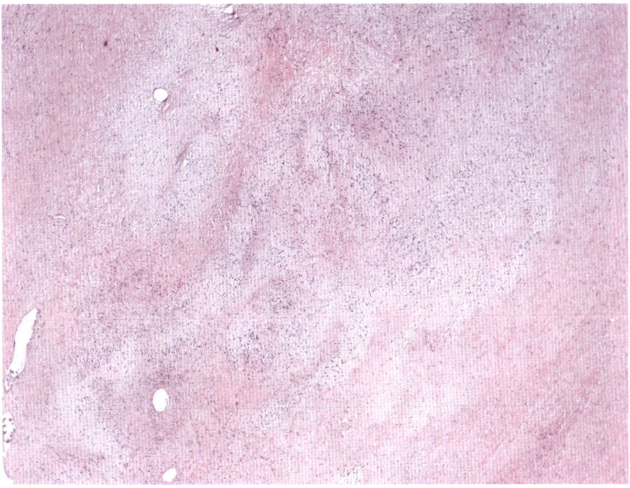

FIGURE 21.18 **Low-Grade Fibromyxoid Sarcoma.** In this area the tumor appears similar to a fibromatosis but differs by having a slightly disorganized swirling architecture rather than uniform fascicles.

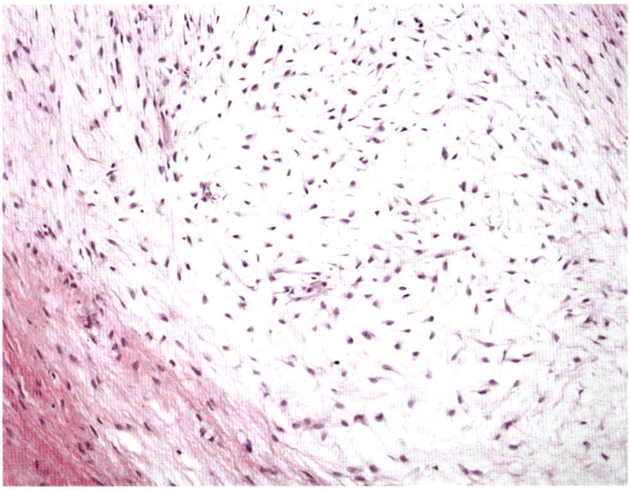

FIGURE 21.19 **Low-Grade Fibromyxoid Sarcoma.** In this area the lesion is reminiscent of a myxoma but the nuclei are more hyperchromatic.

(ACRAL) MYXOINFLAMMATORY FIBROBLASTIC SARCOMA (INFLAMMATORY MYXOHYALINE TUMOR)

"Acral myxoinflammatory fibroblastic sarcoma" and "inflammatory myxohyaline tumor" (IMHT) are terms used to described the same entity. These tumors are usually acral (hands and feet), but not invariably, and thus the World Health Organization (WHO) now classifies them as "myxoinflammatory fibroblastic sarcoma."[26]

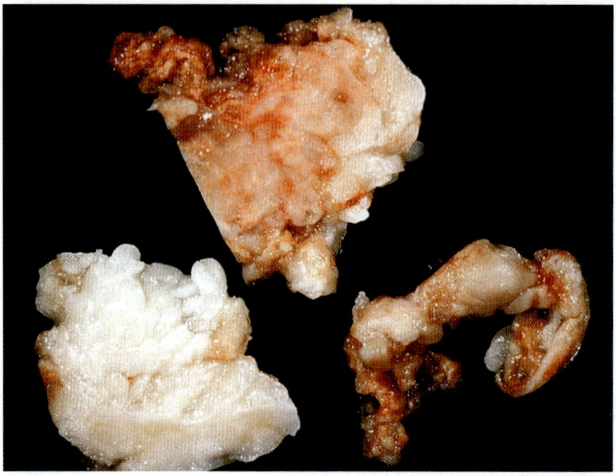

FIGURE 21.20 **Myxoinflammatory Fibroblastic Sarcoma.** These tumors typically arise in the distal extremities and are highly infiltrative, as evidenced by this gross specimen.

Clinical Features

Fifty-one cases of a unique soft tissue tumor with a proclivity for the hands and feet were initially described as IMHT.[51] These occurred over a wide age range (4–81 years; median: 40 years) and affected the sexes equally. Most involved the hands and feet, presenting as painless masses. The wrist/lower arm and the ankles/lower leg were also affected. Recurrences were noted in six of 27 patients (22%) with follow-up. Many of the patients were treated aggressively for their tumors since these cases were initially diagnosed as low-grade sarcomas.

Subsequently, a series of 44 identical tumors was reported as "acral myxoinflammatory fibroblastic sarcoma,"[52] similar to the term (without acral) currently preferred by the WHO, with confirmation of the proclivity for local recurrences and histologic documentation of metastasis in one case. Presumably the finding of metastasis in the second series was a reflection of initial diagnoses of reactive processes; the recurrence rate in this series was substantially higher as well. Subsequent case reports have mirrored the original findings, although occasional aggressive behavior is recorded.[53]

Pathologic Features

Tumors are infiltrative and multinodular (Fig. 21.20, e-Fig. 21.42), characterized histologically by dense inflammation merging with stroma varying from myxoid to hyalinized and containing sheets and small foci of epithelioid spindled cells (Fig. 21.21, e-Fig. 21.43). Some lesions contain foamy histiocytes, giant cells, and hemosiderin. Amid the inflammatory backdrop, scattered bizarre cells having large vesicular nuclei and macronucleoli reminiscent of Reed-Sternberg cells or virocytes are present (Fig 21.22,

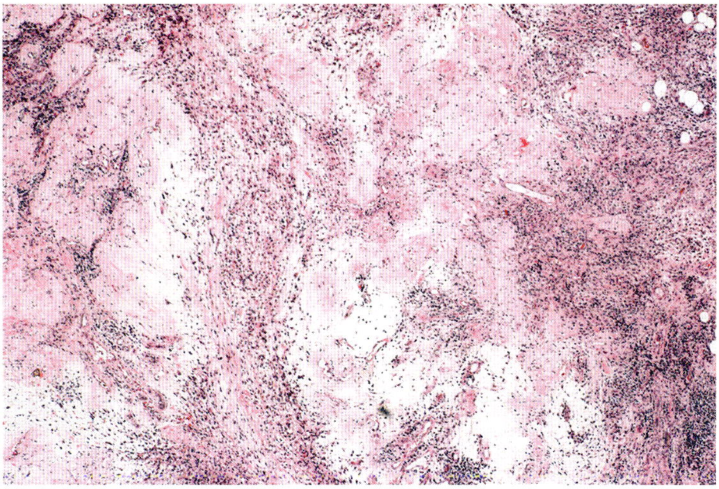

FIGURE 21.21 **Myxoinflammatory Fibroblastic Sarcoma.** This tumor has a hyalinized appearance.

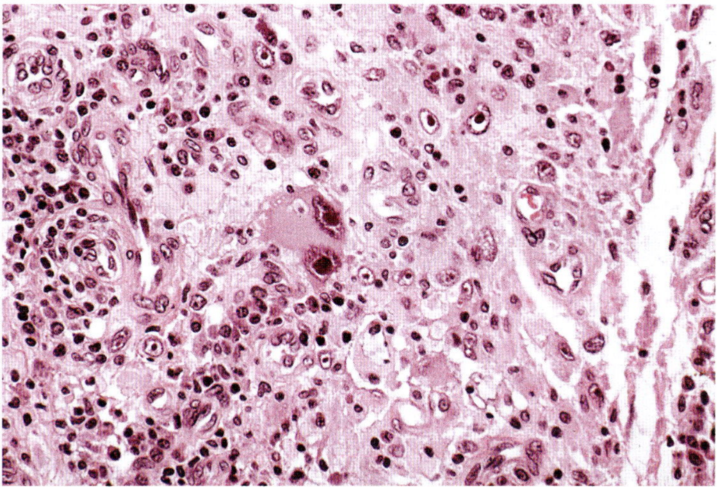

FIGURE 21.22 **Myxoinflammatory Fibroblastic Sarcoma.** The binucleate cell in this tumor is reminiscent of a Reed-Sternberg cell. A background of eosinophils can add to the confusion, but these cells are fibroblastic rather than hematopoietic on ultrastructural and immunolabeling studies.

e-Fig. 21.44). Despite the cytologic atypia, mitotic activity is minimal (mean, 1 mitotic figure per 50 hpf).

Ancillary investigations

Ultrastructural studies demonstrate fibroblastic characteristics.[52]

On immunohistochemical staining, IMHT expresses vimentin and may have focal CD68 positivity. There may be occasional keratin-positive cells[51] or CD34.[52,54] The tumors lack S100 protein, desmin, actin, neuron-specific enolase, epithelial membrane antigen (EMA), and leukocyte markers (CD15, CD30, CD45). Neither CMV nor EBV are detected. They share t(1;10) and amplification of 3p11–12 and some morphologic features with hemosiderotic fibrolipomatous lesion[55] (discussed in Chapter 15).

OTHER LESIONS WITH MYXOID AREAS

As noted previously, almost any soft tissue tumor can have prominent myxoid areas, and such cases are best diagnosed by recognizing the more typical portions of the tumor. However, this can be treacherous on small biopsies and the presence of prominent myxoid areas on small biopsies that are not readily recognizable as a specific entity should always prompt the pathologist to consider a wider differential diagnosis. Neoplasms in which prominent myxoid areas are well known include dermatofibrosarcoma protuberans[56–58](see e-Figs. 20.4–20.9 from Chapter 20), solitary fibrous tumor[59] (e-Figs. 21.45–21.50), leiomyosarcoma[60] (e-Figs. 21.51–21.55), synovial sarcoma[61] (e-Figs. 21.56–21.61), follicular dendritic cell sarcomas[62] (e-Figs. 21.62–21.64), and melanoma, whether primary or metastatic.[63–65] These diagnoses can all be difficult on needle biopsies unless the classic component is also sampled in addition to the myxoid one.

The differential diagnosis of deep myxoid lesions appears in Table 21.2.

TABLE 21.2 Differential Diagnosis of IM, Myxoid Liposarcoma, and Myxofibrosarcoma

Entity	Clinical features	Pathologic features	Ancillary investigations
IM	Deep lesions in middle-aged women	Paucivascular hypocellular myxoid lesion	None useful in differential diagnosis
Myxoid liposarcoma	Deep lesions in young adults, male predominance	Richly vascular tumor in myxoid background with uniform rounded small cells and lipoblasts	Some S100+, Characteristic translocation t(12;16) or t(12;22) and fusion products *FUS-DDIT3* or *EWSR1-DDIT3*
Myxofibrosarcoma	Superficial lesions in elderly adults	Richly vascular myxoid lesion with pleomorphic cells	None useful in differential diagnosis

REFERENCES

1. Kindblom LG, Stener B, Angervall L. Intramuscular myxoma. *Cancer*. 1974;34:1737–1744.
2. Nielsen GP, O'Connell JX, Rosenberg AE. Intramuscular myxoma: a clinicopathologic study of 51 cases with emphasis on hypercellular and hypervascular variants. *Am J Surg Pathol*. 1998;22:1222–1227.
3. Ireland DC, Soule EH, Ivins JC. Myxoma of somatic soft tissues. A report of 58 patients, 3 with multiple tumors and fibrous dysplasia of bone. *Mayo Clin Proc*. 1973; 48:401–410.
4. Wirth WA, Leavitt D, Enzinger FM. Multiple intramuscular myxomas. Another extraskeletal manifestation of fibrous dysplasia. *Cancer*. 1971;27:1167–1173.
5. Meis JM, Enzinger FM. Juxta-articular myxoma: a clinical and pathologic study of 65 cases. *Hum Pathol*. 1992;23:639–646.
6. Antonescu CR, Tschernyavsky SJ, Decuseara R, et al. Prognostic impact of P53 status, TLS-CHOP fusion transcript structure, and histological grade in myxoid liposarcoma: a molecular and clinicopathologic study of 82 cases. *Clin Cancer Res*. 2001; 7:3977–3987.
7. Antonescu CR, Elahi A, Healey JH, et al. Monoclonality of multifocal myxoid liposarcoma: confirmation by analysis of TLS-CHOP or EWS-CHOP rearrangements. *Clin Cancer Res*. 2000;6:2788–2793.
8. Kilpatrick SE, Doyon J, Choong PF, et al. The clinicopathologic spectrum of myxoid and round cell liposarcoma. A study of 95 cases. *Cancer*. 1996;77:1450–1458.
9. Oliveira AM, Nascimento AG, Okuno SH, et al. p27(kip1) protein expression correlates with survival in myxoid and round-cell liposarcoma. *J Clin Oncol*. 2000;18:2888–2893.
10. Spillane AJ, Fisher C, Thomas JM. Myxoid liposarcoma--the frequency and the natural history of nonpulmonary soft tissue metastases. *Ann Surg Oncol*. 1999;6:389–394.
11. Smith TA, Easley KA, Goldblum JR. Myxoid/round cell liposarcoma of the extremities. A clinicopathologic study of 29 cases with particular attention to extent of round cell liposarcoma. *Am J Surg Pathol*. 1996;20:171–180.
12. Tallini G, Akerman M, Dal Cin P, et al. Combined morphologic and karyotypic study of 28 myxoid liposarcomas. Implications for a revised morphologic typing, (a report from the CHAMP Group). *Am J Surg Pathol*. 1996;20:1047–1055.
13. Evans HL. Liposarcoma: a study of 55 cases with a reassessment of its classification. *Am J Surg Pathol*. 1979;3:507–523.
14. Montgomery E, Wilentz RE, Argani P, et al. Analysis of anaphase figures in routine histologic sections distinguishes chromosomally unstable from chromosomally stable malignancies. *Cancer Biol Ther*. 2003;2;248–252.
15. Evans H. Liposarcomas and atypical lipomatous tumors: a study of 66 cases followed for a minimum of 10 years. *Surg Pathol*. 1988;1:41–54.
16. Sreekantaiah C, Karakousis CP, Leong SP, et al. Cytogenetic findings in liposarcoma correlate with histopathologic subtypes. *Cancer*. 1992;69:2484–2495.
17. Sreekantaiah C, Karakousis CP, Leong SP, et al. Trisomy 8 as a nonrandom secondary change in myxoid liposarcoma. *Cancer Genet Cytogenet*. 1991;51:195–205.
18. Paulien S, Turc-Carel C, Dal Cin P, et al. Myxoid liposarcoma with t(12;16) (q13;p11) contains site-specific differences in methylation patterns surrounding a zinc-finger gene mapped to the breakpoint region on chromosome 12. *Cancer Res*. 1990;50:7902–7907.
19. Rosai J, Akerman M, Dal Cin P, et al. Combined morphologic and karyotypic study of 59 atypical lipomatous tumors. Evaluation of their relationship and differential diagnosis with other adipose tissue tumors (a report of the CHAMP Study Group). *Am J Surg Pathol*. 1996;20:1182–1189.

20. Meis-Kindblom JM, Sjogren H, Kindblom LG, et al. Cytogenetic and molecular genetic analyses of liposarcoma and its soft tissue simulators: recognition of new variants and differential diagnosis. *Virchows Arch.* 2001;439:141–151.
21. Downs-Kelly E, Goldblum JR, Patel RM, et al. The utility of fluorescence in situ hybridization (FISH) in the diagnosis of myxoid soft tissue neoplasms. *Am J Surg Pathol.* 2008;32:8–13.
22. Bridge JA, Shaffer B, Neff JR, et al. A complex translocation involving chromosomes 12 and 16 in a metastatic myxoid liposarcoma. *Cancer Genet Cytogenet.* 1988; 34:119–120.
23. Panagopoulos I, Hoglund M, Mertens F, et al. Fusion of the EWS and CHOP genes in myxoid liposarcoma. *Oncogene.* 1996;12:489–494.
24. Hashimoto H, Daimaru Y, Enjoji M. S-100 protein distribution in liposarcoma. An immunoperoxidase study with special reference to the distinction of liposarcoma from myxoid malignant fibrous histiocytoma. *Virchows Arch A Pathol Anat Histopathol.* 1984;405:1–10.
25. Weiss SW, Enzinger FM. Myxoid variant of malignant fibrous histiocytoma. *Cancer.* 1977;39:1672–1685.
26. Fletcher C, Unni K, Mertens FE. *World Health Organization Classification of Tumours. Pathology and Genetics of Tumours of Soft Tissue and Bone.* Lyon: IACR Press; 2002.
27. Angervall L, Kindblom LG, Merck C. Myxofibrosarcoma. A study of 30 cases. *Acta Pathol Microbiol Scand [A].* 1977;85A:127–140.
28. Merck C, Angervall L, Kindblom LG, et al. Myxofibrosarcoma. A malignant soft tissue tumor of fibroblastic- histiocytic origin. A clinicopathologic and prognostic study of 110 cases using multivariate analysis. *Acta Pathol Microbiol Immunol Scand Suppl.* 1983;282:1–40.
29. Mentzel T, Calonje E, Wadden C, et al. Myxofibrosarcoma. Clinicopathologic analysis of 75 cases with emphasis on the low-grade variant. *Am J Surg Pathol.* 1996;20:391–405.
30. Antonescu CR, Baren A. Spectrum of low-grade fibrosarcomas: a comparative ultrastructural analysis of low-grade myxofibrosarcoma and fibromyxoid sarcoma. *Ultrastruct Pathol.* 2004;28:321–332.
31. Nascimento AF, Bertoni F, Fletcher CD. Epithelioid variant of myxofibrosarcoma: expanding the clinicomorphologic spectrum of myxofibrosarcoma in a series of 17 cases. *Am J Surg Pathol.* 2007;31:99–105.
32. Enzinger FM, Weiss SW, Liang CY. Ossifying fibromyxoid tumor of soft parts. A clinicopathological analysis of 59 cases. *Am J Surg Pathol.* 1989;13:817–827.
33. Miettinen M. Ossifying fibromyxoid tumor of soft parts. Additional observations of a distinctive soft tissue tumor. *Am J Clin Pathol.* 1991;95:142–149.
34. Kilpatrick SE, Ward WG, Mozes M, et al. Atypical and malignant variants of ossifying fibromyxoid tumor. Clinicopathologic analysis of six cases. *Am J Surg Pathol.* 1995;19:1039–1046.
35. Folpe A, Weiss S. Ossifying fibromyxoid tumor of soft parts: A clinicopathologic study of 66 cases with emphasis on atypical and malignant variants [abstract 46]. *Mod Pathol.* 2002;15:14A.
36. Minami R, Yamamoto T, Tsukamoto R, et al. Fine needle aspiration cytology of the malignant variant of ossifying fibromyxoid tumor of soft parts: a case report. *Acta Cytol.* 2001;45:745–755.
37. Nishio J, Iwasaki H, Ohjimi Y, et al. Ossifying fibromyxoid tumor of soft parts. Cytogenetic findings. *Cancer Genet Cytogenet.* 2002;133:124–128.
38. Folpe AL, Weiss SW. Ossifying fibromyxoid tumor of soft parts: a clinicopathologic study of 70 cases with emphasis on atypical and malignant variants. *Am J Surg Pathol.* 2003;27:421–431.

39. Miettinen M, Finnell V, Fetsch JF. Ossifying fibromyxoid tumor of soft parts–a clinicopathologic and immunohistochemical study of 104 cases with long-term follow-up and a critical review of the literature. *Am J Surg Pathol*. 2008;32:996–1005.
40. Schofield JB, Krausz T, Stamp GW, et al. Ossifying fibromyxoid tumour of soft parts: immunohistochemical and ultrastructural analysis. Histopathology 1993;22:101–112.
41. Williams SB, Ellis GL, Meis JM, et al. Ossifying fibromyxoid tumour (of soft parts) of the head and neck: a clinicopathological and immunohistochemical study of nine cases. *J Laryngol Otol*. 1993;107:75–80.
42. Fisher C, Hedges M, Weiss SW. Ossifying fibromyxoid tumor of soft parts with stromal cyst formation and ribosome-lamella complexes. *Ultrastruct Pathol*. 1994;18:593–600.
43. Sovani V, Velagaleti GV, Filipowicz E, et al. Ossifying fibromyxoid tumor of soft parts: report of a case with novel cytogenetic findings. *Cancer Genet Cytogenet*. 2001;127:1–6.
44. Ekfors TO, Kulju T, Aaltonen M, et al. Ossifying fibromyxoid tumour of soft parts: report of four cases including one mediastinal and one infantile. *Apmis*. 1998;106:1124–1130.
45. Meis-Kindblom JM, Bergh P, Gunterberg B, et al. Extraskeletal myxoid chondrosarcoma: a reappraisal of its morphologic spectrum and prognostic factors based on 117 cases. *Am J Surg Pathol*. 1999;23:636–650.
46. Enzinger FM, Shiraki M. Extraskeletal myxoid chondrosarcoma. An analysis of 34 cases. *Hum Pathol*. 1972;3:421–435.
47. Antonescu CR, Argani P, Erlandson RA, et al. Skeletal and extraskeletal myxoid chondrosarcoma: a comparative clinicopathologic, ultrastructural, and molecular study. *Cancer*. 1998;83:1504–1521.
48. Domanski HA, Carlen B, Mertens F, et al. Extraskeletal myxoid chondrosarcoma with neuroendocrine differentiation: a case report with fine-needle aspiration biopsy, histopathology, electron microscopy, and cytogenetics. *Ultrastruct Pathol*. 2003;27:363–368.
49. Goh YW, Spagnolo DV, Platten M, et al. Extraskeletal myxoid chondrosarcoma: a light microscopic, immunohistochemical, ultrastructural and immuno-ultrastructural study indicating neuroendocrine differentiation. *Histopathology*. 2001;39:514–524.
50. Okamoto S, Hisaoka M, Ishida T, et al. Extraskeletal myxoid chondrosarcoma: a clinicopathologic, immunohistochemical, and molecular analysis of 18 cases. *Hum Pathol*. 2001;32:1116–1124.
51. Montgomery EA, Devaney KO, Giordano TJ, et al. Inflammatory myxohyaline tumor of distal extremities with virocyte or Reed-Sternberg-like cells: a distinctive lesion with features simulating inflammatory conditions, Hodgkin's disease, and various sarcomas. *Mod Pathol*. 1998;11:384–391.
52. Meis-Kindblom JM, Kindblom LG. Acral myxoinflammatory fibroblastic sarcoma: a low-grade tumor of the hands and feet. *Am J Surg Pathol*. 1998;22:911–924.
53. Hassanein AM, Atkinson SP, Al-Quran SZ, et al. Acral myxoinflammatory fibroblastic sarcomas: are they all low-grade neoplasms? *J Cutan Pathol*. 2008;35:186–191.
54. Fisher C. Low-grade sarcomas with CD34-positive fibroblasts and low-grade myofibroblastic sarcomas. *Ultrastruct Pathol*. 2004;28:291–305.
55. Hallor KH, Sciot R, Staaf J, et al. Two genetic pathways, t(1;10) and amplification of 3p11–12, in myxoinflammatory fibroblastic sarcoma, haemosiderotic fibrolipomatous tumour, and morphologically similar lesions. *J Pathol*. 2009;217:716–727.
56. Mentzel T, Scharer L, Kazakov DV, et al. Myxoid dermatofibrosarcoma protuberans: clinicopathologic, immunohistochemical, and molecular analysis of eight cases. *Am J Dermatopathol*. 2007;29:443–448.
57. Reimann JD, Fletcher CD. Myxoid dermatofibrosarcoma protuberans: a rare variant analyzed in a series of 23 cases. *Am J Surg Pathol*. 2007;31:1371–1377.

58. Frierson HF, Cooper PH. Myxoid variant of dermatofibrosarcoma protuberans. *Am J Surg Pathol.* 1983;7:445–450.

59. de Saint Aubain Somerhausen N, Rubin BP, Fletcher CD. Myxoid solitary fibrous tumor: a study of seven cases with emphasis on differential diagnosis. *Mod Pathol.* 1999;12:463–471.

60. Salm R, Evans DJ. Myxoid leiomyosarcoma. *Histopathology.* 1985;9:159–169.

61. Krane JF, Bertoni F, Fletcher CD. Myxoid synovial sarcoma: an underappreciated morphologic subset. *Mod Pathol.* 1999;12:456–462.

62. Fisher C, Magnusson B, Hardarson S, et al. Myxoid variant of follicular dendritic cell sarcoma arising in the breast. *Ann Diagn Pathol.* 1999;3:92–98.

63. Elliott D, Pitman MB. Malignant melanoma with a myxoid stroma: a diagnostic pitfall on fine-needle aspiration biopsy. *Diagn Cytopathol.* 2001;25:185–190.

64. Bhuta S, Mirra JM, Cochran AJ. Myxoid malignant melanoma. A previously undescribed histologic pattern noted in metastatic lesions and a report of four cases. *Am J Surg Pathol.* 1986;10:203–211.

65. Hitchcock MG, McCalmont TH, White WL. Cutaneous melanoma with myxoid features: twelve cases with differential diagnosis. *Am J Surg Pathol.* 1999;23:1506–1513.

22

PLEXIFORM SOFT TISSUE TUMORS

INTRODUCTION

The term plexiform refers to a pattern of local infiltration in which multiple, interconnected tumor nodules ramify in adjacent stroma or normal tissues and appear discrete in cross section. Thus, plexiform lesions are not circumscribed. Many tumor types can develop a plexiform pattern and some of these form distinct clinicopathologic subtypes. Most are benign but can recur or regrow locally, due to failure to excise all outlying branches of the lesion. In addition, plexiform fibrohistiocytic tumor has metastatic potential. The differential diagnosis is summarized in Table 22.1.

PLEXIFORM FIBROHISTIOCYTIC TUMOR

Clinical Features

Plexiform fibrohistiocytic tumor (PFHT) was first described in 1988 with 65 cases in the original report by Enzinger and Zhang.[1] Subsequent series of 14[2] and 22[3] cases, and most recently a further series of 66 cases[4] have confirmed the original description. PFHT is a slow-growing tumor that occurs mainly in adolescents and young adults, originally with a female predominance but with more equal sex distribution in later series. It forms a painless dermal/subcutaneous nodule, often tethered to adjacent tissues, and mostly on the upper limbs and head and neck region. One case arose in an irradiation field 7 years after treatment for malignant hemangiopericytoma.[5]

In the 2002 WHO classification, PFHT is categorized as a so-called fibrohistiocytic tumor of intermediate (rarely metastasizing) biologic potential. Thirty-seven percent of the original series of plexiform fibrohistiocytic tumor recurred, usually within 2 years, and two cases (3%) metastasized to regional lymph nodes. The overall recurrence rate is 33%, but only 2/16 (12.5%) recurred in one series of 22 patients.[3] However, in this series, one case metastasized to lymph node and two additional cases metastasized to lung. One further example with apparent lymph node metastasis has been reported.[6] There seems to be no correlation between histological features and behavior. A case with cytologic atypia has not recurred after 10 years.[7]

TABLE 22.1 Differential Diagnosis of Plexiform Soft Tissue Tumors

	Clinical Features	Microscopic Features	Ancillary Investigations
Plexiform fibrohistiocytic tumor	Young adults, mostly upper limb, head and neck. One third recur, rare cases metastasizes.	Nodules based on dermal-subcutaneous junction. Rounded cells, multinucleated cells, lymphocytes. Some have branching bundles of fibroblasts. Rarely myxoid or atypical	SMA+, CD68+, CD34–, S100 protein–
Giant cell tumor of soft parts of low malignant potential	Mostly upper limb. Subcutaneous or subfascial. Multinodular or circumscribed. Can recur, no metastases.	Uniformly distributed large osteoclast-like giant cells, bland mononuclear cells. Hemorrhage, peripheral osteoid, or bone formation. Vascular invasion	CD68+ in giant cells
Cellular neurothekeoma	Young adults, upper extremity, head and neck. Recurrence rare, no metastases	Dermal. Rounded nodules of uniform rounded cells. Multinucleated cells rare. Often myxoid. Can show focal nuclear atypia	SMA+, NKIC3 +, MITF+, S100 protein–, HMB45–
Dermal nerve sheath myxoma	Circumscribed multilobulated myxoid lesion, low cellularity	Spindle cells can show focal pleomorphism or multinucleation	S100 protein+ in myxoid areas, EMA+ at periphery of nodules
Plexiform schwannoma	Young adults, extremities, head and neck, GI tract. Deep variant mostly in females	Dermal or subcutis, rarely deeper. Variably sized nodules of Schwann cells. Mostly Antoni A pattern. Nuclear pleomorphism can be seen, but necrosis rare. Cellular variant has hypercellular fascicles, mitoses	S100 protein+, EMA+ at periphery of nodule

Plexiform neurofibroma	Associated with NF-1. Can involve large nerves in deep locations or more superficial ones. Can undergo malignant change. Can extend extraneurally as diffuse neurofibroma	Transitions from normal nerve. Nerve expanded by variable myxoid stroma and increased cellularity. Atypical variant has nuclear crowding, pleomorphism. Diffuse extraneural component in some	S100 protein+ focally
Diffuse neurofibroma	Some associated with NF-1. Children and young adults. Head and neck, subcutaneous infiltrative plaque	Sheets of short spindle cells in loose fibrous stroma, infiltrating between normal structures	S100 protein+ diffusely in nuclei
	Associated with plexiform neurofibroma–extends outside nerve bundles into soft tissue	Wagner Meissner bodies	
Plexiform xanthoma	Adult males, solitary or rarely multiple. Knee, elbow. Hypercholesterolemia rare	Irregularly sized nodule in dermis and subcutis. Sheets of vacuolated macrophages. Occasional giant cells	CD68+
Plexiform ossifying fibromyxoid tumor	Young adults, limbs, head and neck.	Subcutaneous. Each nodule encapsulated. Glomus-like cells with small rounded nuclei and clear cytoplasm	S100 protein+, GFAP+, desmin+ focally
Plexiform leiomyoma	Subcutaneous or female genital tract. No specific clinical features	Nonencapsulated nodules without atypia, mitoses, or necrosis	SMA+, desmin+, h-caldesmon+

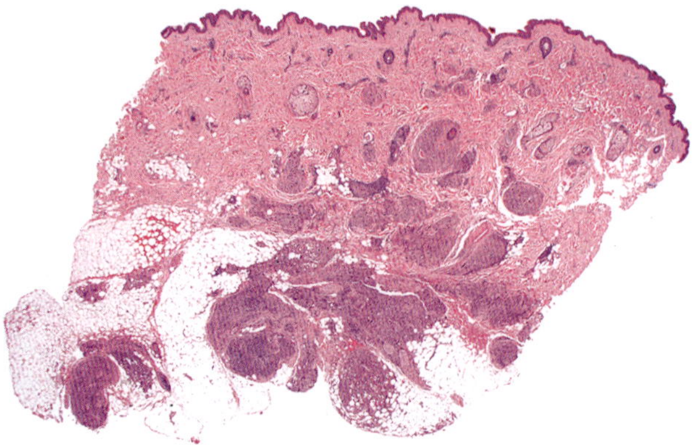

FIGURE 22.1 **Plexiform Fibrohistiocytic Tumor.** The tumor comprises multiple nodules centered on dermal subcutaneous junction and extending into both dermis and subcutis.

Pathologic Features

Most examples arise at the dermal-subcutaneous junction (Fig. 22.1), and can extend superficially or deeply (e-Fig. 22.1), but sometimes are wholly in dermis (e-Fig. 22.2). Two principal histological patterns are described. Forty-three percent display a fibrohistiocytic picture with nodules of rounded or spindled cells with scattered osteoclast-like multinucleate giant cells, chronic inflammation, microhemorrhages, and hemosiderin (Fig. 22.2, e-Figs. 22.3 and 22.4). Twenty-three percent are predominantly fibroblastic with plexiform bundles of uniform spindle cells (Fig. 22.3, e-Fig. 22.5), and 34% have a mixed pattern (e-Figs. 22.6–22.8). Occasional pleomorphic cells are seen, and mitotic figures are described up to 7 per 10 hpf. Myxoid change, bone formation, and focal cytological atypia[7] are rare findings. In older lesions, the nodules are gradually replaced by fibrous tissue (e-Figs. 22.9–22.11).

Ancillary Investigations

Immunostaining for CD68 is positive in rounded cells (e-Fig. 22.12) and in the multinucleate giant cells, which are probably histiocytic and non-neoplastic. The spindle cells have a myofibroblastic immunophenotype with focal reactivity for smooth muscle actin (SMA), and occasionally for calponin, but none for desmin or h-caldesmon. S100 protein, FXIIIa, and CD34 are negative in lesional cells. Ultrastructurally, the few reports variously indicate that the lesional cells comprise a mixture of fibroblasts, myofibroblasts, and undifferentiated mesenchymal cells.[2,8] The findings are similar to those in other benign or malignant fibrohistiocytic tumors.

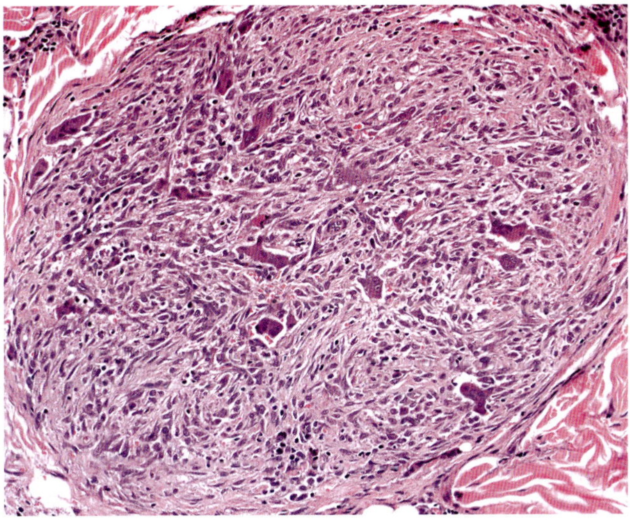

FIGURE 22.2 **Plexiform Fibrohistiocytic Tumor.** The fibrohistiocytic nodules are circumscribed and contain a mixture of bland histiocyte-like cells and osteoclast-like giant cells, with a sprinkling of lymphocytes.

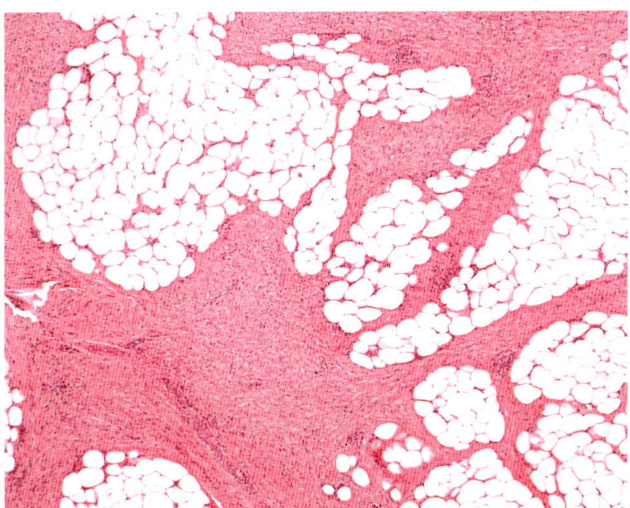

FIGURE 22.3 **Plexiform Fibrohistiocytic Tumor.** Fibroblastic variant. Moderately cellular fascicles of spindle cells in fibrous stroma branch and anastomose in subcutaneous fat.

Clonal genetic abnormalities have been reported in two cases, but no consistent changes have been found. One example had a complex karyotype with numerous deletions[9] and the other demonstrated a simpler karyotype of 46,XY,t(4;15)(q21;q15).[10] All cases examined have been diploid.[3]

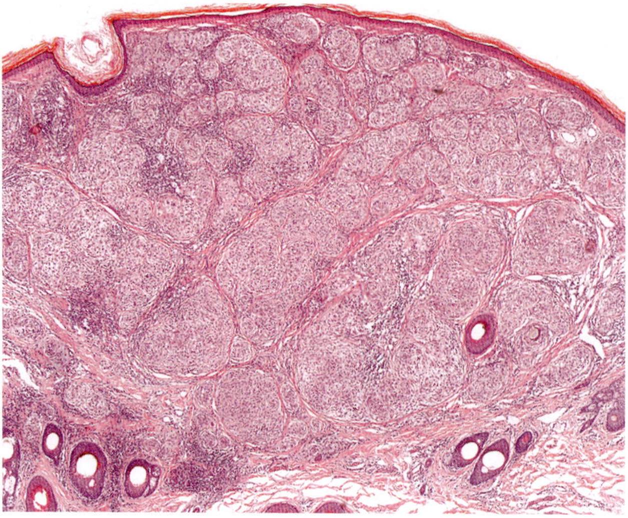

FIGURE 22.4 **Cellular Neurothekeoma.** Low-power view showing an unencapsulated dermal lesion composed of variably sized nests of uniform polygonal cells. The overlying epidermis is thinned.

CELLULAR NEUROTHEKEOMA

Cellular neurothekeoma has many similarities to plexiform fibrohistiocytic tumor. Indeed, in some cases, the distinction cannot be made and it has been proposed that the two entities are closely related if not identical, differing essentially by the plane in which they are located.[11,12] Cellular neurothekeoma was originally thought to be a cellular variant of nerve sheath myxoma, and the term neurothekeoma has included both entities (see Chapter 20). However, dermal nerve sheath myxoma is a circumscribed lesion with multiple myxoid nodules containing S100 protein–positive Schwann cells, with peripheral epithelial membrane antigen (EMA)–positive perineurial cells.[13] This is clearly different from cellular neurothekeoma, a nonneural tumor, even though the latter can show myxoid change.[12] The tumor is usually located in the dermis with occasional extension into subcutis (Figs. 22.4 and 22.5, e-Figs. 22.13–22.15), and comprises ovoid or sometimes spindled cells with eosinophilic cytoplasm in rounded nodules enclosed and separated by variable amount of collagen (e-Figs. 22.14–22.17), and sometimes in sheets. Multinucleated lesional cells can be seen in up to 40% of cases, and moderate to marked nuclear atypia in up to 25% of cases, (e-Figs. 22.18 and 22.19) as well as mitotic activity (e-Fig. 22.20) including abnormal forms. Myxoid change, with cellular spindling, predominates in about 20% of cases, and about 30% of cases are mixed cellular and myxoid lesions (e-Figs. 22.21–22.24). A small number are distinctly plexiform, and osteoclast-like giant cells are seen in up to 30% of lesions. Cellular neurothekeoma differs histologically from plexiform fibrohistiocytic tumor in the absence of fibromatosis-like areas

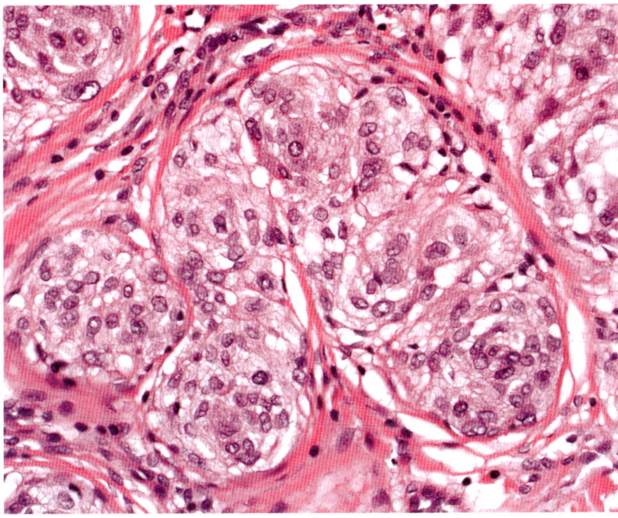

FIGURE 22.5 **Cellular Neurothekeoma.** The nodules contain rounded cells with minimally pleomorphic vesicular nuclei and darkly eosinophilic cytoplasm.

and of nodular hyalinization, in having less hemosiderin, and in the much more frequent occurrence of myxoid change and atypia, but has a similar immunophenotype,[4] expressing NKI-C3[14] and microphthalmia-associated transcription factor (MiTF).[15] S100 protein, and the melanocytic markers melan-A and HMB45, are negative in both tumors.

PLEXIFORM SCHWANNOMA

Clinical Features

This is a dermal or subcutaneous lesion of young adults, involving extremities and head and neck, but also described in GI tract.[16,17] A deeply located variant has been described, which arises mostly in deep soft tissue of extremities, has a predilection for females, and can occur as a congenital lesion.[17] Plexiform schwannomas are usually solitary and occasionally multiple,[18] and are rarely associated with neurofibromatosis type 1 (NF-1)[19] or type 2 (NF-2),[20] or schwannomatosis.[17] Cases formerly described as plexiform malignant peripheral nerve sheath tumor of infancy and childhood[21] are now recognized as congenital and childhood plexiform cellular schwannoma.[22] These occur mostly in females in the lower limb and are unassociated with NF-1. All reported examples recurred locally, but none metastasized.[22]

Pathological Features

Plexiform schwannoma represents about 4% of all schwannomas[23] and is composed of multiple nodules of Schwann cells, usually with Antoni A pattern, with a rim of perineurial cells and a thin fibrous capsule around each nodule (Figs. 22.6 and 22.7, e-Figs. 22.25–22.30). Nuclear atypia is

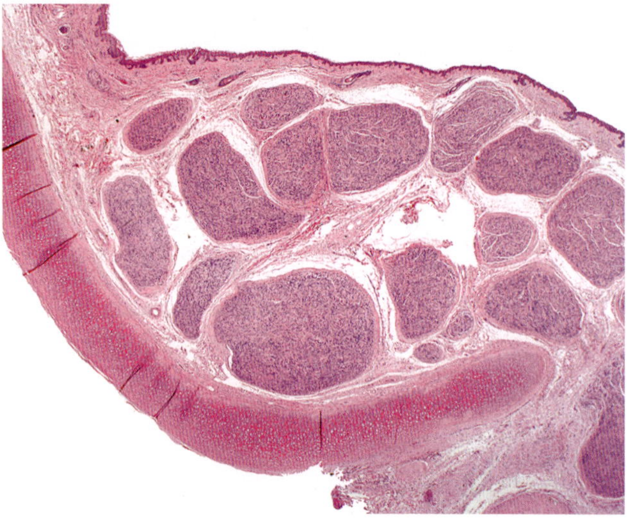

FIGURE 22.6 **Plexiform Schwannoma, External Ear.** The tumor comprises multiple discrete encapsulated cellular nodules within the dermis and subcutis, abutting the cartilage of the pinna.

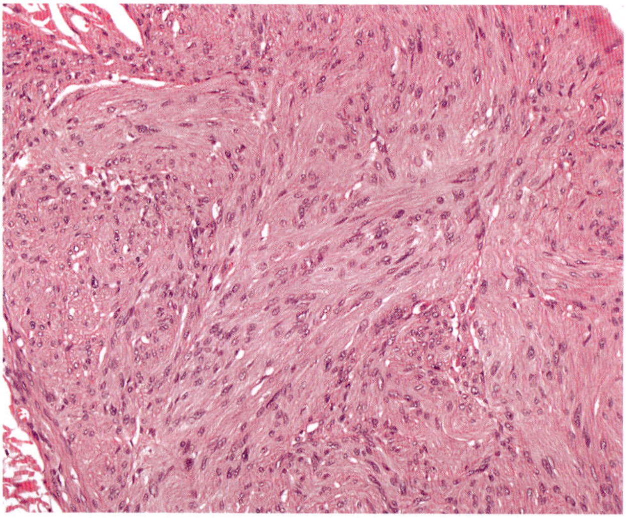

FIGURE 22.7 **Plexiform Cellular Schwannoma.** Each nodule resembles regular cellular schwannoma with fascicles of spindle cells with eosinophilic cytoplasm.

frequently seen (e-Fig. 22.29) and does not indicate malignancy.[24] This lesion differs from palisaded encapsulated neuroma principally in having a more uniform Schwann cell composition and fewer axons. Deep-seated plexiform schwannomas can additionally show necrosis and myxoid change.[17] Plexiform cellular schwannoma is circumscribed or infiltrative and comprises hypercellular nodules of spindle cells with elongated hyperchromatic nuclei and very scanty cytoplasm (e-Figs. 22.30–22.33). This

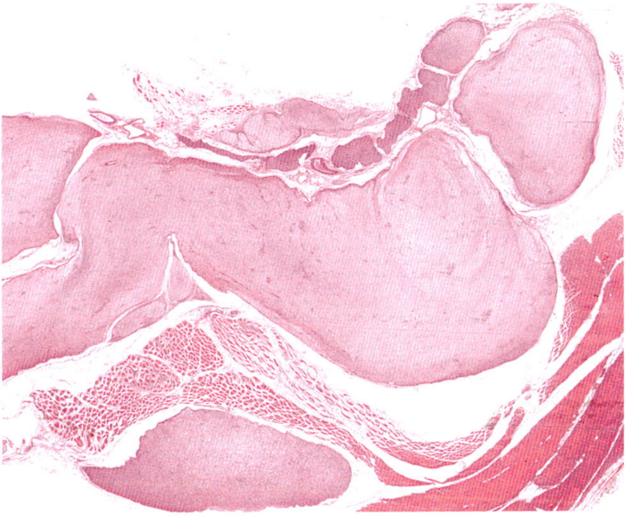

FIGURE 22.8 **Plexiform Neurofibroma.** This lesion comprises several discrete cross sections of expanded nerve bundles. It involves subcutaneous tissue and extends into skeletal muscle.

tumor typically shows mitotic activity that can in rare cases exceed 30 per 10 hpf without being indicative of malignancy.[22]

Ancillary Features

Like regular schwannoma, the Schwann cells show diffuse positivity for S100 protein[25] (e-Fig. 22.33) and variable immunoreactivity for glial fibrillary acidic protein (GFAP). The peripheral perineurial cells can be highlighted by their EMA positivity, and occasional axons can be demonstrated by immunostaining for neurofilaments (e-Fig. 22.34).

PLEXIFORM NEUROFIBROMA

Clinical Features

Plexiform neurofibroma, which is a marker for NF-1, is an intraneural neurofibroma in which the abnormal neural component becomes enlarged and tortuous but remains in continuity with normal nerve. This can involve deep nerve trunks at any site but especially limbs pelvis, retroperitoneum, or mesentery of bowel (with a rare association with ganglioneuromatosis[26]) and presents as a slow-growing mass. There is an increased risk of malignant transformation, often manifest as more rapid enlargement.

Pathological Features

There is a nonencapsulated expansion of the nerve trunk first by increased myxoid stroma, then by proliferation of cells, which can spill out into adjacent soft tissue, resembling diffuse neurofibroma (Figs. 22.8 and 22.9,

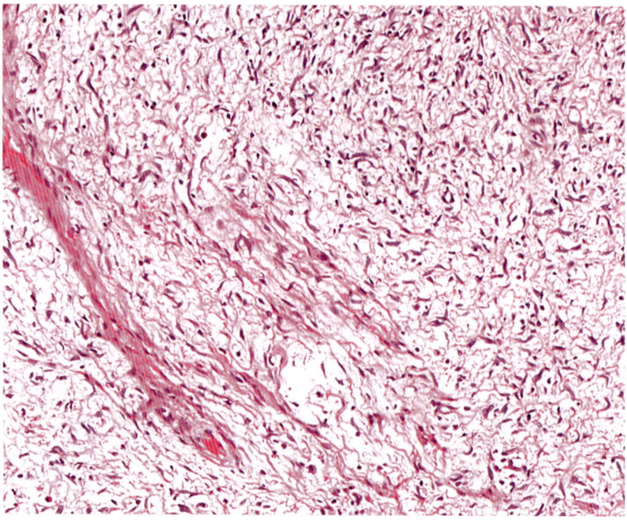

FIGURE 22.9 **Plexiform Neurofibroma.** The abnormal nerves contain increased numbers of cells and an increased amount of collagen and myxoid stroma

e-Figs. 22.35–22.37). The central area of the abnormal nerve can sometimes have more closely packed Schwann cells, here resembling schwannoma (e-Fig. 22.38). These changes are not well demarcated, and there is a gradual increase in cellularity along the nerve trunk. Marked cellularity indicates further observation for features indicative of malignant change–widespread atypia, mitoses, and necrosis.

Ancillary Features

S100 protein highlights Schwann cells, but the staining is less diffuse than in schwannoma (e-Fig. 22.39). In areas of malignant transformation, fewer cells demonstrate S100 protein positivity, which can be very focal. Axons can be demonstrated by immunostains for neurofilament proteins.

PLEXIFORM XANTHOMA

Clinical Features

Plexiform xanthomatous tumor is a rare lesion that can be solitary or multiple and occurs exclusively in males aged between 20 and 59 years.[27–29] The knee and elbow are the most frequent locations, with occasional cases in the hand and foot, but they are very rarely associated with hyperlipidemia. Two patients with multiple lesions experienced recurrences,[28] but none has metastasized.

Pathologic Features

The lesions are located in dermis or subcutis and composed of sheets of xanthoma cells and epithelioid cells, with cholesterol clefts and Touton giant cells in some cases (Fig. 22.10, e-Figs. 22.40–22.42).

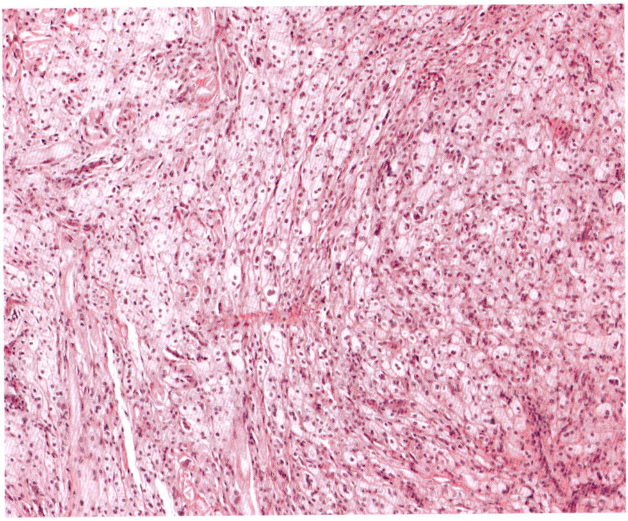

FIGURE 22.10 **Plexiform Xanthoma.** The lesional cells are arranged in ill-defined nests. The cells are small, with clear cytoplasm and rounded, mostly central nuclei.

Ancillary Investigations

The lesional cells are positive for CD68 but lack other markers.

OTHER TUMORS WITH OCCASIONAL PLEXIFORM PATTERN

Leiomyoma (Chapter 6) can sometimes have a plexiform pattern, especially in the female genital tract. A plexiform variant of **granular cell tumor** has been described.[30] This is similar in all other respects to the regular granular cell tumor (Chapter 12). Similarly, plexiform variants of **perineurioma** (Chapter 9),[31,32] **spindle cell nevus**,[33] and **Spitz nevus**[34] are readily identifiable from their other features. **Ossifying fibromyxoid tumor** (Chapter 21) can be multinodular or plexiform especially when located in the dermis or superficial subcutis (e-Figs. 22.43 and 22.44). The nodules are often encapsulated and the small glomus-like cells can be distinguished from cellular neurothekeoma and plexiform fibrohistiocytic tumor by their expression of S100 protein and GFAP, and sometimes desmin. **Giant cell tumor of soft parts (of low malignant potential)**[35,36] (Chapter 23) forms multinodular or circumscribed lesions in superficial or deep soft tissue, commonly in upper limb. Histologically, it is similar to giant cell tumor of bone, with bland mononuclear and short spindle cells and uniformly distributed osteoclast-like multinucleated giant cells (e-Figs. 22.45 and 22.46). Sometimes, there is metaplastic bone or osteoid, usually peripherally, and aneurysmal spaces. Vascular space invasion is common, but none has metastasized, although a proportion recurs.

REFERENCES

1. Enzinger FM, Zhang RY. Plexiform fibrohistiocytic tumor presenting in children and young adults. An analysis of 65 cases. *Am J Surg Pathol.* 1988;12:818–826.
2. Hollowood K, Holley MP, Fletcher CD. Plexiform fibrohistiocytic tumour: clinicopathological, immunohistochemical and ultrastructural analysis in favour of a myofibroblastic lesion. *Histopathology.* 1991;19:503–513.
3. Remstein ED, Arndt CA, Nascimento AG. Plexiform fibrohistiocytic tumor: clinicopathologic analysis of 22 cases. *Am J Surg Pathol.* 1999;23:662–670.
4. Moosavi C, Jha P, Fanburg-Smith JC. An update on plexiform fibrohistiocytic tumor and addition of 66 new cases from the Armed Forces Institute of Pathology, in honor of Franz M. Enzinger, MD. *Ann Diagn Pathol.* 2007;11:313–319.
5. August C, Holzhausen HJ, Zornig C, et al. Plexiform fibrohistiocytic tumor. Histology, immunohistology and ultrastructure. *Pathologe.* 1994;15:49–53.
6. Segura LG, Harris J, Wang B, et al. Plexiform fibrohistiocytic tumor: a rare low-grade malignancy of children and young adults. *Arch Otolaryngol Head Neck Surg.* 2002;128:966–970.
7. Fisher C. Atypical plexiform fibrohistiocytic tumour. *Histopathology.* 1997;30:271–273.
8. Angervall L, Kindblom LG, Lindholm K, et al. Plexiform fibrohistiocytic tumor. Report of a case involving preoperative aspiration cytology and immunohistochemical and ultrastructural analysis of surgical specimens. *Pathol Res Pract.* 1992;188:350–356; discussion 356–359.
9. Smith S, Fletcher CD, Smith MA, et al. Cytogenetic analysis of a plexiform fibrohistiocytic tumor. *Cancer Genet Cytogenet.* 1990;48:31–34.
10. Redlich GC, Montgomery KD, Allgood GA, et al. Plexiform fibrohistiocytic tumor with a clonal cytogenetic anomaly. *Cancer Genet Cytogenet.* 1999;108:141–143.
11. Jaffer S, Ambrosini-Spaltro A, Mancini AM, et al. Neurothekeoma and plexiform fibrohistiocytic tumor: mere histologic resemblance or histogenetic relationship? *Am J Surg Pathol.* 2009;33:905–913.
12. Laskin WB, Fetsch JF, Miettinen M. The "neurothekeoma": immunohistochemical analysis distinguishes the true nerve sheath myxoma from its mimics. *Hum Pathol.* 2000;31:1230–1241.
13. Fetsch JF, Laskin WB, Miettinen M. Nerve sheath myxoma: a clinicopathologic and immunohistochemical analysis of 57 morphologically distinctive, S-100 protein- and GFAP-positive, myxoid peripheral nerve sheath tumors with a predilection for the extremities and a high local recurrence rate. *Am J Surg Pathol.* 2005;29:1615–1624.
14. Sachdev R, Sundram UN. Frequent positive staining with NKI/C3 in normal and neoplastic tissues limits its usefulness in the diagnosis of cellular neurothekeoma. *Am J Clin Pathol.* 2006;126:554–563.
15. Busam KJ, Iversen K, Coplan KC, et al. Analysis of microphthalmia transcription factor expression in normal tissues and tumors, and comparison of its expression with S-100 protein, gp100, and tyrosinase in desmoplastic malignant melanoma. *Am J Surg Pathol.* 2001;25:197–204.
16. Iida A, Imamura Y, Katayama K, et al. Plexiform schwannoma of the small intestine: report of a case. *Surg Today.* 2003;33:940–943.
17. Agaram NP, Prakash S, Antonescu CR. Deep-seated plexiform schwannoma: a pathologic study of 16 cases and comparative analysis with the superficial variety. *Am J Surg Pathol,* 2005;29:1042–1048.
18. Sheikh S, Gomes M, Montgomery E. Multiple plexiform schwannomas in a patient with neurofibromatosis. *J Thorac Cardiovasc Surg.* 1998;115:240–242.

19. Kleinman GM, Sanders FJ, Gagliardi JM. Plexiform schwannoma. *Clin Neuropathol.* 1985;4:265–266.
20. Lim HS, Jung J, Chung KY. Neurofibromatosis type 2 with multiple plexiform schwannomas. *Int J Dermatol.* 2004;43:336–340.
21. Meis-Kindblom JM, Enzinger FM. Plexiform malignant peripheral nerve sheath tumor of infancy and childhood. *Am J Surg Pathol.* 1994;18:479–485.
22. Woodruff JM, Scheithauer BW, Kurtkaya-Yapicier O, et al. Congenital and childhood plexiform (multinodular) cellular schwannoma: a troublesome mimic of malignant peripheral nerve sheath tumor. *Am J Surg Pathol.* 2003;27:1321–1329.
23. Berg JC, Scheithauer BW, Spinner RJ, et al. Plexiform schwannoma: a clinicopathologic overview with emphasis on the head and neck region. *Hum Pathol.* 2008;39:633–640.
24. Fletcher CD, Davies SE. Benign plexiform (multinodular) schwannoma: a rare tumour unassociated with neurofibromatosis. *Histopathology.* 1986;10:971–980.
25. Guarino M. Plexiform schwannoma. Immunohistochemistry of Schwann cell markers, intermediate filaments and extracellular matrix components. *Pathol Res Pract.* 1993;189:913–920.
26. Thway K, Fisher C. Diffuse ganglioneuromatosis in small intestine associated with neurofibromatosis type 1. *Ann Diagn Pathol.* 2009;13:50–54.
27. Beham A, Fletcher CD. Plexiform xanthoma: an unusual variant. *Histopathology.* 1991;19:565–567.
28. Michal M, Fanburg-Smith JC. Plexiform xanthomatous tumor: a report of 20 cases in 12 patients. *Am J Surg Pathol.* 2002;26:1302–1311.
29. Michal M. Plexiform xanthomatous tumor. A report of three cases. *Am J Dermatopathol.* 1994;16:532–536.
30. Lee J, Bhawan J, Wax F et al. Plexiform granular cell tumor. A report of two cases. *Am J Dermatopathol.* 1994;16:537–541.
31. Weidner N, Nasr A, Johnston J. Plexiform soft tissue tumor composed predominantly of perineurial fibroblasts (perineurioma). *Ultrastruct Pathol.* 1993:17:251–262.
32. Zamecnik M, Michal M. Perineurial cell differentiation in neurofibromas. Report of eight cases including a case with composite perineurioma-neurofibroma features. *Pathol Res Pract.* 2001;197:537–544.
33. Barnhill RL, Mihm MC Jr, Magro CM. Plexiform spindle cell naevus: a distinctive variant of plexiform melanocytic naevus. *Histopathology.* 1991;18:243–247.
34. Spatz A, Peterse S, Fletcher CD, et al. Plexiform Spitz nevus: an intradermal Spitz nevus with plexiform growth pattern. *Am J Dermatopathol.* 1999;21:542–546.
35. Folpe AL, Morris RJ, Weiss SW. Soft tissue giant cell tumor of low malignant potential: a proposal for the reclassification of malignant giant cell tumor of soft parts. *Mod Pathol.* 1999;12:894–902.
36. Oliveira AM, Dei Tos AP, Fletcher CD, et al. Primary giant cell tumor of soft tissues: a study of 22 cases. *Am J Surg Pathol.* 2000;24:248–256.

23

SOFT TISSUE TUMORS WITH GIANT CELLS

INTRODUCTION

Many soft tissue lesions have a variable component of benign multinucleated cells of various types. They include cutaneous fibrous histiocytoma (Touton-type giant cells) (Chapter 4), giant cell fibroblastoma (closely packed small dark nuclei in horseshoe arrangement) (Chapter 4), juvenile xanthogranuloma (small wreath-like giant cells) (Chapter 12), pleomorphic lipoma (floret cells) (Chapter 15), plexiform fibrohistiocytic tumor (small osteoclast-like cells) (Chapter 22), and soft tissue chondroma (foreign-body type giant cells, Chapter 23). Some variants of tumors that normally lack giant cells can have such a component on occasion. These include nodular fasciitis (Chapter 3), fibromatosis (Chapter 2), atypical fibroxanthoma (Chapter 4), leiomyosarcoma (Chapter 6), epithelioid sarcoma (Chapter 11), clear cell sarcoma (Chapter 12), and undifferentiated pleomorphic sarcoma with giant cells (Chapter 13). This chapter includes those entities in which giant cells are a prominent and consistent feature. The differential diagnosis is summarized in Table 23.1.

RETICULOHISTIOCYTOMA

Clinical Features

Reticulohistiocytoma is a rare cutaneous lesion that occurs in adults, and can be solitary or multicentric (reticulohistiocytosis). Solitary reticulohistiocytoma (SR) occurs in adults with a male predilection and can occur at any site. Multiple lesions are noted in fewer than one fifth of patients.[1] The lesions are circumscribed yellow-tan dermal nodules. They are benign or self-limiting lesions, and etiologically the lesions are thought to be immunologically driven rather than true neoplasms. Multicentric reticulohistiocytosis is a systemic disease with a spectrum of symptoms, including symmetric arthritis, fever, and weight loss. It is sometimes paraneoplastic, with concomitant malignancies reported in 15% to 28% of cases[2], and can also be associated with autoimmune disorders. Patients develops multiple cutaneous and mucosal papules and nodules along with destructive arthropathy and visceral symptoms.

TABLE 23.1 Differential Diagnosis of Giant Cell Tumors

	Typical clinical features	Microscopic features	Ancillary investigations
Reticulohistiocytoma	Solitary cutaneous or multicentric reticulohistiocytosis affecting skin and synovium of joints	Multinucleated giant cells with ground glass cytoplasm, plump histiocytes, and mixed inflammatory cells	PAS+ (diastase resistant) CD68+, CD163+, MiTF+ (nuclear) in some
Juvenile xanthogranuloma, cutaneous	Infants, head and neck, trunk, proximal limbs. Yellow-brown plaque or nodule	Infiltrative dermal lesion. Sheets of histiocytes. Older lesions have more foamy cells and more Touton giant cells	SMA+, desmin+, h-caldesmon+, S100 protein–, CD163+
Juvenile xanthogranuloma, deep	Infants or young children, trunk, intramuscular	Monotonous sheets of macrophages.	CD68+, S100 protein–, CD1a–
Regenerating skeletal muscle	Damage due to trauma or infiltrating neoplasm	Atrophy of muscle fibers bringing nuclei into close proximity, mimicking giant cells. No cytological atypia	
Localized tenosynovial giant cell tumor	Any age, F > M. Usually in digits, particularly hand, but may involve larger joints. Nodular, circumscribed mass closely related to the synovium of the tendon sheath or joint	Circumscribed. Sheets of small, histiocyte-like rounded or polygonal mononuclear cells, with varying numbers of osteoclast-like giant cells, foamy histiocytes, siderophages, and other inflammatory cells. Hemosiderin deposition	Osteoclast-like giant cells and proportion of mononuclear cells CD68+. Desmin+ dendritic cells in up to 50% of cases

(Continued)

TABLE 23.1 Differential Diagnosis of Giant Cell Tumors (Continued)

	Typical clinical features	Microscopic features	Ancillary investigations
Diffuse tenosynovial giant cell tumor	Young adults. Papilliform lesion within the synovium; can spread into surrounding soft tissue. Extra-articular form has no connection to adjacent joint; usually in periarticular soft tissue but sometimes muscle	Infiltrative margins, sheet-like patterns of mixture of mononuclear cells, osteoclast-like giant cells along with foamy cells, siderophages, and other inflammatory cells. Variable cellularity with looser zones. Cleft-like spaces	Immunophenotype similar to that in localized giant cell tumor
Giant cell tumor of soft parts (low grade)	Typically middle-aged adults, Extremities, trunk, abdomen and pelvis, and head and neck. More common in superficial than deep soft tissue	Multinodular, cellular nodules of multinucleated osteoclast-like giant cells distributed among mononuclear cells. Divided by collagenous septa with hemosiderin-laden macrophages. Mononuclear and giant cells show vesicular, round to oval nuclei lacking atypia. Mitoses. Vascular invasion in some tumors	CD68+ (diffuse and strong in osteoclast-like giant cells, focal in mononuclear cells). Variable SMA+ in mononuclear cells. CK and S100 protein+ (focally in occasional tumors
Phosphaturic mesenchymal tumor	Frequently associated with oncogenic osteomalacia. Soft tissue, particularly limbs. Symptoms abate with removal of tumor	Low to focally moderate cellularity. Sheets of spindle to stellate cells with small, bland nuclei, within calcified smudgy myxoid to myxochondroid matrix. Mitotic activity absent to very low. Thin-walled branching hemangiopericytic vessels. Osteoclast-like giant cells	FGF23+ in most tumors

Tumoral calcinosis	Painless subcutaneous mass near joints or in extremities	Multilocular cyst. Fibrosing granulomatous giant cell reaction around crystalline amorphous or calcified material	
Nodular fasciiti	Young adults, short history, sometimes previous trauma, size <5 cm	Loose fascicles of spindle and stellate cells in myxoid stroma, extravasated erythrocytes, lymphocytes. Small multinucleated cells in later stages	SMA+
Dermatofibroma	Dermal lesions	Epidermal hyperplasia. Storiform pattern of bland spindle cells with foamy histiocytes. Trapping of peripheral collagen bundles. Hemosiderin and mixed chronic inflammation. Touton-type giant cells	Factor XIIIa+, variable calponin and actin+
Plexiform fibrohistiocytic tumor	Children to young adults. F>M. Most often in upper extremities. Small dermal or subcutaneous lesions	Multinodular or plexiform arrangements of histiocyte-like cells, spindle fibroblast-like cells and multinucleated, often osteoclast-like giant cells	Giant cells and histiocyte-like cells CD68+, fibroblast-like cells SMA+
Giant cell malignant fibrous histiocytoma	Older adults. Deep soft tissue of limbs or trunk	Sheets and fascicles of markedly anaplastic spindle to ovoid cells. Giant cells are predominantly osteoclast-like, but atypical tumor giant cells can also be present	Osteoclast-like giant cells CD68+

(Continued)

TABLE 23.1 Differential Diagnosis of Giant Cell Tumors (Continued)

	Typical clinical features	Microscopic features	Ancillary investigations
Giant cell fibroblastoma	Children in first decade. Dermis and subcutis	Loose fascicles of spindle cells in abundant collagenous to myxoid stroma. Variable numbers of scattered multinucleate stromal cells with central closely packed small dark nuclei arranged in wreath-like formations. Pseudovascular spaces rimmed by spindle and giant cells	CD34+
Pleomorphic lipoma	Neck and back. M > F. Subcutis	Admixture of mature adipocytes, bland spindle to ovoid cells, floret cells, and rope-like collagen bundles. Floret cells are multinucleate giant cells with hyperchromatic, radially arranged wreath-like nuclei	CD34+ (strong in spindle cells). Variable S100 protein+
Leiomyosarcoma with osteoclast-like giant cells	Older adults. Retroperitoneum, extremities. Also in skin and subcutis and large blood vessels	Intersecting fascicles of spindle cells with blunt-ended nuclei, paranuclear vacuolations, and eosinophilic cytoplasm	Desmin, SMA, and h-caldesmon+
Carcinoma with osteoclast-like giant cells	Primary site may be evident	Nested architecture, epithelioid cells	CK+

Pathologic Features

Reticulohistiocytoma is a dermal nodular lesion (e-Fig. 23.1) comprising a mixture of mono- and multinucleated histiocytes and fibroblasts, xanthoma cells, and chronic inflammatory cells (Fig. 23.1).[3] The histiocytes are plump with abundant granular eosinophilic cytoplasm. Multinucleate forms are frequent. These are often several times larger than the mononuclear histiocytes and have cytoplasm with a ground glass appearance (Fig. 23.2, e-Fig. 23.2). Nuclear atypia of varying degrees may be present, as well as occasional mitoses. There may be focal nuclear spindling of the histiocytes, but this is rarely extensive, and necrosis is absent.

Multicentric reticulohistiocytosis shows similar features, with nodules in the dermis that may extend into epidermis or subcutis, and can also be present at other sites such as synovium. Typically, there are multinucleated histiocytes of irregular size and shape with prominent nucleoli, with ground glass or foamy cytoplasm, although these tend to be smaller with fewer nuclei than those in SR. Earlier lesions contain a numerous mixed chronic inflammatory cell infiltrate with lymphocytes, plasma cells, eosinophils, mast cells, and histiocytes, while later lesions show larger numbers of giant cells and fewer lymphocytes.[4] As lesions progress, the inflammatory component including giant cells diminishes and fibrosis occurs.[4]

Ancillary investigations

The mono- and multinucleated histiocytes express some monocyte/ macrophage markers such as CD68, HAM56, and lysozyme but are negative for MAC387 and CD13.[5] The plump epithelioid cells express

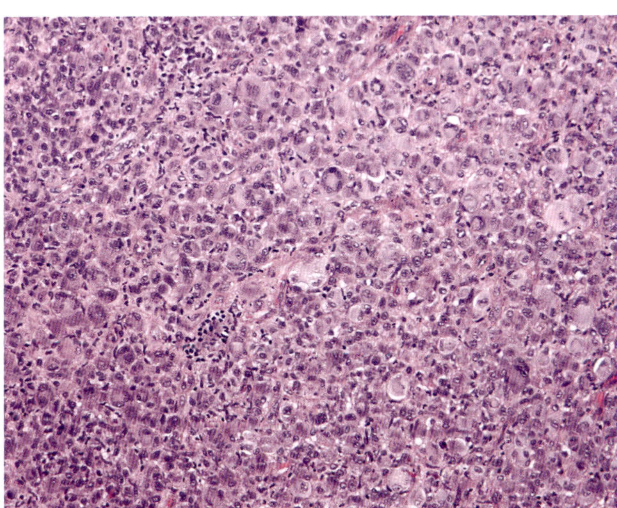

FIGURE 23.1 **Reticulohistiocytoma.** The lesion is nodular, and comprises a mixture of mono- and multinucleated histiocytes and fibroblasts, xanthoma cells, and chronic inflammatory cells.

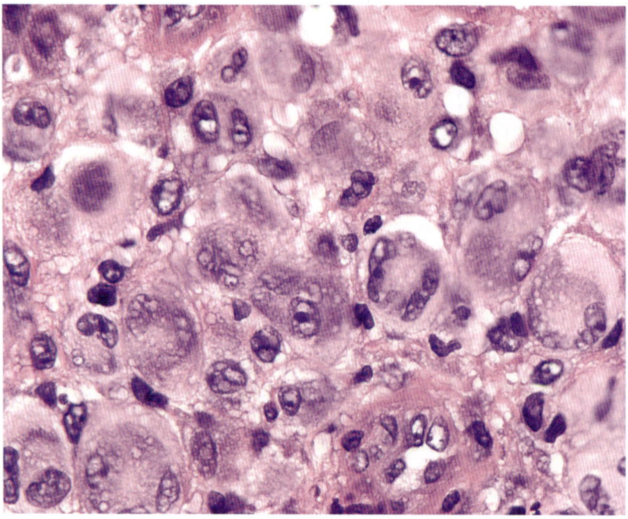

FIGURE 23.2 **Reticulohistiocytoma.** The histiocytes are plump with abundant granular eosinophilic cytoplasm, and there are frequent multinucleated forms.

CD163 and in some cases there is focal nuclear immunoreactivity for microphthalmia-associated transcription factor.[3] Desmin, smooth muscle actin (SMA), S100 protein, and CD34 are negative.[5]

JUVENILE XANTHOGRANULOMA, SUPERFICIAL AND DEEP

Juvenile xanthogranuloma is a benign, stable, or self-limiting non-Langerhans cell histiocytic lesion of unknown etiology. This lesion also has giant cells, but this is not as prominent a feature. A detailed account is given in Chapter 12 (e-Figs. 12.55–12.61). Superficial lesions extend to, although do not infiltrate, the epidermis, and also extend into the subcutis. Deep lesions can involve skeletal muscle. Early lesions show a monotonous infiltrate of macrophages with abundant eosinophilic cytoplasm. The cytoplasm accumulates lipid with time and becomes foamy. Older lesions in addition contain variable numbers of mixed inflammatory cells, including eosinophils, and giant cells of both Touton and foreign body-type. They are usually located at the edges of the infiltrate or within the superficial dermis. Nuclear atypia and pleomorphism and mitoses are rare. Deep lesions appear more monomorphic and less lipidized than superficial ones, and longstanding lesions become fibrotic.

TENOSYNOVIAL GIANT CELL TUMORS

Tenosynovial giant cell tumors can occur as localized or diffuse disease, and arise within (from the synovium of joints, bursae, or tendon sheaths) or outside joints. The clinical subtypes have similar immunohistochemical and genetic features.

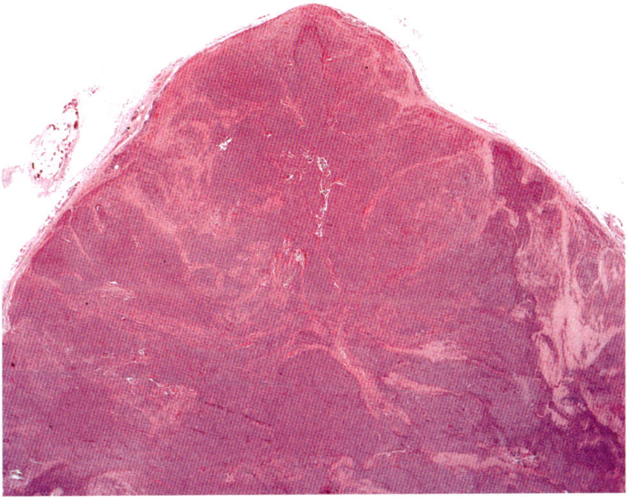

FIGURE 23.3 **Localized Tenosynovial Giant Cell Tumor.** The lesion is circumscribed, with a thin fibrous capsule, and has a multinodular architecture.

LOCALIZED TENOSYNOVIAL GIANT CELL TUMOR (GIANT CELL TUMOR OF TENDON SHEATH)

Clinical Features

This relatively common tumor can occur at any age, but is seen more often in adult females. It usually occur in the digits, particularly of the hand, but may rarely involve other sites including larger joints such as the ankle and knee.[6] It presents as a slowly enlarging, painless, nodular, circumscribed mass closely related to the synovium of the tendon sheath or joint. Tumors may erode into adjacent bone.[7] The tumor is benign and can usually be cured by surgical excision, although it can recur locally.

Pathologic Features

Macroscopically, extra-articular lesions are lobulated and small (<5 cm). Sectioning shows a firm, white, grayish or brown cut surface. Microscopically, the lesion is circumscribed and at least partly surrounded by a fibrous capsule (e-Fig. 23.3). It has a heterogeneous appearance and is composed of sheets of small, histiocyte-like rounded or polygonal mononuclear cells and larger mononuclear cells, with varying numbers of osteoclast-like giant cells, foamy histiocytes, siderophages, and other inflammatory cells (Fig. 23.2, e-Figs. 23.3–23.7). The mononuclear cells are mostly small, with ovoid nuclei and moderate amounts of amphophilic cytoplasm (e-Fig. 23.4). The larger mononuclear cells are more epithelioid with abundant cytoplasm and vesicular nuclei (Fig. 23.3). Giant cells are sparse in some tumors (e-Fig. 23.5). Mitotic figures are usually present (e-Fig. 23.6) with an average of about 5 per 10 hpf, but they can sometimes exceed 20 per 10 hpf.[8] The presence of mitoses does not denote malignancy, but can predict likelihood of recurrence. The stroma is collagenous and sometimes hyalinized (e-Fig. 23.7), and hemosiderin deposition is usually a prominent feature. Necrosis is rare, but can sometimes be seen focally; this is not indicative of malignant potential.

DIFFUSE-TYPE TENOSYNOVIAL GIANT CELL TUMOR (PIGMENTED VILLONODULAR SYNOVITIS)

Clinical Features

This is a locally aggressive neoplasm with significant recurrent potential[3] and which can rarely metastasize. It occurs primarily in young adults, with a slight female predominance. The diffuse form grows as a papilliform lesion within the synovium, most frequently in large joints such as the knee, hip, and ankle, and can spread into the surrounding soft tissue. It can also exist as a wholly extra-articular lesion, without connection to the adjacent joint, usually in periarticular soft tissue but sometimes within muscle.[9] Extra-articular sites include the wrist, knee, thigh, and foot.[9] In contrast to localized giant cell tumor, diffuse tumors are destructive and infiltrative lesions, and can recur after surgical excision. Pulmonary metastases and death have been described in a tumor with sarcomatous change, and nodal metastases have been seen in a case with benign histology.[9]

Pathologic Features

Grossly, tumors are often large. They have a villous pattern when present within the joint. Extra-articular lesions are usually poorly circumscribed. There may rarely be ulceration of the overlying skin. The cut surface varies from rubbery to soft and is variegated with yellow, brown, and white areas. Microscopically, the tumors show infiltrative margins (e-Fig. 23.8), but otherwise display similar morphology to localized tenosynovial giant cell tumor. They are composed of mainly sheet-like patterns of a mixed cell population (Fig. 23.4 and 23.5) of mononuclear cells and osteoclast-like giant cells (e-Figs. 23.9–23.12), along with foamy cells (e-Fig. 23.13), siderophages (e-Figs. 23.14 and 23.15), and other inflammatory cells. The morphological spectrum is wide, due to the variable numbers of each cellular constituent. Although these are cellular tumors, the degree of cellularity can vary within each tumor, with hypercellular areas alternating with looser zones. As in the localized form of giant cell tumor, there are two types of mononuclear cells. Small, histiocyte-like cells with ovoid nuclei predominate (Fig. 23.5), and scattered or clustered larger cells are also present, with bland oval or slightly folded nuclei and abundant pale to eosinophilic cytoplasm and sometimes dendritic cell processes. Cleft-like spaces are common (Fig. 23.6, e-Fig. 23.9) and can be present as synovial-lined spaces

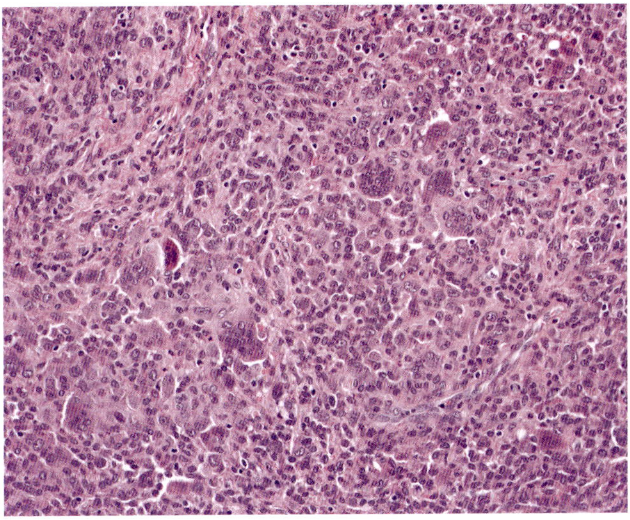

FIGURE 23.4 **Localized Tenosynovial Giant Cell Tumor.** This has a heterogeneous appearance, comprising sheets of small and large mononuclear cells, with varying numbers of osteoclast-like giant cells. Foamy histiocytes, siderophages, other inflammatory cells, and fibrosis are often present in varying proportions.

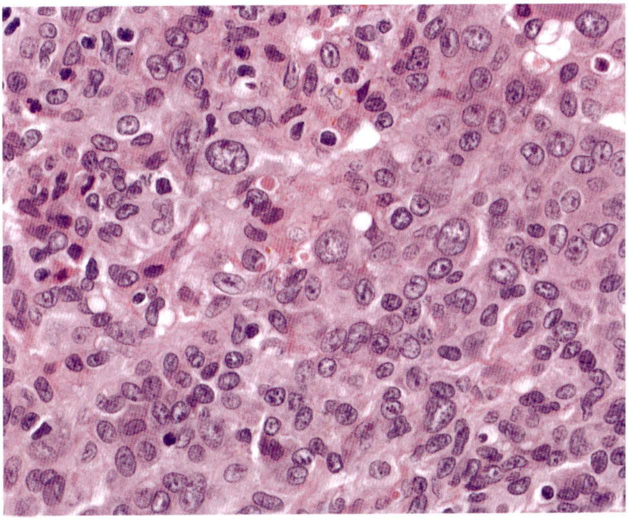

FIGURE 23.5 **Localized Tenosynovial Giant Cell Tumor.** There is a mixture of mostly small mononuclear cells with bland, ovoid or bean-shaped nuclei, as well as larger mononuclear cells that are epithelioid with abundant glassy cytoplasm and rounded vesicular nuclei.

or as apparently artifactual tears. Osteoclast-like giant cells are generally less frequent than in the localized form and in some cases may be sparse (e-Fig. 23.16) or absent. Notwithstanding their similar nuclear morphology, the giant cells are no longer believed to arise from the mononuclear cells and are interpreted as an epiphenomenon. There is a variable degree

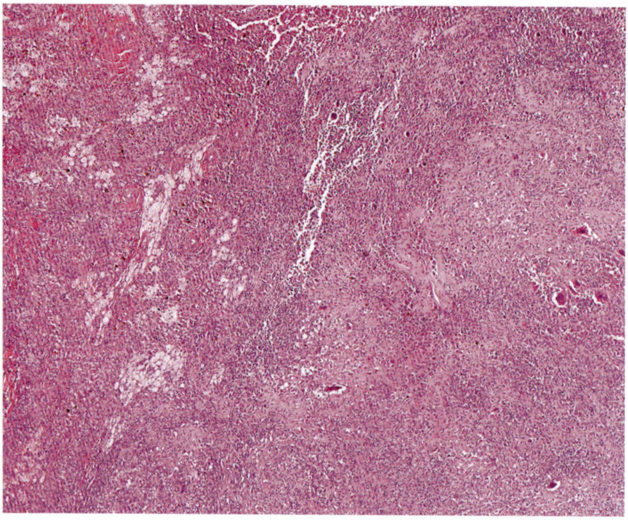

FIGURE 23.6 **Diffuse Tenosynovial Giant Cell Tumor.** This is composed of a mixed cell population of mononuclear cells and osteoclast-like giant cells, foamy cells, and siderophages in a focally fibrous stroma, with irregular cleft formation.

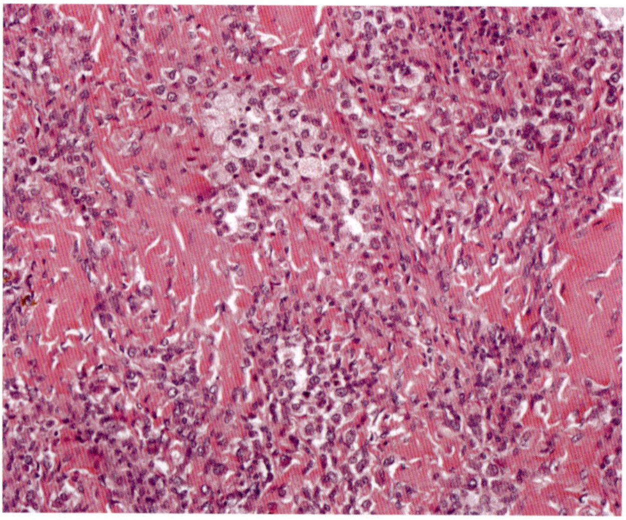

FIGURE 23.7 **Diffuse Tenosynovial Giant Cell Tumor.** The growth pattern is sheet-like, and there is a varying degree of stromal hyalinization. Clusters of lipid-laden histiocytes are also seen.

of stromal hyalinization (Fig. 23.7), with mixed inflammation including lymphocytes (e-Fig. 23.16), hemorrhage (e-Fig. 23.17), and cystic change.

Atypical histologic features such as spindling or cytological atypia of mononuclear cells, increased mitotic activity, and necrosis may be seen,[9] but each morphologic feature is not itself predictive of recurrence. Malignant giant cell tumor of tendon sheath is very rare. The term refers either to the coexistence of benign giant cell tumor with frankly malignant areas (which vary morphologically but which can assume malignant fibrous histiocytoma-like, fibrosarcomatous, or myxofibrosarcomatous patterns),[10] or to recurrence of obvious sarcoma at the site of a previous typical giant cell tumor.

Ancillary Investigations

The findings are similar in localized and diffuse tenosynovial giant cell tumors. Perls stain highlights the abundant hemosiderin pigment (e-Fig. 23.18). Osteoclast-like giant cells are positive for CD45 and CD68,[11] as are a proportion of the mononuclear cells. The mononuclear component also show variable expression of muscle-specific actin (HHF35) and neurone-specific enolase.[12] Additionally, the larger mononuclear cells form a subpopulation of desmin-positive dendritic cells, with long processes interdigitating between adjacent round cells (e-Fig. 23.19).[13] CD163 is also positive in the smaller mononuclear cells.[14,15] A recent study has demonstrated immunoreactivity for clusterin and D2-40 (podoplanin) in the large mononuclear cells.[15] Detection of clusterin, which is also expressed in normal synovial cells, might be useful for diagnosis in problematic cases.

Chromosomal translocations involving chromosome 1p13 are present in a majority of both localized and diffuse-type giant cell tumor. *CSF1*, the gene at the chromosome 1p13 breakpoint, is fused to *COL6A3* (2q35).[16,17] The *CSF1* translocations result in overexpression of *CSF1*,[16] although this has been described in the absence of the translocation, implying the existence of other molecular mechanisms.[18] Sarcomatous change has been associated with nonrandom loss of genetic material at 15q22–24.[19]

GIANT CELL TUMOR OF SOFT TISSUE (LOW MALIGNANT POTENTIAL)

Clinical Features

Primary giant cell tumors of soft tissue resembling those that arise in the bone are rare. They are most frequent in middle-aged adults, although there is a wide age distribution and they can occur in children as well. Presentation is typically as a painless enlarging mass, and the most common sites are the extremities, but lesions also occur on the trunk, and in the abdomen and pelvis,[19] and head and neck. They occur both in subcutaneous and, less frequently, deep soft tissue and vary in size between 1 and 10 cm.[20] Treatment is by surgical excision. Tumors can recur locally, but distant metastasis and tumor-associated death are rare.[20]

Pathologic Features

Grossly, the tumors are circumscribed, multinodular, or plexiform masses that often show hemorrhage and cystic change. Some may show partial

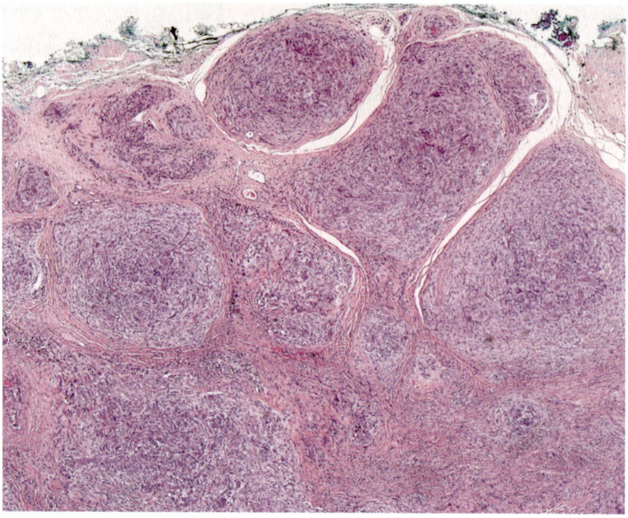

FIGURE 23.8 **Giant Cell Tumor of Soft Tissue.** The tumors are circumscribed, multinodular, or plexiform masses.

circumscription by a shell of reactive bone. Histologically, the appearances are similar to those of giant cell tumors of bone. There is a lobulated or multinodular architecture (Fig. 23.8, e-Fig. 23.20), with cellular nodules divided by collagenous septa (e-Fig. 23.21) that frequently contain siderophages (Fig. 23.9, e-Fig. 23.22). The nodules contain large numbers of multinucleated osteoclast-like giant cells distributed uniformly among mononuclear cells (Fig. 23.10, e-Fig. 23.23). Compared with plexiform fibrohistiocytic tumor, the cellular nodules are larger, the giant cells are more numerous, and a plexiform fibroblastic component is lacking. Both mononuclear and giant cells show similar vesicular, round to oval nuclei that lack atypia or pleomorphism (e-Fig. 23.24). Mitotic figures are usually present (e-Fig. 23.25), varying from fewer than 5 to more than 30 per 10 hpf,[20] and vascular invasion (e-Fig. 23.26) is seen in slightly less than a third of tumors.[20,21] Neither of these features is of prognostic significance. The absence of pleomorphic tumor giant cells and the lack of atypia in the mononuclear cells allow distinction from malignant giant cell tumor of soft parts (giant cell malignant fibrous histiocytoma), even when there is mitotic activity and vascular invasion. The stroma is often vascular and there may be stromal hemorrhage (e-Fig. 23.27), hemosiderin deposition, blood-filled cysts (e-Fig. 23.28), or aneurysmal bone cyst-like areas. The stroma can also show variable fibrosis and collections of foamy macrophages, but necrosis is rare. Metaplastic bone is often present at the periphery and may extend focally into the center of the mass.[19] It is usually of woven or lamellar type but can on occasion display a more immature morphology and include cartilage. The osteocytes are bland without atypia.[19]

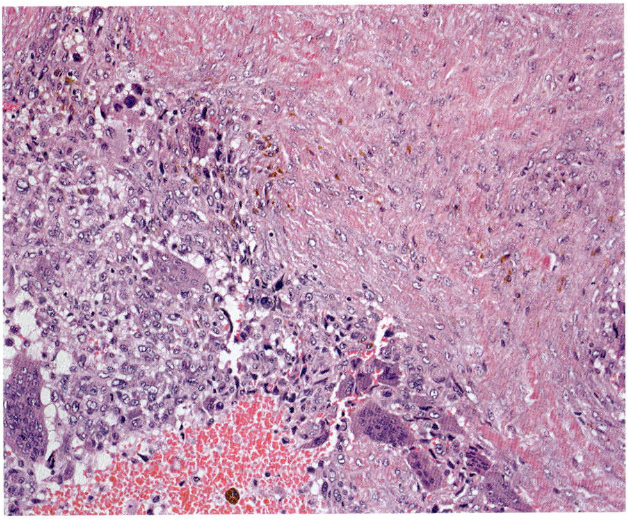

FIGURE 23.9 **Giant Cell Tumor of Soft Tissue.** Cellular nodules are divided by collagenous septa that frequently contain hemosiderin-laden macrophages.

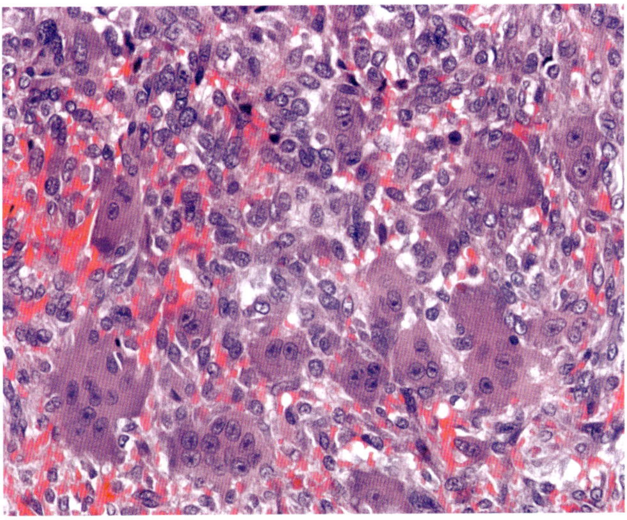

FIGURE 23.10 **Giant Cell Tumor of Soft Tissue.** Large numbers of multinucleated osteoclast-like giant cells are distributed uniformly among mononuclear cells.

Ancillary Investigations

Giant cell tumor of soft parts has an immunoprofile identical to that of giant cell tumor of bone. SMA can be demonstrated in the mononuclear cells,[19] and occasional tumors may show focal cytokeratin or S100 protein expression.[20] CD68 expression is characteristically diffuse and strong in the osteoclast-like giant cells, but only focal in the mononuclear cells.[20]

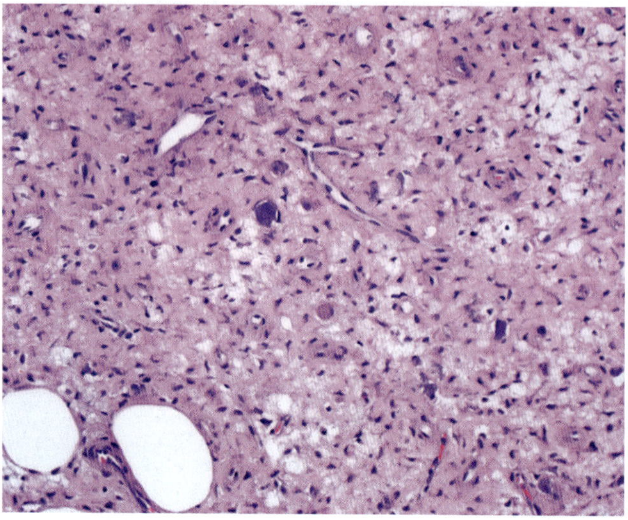

FIGURE 23.11 **Phosphaturic Mesenchymal Tumor.** Most lesions are of low to moderate cellularity, and cells are present within a focally calcified, irregularly granular, or amorphous myxoid to myxochondroid stroma. The thin-walled branching vessels sometimes form a prominent hemangiopericytic pattern.

PHOSPHATURIC MESENCHYMAL TUMOR

Clinical features

Phosphaturic mesenchymal tumor (mixed connective tissue variant) (PMTMCT) is a rare, distinct lesion that is frequently, although not always, associated with oncogenic osteomalacia,[22] a paraneoplastic syndrome due to phosphate wasting. It affects adults of either sex, most of whom present with a longstanding history of osteomalacia. Patient symptoms and biochemical abnormalities resolve with removal of the tumor. The lesion occurs in soft tissue, particularly within limbs, or more rarely bone,[23] and cases have been reported in the sinonasal region.[24] Most tumors are benign, but rare malignant (metastasizing) examples have been described.

Pathologic Features

Tumor size varies between 2 and 10 cm. Microscopically, appearances are very variable. Most tumors have low to focally moderate cellularity, and are composed of sheets of spindle to stellate cells with small, bland, normochromatic nuclei (e-Fig. 23.29). Cells may occasionally be more rounded or glomeruloid (e-Fig. 23.30).[22] The cells are present within a focally calcified, irregularly granular, or amorphous myxoid to myxochondroid stroma (Figs. 23.11 and 23.12, e-Figs. 23.31 and 23.32). Mitotic activity is absent or very low. The vasculature is often

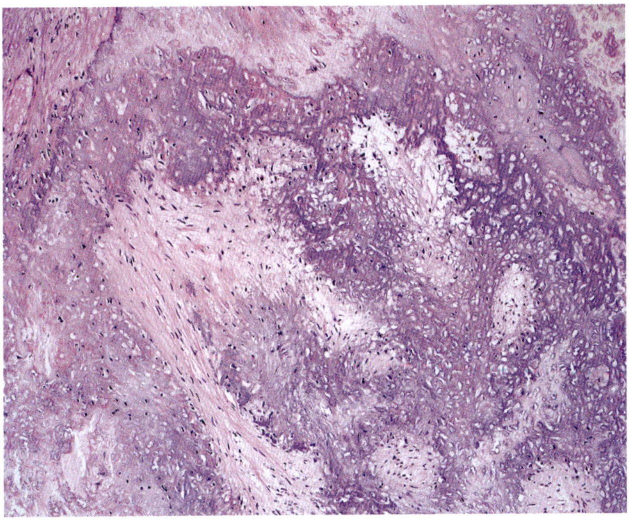

FIGURE 23.12 **Phosphaturic Mesenchymal Tumor.** The amorphous nature of the stroma and the irregular calcification are demonstrated in this lesion.

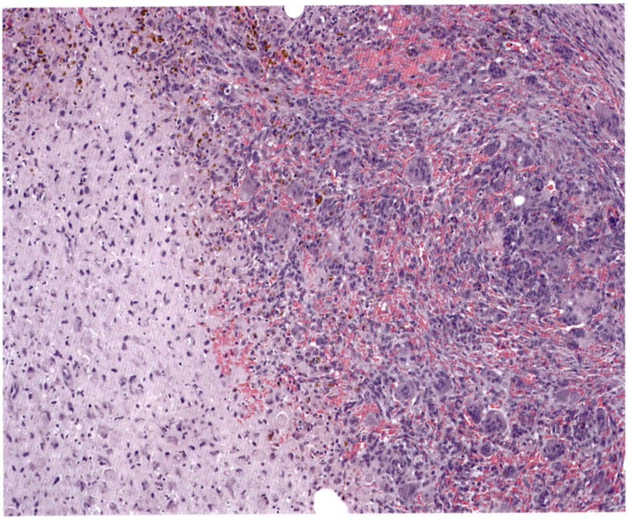

FIGURE 23.13 **Phosphaturic Mesenchymal Tumor.** Osteoclast like giant cells are frequently present, here amid abundant hemorrhage.

prominent, with thin-walled branching hemangiopericytic vessels (Fig. 23.11). Osteoclast-like giant cells are frequently present (Fig. 23.13, e-Figs. 23.33 and 23.34), and there may be hemorrhage[25] (e-Fig. 23.34) and microcysts.[23] Cartilage formation and osteoid-like matrix or bone deposition can occur, sometimes with an incomplete rim of membranous ossification.[22] Although the tumor is circumscribed, there is infiltration of surrounding tissues, including in benign appearing cases.[22] Malignant PMTMCT has at least focal hypercellularity, with atypical cells (e-Fig. 23.35) and a mitotic index of >5 per 10 hpf, and resembles an undifferentiated spindle cell sarcoma.[22]

Ancillary Investigations

Most tumors express fibroblast growth factor-23 (FGF23),[22,26] a protein that is implicated in renal phosphate loss,[22] and this can be detected immunohistochemically or by reverse transcriptase polymerase chain reaction.

TUMORAL CALCINOSIS

Clinical Features

This is an unusual sporadic or familial lesion in which there is extraskeletal deposition of hydroxyapatite crystals with a granulomatous tissue response and subsequent calcification. Some are associated with hyperphosphatemia or scleroderma, and familial examples, which are inherited in an autosomal recessive fashion, have mutations in *GALNT3*, *FGF23*, or *KL* genes. The lesions can be single or multiple, and occur in adults as a painless mass in the subcutis around large joints or spine, often attached to tendon or deep fascia, but not related to bone. A subset involves the extremities. Tumoral calcinosis is a benign lesion that grows slowly but can regrow if incompletely excised.

Pathologic Features

Macroscopically, this forms a poorly defined multilocular cystic lesion. Microscopically, amorphous or crystalline granular material (hydroxyapatite) is surrounded by histiocytes, multinucleated giant cells, and variable fibrosis (Fig. 23.14, e-Fig. 23.36). Later lesions have calcification including calcospherites. Soft tissue chondroma can have similar features but also has a component of differentiated cartilage and lacks the amorphous material.

Ancillary Investigations

Imaging studies show dense periarticular calcification. Serum calcium and alkaline phosphate levels are usually normal although there can be mild hyperphosphatemia.

OTHER LESIONS WITH GIANT CELLS

Damaged or regenerating skeletal muscle fibers, following trauma or infiltration of the muscle by tumor, particularly fibromatosis (e-Fig. 2.35), can be multinucleated, sometimes resembling Langerhans-type giant cells. The nuclei can also be irregular and hyperchromatic when they can be mistaken for tumor giant cells, or for rhabdomyoblasts.[27] The cells are

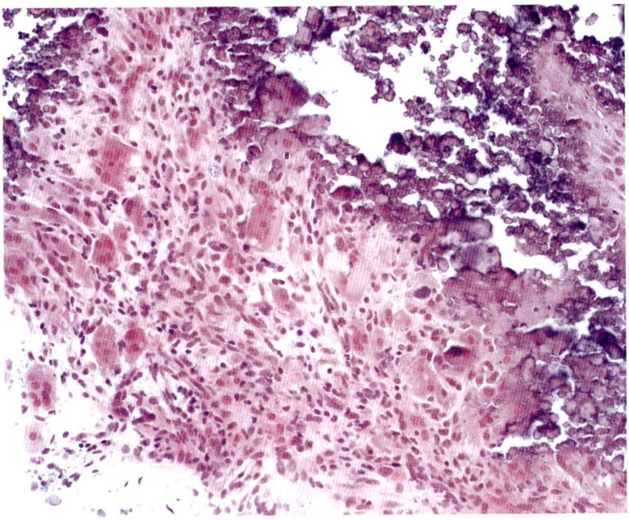

FIGURE 23.14 **Tumoral Calcinosis.** Amorphous or crystalline granular material (hydroxyapatite) is surrounded by histiocytes, multinucleated giant cells, and variable fibrosis.

desmin positive and sometimes focally so for myogenin. However, mitotic activity, prominent nucleoli, and frank necrosis are absent, and awareness of the clinical history and associated lesion, as well as familiarity with the appearances, can prevent error.

Poorly differentiated or undifferentiated carcinomas arising in various sites (chiefly breast, pancreas, lung, or bladder) can have an admixture of osteoclast-like giant cells that can be prominent. These can be identified by clinical features including location and by the demonstration of epithelial antigens.

Leiomyosarcomas with osteoclast-like giant cells form a morphologic subset although they are not behaviorally different from other leiomyosarcomas of similar grade (see Chapter 6).[28]

REFERENCES

1. Purvis WE III, Helwig EB. Reticulohistiocytic granuloma (reticulohistiocytoma) of the skin. *Am J Clin Pathol.* 1954;24:1005–1015.
2. Campbell DA, Edwards NL. Multicentric reticulohistiocytosis: systemic macrophage disorder. *Baillieres Clin Rheumatol.* 1991;5:301–319.
3. Miettinen M, Fetsch JF. Reticulohistiocytoma (solitary epithelioid histiocytoma): a clinicopathologic and immunohistochemical study of 44 cases. *Am J Surg Pathol.* 2006;30:521–528.
4. Tajirian AL, Malik MK, Robinson-Bostom L, et al. Multicentric reticulohistiocytosis. *Clin Dermatol.* 2006;24:486–492.
5. Zelger B, Cerio R, Soyer HP, et al. Reticulohistiocytoma and multicentric reticulohistiocytosis. Histopathologic and immunophenotypic distinct entities. *Am J Dermatopathol.* 1994;16:577–584.

6. Ushijima M, Hashimoto H, Tsuneyoshi M, et al. Giant cell tumor of the tendon sheath (nodular tenosynovitis). A study of 207 cases to compare the large joint group with the common digit group. *Cancer.* 1986;57:875–884.
7. Uriburu IJ, Levy VD. Intraosseous growth of giant cell tumors of the tendon sheath (localized nodular tenosynovitis) of the digits: report of 15 cases. *J Hand Surg Am.* 1998;23:732–736.
8. Monaghan H, Salter DM, Al-Nafussi A. Giant cell tumour of tendon sheath (localised nodular tenosynovitis): clinicopathological features of 71 cases. *J Clin Pathol.* 2001;54:404–407.
9. Somerhausen NS, Fletcher CD. Diffuse-type giant cell tumor: clinicopathologic and immunohistochemical analysis of 50 cases with extraarticular disease. *Am J Surg Pathol.* 2000;24:479–492.
10. Li CF, Wang JW, Huang WW, et al. Malignant diffuse-type tenosynovial giant cell tumors: a series of 7 cases comparing with 24 benign lesions with review of the literature. *Am J Surg Pathol* 2008;32:587–599.
11. O'Connell JX, Fanburg JC, Rosenberg AE. Giant cell tumor of tendon sheath and pigmented villonodular synovitis: immunophenotype suggests a synovial cell origin. *Hum Pathol.* 1995;26:771–775.
12. Cavaliere A, Sidoni A, Bucciarelli E. Giant cell tumor of tendon sheath: immunohistochemical study of 20 cases. *Tumori.* 1997;83:841–846.
13. Folpe AL, Weiss SW, Fletcher CD, et al. Tenosynovial giant cell tumors: evidence for a desmin-positive dendritic cell subpopulation. *Mod Pathol.* 1998;11:939–944.
14. Nguyen TT, Schwartz EJ, West RB, et al. Expression of CD163 (hemoglobin scavenger receptor) in normal tissues, lymphomas, carcinomas, and sarcomas is largely restricted to the monocyte/macrophage lineage. *Am J Surg Pathol.* 2005;29:617–624.
15. Boland JM, Folpe AL, Hornick JL, et al. Clusterin is expressed in normal synoviocytes and in tenosynovial giant cell tumors of localized and diffuse types: diagnostic and histogenetic implications. *Am J Surg Pathol.* 2009;33:1225–1229.
16. West RB, Rubin BP, Miller MA, et al. A landscape effect in tenosynovial giant-cell tumor from activation of CSF1 expression by a translocation in a minority of tumor cells. *Proc Natl Acad Sci U S A.* 2006;103:690–695.
17. Moller E, Mandahl N, Mertens F, et al. Molecular identification of COL6A3-CSF1 fusion transcripts in tenosynovial giant cell tumors. *Genes Chromosomes Cancer.* 2008;47:21–25.
18. Cupp JS, Miller MA, Montgomery KD, et al. Translocation and expression of CSF1 in pigmented villonodular synovitis, tenosynovial giant cell tumor, rheumatoid arthritis and other reactive synovitides. *Am J Surg Pathol.* 2007;31:970–976.
19. O'Connell JX, Wehrli BM, Nielsen GP, et al. Giant cell tumors of soft tissue: a clinicopathologic study of 18 benign and malignant tumors. *Am J Surg Pathol.* 2000;24:386–395.
20. Oliveira AM, Dei Tos AP, Fletcher CD, et al. Primary giant cell tumor of soft tissues: a study of 22 cases. *Am J Surg Pathol.* 2000;24:248–256.
21. Folpe AL, Morris RJ, Weiss SW. Soft tissue giant cell tumor of low malignant potential: a proposal for the reclassification of malignant giant cell tumor of soft parts. *Mod Pathol.* 1999;12:894–902.
22. Folpe AL, Fanburg-Smith JC, Billings SD, et al. Most osteomalacia-associated mesenchymal tumors are a single histopathologic entity: an analysis of 32 cases and a comprehensive review of the literature. *Am J Surg Pathol.* 2004;28:1–30.
23. Weidner N, Santa Cruz D. Phosphaturic mesenchymal tumors. A polymorphous group causing osteomalacia or rickets. *Cancer.* 1987;59:1442–1454.

24. Shelekhova KV, Kazakov DV, Michal M. Sinonasal phosphaturic mesenchymal tumor (mixed connective tissue variant): report of 2 cases. *Am J Surg Pathol.* 2010;34:596–597.
25. Shelekhova KV, Kazakov DV, Hes O, et al. Phosphaturic mesenchymal tumor (mixed connective tissue variant): a case report with spectral analysis. *Virchows Arch.* 2006;448:232–235.
26. Autosomal dominant hypophosphataemic rickets is associated with mutations in FGF23. *Nat Genet.* 2000;26:345–348.
27. Guillou L, Coquet M, Chaubert P, et al. Skeletal muscle regeneration mimicking rhabdomyosarcoma: a potential diagnostic pitfall. *Histopathology.* 1998;33:136–144.
28. Fletcher CD. Leiomyosarcoma with osteoclast-like giant cells. *Histopathology.* 1993;22:94–95.

INDEX

Note: Page numbers in *italics* indicate figures; those followed by t indicate tables.

N

Integrative Clinical Social Work Practice

Essential Clinical Social Work Series

Series Editor: **Carol Tosone**

For further volumes:
http://www.springer.com/series/8115

F. Diane Barth

Integrative Clinical Social Work Practice

A Contemporary Perspective

Springer

F. Diane Barth
New York, NY
USA

ISBN 978-1-4939-0350-4 ISBN 978-1-4939-0351-1 (eBook)
DOI 10.1007/978-1-4939-0351-1
Springer New York Heidelberg Dordrecht London

Library of Congress Control Number: 2014931106

Printed on acid-free paper

Springer is part of Springer Science+Business Media (www.springer.com)

To Joel and Simon, with love and gratitude forever

Preface

In recent years integrative practices have become part of the political and professional landscapes. Not only in medicine and mental health, but also in business, politics, international diplomacy, education, and many other aspects of modern life (e.g., see Fawcett & Hurrell, 2000), the idea of integration, that is, of bringing together parts that may not appear to be connected in order to make a more complete and complex whole, has become part of contemporary thought. In my years as a clinical social worker and psychoanalyst, I have found that many—perhaps most—of my colleagues and students draw from a wide variety of practical and theoretical perspectives in their work. Yet for many clinicians the integrative process is an unformulated and often unacknowledged part of practice. In this book I hope to open up a discussion of this often silent, "unthought known" (Bollas, 1989) component of clinical process. I hope that the book will encourage clinicians to find words for their own unarticulated integrative theory. It has been my experience that there is an important, often unnoticed parallel between clinical work, human development, and clinical theory. Just as contemporary research has shown the importance of talking to another person about what one thinks and feels both as part of development and as a therapeutic tool (e.g., see Fonagy, Gyorgy, Gergely, Jurist, & Target, 2003; Goodman, 2013; Hersoug, Hogland, Monsen, & Havik, 2001; Schore, 2003; Siegel, 1996; Steele, 2008), talking about how, when and, why we bring in different techniques enhances a professional's practice and provides a framework for choosing interventions with each client.

I therefore hope that this book will function as the beginning of a conversation in which readers begin to find words with which to formulate their own thinking about human behavior and what leads to change. Of course, bringing together different ways of thinking also means finding ways of managing conflict. In this book we will look at and attempt to understand conflicting theories, with the understanding that conflicts cannot always be resolved, but that they can sometimes enhance an experience.

Since my own personal and professional values are woven into the fabric of this book, I should probably take a moment to share a little about my own integrative background. Having grown up in a politically active family during a time of great social unrest, I came to social work with strong interests in education and political action. An avid reader, I was fascinated by anything that gave me clues to, as my mother put it, "what made people tick." I chose to become a social worker because the field appeared to honor and weave together these disparate threads. However, my placement in my first year of social work school at the Traveler's Aid Society, an organization that offered financial assistance to travelers stranded in New York City, appeared to address none of the issues that interested me. Neither ATMs nor the Internet existed at the time, and long-distance phone calls were often out of the financial reach of many of the people who presented themselves at the agency's offices. It seemed to me that I would simply be babysitting wanderers stranded until their spouses or parents could wire money to get them on a train or bus back to their homes. Disappointed, I asked my advisor about the possibility of changing placements to somewhere that would be more likely to give me a chance to work psychodynamically with clients. Then as now this was a goal not generally encouraged in social work graduate schools, but my advisor assured me that at the Traveler's Aid Society I would learn more about psychodynamics than I would even at a psychoanalytic institute. Furthermore, she said, I would get a hands-on experience in what Freud called the psychopathology of everyday life.

She was right; the work was fascinating. Clients included paranoid schizophrenics who lived on the streets not because of poverty, but out of fear of being contaminated or damaged. For example, one of those early clients had uncashed checks hidden in her bags but refused to live in an apartment because she believed that people in the building would read her mind and send radio waves to control her thinking. In my dealings with political and war refugees, run-away teens, and a variety of families and individuals from an incredibly broad spectrum of socioeconomic situations, I learned much about the human condition. I also learned that clinical social workers have been bringing together various theories and practices for many years. The idea of an integrative practice, formulated on a theoretical and research base, is more recent. This book offers clinicians, teachers, supervisors, and clients an opportunity to consider the what, when, how, and why of an integrative practice. It is intended to help clinicians think about and evaluate reasons for choosing to utilize specific tools with some clients and not others; and it provides theoretical grounding and evidence for both making and implementing these decisions. Clinical examples throughout illustrate ways that this can be done.

Extremely important to integrative work is the ability to combine flexibility with clear boundaries. One physician I interviewed during the process of collecting material for *Integrative Clinical Social Work Practice* said that underlying any integrative medical practice is a willingness both to recognize when one approach is not working and also to try something else. It is helpful for a clinician to be comfortable with other options in order to respond to what a client needs (Winnicott, 1987) rather than what a specific approach dictates. I believe this is also one of the ideas behind Kohut's (1971) ideas about offering clients "experience-near" explanations of their difficulties, rather than "experience-distant" interventions.

A note about confidentiality: all clinical material in this book is an amalgam of a number of different client/therapist dyads that were working on the issues being discussed. Identifying material has been disguised so that none of the clients or clinicians can be recognized. As I have noted elsewhere, like other authors (e.g., Spence, 1984; Williams & Schaefer, 2005) I have found this to be the best way of communicating important clinical concepts without breaching confidentiality. At the same time, I have sometimes used first names and others used last names because in our field, depending on agency policy and individual preferences, clinicians and clients may be called by either title. In each instance, I have used the same appellation for both client and clinician. Although I am aware that this is not always the case in actual practice, I have done so in the book because I believe it is an indication of respect and mutuality when a clinician and a client address one another in the same way—and can be experienced as a subtle sign of disrespect and inequality when they do not.

Each chapter in this book offers readers a way of thinking about specific aspects of clinical work while maintaining flexibility, theoretical clarity and clear-cut limits. Chapter 1, Integration or Eclecticism: Rationale for an Integrative Theory, explores some of the basic ideas behind developing an integrative clinical practice—what it means and what it entails. It offers three basic organizing principles that anyone who is drawn to such a practice can begin to apply immediately: (1) a clinician's personal and professional values; (2) a client's direct and indirect communications; (3) ongoing consultation, training, and professional education. Integration as an ongoing and developing *process* is discussed, as is the importance of integrating professional training with personal values. This chapter also presents the idea of an interactive approach to the work, which allows a clinician to make use of a wide range of techniques in a way that is meaningful and individualized for each client.

In Chap. 2: Contemporary Psychodynamic Models, readers are introduced to psychodynamic theory as a tool for understanding and making meaning out of what lies behind a client's behavior and experience. To some extent, such meaning-making is about articulating and mirroring a client's personal story, or narrative. Here too, an integrative perspective provides flexibility of approach to exploring and understanding such meaning. Clarifying that a psychodynamic approach does not necessarily mean offering a client such insight, the chapter focuses on eliciting what lies behind some of the thoughts, feelings, behaviors, and symptoms that may not be immediately clear either to a person experiencing them or to an observer. Understanding unspoken, unarticulated, or unconscious meaning can help a therapist determine a client's capacity for insight and as a result can aid in deciding what will be the best therapeutic approach to take.

Chapter 3: Developmental Models, offers a view of developmental theory as an umbrella for both thinking about a client's dynamics and also for thinking about the stages through which a clinical encounter often goes. Erikson's (1980) life stages are adapted to contemporary thinking and used as a model for one way that developmental thinking can be utilized in an integrative approach. In applying Erikson's epigenetic unfolding of different abilities and skills, a clinician may draw from developmental theory to understand both historical and current issues for a client. The idea that developmental theory can both expand and also constrict a clinician's ability to listen to a client's specific needs and concerns is also discussed.

In Chap. 4: Cognitive and Behavioral Models, discuss the idea that many clinicians integrate cognitive behavioral techniques, either intentionally or unintentionally, into work that is done from other perspectives, including psychodynamic and psychoanalytic ones. Similarly, many cognitive behavioral practitioners integrate a variety of theories and techniques into their work. In this chapter we also begin to explore the idea that integrative work can be understood not only as a single clinician bringing in a number of different theories and practices in her work with a single client, but also the work of several clinicians with a single client, in an integrative team. Traditionally, it has frequently been frowned upon when clients saw more than one psychotherapist at a time. Today clinicians are not only accepting, but even encouraging clients to work with other professionals who can offer them more tools for managing their symptoms. For example, a growing number of clients work with both a cognitive behavioral therapist and a psychodynamically oriented clinician at the same time.

Chapter 5: The Body–Mind Connection explores the complex interplay between body and mind, and their mutual interactive influence. Psychodynamic theories increasingly take the body into account Freud (Breuer and Freud, 1893–1895) paved the way for this view in his earliest discussions of the psychological and physiological aspects of hysteria. Conversely, many somatic therapies integrate psychodynamic, developmental, and even cognitive formulations into their premises. While recent explorations of body–mind dynamics have focused on trauma and neuropsychology, this chapter suggests that clinicians broaden the discussion to the interactive nature of body and mind in any therapeutic encounter because of the importance of integrating these aspects of any client's self into a more integrated, well-functioning unit.

Chapter 6: Making Assessments and Choosing Interventions looks at the ongoing nature of both assessments and choosing interventions. It begins with a discussion of the Mental Status Exam (MSE), which can be a useful integrative tool that asks for information about a variety of different aspects of a client or potential client's current and past psychological, social, cognitive, and developmental functioning. The importance of ongoing assessment is noted. Continuing to construct a detailed picture of a client's condition, symptoms, and strengths over the course of the work with any client can help a clinician choose interventions that make sense for that specific client at that specific point in time. Drawing from a variety of different perspectives can be particularly important in assessment. In this chapter we look at ways of dealing with some of the confusion that can also result from looking at a client from diverse and sometimes conflicting perspectives.

Chapter 7: An Integrative Approach to Therapeutic Relationships addresses the question of therapeutic relationships from different perspectives. Given the body of research that suggests that a relationship between therapist and client can be a key factor in therapeutic outcome, no matter what type of therapy a clinician is practicing (e.g., Bacal and Herzog, 2003; Frank, 2004, 2005; Leichsenring, 2005; Parish & Eagle, 2003; Roth & Fonagy, 1996; Schore, 2003; Siegel, 1999; Wallerstein, 2000; Wampold & Brown, 2005), it is clear that clinicians need to pay close attention to the factors involved in such relationships. An integrative approach helps a clinician answer questions such as what sort of relationship leads to change and whether clients with different diagnoses need different kinds of relationships. Further, bringing together developmental and other theories, an integrative approach can help a clinician decide whether to talk about a relationship or allow it to be a background presence, an often important and sticky clinical question.

In Chapter 8: Small Steps and Manageable Goals, we explore the process of goal-setting and evaluation. One key to this process is breaking large, often overwhelming problems and goals into smaller, more manageable components. This activity is presented not only as a tool but as an important part of a therapeutic process and captures an essential aspect of integrative work. Helping clients take small steps toward their goals can address immediate symptoms and engage long-term change, whether using cognitive or behavioral tools, focusing on body–mind dynamics, or working psychodynamically. As part of this process, we clinicians also need to find ways to break our own goals into manageable segments. We want to help our clients feel better immediately even as we help them make changes that will point toward a happier and more productive life in the future. In this chapter we will discuss the way that an integrative position can help us find a place to start that journey.

Chapter 9: Building and Working with an Integrative Team, looks at the idea that teams, whether formally structured or barely linked, can provide support and amplify the effects of any therapeutic experience. Team members can provide different perspectives on dynamics and behaviors, support one another through difficult situations, and provide backup so that a client is never without the support of a known and trusted professional. Research that underscores the importance of such backup, especially with fragile or difficult clients who need extra support or tend to fragment or destabilize when their primary therapist is unavailable, is discussed. Difficulties that can arise as a result of a team approach are also considered. Problems managing conflict are often part of clients' struggles; engaging in and untangling problems that arise in both interpersonal and interdisciplinary aspects of a team can be part of any therapeutic process.

In the final chapter, Working Through and Working On, we take an extended look at two clinical moments to talk about the actual practice of integrative psychotherapy. Recognition of patterns and continuity of experience are discussed. In this chapter, readers have an opportunity to see how the different elements in the preceding chapters can be brought into a practice on a regular and smoothly integrated basis.

Ultimately, of course, the purpose of this book is to engage clinicians in a discussion of how different approaches work, and why they do or do not help clients at any given time. An integrative practice is, almost by definition, a work in process. Hopefully this book will contribute to that work.

New York, NY, USA F. Diane Barth

Acknowledgements

Many, many people contributed to the writing and completion of this book, to all of whom I offer my tremendous gratitude. Clinicians, professors, and students across the United States took time from busy schedules to talk about their work, their training, and how they integrate or, in some cases, do not integrate different theories and approaches in service to clients. The work that these clinicians are engaged in is incredibly impressive. In order to protect the privacy of all clients, I am not thanking these clinicians individually, but my gratitude is boundless. Over and over again, I found myself feeling proud to be part of this incredible community of people, many of whom are working with populations that have been ignored or given up for hopeless by other professionals.

A special thank you to Betty Kramer and Constance Stewart, who provided unstinting hours of editing and support.

Many thanks to Carol Tosone for her encouragement and editorial expertise. Mindy Boslow, Mary Ellen Bowles, Jane Chase, Phyllis Diamond, Janie Eisenberg, Elizabeth Kleinman, Marcia Lavipour, Marilyn Lieberman, Dale Markowitz, Cynthia Medalie, Sherry Moore, Susan Zuckerman Morell, Lois Nachamie, Susan Needles, Christine Peak, Jerry Shapiro, Brian Smith, Cathy Siebold, and Roth Wilkofsky all aided the process. My gratitude to students and supervisees whose open discussions of difficult questions about when and why to make certain interventions and not others have helped me think about the topics in this book.

My brothers, Dr. Richard Barth and David Barth, read my chapters and offered incredibly helpful suggestions, provided endless support and encouragement, and pushed me to think about and expand my ideas in sometimes surprising and always intriguing directions.

Many, many thanks to my husband and son, without whom I could not have done any of this work.

And finally, heartfelt thanks to my clients, who have taught me as much as I have ever taught them, truly exemplifying Erikson's maxim that as we help others grow they do the same—or more—for us. They have often introduced me to parts of myself I did not know, helped me accept qualities I would rather not know about, and have repeatedly shown me the importance and the beautiful complexity of the clinical process.

A note about clinical material: In order to protect confidentiality, all clinical examples in this book are composites of several different people and situations. Following the suggestion of Spence (1984), I have changed names, genders, ages, presenting problems, family makeup, and other identifying information about all clients and clinicians included in these composites. I have similarly disguised settings and professions. Thus, in the telling of the stories, I have distorted and reconfigured facts while keeping dynamics and what Spence calls narrative truth.

Contents

Chapter 1
Integration or Eclecticism: Rationale for an Integrative Theory

Keywords Integrative psychotherapy • Integrative social work • Research • Evidence • Third party requirements • Third party payment • Evidence-based approaches • Personal values • Professional values • Direct communications • Indirect communications • Consultation • Training • Professional education • Therapeutic process • Clients • Clinical social work practice • Psychodynamic • Cognitive • Behavioral • Mindfulness • Body-mind

Once condemned for muddying the waters of clinical theory, integrative thinking is now an important part of the contemporary mental health field. This climate change (Connors, 2011) is partly due to research showing that an integrative approach can be significantly more effective than a single method (e.g. Boulanger, 2011; Busch & Sandberg, 2007; Monti & Beitman, 2009; NIH, 2008; Raja, 2012; Zerbe, 2008). It is also a perfect response to third party requirements and evidence-based approaches. Even more significantly, however, today clients are far better educated about therapy than ever before. Many seek out a clinician who specializes in specific methods, and very few are willing or able to come for multiple sessions a week. Even fewer tolerate a clinician's silence for an extended period of time. Clients quite reasonably want to see results, and to some extent, clinical theory has shifted in order to meet this expectation.

Given these changes as well as the extremely complex world in which clients and clinicians live today, an integrative approach can enhance any clinician's work (e.g. see Fawcett, 1997; Gitterman & Germain, 2008). Perhaps one of the most striking examples in my own experience has been that whereas in the past some psychopharmacologists with whom my clients worked indicated that medication, and not therapy, was the major change factor in psychological issues, today psychiatrists often offer behavioral and body-mind strategies in addition to—and sometimes instead of—medication (see also Fawcett, 1997). Still, with more than 400 different

F.D. Barth, *Integrative Clinical Social Work Practice: A Contemporary Perspective*, Essential Clinical Social Work Series, DOI 10.1007/978-1-4939-0351-1_1,

psychotherapies in practice today (Roth & Fonagy, 1996), most of which now weave in ideas from a wide range of other fields, including biology, genetics, neuroscience, medicine, law, religion, philosophy and history, clinicians often find it difficult to decide what to integrate, when and how. Demands from insurance companies make the process even more complicated. Yet not only do many clinicians spontaneously assimilate a variety of ideas and techniques into their practice, sometimes without realizing or articulating the integration, but, also, as we will see, growing amounts of evidence suggest that an integrative approach may well be the most beneficial to clients. The time has come for us to find ways to talk openly about the integrative process so that we can make use of the wide range of available interventions in an organized, efficient and meaningful manner.

One lesson that has stayed with me from my days at the Traveler's Aid Society is that concrete services and psychodynamic thinking are not antithetical, but that these two approaches to the human experience are deeply and inextricably linked. They simultaneously inform, enhance and explain one another. In social work agencies, psychiatric hospitals and during psychoanalytic training, and in three decades of teaching and supervising, I have seen many clinicians bring integrative practice into their work on a daily basis, almost unconsciously. Consciously, we imagine the voices of teachers and professional "ancestors" telling us not to mix and match: that to offer a mindfulness practice to a psychoanalysand or to be curious about transference with a client who has come for CBT may interfere with and even damage the work. Yet I would suggest that almost any therapeutic offering, whether a psychoanalytic interpretation, a cognitive behavioral exercise, a mindfulness technique, a self-soothing strategy, a prescription for medication or anything else drawn from the deep basket of contemporary psychotherapeutic possibilities, is in and of itself an integration (see Strohle, 2009). Many times we are influenced by ideas that we do not even think of as aspects of different theories. For example, although mindfulness practice may have originated in Buddhist tradition, it has been integrated into dialectical behavioral, cognitive behavioral, psychodynamic and movement therapies (for other examples see Bromberg, 2001; Ekblad, Chapman, & Lynch, 2011; Epstein, 2004; Frank, 1999; Linehan, 1993; and Segal, Williams, & Teasdale, 2012).

Today, with the emphasis on evidence-based and recovery models of treatment in all mental health fields, both in agencies and from insurance companies, it is more important than ever to be able to think in a clear, theoretically informed way about integration, and to have a framework from within which to practice it. In this book, I offer several possible interventions, along with explanations for their application at specific times and with specific clients. I also provide a framework from which clinicians can formulate a choice of interventions within the context of both a theoretical perspective and their own professional values. As often as possible, I will draw from research showing the efficacy of particular interventions with particular symptoms. However, although research can be useful, I also encourage readers, as I encourage my students and supervisees, to read any scientific study carefully.

Statistics can often lead to more than one conclusion, and it is important to understand how any study and any technique does and does not apply to each specific client (for further discussion, see Fonagy, 2002; Leichsenring, 2005; Stern, 2013; Wachtel, 2010; Wallerstein & Sampson, 1971). Experience has shown me that we must be ready to explore various possibilities with every individual with whom we work. Of course, this does not mean practicing techniques for which we are not trained. To do so is not only a violation of The Clinical Social Work Code of Ethics, but is also ethically and pragmatically wrong. With that in mind, let us now turn our attention to some of the practicalities of developing an integrative practice in clinical social work.

Developing an Integrative Practice

In my own work, I have found it productive to think in terms of two organizing principles: one based on Sullivan's (1953) ideas about "*detailed inquiry*" and the other based on the concept of process. Both of these principles help clients live with confusion and begin to explore their experience from the inside. Let us turn first to the detailed inquiry. This is the phrase Sullivan used to describe his belief that the core of an analysand's psychodynamics can be found in the small details of experience. Kanter (2013) suggests that Sullivan's ideas are closely linked to social work assessment, in which a clinician gathers material about a variety of aspects of a client's life. Hirsch (2002) sees the concept as one of the pivotal ways that contemporary psychoanalysis differs from traditional Freudian analysis. I have borrowed from Sullivan's idea to help clients pay close attention not only to the details of their history and personal circumstances, but also to the minutae of daily life, which most of us tend to ignore or write off as unimportant. Not only does a detailed inquiry help clients begin to formulate unarticulated or previously unrecognized or dissociated material, as described by Bromberg (2001) or what Bollas (1989) calls the "unthought known." It also provides an integrative umbrella for the work itself, bringing together an empathic attitude and a sense of professional curiosity. Clients often feel both secure and comforted by the experience that a therapist is trying to understand them.

Process, of course, is the idea that experience, development and therapy unfold over time. As we will discuss in the following chapters, the idea of both psychotherapy and change as process is often unfamiliar to clients today. Expectations, often underscored by both external demands (such as those from insurance companies) and internal needs are for quick change. An integrative approach helps clients find relief from painful symptoms while also recognizing that longterm solutions to difficulties can take time.

According to Roth and Fonagy (1996) many of the 400 different contemporary psychotherapies share common features and few clinicians practice any in pure form. Although merging theories and techniques has been criticized for lacking consistency and conceptual clarity (see Boulanger, 2011) an integrative method can actually be a carefully organized, cohesive and thoughtfully applied synthesis of ideas and techniques (Boulanger, 2011; Connors, 2006, 2011; Fawcett, 1997; Frank, 1999; Wachtel, 1997). Developing such a practice can be daunting, particularly early in one's clinical career. However, it is possible to do so even from the beginning. In this book, I will discuss three basic organizing principles that anyone who is drawn to an integrative practice can begin to apply immediately: (1) a clinician's personal and professional values; (2) a client's direct and indirect communications; (3) ongoing consultation, training and professional education. These are, obviously, broad categories, but they are important components of every clinical approach. Each of the theories discussed in this book encompasses specific and distinct aspects of these issues. As we articulate our professional and personal understanding of each client's needs, we are better equipped to hear what clients communicate about these needs and what will be most useful to each individual. We can also use this understanding to delineate treatment plans for third party payers, a crucial skill in today's world.

Personal Values

It may seem surprising to begin a professional discussion by suggesting that one pay close attention to the personal values which made the field interesting in the first place. However, according to a number of authors (e.g. Smith, unpublished; Stern, 2013; Wallerstein, 2000) clinicians base most professional decisions on personal, often implicit or unarticulated, beliefs. One way to begin to integrate the professional with the personal is to start to articulate beliefs and values. Theory, research and experience gradually come together as we identify and think about personal guiding principles in a professional context.

How does one develop a solidly based synthesis in clinical practice? Integration can be the result of a conscious decision to blend specific techniques, an intuitive response to a client's circumstances and needs at a given time, and/or an attempt to manage external requirements such as agency or government guidelines. A combination of a growing population of clients and increasingly limited resources often leaves clinicians little time to consider more than the most pressing needs that can be legitimately met under the umbrella of specific agency policies. The idea of theory building seems a luxury. Yet although they may not have ever put it into words, most clinicians begin their professional lives with an already existing, albeit often unformulated theory about what motivates human behavior and what leads to change. Researchers have found evidence that talking about what one thinks and feels to another person can actually change the brain and alter feelings and behavior (Busch & Sandberg, 2007; Damasio, 1999; Schore, 2003; Siegel, 1999). Similarly, when a clinician at almost any stage of professional development tries to put into words thoughts that went along with any intervention or choice of technique, this is a step toward clarifying the theory behind that person's practice. In many cases, such choices are based on an unrecognized integrative theory.

Developing one's own integrative theory is a *process* which makes space for both flexibility and firm limits, finding a theoretical grounding (see Bromberg, 2001; Mitchell, 1993; Renik, 2006) while also allowing room to move away from a given platform when necessary or useful. A clinician developing a clinical practice must, therefore, be able to manage contradiction and embrace conflict. I have found over the years that that change occurs best in a climate of understanding, acceptance and curiosity. I have become convinced that no particular approach has a monopoly on these ingredients.

Before describing an example of how this can work, I would like to explain my use of both clinical material in this book. Because confidentiality is paramount when writing and discussing clients, I have chosen to illustrate points by creating examples from components of many different cases described by a wide range of therapists not only during my research for this book, but also throughout my years in practice. Thus no case is based on a single person, family, clinician or agency. All identifying information has been changed to further protect both clients and therapists. Since in our field there are differing practices about the use of first and last names, I have attempted to illustrate this in the examples throughout the book, but because of my own commitment to mutuality and respect, in most instances I have maintained the same format for both client and clinician. That is to say that even though this might not be common practice in some settings, I have usually called all participants (except young children) by either their first name or by their last, rather than the unequal practice of addressing a professional by last name and a client by first.

Let us turn now to an example in which a clinician attempts, with his supervisor, to put his own thoughts and reactions into words in order to help a client begin to think and talk about herself. Like many of the examples in this book, this one does not take place in a psychodynamically-oriented setting, but the process of trying to understand is integrated into and informs the concrete actions taken by the worker. Mr. Andrews was a social worker in a medical facility. When Ms. Robinson, whose seriously ill child was a patient at the hospital, asked for transportation for her own mother and sister to visit her son, he had to make a quick assessment of both the legitimacy of the request and the best response to it. "I could provide the transportation vouchers," he told his supervisor, "but we have had problems with this client from the moment she brought her child into the hospital." Mr. Andrews wondered whether she would even use the vouchers appropriately, but he also thought that there might be a good therapeutic reason to act in good faith to help with her family's transportation, no matter what she actually did with the vouchers. He thought Ms. Robinson might be more cooperative with the treatment team if she felt that she was getting something concrete for herself. Still, Mr. Andrews feared he might be allowing himself to be manipulated into colluding with her acting-out behavior.

When his supervisor asked him to explain his thinking about this situation, he said, "Underneath all that anger and acting out is a frightened, needy woman." He added that on the one hand he thought the mother and sister might provide emotional support for Ms. Robinson in a difficult time. "Except that when they're here, they actually tend to argue and amp up her stress level," he said. Putting these thoughts together with his supervisor, who reflected them back to him, helped Mr. Andrews not only manage his negative reactions to Ms. Robinson, but also to think about what his reactions were telling him about what might be going on with her. Although this was not a setting for insight-oriented psychotherapy, Mr. Andrews's supervisor helped him mentalize (Fonagy, 2005; Fonagy, Gyorgy, Jurist, & Target, 2003; Bateman & Fonagy, 2004) his own unformulated experience, which then helped him formulate an approach to his client. He helped her begin to examine her own conflicting feelings and engaged her in problem-solving. At their next meeting Mr. Andrews asked Ms. Robinson to talk to him about how she felt about her family's being at the hospital and how she thought it affected her and her child to have them there. The ultimate goal was to help her think out and decide whether or not she wanted to provide her mother and sister with transportation assistance.

Ms. Robinson's first response when Mr. Andrews asked if they could speak about the vouchers was, "Oh here we go again. I work my butt off, but nobody wants to help me out." Mr. Andrews held up a hand and said, "You know, that's your automatic response to almost everything I ask you about. But you also know I've been giving you vouchers when you ask for them. I just want to ask you a question about how it's working for you." She seemed surprised at the question as well as at the fact that Mr. Andrews did not respond angrily to her attack. After a minute's thought, she said, "It's been going fine." Mr. Andrews asked if she felt that her mother and sister gave her the kind of support she had hoped to get from them. Again she hesitated briefly, then said that she thought that sometimes they made things harder for her. "They make me feel bad, like I'm not doing everything I should be doing for my baby," she said, tears welling in her eyes. Mr. Andrews nodded. "I had sort of gotten that feeling," he said. "So they don't really provide you with the support you're hoping they'll give you?" She shook her head. "But they're my family. And they're all I've got."

Mr. Andrews had previously asked Ms. Robinson about coming to a support group he ran for family members of children on the unit, but she had refused. Now he repeated that he understood that this was a trying time in her life and that her family was not giving her all the support she needed. He asked if her sister and her mother made it hard to come to the meetings. She nodded but added that she could not tell them not to come. He was silent for a moment and then asked if it would help her if he did not always provide transportation for them. "I don't mind taking the blame. If you like, I can tell you that you can't have the vouchers—maybe on days when you're here for the family group, say?" Ms. Robinson laughed. Mr. Andrews thought some of her laughter was from relief, although he did not ask her to explain it. "Okay," she said. "It's a deal."

When Mr. Andrews talked about his thoughts about Ms. Robinson to his supervisor, he made contact with his own mix of feelings about her request. When he said what he understood to Ms. Robinson, even though he did not offer any insight-oriented comments about her predicament, his understanding helped him communicate something important to her. He empathized with her feelings while also offering help setting limits on one of the external triggers of some of Ms. Robinson's acting-out behavior. Not only did she respond with gratitude and agree to try the support group, but the next day, when she got angry at the doctor for something, she went back to Mr. Andrews for help. "You understand," she said to him. "I thought you could help me know the right thing to say to the lady in charge."

The Role of Theory

Theory is by definition a premise or a hypothesis, not a fact. Good theory is not static, but is an ongoing process. Research and the demand for evidence have become an important part of the theoretical world of psychotherapy, and both can be extremely helpful in professional practice. Yet even research is not finite, but is constantly unfolding, developing and contributing new data to existing stores of information. It is always interesting to me that colleagues, students and supervisees, including many clinicians I interviewed in the process of writing this book, often use statistics as a way of substantiating personal experience. I have seen professionals who have had good experiences as clients in therapy follow their therapists' style of practice and find research to validate their approach (see Wallerstein, 2000; Wampold & Brown, 2005). Similarly, I have seen clinicians turn to research that supports a very different approach from their own therapists.

Johnson (1999) notes that personal experiences can be both powerful instruments and significant problems in our clinical work. Personal knowledge of the difficulties a client is encountering and the long hard road to recovery can make a clinician both empathic and optimistic, which helps some clients through the more difficult parts of therapy. However, if the professional believes that the way he overcame a particular problem is the best way, he may struggle to provide appropriate assistance to a client who, for whatever reason, needs to follow a different path. The integrative approach described in this book suggests not only that diverse theoretical and technical interventions can be useful for the unfolding stages of therapy, as well as with varying groups of needs and issues, but also that two individuals with similar symptoms may not respond in the same way to a clinician's actions. A clinician working from within this framework can devise a therapeutic approach based on each client as a unique individual. Additionally, as I have mentioned, one of the central themes of the integrative process is that every clinician must think about and articulate her own thinking, beliefs and values in the context of her work. This interaction of clinician and client as entities is an important part of the therapeutic work, no matter what approach a clinician takes.

While no single practitioner can—or should—know about or use all of the approaches available to them today, just knowing that there are many approaches underscores the idea that there is no one "right" way to practice. Any form of therapy will unfold based on a number of different factors. A client's temperament, history and current situation; a practitioner's experience, knowledge and personality; the setting in which the work takes place and even current events all influence any therapeutic process. Most clinicians take these elements into account without thinking about it and thereby, without conscious consideration, engage in an integrative approach. Many contemporary clinicians use the term "integrative" to describe their practice of choosing interventions based on what a client needs at a particular time, rather than on a specific theoretical perspective. Even Freud recognized the need for practical intervention before psychodynamic change could be considered. He famously fed the "Rat Man" against his own "austere technical precepts" (Gay, 2006, p. 267), and brought him into his personal circle in a way that would be frowned upon today. Yet clients are best served when pragmatism is integrated with theory. How does one decide when to gratify a client's concrete needs and when to ask a client to delay gratification in order to explore psychodynamics? A consciously integrative practice provides clinicians with a solid base from which to make such a decision.

The plethora of theories of psychotherapy can be overwhelming, making integration feel like an impossible task. As a way of organizing the ideas contained in these widely ranging approaches, I have broken down therapy types into four major categories: psychodynamic, developmental, structural and body-mind. Each of these categories contains a number of different concepts. Unfortunately, putting these complex concepts into categories without oversimplifying them is in itself difficult, if not impossible. For this reason it is important to remember that many of these techniques should only be practiced after a clinician has been trained in the methodology. However, a grasp on the ideas behind these approaches can be useful when a clinician is working with a client who, for example, also seeks help from other experts. An integrative team might offer clients medication in conjunction with supportive psychotherapy, family and individual work and a Dialectical Behavioral Therapy (DBT) group. A bio-psycho-social model offers a broad integrative perspective in which psychodynamic exploration might be integrated with medication and nutritional advice, requiring the client to have a full medical workup.

Therapeutic Models

The following is a brief description of some of the therapeutic models that will be discussed in this book. The overall lens through which all of these models will be viewed sees human behavior as complex and complicated—a function of a variety of influences, including genetic and biological, psychological, socio-cultural and family factors.

Psychodynamic Models: Relational, Intersubjective, Ego and Supportive psychologies

Psychodynamic models are based on the idea that change comes with understanding of some of the psychological forces that motivate actions. This understanding is called "insight" and is based on the idea that behavior and feelings in the present are responses to experiences from the past. Relational and intersubjective theories have emerged as contemporary ways of thinking about some of the ideas presented by Freud and his followers. Instead of viewing all behavior as motivated by an underlying sexual and/or aggressive drive, today's psychoanalysts believe that much of human behavior is motivated by the need for relatedness. Ego psychology, an early offshoot of classical Freudian theory, paved the way for supportive psychotherapy. Although many forms of therapy today have a supportive component, the goal of supportive therapy is to offer a safe setting in which individuals can develop more of a sense of their own abilities. Often there is not an exploratory or insight-oriented aspect of supportive therapy, which utilizes reassurance, advice and encouragement.

While psychodynamic theory is most often practiced as individual therapy, some of the premises can also be applied to group, family and marital work.

Developmental Models

Developmental psychology is interested in the ways that humans change over the course of their lives. The range of developmental issues considered include attachment; cognitive factors, such as problem solving and conceptual comprehension; motor skills; acquisition of language; morality; capacity for interpersonal interaction; sense of self; and identity formation. Some theories focus on infancy and childhood, while others concentrate on adolescence or different stages of adulthood. Perhaps more than any of the other categories in this discussion, developmental theories integrate biological, social and psychological factors, although some to a greater and others to a lesser degree.

Structural Models: Cognitive and Behavioral Theories and Related Techniques

With therapies that include Dialectical Behavioral Therapy (DBT), Acceptance and Commitment Therapy (ACT), Rational Emotive Therapy (RET), Assertiveness Training, Systematic Desensitization and related methods, CBT has been increasingly used in recent years for working with a variety of populations. Because it is both directive and time limited, many clients find it more attractive than some of the longer-term, more abstract forms of therapy. According to one group of authors, (Dobson et al., 2008) three fundamental propositions are the basis of CBT: (1) cognitive activity affects behavior; (2) cognitive activity can be monitored and altered; and (3) desired behavior change can come from cognitive change. Although there are differences in technique and focus, CBT therapists and clients generally work together to identify irrational beliefs and illogical thinking patterns associated with symptoms and behaviors without delving into meanings or historical precursors. Dialectical Behavioral Therapy (DBT) and Acceptance and Commitment Therapy (ACT) both focus on helping patients observe and label their emotional reactions without attempting to analyze, judge or change them. ACT therapists suggest that acceptance of feelings leads to choices in behaviors. DBT clinicians attempt to help clients find a balance (or dialectic) between acceptance and change. Some approaches use primarily group therapy, while others practice with both groups and individuals.

The Body-Mind Connection

Through Freud's earliest work, psychodynamic theories have long recognized the interplay of body and mind, but they focused more on the mind's influence on the body than the other way around. (The controversial radical psychoanalyst Wilhelm Reich was an early exception to this generalization.) In recent decades, complex connections between body and mind have been recognized and become an increasingly significant focal point for therapy. Gordon, Staples, Blyta, Bytyqi, and Wilson (2008) note that the body and the mind are inextricably linked and constantly influencing one another through the brain and peripheral nervous system, the endocrine and immune systems and a variety of chemical interchanges. Body-mind therapies attempt to change problematic feelings and behaviors by altering interactions between body and mind. Growing bodies of research, as well as practical experience, indicate many psychological and physiological benefits of meditation, mindfulness training, yoga and other body-mind practices. A partial list of such practices from the National Center for Complementary and Alternative Medicine (NCCAM) includes behavioral, psychological, social, expressive and spiritual concepts such as meditation, prayer, yoga, biofeedback, tai chi, qigong, relaxation, guided imagery, hypnosis and art, music and dance therapies. Patient support groups and cognitive-behavioral therapy may also be used in conjunction with these practices. Many therapists include some of these ideas in their work, either consciously and purposefully or without realizing that they are integrating body-mind practices. This can be done directly, as when mindful breathing is brought into a psychodynamically oriented therapy or a client is encouraged to seek a movement therapist in conjunction with behavioral work, or indirectly, as when a therapist suggests that there might be a connection between an emotional and a physical state (Table 1.1).

Table 1.1 Therapeutic models and theories

Model	Main concepts	Focus of theory	Theorists	Practice applications
Psychodynamic	Change comes with an understanding of some of the psychological forces that motivate actions	Insight and under-standing	S. Freud Winnicott A. Freud Bowlby Kohut Stolorow Mitchell Fonagy	Understanding and insight, thinking about and explaining personal motivation
Developmental	Human beings change and develop over the life cycle	How and when change occurs	A. Freud Erikson Piaget Mahler Bowlby Beebe and Lachmann M. and H. Steele Fonagy	Understanding problems of childhood and adolescence, understanding how problems of earlier development affect adult experience, understanding adult difficulties as part of adult development
Structural	Thoughts affect behavior and feelings	Behavior can change when thoughts are changed	Skinner Ellis Burns Linehan Chapman Hayes	Looking at thoughts that affect behavior and feelings, altering/accepting/ balancing those thoughts and feelings
Body-mind	The body and mind are constantly influencing one another	Intervene to improve both body health and awareness of body to improve emotional and mental health	Reich KabatZinn Thich Nhat-Hanh Linehan Hayes Chapman Somers-Anderson Knoblach Brown Brennan Kornfield	Enhance the mind's positive impact on the body and the body's impact on the mind to improve physical health, emotional well-being

Many contemporary clinicians have discarded the traditional "medical model" of psychotherapy, in which a client passively accepts treatment offered by professionals. (Even in modern medical practice, patients are encouraged to take a more active role in their own treatment than they were in the not-too-distant past.) Today clients are expected to actively participate in the therapeutic process, both by engaging in the work and expressing their feelings about it. Even therapies that do not view the relationship between clinician and client as a focal point recognize the importance of a working alliance between the two in order for the work to go forward.

Therapeutic Relationship and Working Alliance

I have found, perhaps not surprisingly given the research on the subject, that an important factor tying together many clinical theories is the relationship between clinician and client. As we will discuss in the chapter on assessment, part of any decision about what sort of therapy will be most effective is each individual's personality and needs. But recognizing the significance of the therapeutic relationship—broadly defined as the "collaborative and affective bond" that develops between a therapist and a client (Martin, Garske, & Davis, 2000)—is important to integrative thinking. In a detailed review of studies from 1936 to 2007 of treatment effectiveness, Wampold (2001) finds that the evidence points to the therapist as an extremely significant factor in the therapeutic outcome. When asked to explain why they improved, clients emphasize the relationship with their therapists rather than a particular type of psychotherapy or method of treatment. Carr (2011) suggests that different therapies include different ingredients to help clients change. Like Pine (2006), Carr notes that human beings are extremely complex, which is one reason there are many ways to help someone with emotional distress. He adds, however, that research shows one common theme: all techniques work best when a clinician is both genuinely interested in a client and is also able to form a solid therapeutic alliance with her (Carr, 2011). Yet every therapeutic relationship is complicated and may undergo changes over the course of therapy. A theoretical model can help a clinician navigate and make important choices about interventions and interactions. We will discuss this process more fully in later chapters, but for the moment, let us note here that a working alliance is part of a therapeutic relationship. Hersoug, Hogland, Monsen, and Havik (2001) have delineated four dimensions of a therapeutic working alliance:

1. A client's capacity to work purposefully in therapy
2. A client's affective bond to the therapist
3. A therapist's empathic understanding and involvement
4. Agreement between client and therapist on treatment goals and tasks (Hersoug et al., 2001, p. 207)

In a series of extensive interviews, Wallerstein (2000) found that what a client finds helpful is not always the same thing the clinician thought was helpful. Yet, like Carr, he suggests that a sense of a therapist's empathic understanding, professionalism, experience and knowledge is often important for a client to enter into a working alliance. However, in some forms of psychotherapy, recognizing and acknowledging negative feelings about a clinician are also an important part of the work. Psychoanalytic and psychodynamic theories focus on the relationship itself. Clients are encouraged to put into words not only positive feelings, but also anger, hostility, frustration and/or disappointment in a therapist. The idea is that these feelings may be rooted in early, unformulated and/or unresolved experiences from childhood, particularly in relationships with early authority and attachment figures, who are often a client's parents. A working alliance with genuinely positive affective ties allows client and therapist to examine childhood distortions and conflicts (Freud, 1914; Greenson, 1967).

In his review of a number of studies, Wampold (2001) states something that clinicians learn through experience:linking past with present is meaningful only when it has affective meaning in the here and now. What appears to be most important to the alliance in terms of efficacy of any treatment is a client's sense that his therapist's interventions are directed towards his specific, personal and experienced needs and affective states at a given time (Horvath and Greenberg, 1994). In other words, no one wants to feel that he is viewed as part of a theoretical equation. This finding fits well with Kohut's idea that the most important part of any therapeutic endeavor is the client's sense that the therapist is genuinely trying to understand his feelings (Kohut, 1984). Surprisingly, it can also affirm the opposite view, traditionally taken by many behavioral schools, that talking about the therapeutic relationship can interfere with and/or avoid the actual therapeutic work.

How can two opposing ideas be confirmed by the same research? An integrative perspective offers some insight into this apparent contradiction. What appears to be most important is that a client feels that her needs and concerns are being directly addressed by his therapist. Behavioral therapists may not view the therapeutic relationship as a central topic for discussion, but by addressing a client's immediate concerns, they promote a therapeutic alliance between themselves and their clients. For example, in a discussion of the use of Dialectical Behavioral Therapy (DBT) to treat a heroin addict with borderline personality disorder, Ekblad, Chapman, and Lynch (2010) speak of helping a client learn to work with the paradox of acceptance and change, using the illustration of a therapist saying "I understand why you want to use drugs—they reduce your shame and anger" (p. 15). The point of the understanding is to help the client accomplish the task of managing both his feelings and his behavior. On the other hand, Mitchell (1993), one of the founders of the relational theory of psychoanalysis, suggests that cognitive-behavioral and directive interventions are useful tools for looking at a client's characteristic patterns of relating to others. Understanding how a client engages in relationships is key, he believes, to change.

Managing Contradictions and Conflict

Numerous authors have discussed the importance of contradictions (e.g. Bromberg, 2001; Davies, 1998; Linehan, 1993; Mitchell, 1999; Pizer, 1998) both within any therapeutic process and in life itself. Much of Freud's theory is based on the psychodynamic impact of intrapsychic conflict (e.g. Freud, 1937), but many non-Freudian theories also often view symptoms and problematic behavior as the result of oppositional pulls—for instance, an addiction or an eating disorder may be at least in part the result of a conflict between a wish to feel better (self soothing) and a wish to harm the self. Poor impulse control, mood dysregulation and a lack of self-awareness can make it impossible for an individual to manage these internal conflicts in a healthy or productive way. A variety of therapeutic approaches offer tools for managing these contradictory wishes. On one end of the spectrum of techniques is the psychoanalytic practice of allowing clients to sit with unpleasant feelings in order to learn to both understand their origins and manage them. From this perspective, insight and change comes from allowing uncomfortable and/or unacceptable thoughts and emotions to emerge into conscious awareness. Behavioral approaches view insight as unnecessary for change to occur. Other approaches (e.g. a number of body-mind, developmental and contemporary relational theories) consider that insight comes after a client has learned to tolerate the feelings, and understanding what triggers them is not a prerequisite for change to occur.

Developing the capacity to manage and tolerate internal conflict, bringing with it the concomitant ability to live with strength and vulnerability in oneself and in others is an unspoken goal of many of these different approaches. To this point, I have found that one of the most difficult contradictions for clients and their therapists to manage is the issue of parent blaming. Many approaches to clinical work include developmental theories that look for parental failure, neglect and/or trauma as the cause of clients' difficulties in adulthood. Less often discussed is the role of the same parents in helping their offspring develop strengths, some of which probably make it possible for those individuals to enter therapy. Management of this contradiction is a subject that will be woven through many of the chapters of this book.

And like parents, clinicians must often make decisions about what intervention will be most appropriate and most useful for a given client at a given time without full knowledge of what is happening inside. The best parenting books, in my own experience, offer both theoretical and practical guidance while simultaneously making room for parents to formulate their own ideas about what may be going on with their child. Parents often comment that they have to relearn everything about child development with each subsequent baby, because no two youngsters develop the same way. Erikson once commented that in the process of bringing up children, parents get brought up as well. Children are excellent teachers, and parents learn how to parent by listening carefully to what children "say" both in words and in actions. The same can be said about the therapeutic process. Clients tell us, in behavior and in language, what they need from us.

Neuroscience

Meissner (2007b), responding to criticism of contemporary thinking about and research in neuropsychology, suggests that the reason for learning about neuroscience is not because it necessarily scientifically informs clinical technique, but because it provides yet another way of talking and thinking about what we do in our work with our clients. I would suggest that the same statement could be made about every theory discussed in this book, as well as many I was not able to include. As I address ways of assessing when, why and how to bring in different tools with different clients, I encourage readers to think in terms of these ideas not as a rigid set of guidelines to follow with each type of disorder, but as models of how one can make clinical decisions using an integrative approach. My goal is for readers to learn a process rather than a specific technique.

In numerous interviews with clinicians in a wide variety of settings in cities, towns and communities across the United States, I found this to be one of the most compelling reasons for this book. When clinicians in agencies, clinics, schools, hospitals and other organizations described the specific structure and treatment approach of their settings, an approach for which they often expressed enthusiasm, they still almost universally echoed a longing for, and often actively sought, training in other ways to understand and work with their clients. "It just seems too narrow to think in only one dimension," said one clinician, whose words reflected those of almost everyone I interviewed.

Weaving concepts from one theory into another in practice is part of integrative work. Helping clinicians find ways of thinking and talking about this process is one of the central goals of this book. Choices do not have to be—and in fact should not be—random, but can come from important principles that should guide a clinicians' selection of interventions. I am both a clinical social worker and a psychoanalyst. My shift away from traditional-format psychoanalysis reflects the development of my integrative thinking. If I were to come across a client who I felt would do better by lying on a couch and not looking at me, I might still consider using this technique, but most clients who come into my office tend to need help in the areas of affect regulation, self-knowledge and relationships. In these areas, I have found that face to face interactions allow a client to interact with a therapist as a whole person. Facial expressions and body language are part of the therapeutic process, not something to be filtered out.

What has remained with me from my analytic training is a deeply felt interest in meaning. What does a particular behavior represent for a client? Why this behavior? What thoughts and feelings emerge in relation to a particular event in a client's current life—and what do those feelings and/or thoughts mean? The integrative approach I present in this book offers the interested clinician an opportunity to explore the idea of meaning from a number of different perspectives.

Jane's experience with Alyssa is a good illustration of how this can work. Alyssa was in her early 30s when she began seeing Jane, a therapist, because she had trouble managing her anger at work. In the first meeting, Alyssa and Jane set up a plan for 10 weeks of DBT. In almost every session, Alyssa told Jane that she could not do this "the way you want me to," and that Jane was "pushing too hard." At first Jane tried to understand what this meant to Alyssa and adjust the work in some way, but gradually she realized that their discussions about Alyssa's feeling of being pushed were, ironically, derailing the therapy. She also realized that this was probably a very good example of what was happening at work. Early in the next session, Jane said, "Before we go over the exercises for this week, I think we have to pay attention to what is happening here. I'm trying to do something that I think would be helpful for you. You don't like it, so you get angry at me, which gets me to stop pushing you." She went on to explain that this had a very specific meaning. "You have learned that getting angry helps you avoid things that you don't want to do." And she added that she thought this might parallel what was going on at work. Alyssa said it did, and wanted to talk more about the specifics of the problems at work, but Jane suggested that this was a good motivation for following through on the tasks that were part of the therapeutic process.

This is just one approach a clinician could take. A psychodynamically oriented psychotherapist might look for a different way of expressing and exploring what was happening in the work. While she would also be interested in the probable parallels between what was happening in the therapeutic relationship and Alyssa's difficulties at work, she would likely ask Alyssa to join her in looking for historical and unconscious dynamics that were being played out in this instance. From a developmental perspective, this behavior might be understood as a repetition based on particular unresolved developmental conflicts, while an ego-, self- or resilience-focused therapist might support Alyssa's ability to articulate that she felt "pushed" as an effort to adapt and/or to protect herself. A clinician might express both empathy for the feeling and a desire to understand it better, or he might communicate a desire to respond in a way that would work better for Alyssa. If Alyssa was unable to access any information about the feeling of being pushed or angry, mindfulness techniques might be employed. If she could not manage the emotions without missing appointments or becoming agitated or distraught, self-soothing practices might be taught and implemented.

Perhaps most important of all to an integrative approach is a growing body of data suggesting that many different psychotherapies are useful for a variety of disorders and needs, that even when medication is necessary, psychotherapy improves its effectiveness, and that the therapeutic alliance and the sense that a therapist both understands and is helping is highly predictive of positive outcome (Carr, 2011; Wampold, 2001). In the following chapters we will examine just how this information can be utilized by clinicians who want to integrate different ideas and approaches in their own practice.

Chapter 2
Contemporary Psychodynamic Models

Keywords Psychodynamic approach • Exploration • Meaning • Personal narrative • Clarifying meaning • Integrative practice • Different approaches • Unarticulated or unconscious meaning • Latent • Manifest • Behaviors • Symptoms • Flexibility • Short-term psychotherapy • Long-term psychotherapy • Insight • Cognitive approaches • Behavioral approaches • Prejudice • Blind spots • Integrative social work • Evidence • Research • Mindfulness • Body-mind • Clinical illustrations

Perhaps one of the hardest tasks facing a clinician developing an integrative practice is choosing when and how to incorporate different approaches into the work with each client. How does one develop an overarching approach to guide these choices and bring them together into an organized and complementary whole rather than a mix of a little of this and a little of that? As I noted in Chap. 1, from the beginning, most clinicians have a silent, often even unrecognized frame of reference for our professional work that reflects our personal principles and beliefs. This frame, or base, is often an important but unarticulated part of how we make clinical choices. Putting these principles into words is an important part of developing an organizing theory to guide an integrative practice.

Not surprisingly, theory that supports our personal values and beliefs tends to be the most appealing. As previously noted, these principles often influence our interventions more than we realize (e.g. see Schachter & Kächele, 2007), which is one of the reasons it is important for us to make use of every possible tool for developing self-awareness and managing inevitable prejudices and blind-spots. But it can also be extremely useful—although a bit harder—to think about and incorporate ideas that do not automatically fit into one's professional comfort zone. For example, many of us practice the type of therapy that our own therapists practiced, that is, the kind of clinical work we have experienced as clients. We also model our work on that of supervisors and teachers with whom we feel most comfortable. Yet some of our most powerful learning experiences may come from someone who operates outside of that frame. For many clinicians, a psychodynamic approach seems to be

F.D. Barth, *Integrative Clinical Social Work Practice: A Contemporary Perspective*, Essential Clinical Social Work Series, DOI 10.1007/978-1-4939-0351-1_2,

outside of our personal and professional belief system. Yet even for clinicians with no interest in long-term, exploratory or insight-oriented work, psychodynamic thinking can aid in the development of an integrative practice.

Psychoanalysis has long been criticized for being overly complicated, time and money-consuming, and useful only for a small number of people. The theory, or more accurately *group* of theories is complex and the language often overly complicated. Adding to the difficulty, today there are a number of different schools of psychoanalytic and psychodynamic thought with sometimes contradictory and often confusing approaches. Still, psychoanalysis today has little to do with the stereotypical image of a client lying on a couch and talking to a silent doctor four or five times a week. And psychodynamic theory has a great deal to offer to an integrative practice, even when a clinician's primary approach is not psychodynamic. Furthermore, a growing body of evidence (e.g. Leichsenring, 2005; Leichsenring & Rabung, 2008; Mishna, Van Wert, & Asakura, 2013; Roth & Fonagy, 1996; Schachter & Kächele, 2007; Shedler, 2010) points to the efficacy of psychodynamic work, on its own and in conjunction with other techniques. Because the term "psychodynamic" has different meanings for different clinicians, let us take a moment to define the term. Then we will focus on two concepts from psychodynamic thinking that can help organize an integrative practice: (1) the idea that behaviors, thoughts, symptoms and even feelings can have unconscious or unrecognized meaning and (2) the significance of the therapeutic relationship. These ideas can be useful tools for thinking about and organizing an integrative practice, even for a clinician whose primary interventions are non-psychodynamic in nature.

What Is Psychodynamic Thinking?

Psychoanalytic thinking today is a way of learning about oneself and of using that knowledge to both manage difficult feelings and experiences and enrich one's life. Numerous psychodynamic psychotherapies integrate psychoanalytic concepts, such as exploration of unrecognized reasons for overt behaviors and symptoms, with other approaches, including symptom-reduction and motivational interviewing. Like many of my analytically-oriented colleagues, I have found that psychodynamic exploration can be done very effectively in the context of less frequent sessions and with clients sitting facing their therapists rather than lying on a couch, two of the traditional techniques associated with psychoanalysis. In fact, Schachter and Kächele (2007) make a compelling argument for a revised version of psychoanalysis which integrates a wide range of contemporary techniques. The central goal of psychodynamic exploration, which runs across most psychoanalytic theories, might be said to be to bring together unintegrated aspects of the self in order to allow an individual free access to a wide variety of sometimes contradictory aspects of her internal world. Mitchell and Black (1995) tell us that psychoanalytic thought helps clients bring together different realms of their experience, such as thoughts and feelings, past and present, words and images. Thus psychodynamic theories themselves can be said to have an integrative goal (see Holmes, 1998).

In this chapter, and throughout this book, when we use the term "psychodynamic," we will be referring to the idea that behaviors, symptoms, feelings and thoughts often have more than one meaning, and that some of those meanings may not be manifest, or apparent, at the present time. Exploring unrecognized or latent meanings with a client is only one possible use of this understanding. Simply recognizing the possibility that behaviors, symptoms and even feelings have more than one meaning can help a clinician think differently about what interventions make the most sense at a given time. Here is one example of how that works.

Mr. Nolan came to an outpatient clinic for help with a long-term depression that was interfering with his ability to do his work. His therapist, Ms. Bluen, soon discovered that Mr. Nolan was also an alcoholic whose wife was threatening to leave him if he did not get his drinking under control. Mr. Nolan expressed a commitment to changing his behavior and said that he had begun attending Alcoholics Anonymous already. However, he said, he did not think AA was the right program for him, since he did not feel that he needed to stop drinking altogether. Ms. Bluen, who was a psychodynamically-oriented psychotherapist who specialized in addictions and utilized an integrative approach to the work, considered several possible approaches to the problem. First, she recognized that the client might have a point. Not everyone has to give up alcohol completely in order to become sober. Second, she also knew that he might be wrong, but not yet ready to accept the reality that he did have to give up alcohol forever. And third, she thought that there were probably other reasons for resisting the program, including what she was beginning to see as his fear of feelings that might be emerging as he stops drinking and an intense hatred of feeling controlled by someone else.

Taking these possibilities into account, Ms. Bluen decided to do some educative work about the physiological and neurological impact of alcohol on the brain and the body. She explained that to interrupt what she described as a chemical chain reaction that occurred in his brain every time he drank, he needed to be abstinent for the moment. Utilizing a harm reduction approach, she told him that she thought there was a possibility that in the future the client could begin drinking again in a more manageable way. Motivational interviewing helped them focus on reasons that Mr. Nolan wanted to change his behavior—e.g. to improve his relationship with his wife and his capacity to do his job. Since research has linked addictive and impulsive behaviors with affect management difficulties (Christenson et al., 1994; McElroy et al., 1995, 1998) she also immediately began to address his difficulty tolerating feelings and introduced him to some behavioral, mindfulness and relaxation techniques for managing the unbearable emotions that triggered his drinking and others that would emerge during the process of becoming sober. She also explained that this was one of the benefits of attending AA daily. "They have lots of tools for helping you handle the impulse to drink and the feelings that will make you want to stop being sober." Besides hoping that these tools would help Mr. Nolan get some control over his drinking, Ms. Bluen believed that they would help him stay in therapy long enough to build the internal (ego) strengths that would ultimately make it possible for him to become a "recovering" rather than an active alcoholic.

Although it is generally accepted that insight and exploration is not the treatment of choice for overcoming addictions, especially in the early stages of the work, a psychodynamic perspective can provide a useful frame for this integrative process. For example, as Ms. Bluen worked with Mr. Nolan, she began to hear information that led her to wonder if his complaints about AA were at least partly driven by an unconscious fear that he would fail at the task of abstaining altogether. In such cases, there can be a danger that a client will drop out of therapy in order to protect his self-esteem, so that a therapist might want to address the issue directly. However, clients like Mr. Nolan may not directly present his anxiety about failing, but instead may appear defiant, resistant, and/or as though he just does not care. Based on her knowledge of this population and in response to Mr. Nolan frequently blustery behavior, Ms. Bluen decided not to make a psychodynamic "interpretation" about his fear, but instead spoke in a general and educational way about the idea that drinking often is a way of protecting a person from feelings of embarrassment and shame about not succeeding at tasks that seem ridiculously simple to accomplish. She added that unfortunately the drinking itself also often made those tasks even more difficult, but she said that in her experience people often do fail in life, and that those who stuck with AA and learned the techniques she and he were working on learned to manage those ups and downs in a healthier manner.

In this way, Ms. Bluen made use of a psychodynamic frame to help her decide what aspects of Mr. Nolan' material she should address and how she might best address it. Psychodynamic understanding also led her to the realization that Mr. Nolan was conflicted about the work, even about whether or not he wanted to become sober. Ms. Bluen was able to remind herself and also explain to Mr. Nolan that recovery from an addiction is a process, not something that happens overnight. Even when he stopped drinking, there would be work to do. "You'll need new tools and muscles for coping with the world that you see around you without alcohol," she told him. "It's like working out at the gym. One workout does not give you strong muscles." For an integrative clinician, what is perhaps most helpful about psychodynamic theory is the idea that most behaviors, thoughts, feelings, symptoms and other aspects of experience have meaning (or multiple meanings) that is not immediately obvious, and that efforts to understand some of those underlying or hidden meanings can be key to almost any kind of therapeutic work.

Acknowledging the different aspects of a client's experience can enhance the development of trust in a clinician and at the same time diminish shame and feelings of isolation. Psychodynamic theorists have described this part of the work as providing a holding environment (Winnicott, 1965), selfobject functions (Kohut, 1977), or a "corrective selfobject experience" (Bacal & Herzog, 2003). In all of these situations, the experience of being with an attuned and actively engaged professional is in and of itself therapeutic.

Organizing Principles and Concepts

Psychodynamic thinking has undergone major changes over the years since Breuer and Freud (1957) first described the "talking cure." Numerous schools of thought have diverged from Freud's early conceptualization of conflict over psychosexual and aggressive impulses as the cause of psychological difficulties. Some authors have suggested that psychodynamic thinking today is by definition integrative (see Eagle, 1995; Frank, 1999; Parish & Eagle, 2003; Roth & Fonagy, 1996). Because the human psyche is tremendously complex, Pine (1990) suggests that different schools of thought help us to understand different aspects of experience, which he divides into four major categories: drives (and conflicts), ego, object and self. Today we will want to add other categories. Relational and intersubjectivity theories explore many new issues that emerge in relationships. Current research in attachment, neuroscience and affect regulation have also added to the mix.

Most psychodynamically oriented practitioners, however, would agree on certain basic tenets:

1. Provide a setting in which a client feels safe
2. Help clients recognize ways they avoid distressing emotions and learn to tolerate and become comfortable with a range of feelings
3. Be aware of the importance of relationships
4. Be aware of a client's sense of self and sense of agency
5. Pay attention to the therapeutic relationship
6. Look for patterns of behavior and expectations that have been repeated over time
7. Think about and explore unconscious meaning

Psychodynamic psychotherapy is, of course, "talk" therapy, which means that communicating and listening effectively is an important part of the work. Interestingly, research has shown that simply putting thoughts and feelings into words to another person can be therapeutic over time (see Busch & Sandberg, 2007; Schore, 2003; Siegel, 1999) and can actually make observable changes in brain functioning (Buchheim et al., 2012). Psychodynamic clinicians focus on three central aspects of affects: (1) recognizing, (2) expressing and (3) understanding their conscious and unconscious meanings. Yet for clients who are overwhelmed by feelings or unable to manage them, opening up these emotions prior to building the skills for managing them can be more destructive than helpful. Thus psychodynamically-oriented clinicians learn to listen for resistance and defenses, and to understand these aspects of the psyche as self-protective, not as antithetical to therapeutic progression. Understanding and supporting defenses against feelings can be an important part of psychodynamic thinking, even when it looks like these protective responses are interfering with therapeutic progress. (We will return to this topic when we discuss resistance in Chap. 9).

Self, self-organization, self-representation, and self-esteem are all considered carefully by psychodynamic theorists. Psychodynamic theories are generally focused not only on the inner self, but also on interpersonal relationships. Patterns of interaction and behavior that begin in the past are often repeated in the present and affect current behavior, as well as the ways that new interactions and experiences are understood and responded to. Most psychodynamic psychotherapists attempt to help clients identify and recognize recurring themes and patterns in their lives. There is frequently discussion of both present difficulty and past experiences and attempts to understand what themes link the two.

In my own experience as well as the findings of numerous researchers (e.g. Couch, 1999; Farmer, 2009; Frank, 2005; Freedman, Hoffenberg, Vorus, & Frosch, 1999; Meissner, 2007b) any therapy relationship is important on a variety of different planes. It can, for example, provide what Kohut (1971) calls a corrective emotional experience in which old hurts are repaired and new development takes place. It can also offer clients what Winnicott (1965) calls a holding environment in which difficult or previously unarticulated material can be explored in relative safety. And it can be a setting in which interpersonal difficulties are repeated and worked through over time. By making the therapeutic relationship part of the subject of inquiry, a therapist communicates an interest in understanding feelings and thoughts as they emerge within the therapeutic space as well as outside it. In this way, a clinician provides a safe space for observing and experiencing previously unformulated, dissociated or unthought intrapsychic and interpersonal components of a client's life. I am not suggesting, however, that all of a client's dynamics must or even can be played out within a therapeutic relationship. In my experience, a good therapeutic partnership simply makes it possible for manifest and latent material to be examined, whether it emerges from within the transference or outside of it.

Transference and Countertransference

A therapist's own dynamics are also significant, for example at those times when countertransference may provide information about unconsciously received communications from a client. (However, as I will discuss further in later chapters, I do not agree with theorists who suggest that a clinician's response to a client *always* informs about unconscious or dissociated aspects of the client's experience.) Following the thinking of interpersonal theories, many contemporary practices see each therapeutic relationship as impacting clinical process (e.g. Hoffman, 1996). Mitchell (1988, 1993) suggests that each therapeutic dyad is different, thus questioning the traditional belief that a client has specific dynamics that will emerge with any therapist. From a relational perspective, both manifest and latent meaning continues to be explored through fantasies, dreams, and daydreams.

They are also found in what Sullivan (1953) has called a "detailed inquiry" into the particulars of a client's life (see Barth, 1998; Kanter, 2013). As I have already noted and will continue to discuss throughout this book, I believe that detailed inquiry into all aspects of a client's experience is key to an integrative approach. These details are like the colors and images in a painting, or the background data that gives a reader a rich sense of a character in a novel. The often unnoticed minutiae of daily life not only offer a therapist a special window into a client's reality, but also provide a client an opportunity to put "unthought known" (Bollas, 1989) into words to another person. Numerous studies have suggested that the simple process of saying things to another person can lead to psychological change (e.g. Damasio, 1999; Rustin, 2013; Schore, 2003; Siegel, 1999). The small details, much more than the big ones, are what make each of us who we are.

Some psychodynamic theories still consider that particular material will emerge with any clinician. It has been my experience that certain themes appear consistently throughout an individual's life, but that any relationship, whether with a therapist or another person, will also have unique characteristics related not only to the chemistry of the two individuals involved, but also to the time, place and circumstances in which that relationship unfolds.

When to Use Psychodynamic Thinking and Psychodynamic Interventions

While there are no definitive answers about who responds best to psychodynamic interventions (see Roth & Fonagy, 1996; Milrod et al., 2007; Watzke et al., 2010), it is generally agreed that in order to benefit from psychodynamic exploration a client needs to have enough psychological strength to tolerate the feelings that will emerge during the exploratory process. Some research (see Roth & Fonagy, 1996; Shedler, 2010; Wampold, 2001) indicates that psychodynamically-oriented approaches work best with clients with some self-awareness and psychological-mindedness. However, the presence or absence of these traits cannot always be determined in the beginning of therapy. For example, as I describe elsewhere (Barth, 1998), sometimes highly verbal, thoughtful and apparently insightful individuals are unable to use their apparent self-knowledge for their own psychological well-being. This is sometimes the result of alexithymia, or an inability to process certain kinds of experience with language (Krystal, 1988; McDougall, 1989); but it may also be the result of defenses, personality organization and cognitive impairment. The opposite may also be true, that is, someone who appears to have no capacity for or interest in insight may turn out to be very responsive to a therapist's gentle exploration and offering of possible new ways of thinking about patterns that may have begun in the past and are being repeated in the present. Symptoms of depression and anxiety, inability to enjoy life, and repeating patterns of behavior that limit one's choices have all been shown to respond to these interventions.

Clients who cannot tolerate their feelings, who are in crisis or highly symptomatic, who cannot pay attention to their own thoughts and actions or do not have what is called an observing ego, and who cannot tolerate a developing relationship with a therapist are often not good candidates for psychodynamic exploration, but they often respond to a combination of supportive work and approaches that help them manage these feelings. Some clinicians fear that trying to understand latent or hidden meanings and historical reasons for problematic patterns of behavior will interfere with taking active steps to change behavior. However, understanding meanings can sometimes enhance interventions focused on behavior (see for example Connors, 2006; Frank, 1999; Wachtel, 1997). Kohut (1984) goes so far as to suggest that the simple act of a clinician trying to understand what a client is experiencing is probably more important than an interpretation of unconscious meaning. A number of authors (e.g. Connors, 2006; Frank, 1999; Stern, 1997; Wachtel, 1997) suggest that some active, symptom-focused interventions can be viewed as early stages of psychodynamic work. They may make it possible for a client to begin to feel both hope and trust that therapy and this particular therapist can make a difference in his life.

The following chart can help a clinician decide when to work within the frame of psychodynamic thinking, and when a more active intervention is necessary (Table 2.1).

There are many times when psychodynamic interventions are not indicated, yet psychodynamic thinking can help a clinician make decisions about what is going on and what might be an effective approach. Here is another example of how this can work.

Anna Louise had been hospitalized for a severe depression. She had been stabilized with a combination of medication, individual, group and family therapy. She was highly motivated to return home to her husband and two young children, and did well on a series of progressively longer home visits. However, one day shortly before her discharge Anna Louise began complaining that she was feeling depressed and suicidal again. Her treatment team began to consider the possibility that she needed a higher dose of medication, but her therapist suggested that she was struggling with tremendous ambivalence about going home. "She is afraid," the therapist said. "Here at the hospital she's gotten support and nurturing. When she gets home, she will have

Table 2.1 Psychodynamic interventions

Psychodynamic interventions can be useful when	Psychodynamic interventions are often not helpful when
A client is interested in understanding something about the reasons for their behavior, thoughts, feelings and symptoms	A client's symptoms need immediate intervention
A client can tolerate feelings and thoughts that emerge as the understanding work is going on	A client has little or no access to feelings and/or thoughts
A client who has been participating in a program, doing therapeutic assignments, or otherwise engaged in therapeutic activities begins to resist, withdraw from or otherwise stop engaging in the work	A client is not able to think abstractly (this can sometimes be a temporary condition due to symptoms, and should be revisited periodically in the course of a therapy)
A client has feelings about a therapist that appear to be related to previous relationships, repeat old relational patterns, or seem to reflect a part of the client's self	A client is not interested in understanding or exploring possible meanings of her behaviors, symptoms, thoughts and feelings
	A client is psychotic, confused or suffering from alexithymia (the inability to use language to process feelings)

high expectations for herself, and she will assume that everyone else will have equally high expectations. She will be facing the demands of two small children, a household that needs to be run, a family pet, and her extended family." The team agreed that Anna Louise was not consciously acting depressed and suicidal, but that these feelings had emerged unconsciously as a way of keeping her in a safe and secure environment. With this conceptualization of her dynamics, the clinical team began to work with her and her family to set up a nurturing support system, including having her go into weekly psychotherapy and attend an ongoing parenting support group for young mothers that would help her feel more secure without being infantilized. Anna Louise was able to leave the hospital as planned and moved forward in her life with the support of her family, friends, therapist and support group.

Questions to Ask from a Psychodynamic Perspective

Exploring feelings, the therapeutic relationship and a client's past can stir up many issues for a client and for a clinician, which is one reason that it is so important for every therapist to spend some time in personal therapy. It is also a reason that psychoanalytic training is so rigorous. The work of self-knowledge is an ongoing process, however, which means that every client and every clinician is involved in learning more about themselves in the course of their lives. Interestingly, as McWilliams (2004) has explained, clients also need to learn about the psychodynamic process. Assuming that a clinician has been and is currently working on understanding personal dynamics and feelings that emerge in the work, here are some questions that can bring psychodynamic thinking into almost any clinical contact.

1. Focus on affect and expression of emotion: How are you feeling right now? How are you feeling talking about this topic?
2. Exploration of attempts to avoid distressing thoughts and feelings: How do you usually tend to deal with these feelings? What ways of managing these thoughts and feelings work best for you? What have you tried that doesn't work?
3. Identification of recurring themes and patterns: When have you felt this way in the past? What have you usually done in this kind of situation?
4. Discussion of past experience (developmental focus): What are the similarities between this situation and similar times you've experienced these feelings and thoughts? What makes you think this situation is the same as that one? Are there some of the differences?
5. Focus on interpersonal relations: what is happening in this interaction, with this person, and what does it mean to you? What do you think it means to them? What makes you think this?
6. Focus on the therapy relationship: Am I understanding what you're trying to say correctly? Does this feel helpful? Can you tell me if some of these feelings and thoughts that we're talking about with other people are also occurring in therapy?

Some clients are not able to accept or make use of exploration of their internal conflict and/or confusion. In these instances, even when they are in supportive, cognitive-behavioral, structural or medication therapies, they may enact some aspect of their difficulties and/or behavioral patterns, drawing a therapist into a living experience of their emotional world. As we will see in other chapters, sometimes thinking about possible meanings of the dynamics in which a clinician has become involved can be helpful without necessarily exploring them with the client. In order to do this, discussion with a supervisor or one's own therapist can help untangle a clinician's dynamics from those of a client.

Traditional psychoanalytic theory, often called "one-person" theory because it focuses on the intrapsychic or internal world of a client as the source of all enactments, encourages therapists to push a client to look at these feelings and behaviors as reflective of something about her own history and personal conflicts. The concept of therapist as participant observer (Sullivan, 1953) who unconsciously and frequently unknowingly influences the situation or person she is observing paved the way for contemporary recognition of a clinician's role in the development of any transference dynamic. Our personalities, individual dynamics and history color how we listen to and participate in a client's transference enactments. Mitchell (1993) likens this way of looking at transference and countertransference as going to a party and accepting an invitation to dance. At some point it is a therapist's job to ask, "Why are we dancing this particular step? Why did we choose this music?" Contemporary psychodynamic theories offer a wide continuum of approaches to a clinician's exploration of her role, ranging from a clinician's silent observation of her own thoughts and feelings, to requests that a client articulate what he understands about his therapist's feelings and thoughts, to a clinician's revelations to a client of aspects of her internal world.

A Word About Training

There is a reason that psychoanalytic training takes a long time. Clinicians are asked to understand their own psychodynamic thoroughly, to be able to use themselves easily in the therapeutic process, and to be able to think about and recognize psychodynamics from a variety of theoretical and clinical perspectives. Many analysts and analytically-oriented psychotherapists today consider that a therapist's reactions to a client contain useful information about the internal world and relational patterns of both client and clinician (see, for example, Davies, 2006). Because a clinician's psychodynamics also inevitably impact the therapeutic work, it is crucial to understand one's own dynamics in order to keep them from interfering with the exploration of a client's dynamics—especially in those inevitable moments when a client's struggles, personality or dynamics trigger something in a clinician. Even therapists not interested in doing long-term, psychodynamically oriented psychotherapy can benefit from being in that kind of therapy for a period of time. Given the research showing the importance of the therapeutic relationship to the success of any therapeutic endeavor, it would seem that a therapist's commitment to self-understanding would enhance any kind of therapeutic approach and perhaps should be a requirement in all psychotherapeutic training. That said, however, even the most experienced psychoanalyst continues to evolve and to understand things differently over time. Similarly, psychodynamic theories are continuing to develop as new research and different issues emerge in the culture. They are not finished products that are ready to be applied "out of the package" to each clinical situation. Instead, each moment in clinical practice is an opportunity to explore and learn something new.

Evidence

Until recently, psychodynamic or "insight-oriented" psychotherapy and psychoanalysis were perhaps the least studied forms of psychotherapy, with much of the evidence of their impact coming from anecdotal descriptions and case studies. In a critical evaluation of psychodynamic theories, Eagle (1989) writes that one issue relevant to evidence-based research is that, "psychoanalytic writers attempt to employ clinical data for just about every purpose but the one for which they are most appropriate—an evaluation and understanding of therapeutic change." Recently, this has begun to change. For example, Wallerstein's (2000) study provides fascinating, in-depth data about the experiences of a group of men and women in long-term psychoanalysis, including how successful the treatment was and what the analysands themselves believed to have been the change factors.

It has not just been a lack of research in the field that has led many clinicians and clients to reject a psychoanalytic approach. Shedler (2010) notes that potential clients are often put off by historical images of arrogant and authoritarian psychoanalysts. Others are disturbed by the idea of an analyst sitting in silent judgment as they pour out their inner turmoil. The commitment of both time and money to long-term therapy has also been a problem for many clients and clinicians. Yet despite these negative characterizations of psychoanalysis (and by extension, talk therapy), there is growing evidence that psychodynamic psychotherapy helps many people get better. Some studies have shown that while a number of short term, "evidence-based" techniques have greater immediate impact on clients. Changes that occur in long term therapy (which is usually talk therapy) have a more permanent effect on the individual. For example, Leichsenring (2005), Leichsenring and Rabung (2008), Roth and Fonagy (1996), and Shedler (2010) have reviewed and evaluated research on a wide range of psychotherapies, including a number of both cognitive behavioral and psychodynamically-oriented psychotherapies. Their findings have been consistent: that longer term therapy appears to have longer-lasting results, especially with individuals with personality disorders, and that a variety of therapeutic interventions are effective with different symptoms and difficulties. Further, individuals undergoing long-term psychodynamic psychotherapy showed changes in brain functioning that did not show up in control participants. These changes were accompanied by changes that indicated a lifting of their depression.

According Roth and Fonagy (1996) the belief that specific clients and symptoms respond better to specific therapeutic interventions is not based on hard evidence as is sometimes believed. They write that the evidence about what therapies work for what disorders and groups of clients provides very little consistent guidance for clinicians to go by. Many of the studies have been, they suggest, too small to provide statistically useful results, but even large scale trials (e.g. Crits-Christoph, 1996) have not always been definitive (see also Seligman, 1995). However, like Wampold (2007) and numerous other researchers, they have found that a client's sense of a therapist's knowledge and experience, and interest in what a client is actually experiencing, can play a more important role than the specific therapeutic approach.

Conclusion

Putting thoughts into words out loud, to another person, can sometimes give us a chance to think about our own ideas differently, and leading to growing self-awareness and concomitant psychological change. A psychodynamic approach does not always involve what has traditionally been seen as interpretation or insight. Instead, as numerous contemporary psychoanalysts have suggested (see for just some examples, Bromberg, 2001; Fonagy, Gyorgy, Jurist, & Target, 2003; Frank, 2004; Hoffman, 1996; Holmes, 1996; Mitchell, 1993; Wallerstein, 2000) psychoanalysts today recognize that thoughts, feelings, behaviors and symptoms often have meaning that is not immediately clear either to a person experiencing them or to an observer. Such unspoken, unarticulated or unconscious meaning can play a role in ordinary daily behavior as well as in dreams and impulsive and unexplained actions. They can also impact how a client responds to therapy and therefore how a client uses any interventions, including those that are not psychoanalytically-based. Striving to understand these unspoken and unrecognized aspects of a client's everyday life, as well as those manifested in psychopathology, can be an important clinical intervention itself. This information can also help a clinician decide what other intervention(s) might be most useful for a client at a given time in their lives and in the therapeutic process.

Chapter 3
Developmental Models

Keywords Erikson • Epigenetic • Development • Developmental theory • Integrative practice • Cultural • Psychological • Social • Cognitive • Physical • Biological • Cognitive development • Psychodynamic development • Attachment theory • Emotional development • Teamwork in psychotherapy • Clinical team • Integrative team • Parents • Children • Integrative social work • Clinical illustration • Evidence • Research

Introduction

It is widely accepted today that a child is born with some basic abilities (e.g. the capacity to breathe, to suckle, and to cry) and with many other potential capabilities that will unfold over time. How he will develop will be the result of a series of interactions between that child's genetic makeup and the environment in which he lives. Educators, social scientists, parenting specialists and medical and mental health professionals bring, either implicitly or explicitly, theories of development into their work every day, with every client. However, to many people the idea of development is more theoretical than anything else. For instance, educators and parents alike may fall into a trap of expecting children to be more mature than their chronological or psychological development makes possible. Understanding that development is an ongoing interactive process is useful for both identifying difficulties and formulating an overall approach to a client's therapy. Developmental theory offers an integrative clinician a framework for thinking about the specific life issues that a client is facing (for example, how a college student is dealing with age appropriate issues like separation and identity). This frame, or outline, is not a rigid set of rules, but instead offers a way of organizing one's thinking so that interventions can be chosen thoughtfully. Yet the overwhelming number of developmental

F.D. Barth, *Integrative Clinical Social Work Practice: A Contemporary Perspective*, Essential Clinical Social Work Series, DOI 10.1007/978-1-4939-0351-1_3,

theories in existence today can make it difficult for a clinician to know what areas to focus on.

Developmental theory today cuts across cultural, psychological, social, cognitive and physical/biological fields and is based on extensive studies and observation of children and adults of all ages and at all stages of life. The range of data gathered from infant and child studies in recent decades no longer supports a "blank slate" theory. These studies show that from the moment of birth a child actively engages with the world. Childhood is a time of tremendous physical, cognitive, social and emotional development. Yet clinicians who closely observe and study these processes do not always agree on what they see or understand. In fact, so much has been written on these issues that it would be impossible to summarize in a single chapter (for further elaboration, see Austrian, 2008; Beebe, Jaffe, & Lachmann, 1993; Beebe & Lachmann, 2005; Gedo, 1991, 1997; Piaget, 1969; Rustin, 2012; Schore, 2003).

Because developmental progression does not follow a rigid path and has a wide range of normal variables, it is useful for a clinician to make an effort to become familiar with different developmental and lifecycle theories (see Austrian, 2008, for an excellent summary of developmental concepts that affect an individual's psychological makeup throughout the lifecycle). A practice can also be enriched by the availability of consultants with expertise in a wide variety of issues, including developmental theories. As we will discuss in throughout this book, and specifically in Chap. 9, a team can be formal or informal. In either case, it is useful for an integrative practitioner to have access to other clinicians whose knowledge augments and complements his own.

Understanding developmental theory helps an integrative practice in three different ways. First, it provides a frame for thinking about issues directly related to a client's chronological age. Second, it offers a way of thinking about the psychological themes that emerge at different developmental stages. And third, it helps us think about themes that develop in the course of therapy.

In my own work I have found Erikson's (1980) psychosocial developmental stages useful as a way of formulating developmental themes that are significant in a client's life. Seligman and Shanok (1996) describe in detail ways that they find Erikson helpful in integrating contemporary developmental thinking, including attachment theory. Goldberg and Gedo (1973), Pine (1985, 1990) and Stern (1985) also offer cohesive yet flexible, interactive and epigenetic models of ongoing psychological and emotional development from birth to death. Although many aspects of his thinking are no longer applicable, Erickson's table offers a way of organizing contemporary thinking about attachment, affect regulation and separation throughout the lifespan. Separated from drive/conflict theory, this approach does not privilege one stage of life or one particular set of dynamics or issues, offering instead a conceptualization of continual growth and development throughout the lifespan. As in therapy itself, an individual often revisits and re-works certain themes throughout life. Thus dynamics that are primary in one stage may run through an individual's life and may need to be worked on at various times and within the context of other developmental needs.

Themes and Life Stages

This conceptualization fits with contemporary attachment theory as well as with epigenetic models (e.g. Goldberg & Gedo, 1973). Mitchell (1993) suggests that the unfolding of dynamics both within therapy and throughout the life span can be viewed as alternating figure-ground, that is, that at times a theme plays a central role, and at times it is a background to other material. Similarly, Stern (1985) suggests that certain organizing themes, such as difficulties with attachment or separation, run through an individual's life, albeit in different forms at different developmental stages. Contemporary attachment theory (e.g. Bowlby, 1973; Cassidy & Shaver, 2008; Eagle, 1995; Goldberg, Muir, & Kerr, 1995; Holmes, 1996) and neuroscience research (Bjornsson, Didie, & Phillips, 2010; Lacy & Hughes, 2006; Rustin, 2012) offers tools for thinking about some of these themes.

In this chapter, we will focus on three themes that are frequently re-worked in different stages of development: attachment, separation-individuation (or, as we will discuss, attachment-individuation), and self-regulation, including management of affects and impulses. We will consider these themes as they unfold in three areas of the therapeutic encounter: in a client's past, in his present, and in the therapeutic relationship.

While there is not an exact one to one correlation between interventions and dynamics, a good rule of thumb is that issues related to early developmental issues like impulse control, affect regulation and object constancy require active, symptom-focused interventions, such as behavioral and structural, self-soothing and relaxation techniques. Problems that are tied to attachment insecurity and anxiety often require trust-building and understanding as well as symptom-focused interventions. Clients who are capable of tolerating difficult affects and examining their own thoughts and feelings can frequently make use of insight-oriented, psychodynamically-oriented interventions.

In the late 1930s, ego psychologists (see Hartmann 1939) were aware of and writing about the interplay of psychodynamics and cognitive-developmental processes (see Piaget, 1952, for further elaboration). Erikson introduced the idea that psychological development does not stop, as was once believed, with the "resolution" of oedipal conflict. His thinking that there is an ongoing process to development, with psychological, emotional and social tasks being accomplished at different ages of life throughout the human lifespan, can be a useful tool for an integrative clinician.

Developmental theory posits the existence of distinct developmental tasks that an individual needs to accomplish through the lifecycle. Erikson suggested eight stages of psychosocial development that lead us from birth to death (Table 3.1). While there are several ways in which the theory behind his stages is no longer applicable, including the conceptualizations of male and female development on which some of his thinking is based, contemporary clinical thinkers can still find it a helpful tool for thinking and talking about a client's developmental themes. For example, while most clinicians no longer closely adhere to the psychosexual conceptualization of

Table 3.1 Erikson's eight stages of development

Erikson's stages of development:
1. Trust vs. mistrust (oral-sensory, birth-2 years)
2. Autonomy vs. shame & doubt (muscular-anal, 2–4 years)
3. Initiative vs. guilt (locomotor-genital, preschool, 4–5 years)
4. Industry vs. inferiority (latency, 5–12 years)
5. Identity vs. role confusion (adolescence, 13–19 years)
6. Intimacy vs. isolation (young adulthood, 20–24 years)
7. Generativity vs. stagnation (middle adulthood, 25–64 years)
8. Wisdom: ego integrity vs. despair (late adulthood, 65-death)

development that informs Erikson's early stages, themes of Trust vs. Mistrust can be found in early attachment, and Autonomy vs. Shame and Doubt are useful ways of helping clients understand difficulties related to the initial forays of a young child into separation and individuation (or *attachment* and individuation, as Lyons-Ruth, 1991, calls it). Similarly, while adolescence is today often considered to extend through the 20s (see Amundsen, Borgen & Tench, 1995; Levinson, 1986), some of the crucial issues of this period of life continue to coalesce around identity, role confusion, intimacy and isolation. At the same time, Erikson's model can be used to integrate theories of cognitive development, cultural dynamics, and attachment issues. As Eagle (1995) points out, each theory can also elucidate different aspects of the developmental process.

In an epigenetic model such as Erikson's, development occurs according to genetic potentialities which are constantly interacting with and modified by environmental influences. Each stage is influenced by the way that the stage before it was managed, and also influences the form of the stage to follow. Similarly, issues of development in different realms are mutually impacted by one another: for example, cognitive development influences psychosocial stages and attachment, and vice versa. Each can have an impact on the progression of another. Issues that are primary in an early stage may take a backseat in a later period of life, but they will continue to be worked on and to influence the stages that follow. In clinical work, we often see themes repeating themselves in client's attempts to live their lives. The three themes described at the beginning of this chapter (attachment, separation-individuation/attachment-individuation, and self-regulation, including management of affects and impulses) often recur throughout an individual's life and affect how he engages in his current developmental stage.

Developmental Themes and Developmental Trauma

It is sometimes suggested that a client who shows signs of struggling with particular developmental themes may have been traumatized during the childhood stage associated with that particular theme. Diagnoses are sometimes also made on the basis of a client's developmental themes. However, years of clinical practice have led me to question such one to one correlations, and a growing number of researchers have begun to address these supposed links (see Dozier, Stovall-McClough, & Albus, 2008; Roth & Fonagy, 1996). Although insurance companies often demand that clinicians work within a somewhat rigid frame of diagnosis and treatment requirements, it can actually often be helpful for a clinician to think about developmental issues and interventions from this broader, more integrative perspective without adhering to a rigid one to one correlation between diagnosis and treatment.

Here is an example of how this can work:

Margaret is on the staff of the counseling office in a large university. She loves her work, although she admits that she had imagined it quite differently than it actually is. "I thought I was going to be having deep intellectual discussions with smart young people who were trying to figure out the meaning of life. Instead, I have crisis sessions with depressed youngsters who cannot do their schoolwork, scary encounters with young women who are starving themselves to death or binging and purging several times a day because they think that to be successful and beautiful they have to be a certain body weight, or I'm dealing with a young man who has been hospitalized for the second time with alcohol poisoning but refuses to accept that he has a drinking problem. These are life problems, alright, but we don't have the luxury of exploring what they mean. We are always putting out emotional, psychological and physical fires."

Viewing these symptoms as reflective of developmental themes helps Margaret understand her clients, formulate interventions and also explain their struggles to them and their families.

"These kids are frightened, angry, hurt, sad, depressed, lonely...the behaviors are ways that they have found to manage these feelings and to cope with the very questions I wanted them to be asking in our sessions." These youngsters were struggling with separating from their parents and becoming independent adults in a world that was different from the one in which Margaret and many of her colleagues had grown up. "They have had a different set of pressures and a different set of goals that are part of the high pressure, high achievement world in which they live. Many of them have been so busy trying to get into the 'right' college that they didn't have time to wonder what they might like to do with their lives." College is where many youngsters today do some of the experimenting with identity and roles that high school students did in previous decades. Understanding drinking, eating, gambling, and other problematic activities in this context helped Margaret think more clearly about immediate interventions, which often had to be crisis, symptom and behavior-oriented. It also gave her a frame for addressing longer term goals, including developing a healthy sense of self separate from (although also connected to) family, a capacity to engage in meaningful intimate relationships, and an ability to find meaningful and productive work.

Immediate symptom-focused interventions include referral for medication evaluation, entering a student in a structured psycho-educational or cognitive group, teaching coping mechanisms, including relaxation techniques, addressing the need for nutrition and sleep, and at times making a referral for hospitalization. "I seldom have the opportunity for long-term work with these students," Margaret notes. "But I consider my job to be helping them to get back on a healthy, age-appropriate developmental track. And I also hope that I give them a good experience of therapy, so that they will be comfortable coming back, either to me or to someone else, when and if they need some help at other stages of their lives."

Developmental theory helps parents, educators and government funding sources recognize and address the need for intervention during childhood and adolescence. Attachment research, for example, has been utilized to support government and private programs to aid distressed families in providing an early secure base for their children (see Slade, 2006; Steele, 2008). Other research has shown the importance of active intervention at certain stages of adolescence to help prevent disorders typical of those stages. For instance, Gilligan and Machoian (2002) found that adolescent girls are at highest risk of suicidal behavior in their 13th and 14th years, at the stage of development during which they begin searching for relationships with boys. This is a time when they are feeling hopeful and simultaneously extremely vulnerable.

Attachment and Separation

Although extremely popular, attachment theory is far more complex than is often recognized. Holmes (1996) notes that it is actually not a single theory but is instead an umbrella heading for a number of approaches that privilege the need for secure attachment in the development of a healthy psyche. What has become clear, however, is that attachment is not only a significant early process, but it is a theme that continues to be significant through the lifecycle. It is also amenable to change. Current research also suggests that the separation-individuation process does not stop at a specific point in childhood, but continues to be reworked throughout the life span (see, for example, Bowlby, 1973; Kohut, 1971; Stern, 1985).

Based on observation of infant and toddler and parent dyads, Lyons-Ruth (1991) suggests that we reframe the concept and the tasks involved in what Mahler, Pine, and Bergman (1973) call "separation-individuation." Lyons-Ruth offers the name "attachment-individuation" instead, suggesting that the goal of psychological health is not the development of separateness, but the capacity to be attached to another while also respecting one's own individuated self. Although this is a stage of early development, my experience working with college aged adolescents leads me to agree with Blos (1967) and others that the struggle to separate from and connect to parents in new ways, and simultaneously to develop new relationships in which one is both attached and separate, is a central one in adolescence. While both physical and psychological separation have long been viewed as crucial to the process of individuation and identity building, I, like Lyons-Ruth, have found that it is frequently important to integrate and underscore the importance of healthy, albeit changing, attachment to parents and family as an adolescent becomes independent (see Barth, 1989, 2003). Understanding these themes can be part of an integrative approach in helping young clients and their families recognize and manage separation with connection (see also Chodorow, 1999).

According to Lachmann (2001), one might consider Mahler's view of separation-individuation in a similar light. He suggests that she does not view separation-individuation as a final destination, but rather as part of a process. Similarly, Bowlby, the "father" of attachment theory, writes that attachment itself is a process that goes on throughout life (1973)—an idea reiterated by Kohut (1977), who says that human beings need what he called selfobjects—that is, other people who can understand our thoughts and feelings, and can help us soothe ourselves and manage stressful emotions—just as we need oxygen—from birth to death. Thus, while these developmental issues are part of childhood, they are also revisited and reworked throughout an individual's lifetime. For an integrative clinician, this formulation opens the door to thinking about interventions from a here and now perspective as well as within the context of a client's history. For example, working on attachment needs in the present may be enough to help restore a client to healthy functioning.

Developmental issues of attachment, object relations, affect management and impulse control are often seen in clients with diagnoses in the areas of addictions, impulse control and certain personality disorders (e.g. borderline personality disorder), as well as in some discussions of bipolar disorders (see, for example, Bateman & Fonagy, 2004; Gabbard, 1991; Goldstein, 1999; Linehan, 1993). These formulations do not have to identify historical reasons for a client's current struggle, but thinking in terms of developmental concepts can help a clinician formulate an appropriate intervention. For example, in the case of Mr. Nolan, who was struggling with alcoholism, his therapist decided that he needed help managing his impulses and dealing with his shame about his difficulties. Locating these struggles in the arena of autonomy vs. shame and doubt in Erickson's model helped Ms. Bluen formulate useful interventions that would provide her client with support as he developed the capacity to maintain himself in recovery without causing him undue shame about not being able to do it on his own. They did not, however, mean that Mr. Nolan was stuck at the psychological age of 2–4 years, since over the course of his life he had worked through many of the developmental tasks of both adolescence and adulthood.

Thinking in terms of both ongoing process and managing opposites can seem daunting, but is actually useful in terms of choosing an appropriate intervention. If a client needs help with the kinds of functions usually provided by a secure attachment figure, e.g. self-soothing, time management, coping with overstimulation, and managing emotions, a clinician's first interventions should be directed at shoring up these self-organizing and self-regulating functions. Behavioral, directive and educational interventions might be most appropriate at these moments. Providing food and clean clothing (if appropriate within a specific setting), helping a client find housing, coping with an angry partner, paying bills and finding adjunct services to help with cleaning (for example in the case of a depressed or hoarding client) can be seen as offering not only a "holding environment" as described by Winnicott (1965), but also some of the selfobject functions described by Kohut (1977), as well as some of the attachment functions described by Bowlby (1988).

Table 3.2 Types of issues, interventions, and corrective experience

Type of issues	Interventions	Corrective experience
Early developmental issues: impulse control, affect regulation and object constancy	Active intervention like behavioral and structural, self-soothing and relaxation techniques	Holding (facilitating) environment, containing, corrective selfobject experience
Attachment issues	Trust-building, active interventions, and understanding	Holding environment, containing, affect regulation, corrective selfobject/attachment experience
Issues related to unconscious meanings and repeated patterns in clients able to tolerate emotions and self-examination	Insight-oriented, psychodynamically-oriented interventions	Holding environment, corrective selfobject/attachment experience, new understanding

It is tempting to assume that developmental issues seen in an adult or adolescent client indicate childhood difficulties at a specific age and developmental stage (Table 3.2). Similarly, it is currently common practice to conclude that certain symptoms in adults and adolescents indicate the presence of childhood trauma. While the tremendous amount of work on trauma has added a great deal to our knowledge and understanding of the impact of previously unrecognized or unacknowledged horrors in the lives of many young people, it is also important to remember that other factors may also play a significant role in the unhappiness and problematic behaviors of many clients (see, for example, Mitchell and Black, 1996). For a clinician working to build an integrative practice, the variety of developmental theories available can be a potent reminder that no approach should be applied rigidly or followed blindly. As in every aspect of this work, these concepts are tools for helping us listen to and think about what our clients are communicating to us. As we sort out the verbal and nonverbal messages our clients send, we can select from a wide range of tools to address the specific needs of a client at a given time.

Developmental Organizing Themes

Developmental Organizing Themes are those dynamics from earlier stages of development that a client brings into therapy, no matter what his or her age. For example, for many different reasons, a 29 year old man may come into therapy for help dealing with his dating life. It would appear that he is struggling with issues related to the stage of life Levenson (1989) refers to as transitional, with changes in life structure related to settling down, marrying, starting a family, and moving forward on a chosen career path. But it gradually becomes clear that this young man is struggling with issues related to self-control and autonomy, which emerge each time he begins to move towards a more committed relationship. Developmental organizing issues from early childhood and adolescence color his ability to manage the stress of his actual age-appropriate developmental process.

However, from an integrative position, one would attempt to think in terms not only of developmental and family systems issues, but also in terms of what is actually happening with a client at a specific time in the work. Sometimes it can be helpful to identify repeated patterns as, for example, a struggle between control and autonomy in order to determine what approach might be most useful at a given time. As described by Connors (2006), Frank (1999) and Wachtel (1997), a clinician needs to assess a client's level of discomfort, capacity to tolerate that discomfort, and capacity for self-soothing. When the symptoms are interfering with life functioning—e.g. anxiety that cannot be tolerated, depression that makes it impossible to get out of bed, an addiction or compulsive behavior that is dangerous to physical or emotional life—active, structured interventions are most appropriate. Similarly, if a client is psychotic, acting out, uninterested in exploration or incapable of tolerating or engaging in discussion of these feelings and their antecedents, active work in symptom-reduction is important. For example cognitive behavioral tools can be directed specifically at helping clients gain more of a sense of independence and self-confidence. Mindfulness techniques, ego enhancing work, and some emotional focusing are also helpful.

Interestingly, from the perspective of an integrative approach, Roth and Fonagy (1996), who have reviewed a tremendous amount of research data on the correlation between interventions and symptoms, found that the specific intervention is less significant than a sense that a clinician has confidence in the technique and believes that it is appropriate for what is troubling a particular client. Thus, it is important for a clinician to be trained and supervised. However, even a beginning clinician has access to one of the most powerful techniques possible: trying to understand what a client is feeling and what he needs goes a long way towards helping (see Kohut, 1977; McWilliams, 2004). Like other integrative clinicians I have found that many clients need help learning to soothe themselves and manage emotions before they are capable of exploring distressing feelings. Clients who have been pushed into painful and intolerable feelings without the tools to manage them may become more symptomatic, or may simply leave therapy in order to protect themselves.

On the other hand, having developed the capacity to soothe painful emotions, some clients are able to move more deeply into self-exploration, while others have accomplished what they want from therapy and are ready to move on. Basch (1980) emphasizes the importance of supporting a client in achieving his own goals, even when they are not precisely the same as his therapist's. We will consider this issue further in the chapter on endings. In either case, whether clients are interested in moving more deeply into material or not, helping them learn to manage and structure feelings is, in developmental language, comparable to soothing a crying child. In most cases, a sobbing youngster, no matter how verbal, cannot say what is upsetting about until the crying stops. The pain must be addressed and the child's feelings re-equilibrated before trying to determine what caused the upset. Once the emotions are regulated, the cause may not even be important, but several developmental steps will have taken place: the child will have done some work on developing the capacity to tolerate and the skill to manage the affect the next time and will also have learned that another person can be trusted to help with self-soothing.

Exploring Client History and Current Reality

Developmental concepts offer both clinician and client a way of talking and thinking about some of the difficulties with which a client is struggling. As noted earlier, however, it is important to recognize that there is not necessarily a one to one correlation between the concepts and a client's actual experiences. Instead, thinking in terms of developmental issues can help a clinician formulate interventions that target particular issues. It can be a useful way to talk about dynamics with clients, although it is also extremely important for a clinician to clarify that this does not indicate that a client is acting in a childish manner. Here is an example of how this can work.

After her discharge from the hospital, Anna Louise (who we met in Chap. 1) began to work with Lisa, a psychodynamically-oriented psychotherapist in a clinic affiliated with the hospital. Relatively quickly it became clear that Anna Louise held herself to an impossibly high standard of performance, getting very angry at herself for even the smallest mistakes. She often talked about herself as though she were an imbecile and called herself a variety of names. Lisa silently wondered if she treated her two small children this way as well. There had been no indication of any difficulties with the children—in fact, Anna Louise's husband described her as a wonderful mother—so Lisa decided that she could wait before addressing this question. Still, she carefully considered the most tactful yet direct way to help this sensitive client begin to explore her constant self-criticism. After expressing some curiosity about the ongoing negative descriptions that Anna Louise used to characterize herself, Lisa asked if being so mean to herself helped her get the work done. After a surprised silence, Anna Louise said she had never thought about that. It was just what she did when she was acting so stupid. Lisa said, "You sound like a frustrated mother with a toddler, calling her names because you can't understand that she's really just not capable of managing that task right now." Anna Louise burst into tears and said that exactly captured how she felt about herself. She added that she sometimes felt that way about her children, which made her feel like she was the worst mother in the world.

Since her client had opened up this issue, Lisa took the opportunity to explore a variety of parenting issues. Although Anna Louise worried a great deal about being a bad parent, it sounded like she was doing a pretty good job. Her husband and in-laws confirmed this conclusion, but because of her client's worries, and also as a means to help her develop a support network of peers, Lisa encouraged her to participate in a parenting group as well as her individual therapy. In her individual sessions, Lisa asked about childhood memories. Were her parents critical of her? "Oh no," Anna Louise replied. "My parents are very, very loving. Very gentle and kind." The response may have been a defense against intolerable memories. It may have been a valid description of Anna Louise's parents, although in general descriptions of anything as all good or all bad are seldom complete: few things in life are absolute. Lisa wanted to ask questions to open up who had spoken to Anna Louise in that way, and to suggest that she was treating herself and her children as she had been treated. There are dangers with such a construction, however, since it can be an oversimplification of a complex developmental process and an isolation of a single memory, or cluster of memories. It is important for a clinician to keep in mind that these thoughts exist within the context of a complicated reality. Schafer (1994) calls such formulations "constructions" of history because they are constructed in the here and now and are not necessarily accurate depictions of an individual's past. Mitchell and Black (1995) note that the question of causality of symptoms—childhood trauma or internal conflict—is one of the major controversies for psychotherapists today. Gedo (1991) suggests that the answer is even more complicated: biology, history and conflict are all part of the picture. Even tools like the Adult Attachment Interview, which is often utilized to determine areas of attachment difficulty, need to be assessed with care. Slade (2006), for example, notes that in fact human beings often fall into more than one attachment classification, and furthermore that attachment patterns can change over time.

Attachment themes often contain within them "models of relationships" that clients have learned in early interactions with parental figures, and have carried with them into later relationships. These models lead to both expectations that certain patterns of interaction will be repeated in other relationships, and also to behaviors that may elicit these patterns. Understanding these constructs can help a clinician find a way to talk with a client about both interpersonal and intrapsychic difficulties. For example, it offers an opportunity to begin to talk about a client's implicit, or unarticulated constructions of experience—for example, that to be loved means to be criticized. Talking about Erickson's stage of mastery can help a client understand why certain patterns are repeated without being overly critical of self or of parents, thus maintaining a connection while also developing a separate and healthy sense of self.

Memories and Organizing Themes

A client's memories can be useful tools for thinking about how a client is experiencing and psychologically organizing any interaction. For example, Margaret, the college counselor, routinely asks her clients about previous experiences that might in some way have been painful, difficult or traumatic. For example, she has learned that while some homesick students have struggled throughout their lives with issues around separation—perhaps having been homesick at camp or having problems leaving their mother on the first day of school—it can be helpful to discuss how they managed to master the experiences rather than to focus on their difficulties with separation. If finding a supportive adult or making a new friend helped in the past, the client might be encouraged to think that a similar capacity for mastery will emerge in this process as well. Discussing ways that a client might manage the feelings is another key to the process of both mastery and gradual movement towards a new experience of this ongoing theme. Margaret offers her own ego as support in the process, working together with each client to come up with ideas about managing difficult feelings. One client, for example, might find it useful to become involved in volunteer work organized by a campus group; another decides to have more frequent contact with her parents; while yet another decides less contact with her parents and regular sessions with Margaret would help; and yet another decides that it would be helpful to join a support group at the counseling center.

I have said this before, but it bears repeating: because developmental progression does not follow a rigid path and has a wide range of normal variables, it is useful for a clinician to make an effort to become familiar with different developmental and lifecycle theories. A practice can also be enriched by the availability of consultants with expertise in a wide variety of issues, including developmental theories. This does not mean that members of a team need to be rigidly structured or organized or even consulted in every case, but it is useful for an integrative practitioner to have access to other clinicians whose knowledge augments and complements his own.

Developmental Stages of Therapy

Just as in life, every therapeutic experience is a process that evolves over time, that is, the process of therapy is itself developmental. As questions of basic trust are tested and resolved (and often tested again), old attachment themes are repeated and reworked, leading to an opportunity to find new ways to be connected and separate. Repetition of old organizing themes allows a client to work toward greater security, self-confidence and connection to others. Whether the frame is two sessions of hypnosis, a 12 week course of DBT or a 3 year psychodynamic psychotherapy, there will always be at least three phases of the work: beginning, middle and end, and the work at the beginning will be different from that at the end. Developmental thinking is a useful tool for making decisions about interventions that are appropriate to each phase of therapy. In the beginning of any therapeutic encounter, therapist and client must get to know one another, agree on mutually defined goals, and establish the format in which the work to attain these goals will be done. This introductory phase may include educational instruction from a therapist or be focused on taking information from a client. In some way or another, however, either formally or informally, therapist and client begin the work. In this early stage, a therapist will be looking to see how well a client can tolerate the emotions that go along with engaging in a new activity and learning a new way of thinking.

Connors (2006), Frank (1999) and Wachtel (1997) have each noted that in this stage a therapist often needs to assess the need for immediate and/or structured intervention. Research has shown that clients tend to stay in therapy when they feel that they are getting something from the work (Roth & Fonagy, 1996) and to leave when they are not. Often in the early stages of the work, when symptoms are overwhelming or distressing, it is helpful for a clinician to be more active, directive and/or structured than he might be later in the work, when a client is less symptomatic and has learned some of the techniques and how to apply them. This may also be a time when medication is helpful.

In the middle phase of work, a client is encouraged to try to engage in therapeutic work with some independence. A clinician may continue to offer education and guidance during this period. Sometimes modeling, showing how we might try to work with certain dynamics, whether by exploring the psychodynamic meaning or by suggesting a specific behavioral or mindfulness technique, can be the most useful intervention we can make. If a client has been less symptomatic or has been acting out sporadically, the middle period can be a time for examining some of the triggers of these behaviors, and can also be a time for supporting the strengths that have made it possible for the symptoms to decrease during this time frame.

The final phase of therapy, or the termination phase, is, like the other stages, contingent in part on the type of therapy being done. One of the great benefits of short term, symptom-focused work is that it gives a client a sense of accomplishment. Clinicians who routinely practice longer-term, less focused therapy might do well to incorporate this technique into ongoing work. Basch (1980) says that too often psychodynamically-oriented psychotherapists run the risk of undoing important work they and their clients have done by focusing on work a client still needs to do rather than on the successful achievements already made. As one young client who had participated in a 12 week program of DBT put it, "I really have accomplished so much. I know what to do when I'm having these feelings. I know how to prioritize my activities. And I know how to ask for help when I need it." She was also highlighting a further aspect of the termination phase: to anticipate ahead of time what a client might do should some of the symptoms recur.

Using Developmental Thinking to Help Clarify and Manage Resistance, Defenses, and Issues That Emerge in a Therapeutic Relationship

As noted in Chap. 2, concepts from psychoanalytic theory can be useful for a clinician no matter what approach they are using. Let us return to Margaret, the college counselor, for an example. Margaret found herself struggling with students who resisted her suggestions so often that she sought supervision to see what she might be doing to stir up this resistance. What she discovered was that in many cases, the apparent resistance was developmentally appropriate, if problematic. Many college students, working on the developmentally appropriate issues of individuation and personal agency, are not particularly interested in becoming engaged in a new and dependent relationship to another adult, no matter how much they may like, admire and appreciate that adult. They therefore may forget appointments or avoid making them in the first place. Or, despite being symptomatic and in some psychological pain, they may not seek help because they feel that they should be able to take care of the problem themselves. Understanding this dynamic, a clinician can make a gentle comment about the difference between asking for help and being dependent, to see if a client can engage in a discussion of the issues. Or a clinician might directly address the developmental conflict, for example, "I think you are working hard to be an independent adult, and feeling like you might need help makes you feel like a child again. I wonder if we can work out a way that you could get the help you need without losing a sense of your independence and competence."

It is also common for a clinician to want to "know how the story ends." For those of us who, like Margaret, work with children and adolescents, this desire is often especially difficult, but it also affects clinicians who see adults. While this wish is both normal and comprehensible, it can interfere with the process of helping clients work on issues of separation and self-development. Not only can these endings awaken feelings from a personal developmental stage in which we felt abandoned or rejected, but we may also be left "holding" loving feelings while a client moves on, much as parents sometimes feel when their children work on individuation. Clinicians can feel "stuck" with the caring feelings, while the objects of their attachment get help and move on. Some clients want to move on without feeling that their therapists are trying to hold them back, but others feel more comfortable leaving when a clinician communicates not only positive feelings about the work they have done together, but also good feelings about the client as well. From a developmental perspective, even the ending is part of the process of therapy, helping clients get back on the developmental track and towards achievement of their life goals. We will discuss the complexity of this process more fully when we speak about endings in therapy. For now, let us simply note that this is one of the moments in which an integrative approach offers a range of possible responses, rather than a single technique that is assumed to be correct at all times.

Conclusion

Not surprisingly, sitting with clients as they work through developmental stages relating to attachment and individuation can open up a clinician's ongoing attachment needs. As we discussed in the last chapter, this is one more way that our own personality and psychodynamics can impact our work. For instance, a desire to help others is often accompanied by a desire to make caring connections. I have found that these wishes, which often make us want to stay connected to clients when clients are eager to break the link, can be part of a healthy developmental process in some therapies. Clients sometimes need to know that their therapists will think about them in the future, and will care about how they are doing, even if they are no longer in touch. While I agree with Basch that it is important to support a client's accomplishments, I have also consulted in numerous situations in which it is helpful for a client to know that a therapist believes there is more that can be worked on before they end therapy. Some of these clinicians have agreed to stop the work, despite their professional judgment that it was not the best time to do so, because they did not want to hold on to clients inappropriately. In order to best help each client determine what will be most therapeutic for them at a specific time in therapy, it can be extremely useful to draw from different assessment tools and theories. Let us turn next to bringing cognitive and behavioral interventions into an integrative frame, and then we will talk about assessment as integrative tool not only in the initial phase but also in *any* ongoing therapeutic work.

Chapter 4
Cognitive and Behavioral Models

Keywords Cognitive therapy • Behavioral therapy • CBT • Psychodynamically-oriented psychotherapy • Integrative teamwork • Conjoint therapy • Multiple models • Integrative psychotherapy • Integrative social work • Dialectical behavioral therapy • DBT • Acceptance and commitment therapy • ACT • Mindfulness based cognitive therapy • MBCT • Mindfulness • Self-acceptance • Symptom-focused • Affect regulation • Evidence • Research • Clinical examples • Psychodynamics • Mindfulness • Developmental theory • Assessment • Termination

As I was preparing this chapter, I was also teaching a class on integrating theories to a group of experienced therapists. As we read about some of the contemporary cognitive therapies, one psychoanalytically trained group member commented that she had been practicing some similar techniques for years. "But I always felt like I was looking over my shoulder for someone to accuse me of stepping outside of the analytic frame," she said. "Like it was sacrilege to make a suggestion about a way of coping with certain feelings instead of trying to understand the meaning of those feelings." Another therapist quickly spoke up. "That's pretty funny," he said. "I was trained in Cognitive Behavior Therapy, but there have been many times when I've stopped the training to look at the meanings behind some of the behaviors. And I always felt like the CBT 'police' might come in at any minute and tell me I was breaking that frame!" My own experience and feedback I get from supervisees and students, that most of us integrate many of these techniques without necessarily recognizing that we are doing so, is reinforced by research reported by Roth and Fonagy (1996). I have come to think that there are several possible ways of integrating: (1) to train in more than one form of work and formally practice each of them with the same client; (2) to thoughtfully integrate concepts from different models without formally utilizing the overall practice; (3) to work conjointly with another therapist who offers a different model from one's own; (4) to utilize practices from one model to enhance work in another.

F.D. Barth, *Integrative Clinical Social Work Practice: A Contemporary Perspective*, Essential Clinical Social Work Series, DOI 10.1007/978-1-4939-0351-1_4,

It has been my experience that many clinicians who practice a wide range of therapies integrate cognitive behavioral techniques, either intentionally or unintentionally. In addition many cognitive behavioral theories now integrate not only mindfulness practices, motivational interviewing and other techniques, but they also bring in some previously rejected psychodynamic factors, including concepts such as resistance and consideration of the therapist-client relationship. Traditionally, it has been less acceptable for clients to see more than one psychotherapist at one time, but in contemporary practice more and more clinicians not only accept, but even encourage clients to work with other professionals who can offer them more tools for symptom management. Let us turn to a brief example of one way that cognitive behavioral work has been integrated with other approaches, and then we will discuss some of the theory that informs these interventions.

Clinical Illustration

Ms. Robinson (the mother of the ill child described in Chap. 1) was struggling with feelings of inadequacy and anxiety. As her social worker, Mr. Andrews, got to know her better over the course of her son's illness, he became convinced that her difficulties preceded the illness and were in part due to a number of difficulties she had managing her thoughts and affects. The hospital offered Dialectical Behavioral Therapy (DBT) groups for clients who were having difficulties managing some of the feelings related to their children's illnesses. However, many clients found it useful for dealing with other, longer term issues as well. Mr. Andrews felt that the group, which he ran, would provide some tools that Ms. Robinson might find helpful for managing the often disruptive anger that seemed to explode in her household. With his encouragement, she began coming to the group and found herself enjoying the sessions tremendously. She liked the contact with other parents, the sense that she was appreciated and even admired by some of them, and the feeling that some of the things she had to say to them were helpful. She also found that the tools the group had to offer—including beginning to find words for feelings, paying close attention to her own thoughts, feelings and physical sensations, as well as breaking down large difficulties into smaller segments—were all extremely helpful.

Despite having to travel for over an hour and take two buses and a train to get to her sessions, Ms. Robinson initially got to the group meetings on time or even a little early. After a few weeks, however, she began arriving at least 20 min late, which of course cut into the work and left her, the group and Mr. Andrews feeling frustrated. A psychodynamically-oriented therapist might have examined her reasons for being late and perhaps explored unconscious motivations. An integrative perspective would lead a therapist to ask whether such an exploration would be the most effective. Because Ms. Robinson had shown little interest in or ability to explore her own psychodynamics, and also because the behaviors were having immediate negative consequences that Mr. Andrews did not want to see reinforced, he chose to meet with her individually for a few sessions to try to stop the pattern.

Not surprisingly, Ms. Robinson arrived late for her appointment. Using a combination of what cognitive behavioral therapists call chain analysis and motivational work, and what Sullivan (1953) calls "detailed inquiry," Mr. Andrews asked her to go over what had happened from the moment she began thinking about getting ready to come to her session to the moment that she actually got on the first bus. Ms. Robinson explained that she had been getting ready to leave when her mother called to her from a back room and asked her to bring home some bread from the grocery store on her way back from the hospital. Ms. Robinson was upset with her mother for stopping her, but she also knew that they did need bread and a few other groceries, so she stopped to check to see if she had any money in her wallet. She discovered that she did not have money and had to go into her mother's room to ask for some. Her mother then began to criticize her for always needing cash. Ms. Robinson began to defend herself, which delayed her departure even further. By the time she got out the door she was too upset to immediately get on the bus, so she stood outside for a few minutes trying to pull herself together.

After Ms. Robinson described this incident, Mr. Andrews empathized with her frustration and said that it made sense that she had been late. He asked if this kind of interaction with her mother happened often. At first she said no, but then, as they continued to unpack her tardiness, she acknowledged that she was late to many activities, and often felt so ashamed of being so late that she did not even attend events and activities that she had been anticipating with pleasure. Mr. Andrews asked if she could think of any other ways to deal with her mother's frequent last-minute requests. As they came up with some possible responses, Ms. Robinson spontaneously commented that she thought that her mother was jealous of all of the attention she was getting at the hospital. "It's crazy," she said. "I don't want to be coming here. I want my baby to come home." Fonagy, Gyorgy, Jurist, & Target (2003) view the process of imagining what someone else is thinking and feeling (what they call "mentalizing") as an important step in the development of the self. Mr. Andrews integrated this idea into his work as well, asking Ms. Robinson to talk a little bit more about how she understood what her mother was feeling. As a result of both understanding her mother's feelings and simultaneously becoming more comfortable setting limits with her mother (with Mr. Andrews' support and specific suggestions), Ms. Robinson began to feel that she had more control over the process of leaving the house and began arriving on time for her appointments. Furthermore, she spoke of feeling more comfortable setting limits with her boyfriend and with her children, something that had been an unspoken problem for her.

One day Mr. Andrews walked into the boy's hospital room and found Mrs. Robinson and her mother, the child's grandmother, engaged in a quiet although intense conversation. Her mother spoke pleasantly to Mr. Andrews, then left the room, giving her daughter a hug. Ms. Robinson looked at the clinician. "We could never have done that before," she said. "I don't know exactly what has happened, but I feel like a very different person from when my son came to this hospital." She hesitated for a minute, then said, "That's not quite right. I think I feel like myself—only more." When Mr. Andrews encouraged her to say more, she said, "It's kind of hard to put into words. And it feels a little silly to say. But I sort of feel like I know what I'm feeling now, and I know what to do with those feelings. And that means…I'm just more okay being who I am. I don't have to defend myself to anyone anymore—not to my mother, not to my sister, not even to you. And I guess that makes me less prickly. And makes it easier to be me."

Integrating these different approaches sometimes seems almost spontaneous, which is one of the reasons integrative therapy is often called eclectic. However, it often only takes a moment for a clinician to recognize why he has "shifted gears" with a particular client at a particular time. Understanding why we make some of these spontaneous shifts can lead to a practice in which we make thoughtful and well-reasoned decisions to bring in a different technique at any given time. Let us turn briefly to an overview of the major cognitive behavioral therapies in order to see more clearly how and when they can be utilized in an integrative practice.

Overview

There have been several phases of development in cognitive and behavior therapy, which have been an important part of the therapeutic community's repertoire since the 1950s (for an extensive discussion of the development of and similarities and differences between these theories, see Hayes, 2004). In a very general way, cognitive therapies are based on the idea that thoughts can influence feelings and that emotional responses to a situation can come from thoughts about that situation, including how one might interpret or explain it to oneself, while behavioral theories tend to view problematic thoughts and behaviors as the result of reinforcement from a person's environment. As we consider the history of these approaches, it becomes clear that an integrative process has been going on in the development of contemporary cognitive and behavioral techniques. Early behavioral therapy focused on altering the results of this spontaneous or accidental rewarding of behavior (Skinner, 1957). Critical of a psychodynamic search for unconscious meanings to explain problematic behavior, early behavioral therapists suggested that psychological problems could be understood as the result of positive and negative reinforcement (see Bandura, 1986). Thus behavioral therapies tended to focus on helping clients try new behaviors and to stop allowing negative reinforcement to dictate how they act and what they do. However, Ellis (1961), with his Rational Emotive Behavioral Therapy, or REBT, integrated cognitive concepts aimed at helping clients change critical and self-defeating thoughts and behaviors through recognizing the problematic beliefs that are linked to these thoughts and actions. For example, an REBT therapist would try to help a client change thoughts that he "should" or "must" do certain things or "be" certain ways into thoughts of self-acceptance and self-empowerment. Following Ellis, Beck (Beck, 1976; Dozois & Beck, 2010) developed Cognitive Therapy in the 1960s. There are many similarities between REBT and CT, including the attempt to identify what Beck calls "automatic thoughts" that contain distorted and problematic information which contributes to depression, and to change those thoughts into more realistic and self-empowering ones. Beck (1976) also discusses the importance of "core negative thoughts" that are often part of the automatic thought process and that lead to depression. Such thoughts may include things like "I'm a failure" or "I am stupid," that a client may automatically think in response to disappointment and other problematic experiences. In other words, clients may blame themselves for something for which they actually bear no responsibility, thus adding to a sense of depression and self-defeat. CT today uses a combination of behavioral approaches to improving self-care and building confidence and verbal techniques for changing negative and automatic thoughts into more realistic and positive concepts.

Integrating Cognitive Behavioral Therapies

In what Hayes (2004) calls the "second wave," the focus turned more specifically to the maladaptive thoughts instead of problematic behavior. In his classic book on cognitive behavior therapy (CBT), Beck (1976) elucidates how altering certain maladaptive ideas and beliefs can lead to changes in behavior which then leads to improvement in both mood and self-esteem. Focusing initially on depression, Beck (Beck, Rush, Shaw, & Emery, 1979) suggested the disorder was often preceded by a series of negative thoughts. He found that by first identifying and then questioning the validity of these thoughts, clients could learn to change habitual patterns of cognition that led to the depressed state. Beck and his followers (e.g. Burns, 1999) continued to critique insight-oriented work as both inefficient and also based on invalid assumptions. From their perspective, trying to explore psychodynamic meaning could actually interfere with a client's therapeutic progress.

However, like Connors (2006), I have found that it can be extremely useful to integrate some of these ideas into a more psychodynamic approach. For example, a detailed inquiry (Sullivan, 1953) into the apparently insignificant and often concrete aspects of experience that a client feels are too silly to talk about can lead to a discussion of some of the assumptions a client makes about what certain behaviors—his own and those of others—mean. In a detailed inquiry a clinician engages with a client in a conversational and non-threatening manner in order to gather information about a wide range of features of that client's current and past life. Some assumptions that a client has made and taken for granted may be part of the reason that he feels self-critical, hopeless or anxious. A clinician can have a surprising impact on the chain of thought that leads to these feelings by commenting that he has a different perspective on the situation and asking if a client would like to hear it. Further, one can also expand a client's repertoire of reactions by bringing in the idea of mentalization (Fonagy, Gyorgy, Jurist, & Target, 2003). For example, asking for an elaboration of a client's understanding of what might be going on in the mind of the other person involved in a certain interaction can both help stimulate mentalization and also broaden a client's perspective on a situation.

However, clients cannot always simply "let go" of these assumptions. One of the difficulties with CBT as it was practiced during this period arose when clients felt self-critical because they could not follow through on the assigned goal of changing problematic thoughts. For example, Elaine, who sought help for low self-esteem and difficulties in relationships, talked about crossing the street when she saw a colleague "so that he did not have to say hello to me." She also described phobias based on fears that she said she knew were irrational. The cognitive behavioral therapist with whom she worked helped her focus on changing the maladaptive thoughts that went with each of these symptoms. For instance, he suggested she tell herself that there was no evidence that the colleague did not want to speak with her, or that the elevator she was getting on would get stuck between floors. The therapist taught her to remind herself that her feelings of poor self-esteem or anxiety were due to problematic thoughts, not to facts or reality. Yet because she was unable to master her thoughts, Elaine became even more self-critical and despondent. "There's really something wrong with me," she said to herself. "I can't even get the assignment right."

Cognitive behavioral therapists now view such maladaptive thoughts as common and frequently difficult to alter. Because many clients like Elaine reported feeling even worse when they could not change their thinking as instructed, contemporary CBT techniques have shifted significantly.

Recent Developments in Behavioral and Cognitive Therapies

In what Hayes (2004) calls the third wave, which he says draw from both the cognitive and behavioral "wings" of the earlier approaches, therapists emphasize changing a client's relationship to his thoughts rather than changing the thinking itself. Dialectical Behavioral Therapy (DBT), Acceptance and Commitment Therapy (ACT) and Mindfulness Based Cognitive Therapy (MBCT), for example, have addressed some of these issues by integrating ideas about self-acceptance and mindfulness into the work of disrupting and shifting rigid thought patterns and concomitant behaviors and feelings. Problematic thoughts and feelings are now observed and accepted in a mindful manner as part of the change process. However, Dozois and Beck (2010) suggest that some form of acceptance has always been part of Beck's formulations of cognitive therapy and that despite some philosophical differences between mindfulness and acceptance-based and traditional cognitive approaches, the two styles are both compatible and complementary. Similarly, Burns (1999) proposes that by focusing on and labeling "automatic thoughts" one develops the ability to become aware of those thoughts in ways that are compatible with ACT.

DBT, which focuses on the dialectic between acceptance and change, was developed by Linehan (1993) in the 1990s to help people with Borderline Personality Disorder who are often overwhelmed by their emotions and find traditional therapies less than helpful for managing their feelings and their often problematic behaviors. Linehan added a number of emotionally soothing, self-accepting, and relationship-building practices to cognitive therapy, making the practice useful for clients with a wide range of symptoms involving difficulties managing intense emotions.

DBT is a highly structured approach that often integrates individual therapy sessions with skills-building groups (see Ekblad, Chapman, & Lynch, 2010). Mindfulness practices from the Zen Buddhist tradition are also integrated into a DBT practice. Although Linehan was one of the early leaders in this direction of integrating mindfulness with CBT practice (see also Kabat-Zinn, 1990), today some form of mindfulness practice is part of many CBT techniques.

Another recent addition to the CBT repertoire is Acceptance and Commitment Therapy (ACT) developed by Hayes (2004). Like Dialectical Behavioral Therapy, ACT integrates meditation-oriented mindfulness practices into a therapy which is aimed at helping clients observe what they are thinking without making judgments (acceptance) and learning to distance themselves from distressful and unhelpful beliefs (cognitive defusion) rather than getting caught up in the beliefs that accompany those thoughts (cognitive fusion). Mindfulness Based Cognitive Therapy (MBCT) (Segal, Williams, & Teasdale, 2012) offers an 8 week program for using mindfulness and other cognitive techniques to help clients with depression and encouraging mindfulness on the part of clinicians as part of the therapeutic approach.

Today CBT is often used as a broad or general label for a variety of focused and structured psychotherapeutic approaches for dealing with difficult emotions, behaviors and thought processes. These approaches often utilize specific activities and techniques to help clients identify and then make shifts in how they handle thoughts, feelings and actions that have created and maintained difficulties in their lives. In contrast to more exploratory, open-ended psychodynamic models, behavioral interventions tend to be activity-based and goal-oriented. They also focus more on the here and now than on a client's past.

Behavioral and cognitive therapy is currently utilized for a variety of conditions and diagnoses, including mood, anxiety, personality, addictions and eating disorders. It also frequently targets specific symptoms, such as phobias, fears, sleep problems and impulsive behaviors. The new approaches incorporate a contemporary understanding that clients often need help developing tools for regulating and managing disruptive emotions. One of the "dialectics" of DBT is actually shared by many integrative approaches: simultaneously helping clients begin to recognize and accept themselves and the reality of their lives (sometimes called radical acceptance) while also working to learn new ways to manage their own feelings and behaviors. Like a wide range of psychodynamic, Buddhist and mindfulness practitioners (e.g. Bromberg, 2001; Epstein, 2004; Kohut, 1971, 1977; Nhat Hanh, 1992), these clinicians have found that acceptance itself can actually lead to change.

Although many clinicians and theorists point to the evidence that cognitive behavioral therapies are highly successful treatment techniques, some recent research (e.g. Wachtel, 2010; Wampold & Brown, 2005; Watzke et al., 2010) has questioned whether contemporary beliefs that one treatment is more effective than another for specific disorders is completely accurate (Table 4.1). For example, although panic disorders were once believed to respond best to behavioral and medical interventions, Westen and Morrison (2001) report that a mix of interventions, including psychodynamic therapy, appears to be the most beneficial in the treatment

Table 4.1 Behavioral and cognitive therapies

Type of therapy	Basic concepts	Founding theorists
Classical conditioning	Introduced concepts of learned conditioned responses	Ivan Pavlov, John Watson
Behavioral therapy	Positive/negative reinforcement of behavior	B.F. Skinner
Rational emotive behavioral therapy	Through structured activities, change distress-producing beliefs to empowering new beliefs	Albert Ellis
Cognitive behavior therapy	Identify "automatic thoughts," recognize the distortions contained in them, and work towards developing more realistic and self-empowering new thoughts	Aron Beck, David Burns
Dialectical behavioral therapy	Through behavioral and mindfulness techniques find a balance (dialectic) between acceptance and change	Marsha Linehan
Acceptance and commitment therapy	Using self-acceptance and mindfulness practices, step back from thoughts and observe and accept them without buying into them	Stephen Hayes
Mindfulness based cognitive therapy		Zindel Segal

of these disorders. These findings fit far more closely with my own anecdotal and clinical experiences over the past 30 years in the field. From this perspective, rather than focus on a particular type of therapy as more effective than another, it seems that a more useful approach is to try to determine what interventions will work best for a particular client at a specific time (see also Stolorow, 1975)—and what interventions a particular clinician is most successful at using, Such a pragmatic, integrative and realistic approach would directly counteract the concerns I have heard expressed by more than one client over the years, but most succinctly by a client who said, "If this therapy is supposed to work so well, and I'm not getting better, then either you're a lousy therapist or I'm a lousy patient."

Of course, this is exactly the conclusion one hopes a client will not draw, yet at times it is true that a therapist may not be applying techniques correctly and a particular approach may therefore be compromised. Obviously, some symptoms can take far longer to ameliorate than others. A client's goals, motivation, compliance and capacity for change can dictate the speed at which they start to see differences. In other words, someone who wants to make deep personality change in the course of therapy will need to wait longer to see results than someone who has a specific behavioral shift in mind. However, it seems to me that any client should have a sense that *something* is happening in the therapy within 2–3 months, even if it is only a minor or small modification in their mood or circumstances. When this does not happen, both therapist and client should take stock together and separately to determine either what might not be working or what they might be missing. When it seems that the particular approach that a clinician is best trained for is not going to bring about change, at least without further help from other sources, a therapist may refer a client to a professional who specialize in a technique that they believe will be helpful but that they do not practice themselves. When this occurs, both therapist and client need to agree on the way that they are going to integrate these approaches. In some cases, clients will stop seeing one therapist while working with the other. At other times, the therapists will work together as a team. In either situation, as we will discuss further in Chap. 9, both therapists will need to be sensitive to issues such as splitting and competition that can interfere with the therapeutic process, even in the best of teamwork.

Clinical Example

In the following example, all of the above difficulties emerged at different times, but because the therapists worked closely with one another, they were able not only to defuse a possibly explosive situation, but also to utilize their interactions with one another and with the client to enhance the therapeutic work.

Ms. Conrad, a primary school teacher, was in her mid-twenties when she sought help for her obsessional thoughts and compulsive, ritualistic behavior. For example, she had a morning routine of prayers, yoga and "checking" her house before she left for work. Initially a soothing way to start her day, the rituals had become so involved that she was often late for work. "I've tried getting up early to give myself more time," she said, "but I ended up adding another ritual to the routine. Instead of walking around the house three times, now I have to do it a fourth time. So I'm still late." She had been told that a combination of cognitive behavioral therapy and medication were considered the most successful techniques for the kinds of symptoms she was struggling with, and she felt lucky to have found Dr. Aikens, who was both a psychopharmacologist and a CBT practitioner. After doing a thorough psychosocial assessment and requesting that Ms. Conrad also get a complete physical checkup, Dr. Aikens started her on a low dose of the antidepressant Paxil and asked her to keep a record of some of the rituals and obsessional thoughts she had described as most problematic. He then asked her to choose one behavior that she would be willing to work on shifting. He gave her some assignments and worksheets to follow, and she eagerly began the work.

Ms. Conrad, who was charming, smart and very likeable, seemed to be trying her best to follow the routines. She filled out her daily worksheets and brought them to her therapy sessions without fail. She described her attempts to follow the routines. She did her homework. But she did not seem to be getting better. Dr. Aikens raised her Paxil, but Ms. Conrad hated how she felt on the medication. "I'm tired all the time," she said. "And I don't feel like myself." Dr. Aikens asked her to try to stay on the medication a little longer and to keep working on her homework assignments. Ms. Conrad did so, but complained that she was having difficulties concentrating. Dr. Aikens liked Ms. Conrad a great deal, but was becoming somewhat frustrated. He wondered if she was truly being compliant with her homework and with her medication. He had just decided to push her a little bit harder when she came into a session and said that she was worried that she was not doing the work the right way. "I mean, shouldn't I be feeling better?" she asked.

"I'm sure it's something I'm doing wrong," she added. "You're wonderful, and I know I could be feeling better if I would work harder." Dr. Aikens asked her how she thought she might work harder. "I don't know. I was hoping you would have some suggestions." He asked if she was doing her homework. "Oh yes," she said. "But I know you must be feeling frustrated with me." Dr. Aikens attempted to look at some of the ways in which Ms. Conrad might be avoiding the work. Like Mr. Andrews, he worked to help Ms. Conrad be clearer about her motivation to change, and at the same time he attempted to unlink her thoughts and behaviors from the patterns into which they had fallen. But nothing he did seemed to work. He consulted with a colleague who suggested that Ms. Conrad did not want to get better. He thought this might be part of the picture, but he also thought that she did want to get better at the same time. Finally, he decided that it might be useful for her to work with a psychodynamically oriented psychotherapist to try to untangle her conflict about disengaging from her symptoms. When he presented this idea to Ms. Conrad, she initially expressed concern that she had disappointed Dr. Aikens. He told her that she had not, but that he was concerned that he was not helping her. He also said that, if she was willing to do so, he would like to continue to work with her as she worked with the new therapist. He could see her visibly relax as he clarified that he was not rejecting her, but that he was seeking further help for her.

Therapist/Client Relationship

Authors who have described integrating cognitive behavioral techniques with psychodynamically-oriented ones have focused on the importance of the relationship between therapist and client (Connors, 2006; Frank, 2004, 2005; Wachtel, 1997). As we have noted earlier, research (e.g. see Freedman, Hoffenberg, Vorus, & Frosch, 1999; Norcross, 2002; Roth & Fonagy, 1996; Wampold, 2001; Wallerstein, 2000) has also indicated the importance of this relationship in any therapeutic endeavor. Dr. Aikens' training had not focused on this aspect of the work, but he recognized that he had become important to Ms. Conrad and that her apparent resistance to the work was neither a rejection of him nor a commentary on the efficacy of the treatment technique. He referred Ms. Conrad to a colleague with whom he had both consulted and worked on other cases, a woman who he knew would focus on some of the issues that might be emerging in Ms. Conrad's feelings towards himself and, possibly, over time, towards her as well.

Connors (2006, 2011) describes a two-pronged approach based on the need for "self-regulation" and "self-initiated behavior change." I think of this as the need for help with self-regulation and self-soothing in order to do whatever other work one has in mind—whether it is exploration of meaning (psychodynamic), acceptance (mindfulness), body work, motivational interviewing, harm reduction, group or family therapy, or compliance (with medication, clinic or agency rules and regulations, therapeutic goals, etc.). Wachtel (2010) integrates the relational aspects of the therapeutic interaction with specific cognitive and behavioral tasks, and Frank (2001) describes integrating understanding and exploring with behavioral techniques. Mitchell (1993) offers an example of this, noting that he often gives clients concrete "homework" assignment that they do not complete. According to him, what is most important is not the work itself, but the use of it in a psychodynamic exploration of the reasons that they failed to follow through.

I have discussed integrative work with therapists who have many different perspectives on cognitive behavioral work. Among the therapists with whom I spoke, I found that many felt that they integrated a number of other techniques and theories into their work, including psychodynamic, mind/body, and mindfulness concepts. Often psychopharmacological intervention is considered an adjunctive treatment as is working as part of a team with clients who were being seen for long term psychodynamic work as well. I also found among psychodynamic, body/mind and developmentally-oriented practitioners that behavioral techniques were often integrated into the work. It is often difficult for a clinician to tell whether the mixture of techniques is intentional or pragmatic. In fact, it is sometimes only after the fact that one realizes that one has been working behaviorally or educationally or psychodynamically at all. In my own work, I have found that offering cognitive and/or mindfulness techniques or even simple suggestions for self-soothing—such as going for a walk, listening to music, taking a bubble bath, calling a friend, watching a TV show—brings the question of managing affects into the therapeutic conversation in a concrete and manageable way. In much of the work in which psychodynamic work is integrated with behavioral techniques, the relationship is considered to be a crucial component of the work even though, as discussed above, when it comes into cognitive behavioral work it is generally considered in very specific ways.

One study (Westra, Aviram, Barnes, & Angus, 2010) found that clients often are surprised by aspects of their CBT experience. According to the study, 84 % of respondents said that they had expected more direction and less responsiveness from a therapist and were pleasantly surprised by their therapist's interest in making it a collaborative experience in which they could choose the therapy's direction rather than being told what to work on. These respondents also were pleased that their therapist was less judgmental than they had expected. In other words, clients were more comfortable with the process and learned more than they had anticipated. There was also some sense that it could be helpful to discuss the past, even though many clients were happy to focus only on the present. The majority of respondents also said that they had worked harder in therapy than they had assumed they would.

Most cognitive behavioral techniques, however, focus on helping a client become capable of doing the work him or herself. While in psychodynamic approaches, delving into the relationship with a particular therapist is considered an important part of the therapeutic process, in cognitive behavioral work the relationship is important in that it aids a client in learning new ways of thinking about his own ideas and feelings. Traditional techniques that focus on a client's distorted thoughts about therapy or his therapist can rupture the work by damaging the therapeutic alliance (Castonguay, Schut, Aikins, & Constantino, 2004). In both cases, the relationship is a tool, but the ways in which that tool is used are somewhat different. We will discuss this in more detail in Chap. 8 when we look more closely at the role of therapeutic relationships, but for the moment let us note that these different approaches each have value in an integrative practice. Sometimes it can be useful to explore some of the thoughts and feelings a client has about her therapist, but sometimes to do so can interfere with the work, even in a psychodynamically-oriented approach (see, for example, Bromberg, 2001; Kohut, 1977).

One place that these two approaches can converge is in the area of resistance. Working to build a strong therapeutic alliance, and utilizing both motivational interviewing (that is, helping clients recognize why they might want to change), acceptance (change is hard), and specific tools for making those changes, cognitive behavioral therapists work to manage this resistance without focusing on a client's history or unconscious conflicts. Resistance, or therapy interfering—behavior, such as failure to do assignments or to show up for sessions, is an important part of the process for cognitive behavioral therapists just as it is for psychodynamically-oriented therapists. When a client fails to carry out assignments or to follow through on activities or is consistently late for appointments, a psychodynamically-oriented therapist might ask questions meant to open up why the client might be behaving in this way, and a cognitive behavioral therapist might use motivational interviewing techniques to open up why the client wants to change. A DBT approach is also to highlight the behavior and then do a chain analysis, which Chapman (personal communication) calls "talking the behavior to death." This is a minute and detailed discussion of what led up to the moment—a "mini-analysis" of the events and experiences that led up to an incident. The idea, from both ACT and DBT, is that one talks the incident to the point of removing the instigating factors from the equation (see Hayes, 2004) so that a client begins to do the necessary tasks, to get to therapy on time, or to do the homework. In motivational interviewing, however, resistance is believed to be the result of a disparity between a client's current stage of change (DiClemente, 2006) and a clinician's expectation or belief in how ready that client is or "should be" to change. A clinician's task is to deal with this disparity separately from the therapeutic work—for example, when a therapist is feeling overburdened by too many client phone calls, bored or simply not invested in the process, it is the therapist's responsibility to work on those problems, perhaps by going for further training or by using some of the therapeutic tools personally.

Interestingly, although there are philosophical, theoretical and technical differences between a chain analysis and Sullivan's (1953) detailed inquiry, there are also many similarities. More importantly, many of these ideas can be integrated in order to work with different aspects of a client's needs at different times—or with different clients with similar symptom pictures but different personalities. For instance, when a client is either consistently acting out or having difficulty moving more deeply into the therapeutic work, a clinician may ask for specific details about where that client lives, what his living situation is (e.g. who else lives with him), how he gets to work, what time he has to get up in the morning to get to work on time, and what his morning rituals consist of. As I have described elsewhere, such detailed inquiry into the daily activities of someone with an eating disorder or other addictive or compulsive behavior can reveal useful data about how a client manages affects and what routines (or lack thereof) complicate her life (Barth, 1998). Kanter (2013) notes that a detailed inquiry offers a therapist an opportunity to begin to note patterns and inconsistencies that can help in the formulation of interventions and tools that will be most useful to that client. And as we have noted throughout this book, an integrative practice is a practice that attempts to match therapeutic interventions with client needs and clinician's abilities.

Chapter 5
The Body-Mind Connection

Keywords Body-mind • Alternative therapies • Mindfulness • Cognitive • Behavioral • Development • Therapeutic openness • Therapeutic curiosity • Clinical illustrations • Research • Evidence-based • Acupuncture • Yoga • Drug addiction • Headaches • Somatic complaints • Hypochondria • Defense • Couples therapy • Referrals • Teamwork

The intricate interplay between a human body and the mind that inhabits it perfectly illustrates an integrative process in action. Although at times they have been viewed as distinct and separate entities, today we consider body and mind to be mutually influencing, collaborative components of an overall whole. Physicians, mental health clinicians and clients themselves have become increasingly aware of the relationship of body and mind in both physical and psychological health and distress (e.g. Eccleston, 2001; Wolsko, Eisenberg, Davis, & Phillips, 2004). Almost two thirds of patients seeking aid for neurological distress like migraines also try "alternative and complementary medicine" (Wahbeh, Elsas, & Oken, 2008, p. 2321). Barnes, Bloom, & Nahin (2008) provide a chart (reproduced below) of the ten most common alternative treatments sought by patients. These included natural alternatives, breath work, meditation, chiropractic and osteopathic, massage, yoga and diet-based therapies, progressive relaxation, guided imagery and homeopathic treatment.

F.D. Barth, *Integrative Clinical Social Work Practice: A Contemporary Perspective*, Essential Clinical Social Work Series, DOI 10.1007/978-1-4939-0351-1_5,

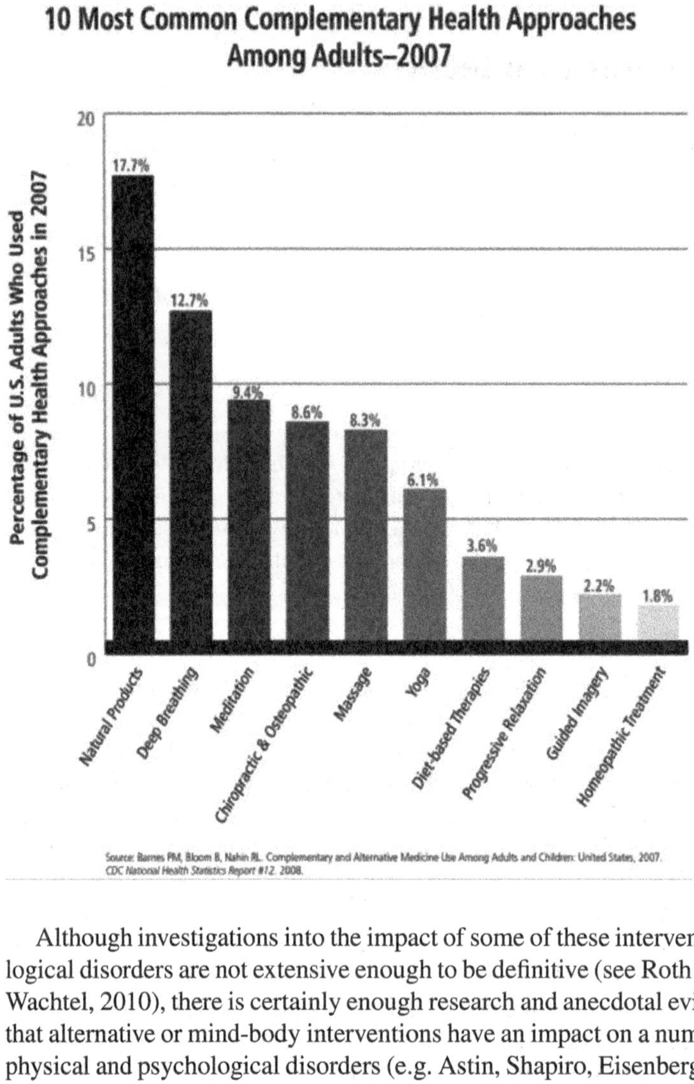

Although investigations into the impact of some of these interventions on psychological disorders are not extensive enough to be definitive (see Roth & Fonagy, 1996; Wachtel, 2010), there is certainly enough research and anecdotal evidence indicating that alternative or mind-body interventions have an impact on a number of aspects of physical and psychological disorders (e.g. Astin, Shapiro, Eisenberg, & Forys, 2003; Brown & Gerbarg, 2012; Barnes, Bloom, & Nahin, 2008; Damasio, 1999; Levine, 1997; Linehan, 1993; Rustin, 2012; Schore, 2003; Siegel, 1999) to warrant our thinking about these ideas in our clinical work. Straker (2006), for example, writes that helping clients learn to notice and listen to their bodies can be extremely helpful for suicidal clients. Stolorow's (1975) idea that self-harm can be an attempt (among other things) to make contact with the physical self has interesting implications in terms of working with this population (see also Gilligan & Machoian, 2002).

This does not mean that we need to actively engage in these alternative forms of treatment ourselves. In fact, as is true with other techniques discussed in this book, one should be trained in any intervention that one makes with any client. An integrative practice makes room for a client to explore alternative possibilities, with a clinician finding ways to be both interested in and curious about what these adjunct therapies might mean to our clients. Here is a brief example of how this can work. I was seeing a businessman in his forties for traditional psychodynamic psychotherapy. As a result of some family issues, he also began working with a DBT clinician, who taught him some mindfulness techniques. He was particularly impressed by the idea of taking a moment to pay attention to his physical experience. "I never in my life thought to simply stop and ask myself what I was feeling in my body," he told me as we discussed the experience. This man had a history of impulsivity which we had been exploring in his individual therapy. I asked him if he thought he could use the mindfulness technique he was learning in DBT in his individual work with me. Hesitant at first, he found that it was extremely useful as we opened up material that had previously been too overwhelming for him to tolerate and that had sometimes led to impulsive acts after a particularly difficult therapy session. Like many clinicians, I had long been aware of the importance of encouraging clients to pay attention to physical manifestations of emotions, but this was a reminder that sometimes clients need to be taught simply to pay attention to their physical experiences as a goal in and of itself. I would suggest that this is one of the crucial and often unarticulated components of integrating body and mind in clinical work: that is, the body is not simply a metaphor or a symbol, but is also an actual meaningful reality. Let us turn now to some ways that a clinician can think about and organize the integration of both symbol and reality of body and mind into clinical work.

It is outside the scope of this chapter to try to detail all of the body-mind therapies available today. Putting aside homeopathic and alternative medications as being outside the purview of this discussion, we will look instead at five general groupings suggested by the alternative therapies listed above: (1) breathing and relaxing techniques; (2) direct body-based intervention; (3) diet and nutrition; (4) exercise; and (5) meditation and mindfulness. There are a number of ways in which these categories overlap with one another, but taken together they provide a useful outline for exploring the integration of body and mind in clinical social work practice. Much of the evidence that we have discussed throughout this book points to the role of several key themes in any therapeutic process: affect regulation, self-awareness, supportive relationships, self-esteem and a sense of security and safety. In this chapter we will look at some ways that body-mind issues can help enhance therapeutic work with these issues.

It is my hope that the chapter will help clinicians become more comfortable discussing a variety of the links between body and mind that are not always brought into talk therapy. Referring clients for adjunct work—e.g. yoga, meditation, acupuncture, nutritional advice and so on—is already part of many clinicians' practice. In this chapter we will consider ways to make use of these experiences—to paraphrase Freud (1893–5)—to bring both body and psyche into the therapeutic conversation (p. 296). Helping clients talk about nonverbal and/or physical experiences that they may not have previously considered part of their psychological or emotional experience can be an extremely important integrative practice. For example, a clinician's encouragement for a client to exercise, get massages or even to take a warm bath to self soothe in times of physical and emotional stress underscores the link between the physical and emotional aspects of experience. Discussions not only of possible ways of utilizing such activities for self-soothing, but also of a client's sometimes surprising resistance to these suggestions can be can be an invaluable addition to any therapeutic process. In some cases these conversations can awaken old and deep connections between body and psyche. In others, new skills for self-management become quickly integrated into a client's emotional repertoire.

Another brief example, this time from my own initial foray into therapy, illustrates that a clinician doing "nothing more" than talk therapy can integrate body-mind material into the therapeutic process.

I was a recent college graduate with a low paying job. I wanted to start psychotherapy but had no idea about how to find a therapist I could afford. A new roommate offered a key not only to that door, but also to another unmet wish that I did not, at the time, realize was connected to the first. She told me about a clinic near our apartment where she was seeing a therapist, and when I expressed an interest she encouraged me to call for an appointment. When I also expressed my admiration that she was taking a ballet class, she invited me to come with her to try one out. I was quickly hooked on both experiences, and although I did each only once a week, within a few months I told my therapist that I felt like I had received a blood transfusion, like blood filled with oxygen and nutrients was flowing through my body and my brain. "It's like I can feel the tips of my fingers and toes for the first time," I told her. My therapist asked about the feelings, and we talked about many different aspects of the dance classes, including not only what we actually did in them, but also many complicated feelings (e.g. of simultaneous admiration, competition, and envy) that emerged in relation to my classmates. Psychotherapy and dance soon became entwined components of my personal and professional therapeutic development even though they were never actually physically combined (I never did dance therapy, for example).

In the years since then, I have heard comments about the interaction of psyche and bodywork from many clients. One client who began psychotherapy, meditation and yoga simultaneously told me, "I actually feel like I can see colors and hear sounds more clearly, but it's more than that. It's like I can hear my thoughts and feel my feelings more distinctly…like I'm wearing internal glasses and things that were once blurry are now distinct and sharply outlined." Although I might have wished to take full credit for this experience, I believe it would have been a false assumption on my part. It seemed to me that her sense of clarity came from opening up channels of communication between her body and her psyche, and that the talk therapy, yoga and meditation had all contributed to this process. I would suggest that this is one of the goals of any body-mind work—to open channels of communication between body, mind and psyche. There are a number of ways that this can be done. As the previous examples suggest, the work can be done by a clinician who recognizes and verbally explores links between a client's physical and psychological or emotional experiences. But with some clients, it is also helpful if a clinician is familiar with some techniques for managing body-based affects in the clinical process (for some useful examples, see Connors, 2006; cancer.org 2008, 2011; Frank, 1999; Linehan, 1993; Wachtel, 1997).

Before turning to a discussion of some of the ways that an integrative practice can bring body-mind dynamics into the clinical work, let me address one other component that is crucial to all therapy, but that stands out as particularly significant when working with body-mind issues.

Boundaries and Training

As in all therapeutic work, it is extremely important that clinicians observe professional and ethical boundaries with clients at all times (see Gabbard & Lester, 1995 for further discussion of this extremely important issue). Not only must any hands-on work be completely professional, but it must be well-thought out and thoroughly discussed with a client before it is put into practice. It might seem that a tense and frightened client would benefit from a gentle massage of neck and shoulders, for example, but the contact could be experienced as a sexual overture and/or a potential repetition of childhood abuse to which the client has no recourse except to submit. Even when clients request body work, their current psychological state and past history must be thoroughly assessed and factored into any decision to implement such work (e.g. Craige, 2013). Ongoing discussion of a client's response to the therapy is also crucial in order to determine if he is having any sort of problematic reaction to any intervention.

Again, it is important for a clinician to be thoroughly trained in any area in order to integrate it into the work. As in my own experience of spontaneously integrating experiences from dance class into my work with a traditional talk therapist, and as I further discuss in Chap. 10, an integrative approach can consist of a clinician's active incorporation of different techniques. It can also be reflected in work with a more or less structured team which, along with a clinician, addresses different aspects of a client's dynamics and/or needs. Thus a referral to a specialist in body therapies, like a referral to a psychopharmacologist, nutritionist, art therapist, DBT or ACT specialist, can be viewed as part of integrative work.

Let us turn now to some of the different types of body work that have been integrated into talk therapy over the years. The following table will provide an overview of some of the major areas of thought in this area (Table 5.1).

Before turning to the specific headings in the table, let us discuss one topic that can be seen in almost all of the categories: trauma theory.

Trauma Theory and the Body

Trauma theory looms large in any discussion of body and mind therapies and techniques. It is the one area in which body and mind are most commonly and regularly brought together in clinical work, and the recent expansion of and focus on trauma

Table 5.1 Body-mind concepts and therapies

Model	Basic concepts	Focus of theory	Theorists	Practice applications
Breathing and breath-work	Breath is the "portal" to the body-mind system (Brown & Gerbarg, 2009)	Using breathing to change open inner awareness	Brown & Gerbarg; Chapman & Linehan; Descilo, Vedamurtachar & Gerbarg, et al. Hayes; Raja; Connors; Wachtel; Ogden; Elliot	Breath counting and monitoring to relax, manage anxiety, aggression and other strong affects
Meditation and mindful-ness	Meditation opens the mind to all thoughts without judgment or criticism, mindfulness focuses the mind—both promote self-awareness and relaxation	Slowing down and becoming more accepting of self	Benson; Kabat-Zinn; Chapman & Linehan; Epstein; Hayes; Linehan; Siegel; Thich Nhat Hanh; Van der Kolk Kabat-Zinn	Meditation is used to help clients relax and become less critical of their thoughts and feelings. Mindfulness is used to help clients recognize feelings for what they are
Energy work	Various techniques for opening physical and emotional energy flow, which may be blocked because of fears, anxieties, and other causes	Releasing and rechanneling energies for healing mind and body	Alexander; Callahan & Trubo; Eden & Feinstein; Fehmi; Feldenkreis; Kabat-Zinn; Shapiro; Numerous others	QiGong, Reiki, Bilateral stimulation, Sensorimotor work, therapeutic touch, Feldenkreis, Alexander technique, Biofeedback, Acupuncture, Acupressure, Massage, Zero-balancing, lights (e.g. for depression), and a variety of other methods attempt to open blocked energy and rebalance the mind

Diet, nutrition exercise and movement	Nutrition, diet, & exercise have an important impact on mental health	Balancing physical well-being to help psychological health	Linehan, Hayes, McClintock Greenberg, Connors, Buyback, Blumenthal, Herman, Kari; Burks & Kelley; Strophe; Brown & Gerbarg, Numerous others	Some, such as DBT, theories of eating disorders, addictions, and other impulse and affect regulation disorders, and geriatric work actively integrate these ideas into the therapeutic process. Others, such as psychodynamic psychotherapies, discuss the links and encourage clients to make use of this knowledge
Physical manipulation of the body	Unexpressed Or unrecognized emotions are the cause of certain physical symptoms. The body "holds" unformulated or Unverbalized experiences		Feldenkrais; Janov; Levine; Lowen; Ogden; Reich; Rolf; Traeger; Numerous others	Alexander technique, Rolfing, Primal Scream, Traegerwork, Feldenkrais, Sensorimotor psychotherapy

theory (perhaps a sad commentary on the world in which we live) has ultimately brought body and mind work to the attention of many more clinicians. Almost all of the categories listed in the chart above have been integrated into some aspect of contemporary trauma theory. The treatment of trauma is an important specialty, one to which even a brief summary cannot do justice. Research into the most effective tools for working with a wide range of traumatic experiences is ongoing. For the purposes of this chapter, I will simply note that almost every theoretical approach to clinical work has addressed questions of trauma in some way (see also Brandell & Ringel, 2011). However, there are still ongoing controversies and questions about the best ways to address trauma (e.g. see Boulanger, 2007; Mischel, 2009; Shedler, 2010). Because research is not always definitive (see also Burks & Keeley, 1989; Carr, 2011; Gaudiano & Herbert, 2000; Roth & Fonagy, 1996), we are clearly in need of further data on the subject. Rather than try to summarize the wide range of thinking on the topic, what I will focus on in this chapter is that this is an area of clinical work in which integration, not only of body and mind but also of interventions, is recognized as paramount.

Bringing the Body into a Therapeutic Conversation

Most of us do not need research to convince us of what we have learned from experience: that diet, nutrition and exercise can have a positive impact on a number of psychological and emotional issues and disorders, ranging from depression to anxiety, to eating disorders to addictions and other disorders of affect regulation and impulse control, and from populations ranging from childhood to the elderly. There is, however, research underscoring this belief (see e.g. Babyack et al., 2000). Because these issues are also part of the popular culture, they are relatively simple to bring into almost any therapeutic conversation. Traditionally, when clinicians have addressed these issues they have had brief discussions about a client's exercise and eating habits. In more recent years, perhaps in part due to the growth of eating disorders, which may have made exploration of diet and exercise almost mandatory, clinicians have become more alert to the importance of more intensive exploration of these behaviors. Linehan (1993) offers specific suggestions of physical activities to be utilized for self-soothing, but a growing number of clinicians now integrate a discussion of how a client might begin to use exercise and food constructively in the management of psychological and emotional difficulties. What clinical knowledge adds to the mix is the understanding that following through on such commonsensical recommendations is not always as straightforward as one might expect.

This is how it worked for Mr. Nolan, who we met in Chap. 2. As his therapist, Ms. Bluen, got to know him better, she began to understand that it was extremely important to him to feel that he was in charge—at home, at work, and even in therapy. She learned that it was much more productive to ask him to explain his own thinking about himself than it was to try to tell him what she understood about him, even if she felt that she had something that might help him deepen his self-perception.

Like some of the clients described by Kohut (1971, 1977, 1984), Mr. Nolan needed her to operate as though she were an adjunct to him rather than a separate person. During one series of sessions, for example, he spoke of his difficulty getting any kind of exercise.

"I used to run," he said. "I really did enjoy it. But now I keep telling myself I'm past that. I don't need it. I don't know what that's about." Ms. Bluen knew from previous interactions with Mr. Nolan that this was not a request for her to give him her thoughts. At some point it might be useful for them to explore this dynamic, but for the moment Ms. Bluen thought it might be more productive to help him articulate his own ideas about this rather unusual idea, that he was "past that." She said, "I know you don't know, but do you have any guesses about what it might be about?" she asked.

"I know I'm a perfectionist," he replied. "I don't like to do anything if I can't do it right. And running…I used to do it really well. Now, I'll have to start from the beginning again…"

Ms. Bluen had several choices. She could have reflected back what she was hearing, that Mr. Nolan did not want to start at the beginning again. She could have asked what would make that so painful. Or she could have suggested that it might not be as painful as he was imagining. Instead of any of these, however, she chose to put what she heard as a dilemma into words. "You seem to want to run again," she said. "It sounds like it really makes you feel better, and maybe works almost as well as a drink to calm you down." He nodded and said, "Maybe better, sometimes." She continued, "But it sounds like to start at the beginning again would be so frustrating for you that it might almost make you feel like you need a drink!"

He grinned. "Bingo. That's the problem in a nutshell." He then went on to elaborate on the difficulties, again almost as though he had made the comments himself. Ms. Bluen encouraged him to talk more about how he felt when he was running, how his body felt, and what was the difference between when he was in shape and how he imagined it would be if he were to run now.

"That's interesting," he said. "My first reaction is that it wouldn't be so very different. One of the things I'm learning in here with you is that there is a process to things. That I can start in one place and gradually move to another. It makes it a little easier to tolerate that gap between what I want to do, what I think I should be doing, and what I can actually do at any given time."

He was silent for a moment and then added, "I have a kind of funny relationship with my body." Ms. Bluen remained silent, waiting for him to continue with his thought. "I don't always believe myself. I mean, sometimes, I think I don't feel so well. And then I start to think that I'm fine, I'm just making a big deal out of nothing. And then I think, 'well, but maybe it's not such a nothing.' Like when I have a headache and don't want to go to work. I'm not ever sure whether I should make myself go and work through it, or stay home and do what I've learned to do till it goes away. Which way will make it go away faster? Sometimes ignoring it is the best thing. Sometimes I'm dehydrated, and I need some quiet space and some silence, and then I'm good to go."

The Body as Container of Unarticulated or Unknown Emotional Experience: Talk Therapy, Breath Work, Energy Work, and Physical Manipulation

The idea that the emotions are influenced by unrecognized or unknown experiences within the physical self can be found in both Eastern and Western traditions. In traditional Ayurvedic practices from the Indian subcontinent, Chinese medicine, and in the work of the Greek Hippocrates, medical interventions took into account an accepted interplay and interconnectedness of people and the universe. Each links temperament, mood and health related to physical elements in the world—for example, air, earth, fire, water, wood and metal (the actual elements are different in different traditions) (NIH, 2013; Reichstein, 1998). Hippocrates believed that health, both psychological and physical, was based on the four "humors" that he considered the human manifestation of the four basic elements of the physical world being in balance (Hansell & Damour, 2008). These beliefs impacted Western treatment of emotional and physical disorders (e.g. the practice of bleeding an ill patient was derived from the theory of the humors). Ayurvedic and Chinese medicine practices have become more popular in Western cultures in recent years, although there are some serious concerns that some of the herbs used to balance the system can themselves be harmful when not properly monitored or prescribed (e.g. NIH, 2013).

An integrative approach recognizes that it is important for clients to process experience both verbally and nonverbally (see for example Connors, 2006; Frank, 1999; Hayes et al., 1999; Linehan, 1993; Greenberg, 2009; Wachtel, 1997). Meissner (2007a) makes the case that this is not a new idea even in the realm of talk therapies. He says that the body has always been and continues to be a crucial part of any psychoanalysis. Freud's ideas about drives were derived in part from his work as a neurologist and his deep belief in the subtle and often unrecognized mutual impact of body and mind (Sulloway, 1979). Not only did he believe that hysterical symptoms were the result of the mind's utilizing the body to avoid unacceptable memories and emotions, but in some of his earliest work on hysteria, Freud (1893) also described a client's body "joining" the therapeutic conversation (p. 296) when a clinician got too close to some of those intolerable feelings and thoughts. Although he was by no means the first to come to this conclusion (see also Gay, 2006, for further discussion of this phenomenon) he brought the idea to popular contemporary culture with his prolific writing, linking non-organically based physical symptoms such as blindness, lameness and an inability to feel or swallow with specific emotion-laden events. His early therapeutic work centered on bringing the unrecognized or unconscious emotions into conscious awareness by having a client talk about what had happened until it no longer remained buried in the body, leading to what his colleague Breuer dubbed "the talking cure" (Breuer, 1895).

Freud soon learned that the path from talk to symptom release was not always a straightforward one, leading to the theory of defense and resistance that has been further explored and elaborated on by numerous psychoanalytic thinkers over the years. Wilhelm Reich, one of Freud's followers, transformed these ideas into a theory of body armor which both reflects an individual's basic personality and has to be pierced through physical manipulation in order to change a client's psyche (Reich, 2013). Although Reich took these ideas to an extreme, some of his ideas may have influenced numerous body-mind theories. The idea that the body is the site of unexpressed emotion is also significant in contemporary trauma theory. Sifneos (1996) and Krystal (1988) elaborated on the concept of alexithymia, or the inability to utilize language to process emotions created during a time of trauma. Levine (1997) further explored the idea that the body "holds" memories, thoughts, and feelings outside of conscious awareness, and numerous other trauma theories continue to explore these ideas. The assumption is that these aspects of experience are not verbal and that they affect a client's behavior and overall sense of well-being. They are part of the "unthought known" (Bollas, 1989) or unformulated or dissociated thoughts and feelings (Bromberg, 2001; Stern, 1997; The Boston Change Process Study Group, 2010).

Numerous techniques have been developed in recent years to help clients who cannot speak about or use words to help remember and/or process trauma contained in the body. These range from bodily manipulation to bilateral stimulation (e.g. EMDR, EFT), and also include hypnosis, meditation, mindfulness, yoga and breathing practices. While many of these techniques may offer hope of immediate change in symptoms, some of them can also open up unexpected material and distressing reactions in vulnerable clients, which again points to the need for a clinician to be well-trained and supervised and a client thoroughly assessed before undertaking these techniques. While many clinical theories have drawn attention to previously neglected nonverbal cues as a source of significant information, it is important to recognize that both verbal and nonverbal material can sometimes be misleading.

Nonverbal communication is not necessarily an accurate reflection of unconscious or unformulated material simply because it is not expressed in words. What we perceive, hear or think we understand about another person is not always what is being felt or communicated by that person, whether by verbal or nonverbal means. For example, in recent studies of interpretation of facial expressions, scientists have found that many factors can influence a client's facial expressions, including even something as simple as how many times a person blinks in a minute, which in turn colors how others interpret those expressions. Even trained observers can draw inaccurate conclusions based on movements of the face, body and extremities (e.g. Girard et al., 2013). It is therefore extremely important that a clinician constantly utilize both verbal and nonverbal exploration to try to clarify a client's condition rather than drawing conclusions on the basis of either set of "data."

Symbolic Meaning and Body-Mind

For an integrative clinician, it can be sometimes be enough to find ways to talk and think about a client's physical reactions in relation to his psychological and emotional experiences. Let us return to Mr. Nolan for an example of how this can work:

Mr. Nolan had suffered a serious illness as a child. He and Ms. Bluen had spoken about a number of different aspects of the illness. Now, in relation to his ongoing uncertainty about how he felt, both physically and psychologically, Ms. Bluen began to explore what he had understood and known about himself during the illness, from which he had taken nearly a year to recover. "I still don't even know if I was really sick," he said. "Was I just faking it? Could I have gotten better faster? Could I have gone back to school? What was really the matter with me? Was it in my head? Or in my body?"

While it was tempting to suggest that Mr. Nolan find out the "truth" about his illness, his medical records could only offer partial assistance to the work. A traditional either/or approach is captured by the phrase "it's all in her head," the implication being that physical pain is either "purely" psychological or "purely" physical (or, as it is technically termed, "organic"). Physical symptoms can take on a life of their own (for another interesting discussion of this issue, see Grzesiak, 1994; also Aron & Anderson, 2000). An integrative clinician's task is to help a client find ways to address both the realities of any physical experience (e.g. what does it feel like, what does it do to the body?) and, not necessarily simultaneously, the realities of linked emotional and psychological experiences. Only in this dual track, as it has been called (Connors, 2006; Frank, 1999; Wachtel, 1997) can a clinician address the idea that body and mind are not really separate entities, but are mutually influenced and influencing parts of the same bio-psycho-social system that makes up human experience.

The interplay of symbolic meaning and regulation of affect through physical experience is often central to our work, although it is not always spelled out so clearly. Connors (2006) provides some excellent examples of this process, as do Frank (1999), Freis (2012), and Wachtel (1997). I have found that an integrative approach offers a clinician the opportunity to work with both aspects of this equation. In my experience, when a client is not able to engage in exploring meaning, for example, it often signifies that they do not yet have the tools for self-soothing in the face of some of overwhelming feelings. Rather than focusing on resistance to knowing or feeling, I find it useful first to focus on how a client manages painful or distressing affect. In my work with clients with eating disorders, for example, I often find myself moving back and forth between concrete discussions of specifics like using exercise, diet and other body-related tools to manage physical and emotional discomfort, and exploring some of the reasons behind both areas of discomfort. However, sometimes in the initial phases of work, the main focus will be on the physical soothing of both body and mind.

An example of how this might work in therapy can be seen with Hank, a young emergency worker who came from a long line of emergency workers. His father, uncles, cousins and siblings were all first responders of one sort or another. Hank had learned from an early age to ignore both physical and emotional pain. Heavy drinking, hardy eating, physical action and good sex were antidotes to life's problems. However, shortly after assisting a colleague who had been badly injured, Hank began to suffer from debilitating back pains. He appeared to have strained his back slightly, but there were no clear organic explanations for the severity of his pain.

Hank's physician thought he needed psychotherapy, but also knew that it was unlikely that he would follow through on a referral, since psychotherapy was not part of his culture and would probably have been viewed as a sign of inadequacy or weakness on his part. However, she had learned of an organization that was offering an integrative approach to helping first responders with physical and psychological issues. This organization offered body work, including yoga and acupuncture, along with some psychotherapy for those who might make use of it. It had been recommended by Hank's union, which made it more acceptable to Hank, as did her statement that they would help him deal with the physical symptoms. Hank actually knew of an older colleague who had been there and found it helpful, so he accepted the referral without the resistance he would have presented to a referral for talk therapy. Still, with some reluctance, Hank began to take a yoga class at the center. The teacher explained that her focus was not only on helping her often physically powerful students relax and stretch some of their muscles, but also developing a different kind of muscle strength. She also explained that some of the work they were doing could help some of their muscle-related tension. To Hank's surprise, he found that within a short time of beginning the classes he was sleeping better. "I'm not sure how that works," he told the physician who had referred him. "But it's really nice."

Similar results can also be seen in clients who are making good use of talk therapy. For example, to return to Mr. Nolan, Ms. Bluen suggested that a yoga class might be worthwhile for him. A physically active man who regularly ran for exercise and pleasure, Mr. Nolan initially responded that yoga was not his kind of activity. "I don't think it can help me," he said. Ms. Bluen said that she did not want to pressure him into it, but asked if he could talk to her a little bit about his resistance. They did not spend much time on it, but in their brief discussion Mr. Nolan described not only his reluctance to participate in something "alternative," but a lifelong distaste for engaging in any activity that he would not be good at. This dynamic was obviously an important one, which they returned to over time in relation to a variety of different issues. At one point, Mr. Nolan decided to take a yoga class as an experiment, to see if it actually helped him calm down and also to open up more of the discussion about his discomfort with new things. Not only did it turn out to be an activity that over time gave him a great sense of comfort, but the experience allowed him and his therapist to further explore his anxiety about doing anything new, opening up a lifelong fear of failing that contributed to his feelings of isolation and loneliness.

Talk Therapy for Physical Issues

Clients with physical difficulties, whatever the origins of the problems, often benefit from a combination of interventions, including when appropriate, medication, biofeedback, acupuncture, meditation, physical therapy, exercise and massage, among others. Group and individual work together are often useful as well. It is therefore important that a clinician be sensitive not only to clients like Hank, who might do better with physically oriented therapies, but also to the possibility that, as with Mr. Nolan, even talking about physically based activities can open up previously closed off areas of an individual's psychodynamics.

As I have discussed throughout this book, my use of Sullivan's (1953) concept of a "detailed inquiry" into the minute aspects of a client's daily life is part of my own integrative approach. Asking about small details such as where a client sat or stood to eat breakfast or even what color the room was painted, or who else was present and what time was it when bad news was received, can provide invaluable information about unarticulated experience. For instance, I have found that eating disorders in college students can be reflective of struggles to manage the sometimes contradictory and often confusing tasks of this developmental stage : finding a path towards independence, creating an adult identity, and simultaneously learning to be connected to others (Barth, 2003). Physical changes in the body, including both gaining and losing weight, can be symbolic, symptomatic and reflective of some of the emotional and developmental struggles in which these young people are engaged. Close attention to the details of a client's story can help a clinician determine what aspects of the difficulties to focus on at a given moment in the work. For example, Margaret, the college counselor we met in Chap. 3, has found that when she listens closely to the details of a student's daily life, she may find surprising reasons behind problematic eating. "Like one student who had grown up in a different culture and who was literally starving for her native foods, which we didn't have anywhere on campus—or even in town! I helped her make a phone call home and encouraged her parents to send care packages of food and to get other relatives to do the same. I'm not sure whether it was the food, or making her parents aware that she was feeling so fragile, or just my having understood her and being an ally. Maybe all of the above. But she started to get better."

A Damaged or Suffering Body Can Affect Psychological Well-Being

Not only does a healthy body promote a healthy mind, but a damaged or suffering body can affect psychological well-being (e.g. Greenberg, 2009) and can make it difficult for a client to heal emotionally. In my work with clients with eating disorders, for example, I have repeatedly seen evidence that starvation from both anorexia and bulimia can interfere with a client's ability to think or work productively in therapy. Similarly, in interviews with clinicians across the country, I heard repeatedly that it was crucial to take care of the physical needs of clients who were ill, dirty and/or hungry, as well of course as those who were physically debilitated by alcohol and drugs before psychological and emotional issues could be addressed. Not infrequently, as clients begin to pay attention to their physical experience, they may begin to exercise regularly and even pay better attention to their eating and sleeping habits without active guidance from a therapist. Some clinicians work directly with the body in the belief that emotional issues will begin to emerge and be worked through in the body. Meissner (2007a) writes that even when the body is not part of the conversation, it is participating in the therapeutic process, since a clinician's empathy is in part due to unarticulated and unformulated physical attunements (see also Davies, 2005; Fonagy, Gyorgy, Jurist, & Target, 2003). An integrative clinician will not assume that all physical disorders have psychological causes any more than that they are all simply physiological. Sometimes doctors can misdiagnose a physical symptom as psychosomatic, or sometimes a physiologically based illness will have emotional ramifications (Greenberg, 2009) Even a psychologically-caused physical illness can impact the body's chemistry and physiology.

Integrating body and mind can sometimes be as simple as noticing that a client is hungry, dirty, tired or "strung out." Some of the clinicians I interviewed worked in agencies that provided showers, clean clothes and food for homeless clients. Clinical work was done both with the offering of these concrete physical comforts and also in the form of talking afterwards. As one worker put it, "You can't do any kind of insight therapy with someone who is starving or exhausted. But getting food in their stomach and making sure that they get a chance to sleep on a cot in a room where they feel safe does wonders for getting the therapy going."

Conversely, many clients who one might expect to be particularly aware of their bodies are surprisingly disconnected from their physical sensations. Athletes and dancers for example, are taught to play or dance through pain rather than to view it as a signal from their bodies to protect the injured body part. Cultural focus on thinness supports a general attitude of ignoring or misreading cues about hunger, and at times our punishing work ethic leads to sleep disorders, many of which are the result of ignoring the body's need for sleep, rest and relaxation. I have worked with many athletes, dancers and other physically active individuals who come in for a session after a big competition, a marathon or weeks of intense rehearsal for a dance performance and complain of feeling irritable and unhappy. Although there are often psychological aspects of their emotional state, of course, including let-down when an event is over, conflicts about both winning and losing, and so on, there is also a simple physiological component that many of them have missed. Many of these clients are taken by surprise when I ask what they have done to repair their bodies after putting so much stress on them. They are even more surprised when I suggest that some of their emotions may be the result of the toll taken on their physical selves.

As we discuss in Chap. 6, a clinician needs to include an ongoing evaluation of every client's physical condition and relationship to his body in her thinking about that client. A surprisingly large number of clients, even those with physical concerns, come into therapy not having consulted with a physician for an extended period of time. A complete physical checkup by a qualified physician is required by many agencies and is part of my own initial expectation of all clients. Explaining that making sure that a client's physical health is taken care of is part of an initial assessment process and also introduces the idea of important and often subtle links between psychological issues and the physical self early in the therapy. The discussion often also quickly flushes out some of a client's concerns and anxieties not only about seeing a physician, but also about his body. It also provides an early opportunity for learning more about a client's exercise and diet practices, history of illness and general relationship with her body. Eventually this information will help a clinician determine what, if any, body-mind interventions might be most useful with a specific client at a given time in the therapeutic process.

Focus on Physical Health Can Also Be Resistance

Ironically, sometimes physical activities can block links between different parts of a person's self. Even healthy athletes may actually be using their bodies to shut out their feelings. In fact, exercise is an adaptive tool for managing emotions that clinicians often try to encourage clients to begin to use. But at times such behaviors are incorporated into resistance to actually experiencing important, albeit unpleasant, feelings. As we will discuss in Chap. 7, an integrative practice can be enhanced by a therapeutic team, whether formally or informally structured. In working with body and mind, nurses, doctors, psychopharmacologists, physical trainers, and a variety of professionals who teach and work with the body can become part of the therapeutic process. A clinician's task in such a situation is often to help a client integrate this varied team's input, even when it is contradictory and/or confusing.

Alexithymia

Feelings often occur without being named or thought about. Some people manage these kinds of feelings or sensations comfortably, but for others, this inability to know one's feelings in words is related to alexithymia, or the inability to use language to help process emotions (Barth, 1998, 2008; Bromberg, 2001; Krystal, 1988; McDougall, 1989; Sifneos, 1996). Some individuals who suffer from this difficulty are actually quite verbal and skilled at talking about their emotions and even explaining the historical precedents for them. Their apparent insight may give the appearance that they are able to use their often psychologically astute explanations to help them manage or regulate their feelings when this is actually not the case (Barth, 1998, 2008). It is important for a clinician to keep in mind that many verbal and intelligent clients suffer from this difficulty. Many of these clients have spent their lives disappointing others—parents, teachers, and so on—whose expectations were based on their high level of intelligence. Recognition of the presence of alexithymia can help a clinician choose appropriate interventions that reinforce a client's ego strengths and help build up areas of weakness instead of repeating these previous experiences.

This is how it worked with Anna Louise, who we met in Chaps. 2 and 3. As the therapist gently explored Anna Louise's feelings in a number of different situations, she concluded that the young woman was suffering from a very subtle form of alexithymia. Based on this conclusion, she began to work with her to develop a capacity to recognize some of her internal emotional cues. However, there were several different aspects of this work. On the one hand, they needed to work on Anna Louise's capacity to tolerate the emotions she began to contact. On the other, because Anna Louise had a history of "not living up to" her potential, her therapist needed to be sensitive to both her possible embarrassment about what she might see as a failure and her anxiety about not living up to the therapist's expectations.

For many of us, even those without alexithymia, it can be easier to make contact with physical sensations than with emotional ones. Because she thought this was probably true of Anna Louise, who had always been physically active and therefore in some ways attuned to her body (although as with many individuals with eating disorders, the attunement was not complete or even always accurate), the therapist suggested they begin with some simple physical data.

"Close your eyes," she said, "and just sit comfortably." She waited till Anna Louise seemed somewhat comfortable. "Now, let your mind's eye wander around in your body. Pay attention to any physical sensations you might have. Breathe gently while you are noticing what you are feeling physically." Because Anna Louise was not used to paying close attention to many of the communications from her body, the therapist did not want to stir up any material that might be potentially overwhelming or distressing. She wanted Anna Louise to feel comfortable about this initial foray into the realm of her physical self, and hoped she might also learn something new about herself in the process. Not wanting to arouse too much anxiety, she did not ask Anna Louise to remain with her eyes closed for more than a few minutes. "Now slowly open your eyes," she said. She had her take some counted breaths—breathing in for a count of three and out for a count of three—and then asked her to return to breathing normally.

"Can you tell me what you noticed?" she asked.

Anna Louise smiled. "I could feel my heart beating," she said.

"Excellent," said the therapist. "Tell me all about it."

Anna Louise looked at her blankly. Gently, the therapist asked, "For example, did it seem to you to be beating fast or slow?"

"Oh…I'm not sure…slow I guess…"

The gentle questioning continued for a few moments, after which the therapist suggested to Anna Louise that she try doing this exercise—closing her eyes, breathing evenly, and paying attention to some part of her body—for a few minutes every day. "Let's just see where it takes us," she said.

Integrating body and psyche can sometimes begin with nothing more complex than a simple exercise like this one. In fact, Brown and Gerbarg (2012) call the breath the "portal" to the mind-body system. They are among a number of body-mind synthesizers who offer readers techniques for breath counting. They also describe some of the obstacles that can interfere with a client's use of these techniques. Clinicians also often feel uncomfortable bringing breath work into other forms of therapy. DBT and ACT incorporate some breathing and mindfulness tools into the work almost as a matter of course, but many psychodynamically-oriented therapists worry that it will interfere with the opening up of transference and other unconscious dynamics. In my experience the opposite is often true. For Anna Louise, for instance, the breath work opened the door to a discussion of her dependence on her therapist and her fear that her therapist would eventually tell her that she was finished. "I'll have to leave. I'll be on my own. I won't know how to function without you."

As her therapist sensitively explored these ideas, Anna Louise began to sob and was once again unable to catch her breath. The therapist asked if it would be helpful to do the breathing exercise again. Anna Louise nodded. They went through the steps again. When Anna Louise was feeling more stable, the therapist asked if she could stand to think about other times in her life when she had felt so destabilized. Anna Marie was hesitant, but said, "If you'll help me when I get frightened. Maybe we could stop and do the exercise again each time?" The therapist agreed, and for months afterwards they gently probed and discussed memories and fears. At one point in the process, Anna Louise said, "You know what's incredible. I've started doing this myself sometimes! I got really upset the other day and realized that I could stop and breathe. And I did. And I felt much better!!!"

She then looked worried. "This doesn't mean I have to stop therapy, does it?" Her therapist replied, "Not at all. It just means that you're starting to take in some of the work we're doing and making it your own. That's terrific, but I think there are other things you'd like to work on, right?" Anna Louise nodded. "So we'll keep working on them," the therapist said.

A number of clinicians I interviewed in the process of writing this book told me that they use some of these techniques in their work with acting out, impulsive and sometimes cognitively impaired clients. They shared stories of clients who had historically become involved in physical fights and were able to "check" themselves and interrupt their own impulsive action by using breathing and body awareness techniques they had learned from therapy. One therapist told me that she saw a young man start counting his breaths with his fingers in a situation that would previously have devolved into a fight. "And when he stopped counting, he turned around and walked away!" she said. Another, whose client reported a similar situation, asked him if he could explain what had felt different in this case. He replied that he could not say, but that it was fun. He had never felt so powerful before.

Research has shown that talk therapy changes the brain (see Busch & Sandberg, 2007; Rustin, 2012; Schore, 2003) which in turn changes the self. Similarly, systems theory tells us that changes in behavior can impact the system in which a client lives (see Gitterman & Germain, 2008) which in turn reinforces the alterations in activity. Yet clients and clinicians often resist doing the work that leads to these changes. I have often found that clients reject my offer to teach them a short breathing exercise. When this happens, I try to respect their refusal while also asking if they can talk about what makes them uncomfortable about my suggestion. Exploring these obstacles can be extremely useful, providing surprising details about a client's internal world. One client, for example, told me she felt too vulnerable when she closed her eyes and followed my instructions. Like Anna Louise, this interchange opened up her fears of being dependent and abandoned. While exploration of the material can sometimes remove the resistance, it is important for a clinician to accept a client's reluctance. In another case, a young man never did a breathing exercise I suggested, but our exploration of his discomfort opened up some important previously unarticulated areas of his struggles to manage his feelings in the presence of others. Sometime later, he told me that after our discussion he decided to take some classes in meditation, which he found very soothing and ultimately extremely helpful in dealing with his anxiety. Even though he had not wanted to do any breath work with me, he told me that the suggestion was what had inspired him to look into meditation.

Conclusion

An integrative practice is a balancing practice. One pays attention to different aspects of any client's experience and attempts to balance different needs with different interventions at different times. For example, there is evidence that psychiatric medications work better when a client is also in talk therapy (Busch & Sandberg, 2007), but sometimes resistance to one or the other of these interventions means that a clinician cannot integrate them. At these times, a clinician must decide whether to insist (e.g. if there is danger to a client or to others because he is refusing to take medication), or to work with the resistance in hopes of either removing obstacles to the integrative work or reducing the problem without medication. Similarly, a psychiatrist with whom I often work closely has a policy that all patients on medication must also be in talk therapy. When a client is unwilling to do so, this psychiatrist sometimes works with them on understanding their reluctance, or, if they have been in therapy for a long period of time and the work seems to have reached an appropriate conclusion, he will continue with medication alone. Thus his policy is integrative and also flexible, depending on the needs and dynamics of specific patients.

In conclusion, another aim of an integrative approach is to find ways to think and talk about the interplay of affective and physical experiences (see Anderson, 1998; Greenberg, 2009). This helps clients integrate into a whole (albeit not always smoothly functioning) system, rather than disconnected part-selves.

Chapter 6
Making Assessments and Choosing Interventions

Keywords Mental status exam • MSE • Evaluations • Assessments • Integrative tools • Multiple perspectives • Detailed inquiry • Ongoing process • Cognitive • Behavioral • Development • Clinical illustrations • Research • Integrative social work • Evidence-based • Acupuncture • Yoga • Drug addiction • Headaches • Somatic complaints • Hypochondria • Defense • Referrals • Teamwork

In order to decide how to best help a client make constructive change, a clinician must first understand not only the problems that client presents for help, but also what has created those problems, what clinical interventions can be most effective, and what kind of work a client is actually capable of engaging in. From an integrative perspective this means understanding something about a client's developmental needs and level of functioning, cognitive capacities, and self-awareness, as well as his external support system. One tool which has traditionally been utilized for making an initial assessment of a client's psychological state is the Mental Status Exam (MSE). Although not described as integrative, by asking for information about a variety of different aspects of a client or potential client's current and past psychological, social, cognitive and developmental functioning, this exam incorporates two keys to integrative work: detailed inquiry and an understanding of process. It can be given both formally, as is often required in an agency setting, or informally, as may be the case in private practice when a client details reasons for seeking professional help at that time. Some of the questions are not meant to be asked directly, but are general guidelines for clinicians as they listen to and observe a new client—for example, a clinician can note how clients hold themselves as they walk into the consulting room, whether or not they make eye contact, their general physical appearance and condition, and their initial social skills. Information about a client's history and environmental support system (e.g. family, friends, school, work, and living situation) is sometimes taken separately, as part of a social history. From an integrative perspective, this information as well as data about medical conditions and previous psychiatric interventions is part of a thorough initial assessment.

F.D. Barth, *Integrative Clinical Social Work Practice: A Contemporary Perspective*, Essential Clinical Social Work Series, DOI 10.1007/978-1-4939-0351-1_6,

It is important to remember that assessments require ongoing work on the part of a clinician. In my opinion, the central issues of a client's psyche are seldom revealed in a single interview. Every assessment is silently influenced by a number of other factors, not all of which are directly related to a client's presentation or needs. A clinician's experience and personal and professional biases, the setting in which the interview is done, and the treatments available at that setting are all factors in any assessment. The following is a somewhat extreme example of what can happen when an assessment is based on a client's appearance, intelligence and description of her needs:

Laurie, a young dancer, went into therapy for help with her eating disorder. She liked her therapist, Mrs. Herman, but she was concerned that because she was older and traditionally-oriented, the therapist would not quite "get" a performer with a cutting edge modern dance company. Mrs. Herman was kind and empathic, but in many ways the polar opposite of Laurie, whose "edgy" clothes, spiked hair, piercings in various parts of her face and body, and tattoos were open communications of her very different attitude towards life. Laurie did not take drugs, but deciding that her problem was "an addiction to dieting," she went to a drug treatment center to see if they could help her.

An inexperienced intake worker accepted Laurie without finding out exactly what disorder she was concerned about. This mistake could have been rectified by some simple questions about her symptoms, her history and her specific hopes about what therapy might do for her. Only when she was in her first group session did it become clear that she was not using drugs or alcohol and that her addiction was in many ways significantly different from those of other group members. The treatment team's creative response was to help her to integrate the work she was doing with her individual, psychodynamically-oriented psychotherapist with their treatment approach, which included cognitive behavioral, motivational and peer group work. Although some of the peer-counseling and confrontational group sessions were distressing to Laurie, her overall sense was of being understood and of having her needs and wishes recognized and reflected by the staff and other group members.

Many MSE protocols integrate a social as well as a medical and psychological history (see, for example, Lukas, 1993; Martin, 1990; Waldinger & Jacobson, 2001) and therefore are almost automatically part of an integrative process. Martin (1990), whose list of factors to be included in a MSE can be found below, calls the mental status examination "a structured assessment of the patient's behavioral and cognitive functioning" (Martin, 1990, p. 924). He includes factors such as a client's physical appearance and behavior, degree of attentiveness, motor and speech activity, mood, affect, ability to speak of his thoughts and perceptions, his attitude toward the examiner and his insight into his problems. Martin also considers an examiner's reaction to a client to be an important source of information about that client's current mental functioning.

Because there is much data to be gathered, therapy often begins before an assessment is completed. As the work progresses, further information can be utilized to help fine tune interventions to a client's needs. Even in long-term psychotherapy, ongoing evaluations of a client's mental status and social functioning can help both clinician and client recognize where therapy is helping and where changes in therapeutic approach might be useful. However, the integrative approach begins the moment a client asks for help or is referred for assistance, whether by an authority, an agency or another individual. Clinicians immediately begin to assess both the specific request and that client's capacity to utilize the particular treatment requested. Putting together a rich, detailed picture of a client's condition, symptoms, and strengths helps clarify interventions that make sense for that specific individual at that point in time.

Following is a table of Martin's list of factors to be considered in a Mental Status Examination, which we will then discuss as guidelines for an integrative perspective (Table 6.1).

There are a number of thorough and detailed discussions of the elements of the MSE (e.g. Lukas, 1993; Martin, 1990; Waldinger & Jacobson, 2001). It is important to remember, however, that the MSE is an instrument, not a set of hard and fast rules. In this chapter we will look at how these concepts can be understood from the perspective of the four categories of integrative work. Some key concepts from each category can help a clinician begin to think about the elements of an MSE in an integrative process. We will look at each of these categories in more detail in later chapters (although readers are welcome to turn now to those four chapters and then to return to this one, or to consider returning to the discussion of assessment after having completed the other chapters). The following is a brief outline of concepts to be considered under each integrative heading, and a list of questions a clinician might ask from each perspective.

- A *psychodynamic perspective* alerts one to manifest and latent material. Manifest material is that which we know and can talk about. In a dream, for example, manifest material is what we remember about that dream when we wake up. Latent content is material that is hidden from our conscious awareness,

Table 6.1 Factors to be considered in mental status examination

Level of consciousness
Appearance and general behavior
Speech and motor activity
Affect and mood
Thought and perception
Attitude and insight
Cognitive abilities
Attention
Language
Memory
Constructional ability and praxis
Abstract reasoning
Examiner's reaction to the patient

Martin (1990, p. 924)

often containing psychological meaning that we are either unaware of or uncomfortable knowing. In a dream, it is the symbolic meaning of the dream's manifest, or known, content.

- A *cognitive-behavioral perspective* alerts a clinician to a client's potential capacity to modify behavior, to carry out instructions, and to delay impulse gratification long enough to do the work that will lead to behavioral and cognitive change. This framework is less interested in hidden meaning and more interested in motivating a client to carry out specific behavioral tasks.
- A *developmental model* is useful for both psychodynamic and behavioral interventions, in that it provides information about a client's current stage of psychological, emotional, cognitive and behavioral development. An assessment will also include information about a client's history, his highest level of developmental achievement, and experiences in his life that may have enhanced and/or interfered with his ability to move through the developmental stages leading to psychological and emotional health.
- *Body-mind models* pay close attention to the interplay between the physical and the psychological, emotional, cognitive and developmental aspects of an individual's life and functioning. For example, someone who is suffering from a debilitating physical illness or from a psychological disorder with physical consequences, such as an eating disorder or drug or alcohol addiction, may have difficulties accessing her potential developmental and cognitive skills, despite high levels of achievement and apparent capacities.

The following chart provides a simple list of questions a clinician might ask herself while making an assessment that includes all four of these perspectives (Table 6.2):

As will become clear, there is a certain amount of overlap in the elements, which an integrative approach takes into account. Because almost any form of categorization is, to some extent, both arbitrary and individual, readers may find themselves looking at some of these concepts from a different perspective. Indeed, to do so is not only desirable, but also part of an integrative process in which a therapist works to understand a client's dynamics. Our point of view is part of what helps each clinician determine what intervention might be most useful to a particular client in that situation and with that therapist. An integrative perspective recognizes also that these choices will be influenced by the policies and expectations of the institution or agency in which client and clinician are working and by the specific relationship developed within a particular therapeutic dyad and by the interactions that emerge between a specific client and clinician. Other factors, for example the gender, age

Table 6.2 Questions to ask from each of the four integrative perspectives

Psychodynamic: What is the underlying meaning of the behaviors, symptoms, feelings and thoughts?
Cognitive-structural: What thoughts and feelings are contributing to these behaviors or symptoms?
Developmental: What developmental issues are expressed in these behaviors, thoughts and feelings?
Body-mind: What are the links between physical and psychological symptom and behaviors?

and background of both participants, a therapist's training, experience and skill in different techniques, and a client's immediate need and capacity to experiment and/or tolerate uncertainty, as we will see, also play a role and must be taken into account in the assessment process.

A thorough assessment of a client's current and past psychological, social, physical and general functioning can be especially important to a clinician trying to choose from a variety of possible interventions for a specific client. An integrative assessment begins with the first contact with a client—a voice on the phone, a new face in the agency's waiting room, even an initial glance at a prospective client's folder. A clinician takes in and begins processing information almost without conscious thought—as in any social interaction with another person. Concrete and subjective information about a client's appearance—sex, age, race, and ethnic background, physical condition (e.g. under- or overweight, malnourished, sleep deprived, physically agitated, calm, etc.), hygiene and grooming, clothing (whether or not clothing is appropriate for the weather and for client's age and situation)—which is often registered automatically, contains important details for both initial and ongoing assessments. Is there good eye contact? Is affect, or expression of emotion, appropriate and consistent with what a client is talking about? It is extremely important to remember that assessment is a process. An initial evaluation tells a clinician a number of things, but what it does not reveal is how a client will appear on another day or at another time. Since assessment is an ongoing process as a client changes over time in the course of therapy, it is important to continue to integrate these spontaneous observations into a conscious and purposeful assessment of any client, whether it is the first or the hundredth meeting.

Despite the technical language, many of the concepts listed in both of these tables are already part of every clinician's day to day, automatic way of participating in any interactive situation. Even integrating the different perspectives into an initial assessment is part of our day-to-day vocabulary. Therefore a formal evaluation of a client from an integrative point of view is less complex than it may seem at first. For example, when I was recently introduced to a well-dressed young woman at a professional gathering, I was surprised and curious when we shook hands and I felt her rough, callused palms. Without even noticing what I was doing, I found myself doing a mental search for an activity that might cause such a texture. I wondered if she was a farmer, but discarded that idea, based on knowledge of where she lived—a large urban area—and her city style of dress (revealing an unrecognized preconception about farmers and their style. If she had been a client, I would have wanted to explored this response in order to see what impact it could have on the work.). I thought she might be a sculptor or potter, but again discarded the idea based on initial impressions. Such informally gathered data is an automatic part of the initial phase of any social or professional interaction, but a clinician needs to pay close attention to his or her personal and cultural biases which, if unexplored, can lead to unconscious parallels to "racial-profiling," in which spontaneous judgments about an individual's criminal intentions are based on such physical characteristics as skin color and apparent racial features (Gabbidon, 2003).

We will return to this issue when we discuss a clinician's response to a client in the Mental Status Exam. For the moment, however, let us turn to the table at the beginning of this discussion. Many aspects of a mental status exam can be evaluated at least in part through careful observation and attentive listening on a clinician's part. For example, level of consciousness (whether a client is awake or not, and how alert and aware of his surroundings he is), appearance and general behavior, speech and motor activity (how clear, organized and appropriate is his speech, and how well is his movement coordinated, and how comfortable does he feel in his body) can be initially assessed as a client walks into a room, responds to a clinician's greetings, and sits down in an appropriate chair. A clinician will almost spontaneously ask herself questions from each of the four categories while observing this early behavior, as I did with my colleague in the example I have just described.

For example, Lily was 10 years old when she was referred by her school for an assessment of possible sexual abuse. A normally quiet, well-behaved and unremarkable child, she had recently begun acting out in class and on the playground. Of particular concern were repeated demands that boys from her class kiss her on the lips and put their hands on her breasts. The referring guidance counselor had already begun the evaluation process by making the assumption that these behaviors had underlying meaning and wondering if they were signs of sexual abuse. Mrs. Warren, the intake worker, observed that Lily was a small but physically developed girl, with obvious breasts and hips. At the interview her thick hair was pulled back into a tight, uncomfortable looking pony tail and her clothes were noticeably too small and tight, as though no one had noticed that she was growing. Mrs. Warren asked herself if the clothing and hairstyle had meaning—for example, were they signs of neglect, poverty, a mother's dislike of her daughter, and/or a wish to simultaneously hide and reveal her daughter's sexuality. Mrs. Warren knew from years of experience that her evaluation of Lily would need to include Lily's mother and possibly other important people in her life, taking into account environmental and relational aspects of Lily's situation even as she began to observe and process the details of her appearance and behavior in the consulting room.

After making Lily and her mother as comfortable as possible, she asked what they understood about why they had been sent to her. She also asked how they felt about the referral. Listening carefully to their answers helped her deepen her initial ideas about what thoughts and feelings might have been behind Lily's recent behaviors. Lily's mother commented that she had a new boyfriend and that Lily had walked in on them having sex shortly before she began acting out at school. Mrs. Warren accepted the manifest, or concrete explanation of Lily's sexual acting out, but remained curious about how and why this experience might have led to these behaviors. As she continued to ask gentle questions and listened to both Lily's and her mother's descriptions of the new boyfriend, she was also taking note of how they spoke, how they interacted with her and with one another and how well they explained their ideas and thoughts. This information helped her begin to have an idea of the psycho-social developmental issues they were each dealing with as well as the underlying meanings and the thoughts that led to the activities that had created problems for Lily. She was also paying close attention to any information that might give her some sense of both mother's and daughter's relationships with their own and one another's bodies, which could both inform her understanding in each of the other areas and also help her develop an appropriate plan for intervention.

This approach is derived in part from Sullivan's (1953) concept of "detailed inquiry," which we have been discussing throughout this book. Sullivan believed that we can never actually get into another person's mind and "know" what they experience, but by asking questions about the concrete details of an experience, the "who said what to whom" (see Mitchell, 1999), we can learn what an individual thinks and feels about different aspects of his life. Through this in-depth exploration of the obvious, a clinician can gradually begin to put together answers to each of the four questions listed in the table above. It is important to keep in mind, of course, that beginning to build a working alliance with a client is often as important to an assessment as is getting all of the details. An effective detailed inquiry requires that a client trust a clinician, and genuine trust only develops over time.

While conducting an initial interview, a clinician is also listening carefully to information about other aspects of a client's mental status. For example, mood can be viewed as the feeling a person has most of the time, and affect as the way a person shows the feelings (see Lukas, 1993, for further discussion of this distinction). Inappropriate affect involves a dissonance between a client's expression of feelings and what he or she is talking about, as when a client laughs while telling a sad story. Lily's silly grin while speaking to Mrs. Warren appeared to be an expression of inappropriate affect. Such behavior can represent any number of issues, ranging from serious emotional problems to nervousness or anxiety at a given moment. Most practitioners conducting MSE's automatically take an integrative approach, recognizing that both affect and mood can be affected by external and internal circumstances, and that an initial interview only provides a brief snapshot of a client's full emotional state.

Martin (1990) tells us that it is extremely difficult to assess a potential thought disorder. Because experience is one of the most useful tools in such evaluations, when one suspects a thought disorder is present it can be extremely important to consult with and perhaps have a client seen by a more experienced colleague. Seeking such counsel from others is not a sign of weakness. Conversely, it reflects a genuine capacity for this very difficult work. Disordered thinking, which may range from overt hallucinations and paranoia to severe confusion and disorientation, can signal the existence of severe psychiatric disorders such as schizophrenia and bi-polar disorders. Because the signals that a client is suffering from psychotic thinking can be subtle, it is not unusual for a clinician to miss them. The setting in which a clinician works may also influence his ability to recognize signs of disordered thinking. For example, in a clinic that treats mainly overweight women struggling to control compulsive eating behavior, a thin woman's complaints about her body weight may be seen as neurotic, but not seriously disturbed. The delusional nature of her thoughts may be missed because of her high intelligence, her high level of functioning and her articulate descriptions of her psychological state. A clinician with more familiarity with anorexia, however, will know to look more carefully for body dysmorphia and starvation-induced psychosis. The interviewer will be on the alert for signs of such thinking, paying attention to symptoms of psychotic thinking as they discuss the need for weight gain, and gradually attempting to determine whether such thoughts are secondary to the anorexia or symptoms of a primary psychosis.

Because no clinician can be an expert on every diagnosis, consultation with other professionals and the development of a treatment team is an extremely important part of integrative work. The topic of teamwork is one that we will return to as we discuss interventions, as it has important implications for any integrative work. It can also be helpful to distinguish between process, which can be viewed as *how* a person thinks, and content, which is what a person thinks *about* (again, see Lukas, 1993, for elaboration of this difference). Thinking in these terms helps an integrative clinician understand another aspect of the complex mix of issues that can be creating problematic behaviors and symptoms that lead a client into a clinician's office.

An important goal of the initial interview is arriving at an empathic understanding of how the patient feels. When the clinician listens carefully and then communicates an appreciation of the patient's worries and concerns, the patient gains a sense of being understood. This sense of being understood is perhaps the bedrock of all subsequent treatment, and allows the clinician to initiate a relationship in which an alliance for treatment can be established.

Medical history and psychological reports, work history and family history are all extremely important in helping tease out what a client needs and what services and interventions would be most useful. A history of previous therapeutic experiences can also help a clinician determine what may be most useful in the current situation. For example, if a client has had a good experience with group therapy, but did not like individual sessions, it may be preferable to start them in a therapeutic group. Similarly, if someone has been in a rehabilitation setting for alcohol or drug use several times in the past and is currently being referred for the same problems, it can be extremely useful to do an extensive exploration of what helped and what did not in the previous settings prior to making a decision about what form of work to offer the client this time.

Let us turn now to a key element in the evaluation process: assessing a clinician's reactions to a client.

Clinician's Reactions to Client

As I have mentioned in earlier chapters, studies have found that the quality of a therapeutic experience can be a better predictor of a successful therapy than almost any other criterion (see e.g. Connors, 2006; Couch, 1999; Farmer, 2009; Roth & Fonagy, 1996; Wachtel, 1997; Wampold, 2001). What is important for this discussion is that this finding does not mean that a therapist and a client have to become best friends—or even to like one another. Salter discovered many years ago, for instance, that a good attachment object is not necessarily warm and friendly or even obviously loving (Main, 1999). A good clinician is not a buddy. Changing habitual patterns of behavior and ingrained beliefs and attitudes is hard work, no matter what technique is utilized. From an integrative perspective, the therapeutic relationship can be seen as the scaffolding which supports the therapeutic process, or what Winnicott (1965) calls a holding environment that supports a client as he engages in the difficult task of changing.

To this end, the initial interview is not just for the purpose of evaluation, but can also help set the groundwork for a positive relationship with both a clinician and a clinic or agency. However, at the same time that we are working to both engage a client and make a preliminary evaluation of their current functioning and needs, a clinician will be paying attention to our own reactions to that client. Originally called "countertransference" by Freud (1914), such reactions were once viewed as the result of a patient's influence on a physician's unconscious. Freud and his followers saw these reactions as the result of an analyst's unresolved psychological issues and believed that they were problematic, because they interfered with an analyst's ability to be objective about an analysand's problems. Beginning with Jung (see Samuels, 1985) and Racker (1957) countertransference was viewed as having some positive components, including the possibility that it might actually help an analyst begin to understand something about an analysand's unconscious process.

While some analysts (e.g. Langs, 1981) took this concept to the extreme of suggesting that every reaction an analyst has is caused by an analysand and therefore information about the analysand's dynamics, most contemporary analysts agree that analysts have their own dynamics that must be understood in order to sort out what is happening in the interactive space. Contemporary psychoanalysts generally believe that therapy is an interactive process in which both parties play a significant role (see, for example, Davies, 2002; Mitchell, 1999). These theorists have looked for inroads to make use of this potentially rich interactive dynamic. Our reactions may therefore reflect something about ourselves and also about a client (see Feiner & Epstein, 1993; McWilliams, 2004, for extremely useful discussions of this subject). The process of separating one's personal feelings from information about a client is one of the reasons it is extremely important for a clinician to undergo a personal psychotherapy.

Clinicians learn, over time, to ask themselves questions about how they are feeling in the room with a client, whether or not they are following what the client is telling them or are feeling confused and disorganized, and whether their own mood has shifted in some way during the course of the interview. These and other internal communications frequently capture something significant about a client. An integrative approach requires that a therapist be alert to her or his own dynamics, as well as to unspoken or unacknowledged prejudices and cultural and religious biases that may color how a client's presentation and/or issues are perceived and assessed (see, for example, Burch, 1993; Campbell & Morrison, 2007; Ganzer and Ornstein, 2002).

Let us return to Laurie, who we discussed earlier in this chapter. Interestingly, she was able to use the support of Mrs. Herman, who turned out to be far less conservative in her approach than Laurie had thought, to explore some of the issues that arose in the drug treatment community. It turned out that many of these experiences paralleled some of her conflicts and struggles with friends and family in "the real world." Interestingly, not only Laurie, but everyone involved in her treatment found themselves reconsidering an important part of the assessment process. As she put it one day in a session with Mrs. Herman, "I didn't turn out to be who they thought I was when they took me into the drug treatment program. And you didn't turn out to be who I thought you were. I guess we're all learning that it's really true that you can't judge a book by its cover..."

Assessment of Violence

It would be irresponsible not to discuss the potential for client violence in a chapter on assessment. Because aggressive and violent clients can be extremely difficult and in need of careful management, anyone working with potentially violent and/or aggressive clients needs to be specifically trained to deal with this population. Inexperienced clinicians sometimes feel badly about not being comfortable with certain clients, yet their discomfort may very well be a communication that there is something happening which they are not equipped to handle. This is not a sign of incompetence. In fact, asking for help when one is unsure about how to manage a difficult client is part of the teamwork approach that we will discuss in Chap. 10. A team, as we will consider in that chapter, may be made up of only two people: a clinician and his supervisor, for example. But asking for help is crucial not only to assessments but also to ongoing work. Here is an example:

For example, Margaret, the college counselor whose work I described in earlier chapters, sometimes has to assess students at a variety of levels of psychological functioning. Peter was a brilliant student who had been hospitalized for paranoid ideation and violent fantasies at the beginning of the winter semester. He had been given a leave of absence and was now requesting that he be allowed to return for summer school. His treatment team had been in close contact with Margaret and school officials and reported that he was doing better, but that he was still somewhat volatile and that they were not sure that he was being compliant with medication. Margaret requested that his parents come with him to the interview, but even with them present he seemed anxious and somewhat disorganized in his thought processes. Suddenly he started speaking in an increasingly loud voice, and then simply stopped talking and looked pensive. Margaret was concerned, but as an experienced clinician, she was able to help him calm down, speaking quietly and firmly with him about what she thought might be going on with him. When she told him that she needed to make sure that he was taking his medication and following through on all of his therapy, however, he became more agitated.

It turned out that he was hallucinating while Margaret was talking and had stopped shouting in order to listen to an "order" from one of the voices he was hearing. Minutes later, he stood up, shouted obscenities and threw his chair across the room.

Margaret had prepared for this possibility by arranging to have a campus security guard wait outside her office during the interview. When he heard Peter's raised voice he quietly came into the room and asked if Margaret needed him. She turned to Peter and his parents and said that she had needed to call for backup help because of Peter's actions. The security guard stayed with them until an ambulance arrived to take Peter back to the hospital. Although Peter continued to speak to himself, he remained calm in the presence of the large guard.

When the paramedics arrived, Margaret told Peter that she hoped that he would start taking his medication regularly. "We want you to be able to come back to school," she said. "But we want to be sure that it will be a good experience for you. You need to be as healthy as you possibly can be." Peter was mumbling to himself and she doubted that he had taken in what she said. His mother was crying. Margaret said, "Please call me and let me know what happens. And let's talk about what the next steps should be."

Newhill (2004) offers an extremely useful perspective on violent clients in clinical settings. Providing a number of strategies and ideas about how to assess and work with potentially violent clients, she also encourages agencies where such clients are treated to provide their staff with ongoing training in risk management and assessment. She says that only when such agencies both acknowledge client violence as a concern and provide a safe workplace for staff, can clinicians actively provide help to these individuals.

Assessment of Strengths

Clinical assessments often focus on what is wrong in a client's life, however, from an integrative perspective, clients strengths can sometimes be even more important than their weaknesses. Theories that focus on resilience recognize the importance of a client's strengths, which may not always be evident in an initial assessment (see, for example, Gitterman, in press). Once strengths have been recognized and noted, it is also important to assess how best to make use of them in the therapeutic work (see Cowger, 1994; Martin, 1990). Cowger (1994) writes that looking at a client's strengths reinforces feelings of competence and agency. Paradoxically, recognizing a client's competence can sometimes interfere with a clinician's ability to identify a client's vulnerabilities. To see how this can work, let us return to Ms. Conrad, who we met in Chap. 4.

In her late twenties, Ms. Conrad had begun working with Dr. Aikens for problems with obsessional thoughts and ritualistic behaviors. Dr. Aikens had become frustrated with Ms. Conrad's difficulty in following through on her assignments with him. When he referred her to a psychodynamically-oriented clinician to work on the problems that might be causing her to resist the work, he made it clear to her that he was not rejecting her and that in fact he would like to continue to work with her if she wanted to. He also told her that he would be willing to speak with the new therapist. When the other clinician did call, Dr. Aikens was surprised when she asked if he really was willing to continue to work with Ms. Conrad. When he said that he was definitely happy to continue with Ms. Conrad, but he felt that he was not getting through to her, the clinician said, "I think you've gotten through to her. She's very attached to you. But I have a hunch that her obvious strengths have made you expect more from her than she is actually able to do right now. I think that may be true in her life in general. I'm wondering if you would be able to keep working with her, and to help her start with smaller steps, smaller goals that she actually could accomplish."

Dr. Aikens realized that Ms. Conrad's competence had indeed hidden some of her vulnerabilities from him. Re-visiting her history and her symptoms, he realized that he had been expecting her to accomplish more than she actually could. He agreed with the other clinician that this might be true in other aspects of her daily life. Teaching her to break large goals into smaller, more easily achieved tasks would probably be very useful for her and might actually help with some of her symptoms. He knew that obsessive-compulsive symptoms were some of the most difficult to treat (Jakubovski et al., 2011) and wondered if he had actually overestimated not only Ms. Conrad's abilities, but also his own.

In his next meeting with Ms. Conrad, Dr. Aikens shared with her that he thought they might want to start with some smaller goals. She was distraught. "I've failed," she said with tears in her eyes. He tried to reassure her that she had not failed at all, but explained that they were simply working on things a little differently. "I'm so sorry," she said. "I'm making your work so hard."

Dr. Aikens suggested that her reaction was probably an example of one of the things that fed into her symptoms. "You're going from 0 to 60 miles an hour in nanno-seconds," he said. "Let's see if we can break this down into smaller increments. You are assuming that you have failed because I want to start with smaller goals. Maybe the problem is that you feel disappointed and you don't know how to manage that feeling?"

Ms. Conrad nodded and added, "Yes, and I feel like I've disappointed you."

Although in other circumstances Dr. Aiken might not have addressed this statement directly, not wanting to distract them from the work at hand, he decided in this situation to ask Ms. Conrad to talk about her thought that she had disappointed him. Encouraging her to mentalize (Bateman & Fonagy, 2004), he hoped to help her begin to find words for some of her own confused and distressing feelings when she disappointed someone and when she was disappointed herself. Becoming more comfortable talking about these feelings would be a step towards helping her learn to manage them with a variety of tools other than the OCD rituals that had been driving her life. At the same time, he did not want to let her get so caught up in the feelings that she did not take the next step towards managing them. After encouraging her to talk about these thoughts for a few minutes, he then suggested they try one of the exercises they had been working on. She had, he said, just been exposed to one of the experiences that he thought worked as a trigger—the experience of disappointment in herself and fear that she had disappointed someone else. Now he suggested they try one of the cognitive behavioral techniques they had tried before. Ms. Conrad took a deep breath and nodded. As they went through the exercise, Dr. Aikens had a sense that for the first time in their work together, she was actually taking in the ideas he was trying to teach her.

Conclusion

In an integrative practice, assessment is an active, ongoing process that is part of every intervention. Humans are complex and complicated beings. The fact that we are capable of changing is what makes therapeutic intervention useful, yet this is also sometimes confusing. A client may change not only in the course of months or years, but even within the course of a single hour. In the following chapters we will discuss how integrative theory can help clinicians decide which of their therapeutic tools to use at any given time with any given client.

Chapter 7
An Integrative Approach to Therapeutic Relationships

Keywords Therapeutic relationship • Transference • Countertransference • Research • Evidence • Clinical examples • Psychodynamic • Integrative practice • Small steps • Detailed inquiry • Affect-regulation • Attachment • Developmental • Holding environment • Secure base • Integrative approach to therapeutic relationship • Teamwork • Termination • Ending

As I have noted throughout this book, a growing body of research has found that a relationship between therapist and client can be a key factor in therapeutic outcome, no matter what type of therapy a clinician is practicing (e.g. Bacal & Herzog, 2003; Eagle, 2000; Frank, 2004, 2005; Leichsenring, 2005; Parish & Eagle, 2003; Roth & Fonagy, 1996; Schore, 2003; Siegel, 1999; Wallerstein, 2000; Wampold & Brown, 2005). But this finding actually leads to more questions, such as what sort of relationship leads to change? Do clients with different diagnoses need different kinds of relationships? Do these relational needs change over time, as they do with children and their parents? How does a clinician go about providing the right kind of relationship for each client? And is it better to talk about the relationship or to allow it to unfold silently as a background to the work?

To answer these questions, I have found that clinical theory and research results must be combined with a close reading of an individual client's specific needs and experiences at any given time. Furthermore, the relationship between each client and each clinician is, as we now understand, based not only on a client's but also on a clinician's personality. Much has been written about various aspects of therapeutic relationships (for just a few examples, see Feiner & Epstein, 1993; Frank, 2005; Gabbard, 1995; Hausner, 2000; McWilliams, 2004; Meissner, 2007a, 2007b; Norcross, 2002; Novick & Novick, 2006; Parish & Eagle, 2003). In this chapter I will focus on some specific relationship issues that frequently arise in clinical work in order to discuss ways that a clinician might respond to them in an integrative practice.

F.D. Barth, *Integrative Clinical Social Work Practice: A Contemporary Perspective*, Essential Clinical Social Work Series, DOI 10.1007/978-1-4939-0351-1_7,

Interventions Based on Diagnosis

Although research seems to indicate that certain techniques are more successful than others with specific diagnoses, close reading of some of the data as well as anecdotal evidence underscore the idea that these findings are not necessarily as definitive as we might like to think (Goodman, 2013; Roth & Fonagy, 1996; Wampold & Brown, 2005). There are a number of reasons for this discrepancy, including both problems with measurement tools and with clear adherence to specific techniques (Goodman, 2013). In other words, even in research situations, clinicians often unintentionally integrate techniques and theories. While this may muddy the waters of the research, it contributes to our understanding that each therapeutic dyad will have both similarities to, and differences from, any other clinical relationship. Similarly, clients with the same diagnosis may still have personality differences and need slightly different interventions. An integrative approach takes into account research that suggests that certain interventions are more useful for certain diagnostic categories, but also pays close attention to each client's needs as they become apparent in the clinical situation.

For example, while there is evidence that clients with addictions need structured interventions to deal with their behaviors, there is also evidence that many of these clients have co-morbid disorders and therefore need a combination of interventions, including medication and social and psychological support, as well as structured tools, limit-setting, and motivational interviewing (Sonne & Brady, 2002; Weiss, Kolodziej, Najavits, Greenfield, Fucito, 2000). My own experience, both in my practice and with therapists I have supervised, has been that motivational interviewing and an ongoing relationship with a clinician who both sets limits and provides an opportunity for exploring issues that interfere with the work can enhance this process. Similarly, Goldstein (1999) and Goodman (2013) offer evidence that some of the preferred treatment techniques for Borderline Personality Disorder are in and of themselves actually integrative practices. In the process of setting limits and helping a client with self-regulation, a clinician offers a client an opportunity to work through old attachments and relational patterns and learn new ones (e.g. Connors, 2006, 2011; Frank, 2001, 2005; Goldstein, 1999; Goodman, 2013; NIMH, 2013; Wachtel, 1997).

However, while understanding a client's diagnosis can be extremely useful, thinking exclusively in terms of diagnostic categories can lead to problems in the therapeutic work.

Developing a Working Relationship

Clients come to therapists for a number of explicit reasons and often with an equal number of unformulated or unrecognized ones. Sometimes they have agendas that they purposely hide from a clinician—for example, court mandated clients may not reveal that this is the reason they are coming for therapy (although, conversely, some will deny any need for help and will say that are only coming because they have to). Clients may hide symptoms, such as addictions and compulsions, and also the degree of their dysfunction until they feel safe with a clinician. While a client may not always be completely forthcoming about what he wants from therapy, it is part of a clinician's job to attempt to make sense of the request, as much as possible. Therapy begins when that clinician makes an honest attempt to both understand and respond to what a client is communicating.

Attempting to put into words why we might be doing what we are doing is an important part of any therapeutic work for several reasons, some of which we have already discussed. A clinician's attempts to talk about why a client has come, and what help the therapist is able to offer, can partially alleviate initial anxiety about asking for help as well as fears that a client's request will be misunderstood or rejected. By verbalizing and asking clients to confirm or further clarify what they are asking for, a clinician also models a process of communication that will be crucial to any ongoing work. This modeling also immediately invites a client to be a partner in the therapeutic process.

A client's engagement in the work is so important to an integrative practice that I choose to avoid the terms "patient" and "treatment" whenever possible, in order to avoid the implication that something is about to be done to them, or that they are passive recipients of my clinical interventions. Over the years some clients have struggled to find a better word to capture our relationship. They have told me that "client" does not work for them because it turns what is a deeply meaningful, personal and interactive process into a business association only. One woman who has participated in a very successful long-term psychodynamic psychotherapy with me suggests "therapeutic partnership," but this term also has problems, in that it implies an equality of sharing and expertise that in itself disguises the complex reality of the relationship. Although I am still searching for a term that captures all of the complexities and emotions that can be woven into even brief therapeutic partnerships, for the moment I am still using "client" as the operating term.

All of which is to say that making a contract with a client is often not as simple as the word might imply. I have written about an apparent contract change when clients share hidden symptoms after a long period of therapeutic work (Barth, 2008). I find that sometimes this contract change comes because a clinician has passed some important tests that a client sets, either consciously or unconsciously. Such tests can come in the very beginning of therapy—even in the first phone call. For example, years after she had started therapy, Laurie, the young dancer described in earlier chapters, explained why she had stayed with her therapist, Mrs. Herman, even while she was looking for a therapist who would focus more directly on her eating disorder. She was impressed in their first phone conversation, before they had even met, when Mrs. Herman expressed concern about Laurie as a real person. "You told me that you were going to a conference," she said, "so you couldn't see me right away. You asked me if I was okay waiting until you got back, or if I needed you to ask another therapist in the clinic to see me sooner." Mrs. Herman's openness about the process, her clearly expressed concern about Laurie, and her invitation to her to express what she needed from the outset of the work set the stage for her to become a secure attachment object even before they met.

The story was somewhat different with Laurie and James, her primary worker at the drug treatment program. In their first few sessions, Laurie shared a great deal of personal information with James, which led him to believe that they were developing a good therapeutic relationship. Based on his initial assumption that she was an addict, James drew a number of conclusions about issues Laurie raised. Hearing that she was having some difficulties with other members of her dance company, he attempted to provide her with tools for managing her feelings and the often impulsive behavior that went with them, but she was resistant to almost any intervention he made. He then began to use motivational interviewing to try to help her formulate reasons she might want to make change, even though she was also resistant to it. He thought they were making some headway, when she called to tell him that she was canceling therapy for good. "This stuff is worthless," she said. James felt overwhelmed and incompetent at first, and later he began to feel angry with Laurie. "She's a borderline and an addict," he said to a colleague. "I guess I should have been prepared for her to act out on me."

Diagnoses are helpful tools in assessment of a client's dynamics and level of engagement, but they can also pose obstacles to the therapeutic work. Davies (2006) and Bollas (1989) both illustrate ways in which diagnostic categories can, ironically, be ways of avoiding painful material that is emerging in a client-clinician relationship. In a consultation with a colleague, James began to ask himself what might be going on for him in this process. He started to look into his own history for some personal factors that might be influencing his response, but his colleague stopped him. "Most of us have some kind of reaction to clients with borderline dynamics," he said. "But what's going on here seems to be that you're taking Laurie's response personally. That may be a problem you have in general in your life, and might be something you want to look at in your own therapy; but in terms of Laurie, if we just get you to step back and not take her behavior personally, what could we learn about what it means to her?"

Taking It Personally

James was struggling with a common dilemma. A therapeutic relationship is often simultaneously professional and personal. Part of a clinician's task is to recognize that behavior that appears to be directed specifically at a clinician is actually reflective of that client's patterns of interpersonal interactions. In some therapies, generally psychodynamically oriented ones, these patterns are often explored as they arise in the transference. Contemporary relational theorists (e.g. Aron, 1991; 1996; Bromberg, 2001; Davies, 2002, 2006; Mitchell, 1999) have also brought to our awareness the importance of the interplay of a clinician's psychodynamics with a client's in any transference/countertransference interaction. On the other hand, there is ongoing dispute about how much the therapeutic relationship itself should be the focus of therapeutic exploration. While some clients find it useful, others find it disturbing and/or distracting from the "real" work of therapy. Novick and Novick (1998) caution against confusing a professional alliance, which has specific therapeutic goals, with a more general, personal relationship. Yet a therapeutic relationship is also an interaction between two people that can make both members of a therapeutic dyad feel vulnerable (see Gabbard & Lester, 1995).

Within the context of a professional relationship a client can and should feel seen (or recognized) and understood by her therapist. It is this feeling that clients often report when asked what was most helpful in their work with a particular therapist (see Wallerstein, 2000; Wampold & Brown, 2005). Some clients want to know more about their therapist as a person, and some prefer to have no extraneous information about her, even sometimes becoming irritated when something personal inadvertently enters the frame. The more clinicians know about themselves, the better able they will be to both recognize their roles in the mutual interaction and to simultaneously refrain from taking a client's responses to heart, and the better able they will be to explore what these responses mean to and about that client.

Recognizing our own role in any therapeutic encounter and the ways in which our engagement with clients may replicate old patterns of interacting for us as well as for them can lead to powerful shifts in our ability to choose interventions that will help clients work through some of their underlying issues. This does not necessarily mean sharing personal information with clients. It is important to have a colleague, therapist, or supervisor with whom we can explore these issues for ourselves in order to have more clarity about how to proceed with a client. Kohut (1971) suggests that clinicians need selfobjects in order to avoid making clients serve those functions. He further notes that clients respond to a clinician's genuine attempts to understand their experience. When we recognize that even a rejection by a client is not usually about us personally, it makes it easier to think about what the behavior means and thereby to understand it.

When James was able to ask himself what Laurie's rejection of therapy meant, he realized that she had exposed herself to him, a stranger, albeit a professional whose goal was to help her. He did not know a great deal about her history other than that she described her parents as overprotective and intrusive. She was not close with her older brother, who was often in trouble and who James suspected was a drug user himself. Her younger brother was autistic and Laurie was very close to and protective of him. When Laurie was a young teen her parents had put this brother into a residence for autistic children. She said that it broke her heart. "Why couldn't we take care of him at home?" she asked with tears in her eyes. This was when she began restricting her food intake and cutting herself. "No wonder she rejected me," James said after discussing this material with his colleague. "She was probably prepared for me to either hurt her or abandon her, so she beat me to the punch and rejected me first."

The Role of Understanding

Understanding alone is, in my experience, generally not enough to make change happen, but it is an invaluable tool in an integrative practice. One recent study (Goodman, 2013) underscores Kohut's (1984) belief that attempting to understand a client's experience from his perspective is a key—not often recognized—to a variety of different therapeutic techniques. One important tool in the work of understanding is to encourage clients to explain to us what they are thinking, and to ask them to tell us what they think we or another person might be experiencing. This is not only a tool for exploring transference and countertransference material, but also a practice of encouraging mentalization (Fonagy, Gyorgy, Jurist, & Target, 2003; Goodman, 2013) as well as an observing ego (see, for example, Gabbard, 1993). Renik (2006) has also pointed out that as clinicians try to put into words for clients what we understand about them and how we came to those conclusions—for example, based on what they have told us about their history, or in response to a particular facial expression or body position—we are modeling the process of self-reflection. Done in ways that are tolerable and manageable for each client, talking about what we understand and helping them put their own thoughts and feelings into words can be an important part of any therapeutic endeavor. Research in neuropsychology has shown that verbal clarification is one way in which therapy helps clients develop the capacity to both tolerate and manage their affects (Rustin, 2012; Schore, 2003; Siegel, 1999).

This explicatory process also has tremendously useful implications for a client and clinician's agreement about what they are working on and how that work will proceed. Although even at the beginning many clinicians do not overtly spell out what this agreement may be, therapy is a mutual agreement to work on particular issues in a particular way. But what each member of the therapeutic dyad has agreed upon may actually be quite different. Recognizing that there is a contract, albeit often unspoken, and clarifying what that contract might be is an important part of any therapeutic encounter. Often, such contracts are renegotiated several times in the course of therapeutic work—again, sometimes without ever being articulated overtly.

The Therapeutic Contract

Contracts are not always so easily made, nor are they always direct. Often, for a variety of reasons that neither clinician nor client can control, they have to be broken. It is the process of establishing and working within a therapeutic agreement that is important. The arrangement does not have to be formal (I am not speaking here of the kind of written contract that some clinicians have suicidal clients sign, which by their very nature need to be formalized). If a clinician models an open and honest attitude towards establishing an agreement of sorts with a client from the beginning of therapy, renegotiation is more manageable and in fact can be seen as part of the work. A contract can therefore be both firm and flexible—one of the many contradictions present in life and echoed in the therapeutic process. By establishing and re-establishing what both client and clinician believe to be the goals of their work and the ways that these goals may be met, a clinician may be handed all of the tools she needs for making decisions about what interventions will be most useful at a particular time with a particular client.

This is how it worked, for example, with Hank, who we met briefly in Chap. 5. Hank was an emergency worker whose physician referred him to an agency that provided body work like yoga, acupuncture and nutritional guidance for first responders. The agency also provided psychotherapy, marital counseling, and help with addictions, including regular meetings of several twelve step programs. The intake worker listened carefully to Hank's request for help with his back and recommended acupuncture and yoga to begin with. She also explained the availability of other help, but quickly accepted Hank's rejection of everything other than those two approaches. She also discussed his doubts about both techniques and suggested that he talk to some of the other clients who might be sitting in the drop-in area, where coffee and pastries were available, to see what their experiences had been like. To his amazement, Hank found an older colleague in the lounge. When he told Hank that this place was terrific, that they had helped him with back troubles and also with problems sleeping, Hank was sold. But when the acupuncturist with whom he started working suggested that he might also consider talking to a therapist, Hank made it clear that he was not interested. She accepted this and worked with him for several months until his back pain diminished significantly and he stopped coming for help. Some months later he referred a colleague to the center, saying, "You won't believe how much they can help."

Manifest and Latent Material in the Relationship

As we discussed in the previous chapter, an initial assessment is extremely helpful to a clinician's decisions about what will be the most useful intervention for a particular client. Because clients have different relational needs and dynamics, it is useful for clinicians to be able to think about the specific needs of each client. For example, clients who are quite anxious or having difficulty managing their impulses may need a therapist to be actively engaged, asking questions, guiding the therapeutic conversation and offering suggestions and direction. Someone who is depressed or simply more methodical might prefer a therapist who acts more as a witness than as a guide. They may need a clinician who can sit quietly with them while they attempt to think their thoughts rather than one who makes suggestions or asks questions.

No matter whether or not one works directly within a therapeutic relationship, it is useful to have some understanding of how a client's feelings about his therapist can impact the work. Further, it is helpful to have some ideas about obstacles that might interfere with this relationship and thereby negatively affect therapy. Resistance, for example, may appear to be related to some aspect of the work itself, but it may also be motivated by latent or unformulated issues from the therapeutic relationship itself. Such issues may derive from a client's history and/or background, of course, but they may also be related to a clinician's unrecognized or unarticulated dynamics. In an integrative practice a clinician keeps both sides of a relationship in mind, even though he may never bring a discussion of these dynamics into the therapy office.

For instance, both a person with borderline personality disorder and an individual with a generalized anxiety disorder may both need active intervention, including not only question-asking, but also guidance about what to talk about and even some limited self-disclosure from a therapist. For a person with borderline personality disorder the clinician's activity could help limit impulsive acting out, while an anxious person might use the interaction to help manage disturbing thoughts and feelings that he cannot yet handle alone. And while one person struggling with depression may want to sit with a therapist because, as one client once said to me, "it's the only time it's safe for me to think," another may long for input into what feels like a dark and empty space from which he cannot emerge alone.

An assessment of a client's specific developmental issues and conflicts, both historically and in the present, can also help a clinician consider how best to approach particular issues. This can include not only a client's history, but also the history of the therapeutic work. For example, many clients need more active intervention at the beginning of therapy. As they become more comfortable with a clinician and more familiar with the process of self-examination, they may require less activity from their therapist. Similarly, as we will discuss in the chapter on endings, a client who has been capable of self-initiated exploration but is preparing to leave a meaningful clinical relationship may need more support and guidance in this final period of the work.

It is crucial for clinicians to be attuned to our own dynamics as they unfold within each therapeutic relationship in order to avoid allowing these personal responses to interfere with the therapeutic process. These responses can also be clues about important, unarticulated material about a client. Mitchell (1998) offers the image of transference and countertransference as a relational "dance." Much of the therapeutic work, he suggests, involves being curious about why we and a client have chosen a particular dance step and music at a particular time. This sometimes means paying close attention to reactions which involve parts of ourselves that we do not like, or of which we are critical, ashamed or embarrassed.

These feelings can interfere with therapists' ability use our reactions to help us understand something about our clients' unconscious or unformulated experiences. They can also lead to an inability to manage our own unconscious and unformulated dynamics, important in order not to induce or project or issues in a client. Since, as Greenberg (1991) notes, we all have blind spots which by definition we cannot see, these events cannot be completely avoided. Handled with humility, empathy and tact, these situations can be powerful learning events in any therapeutic work, whether the frame is cognitive and behavioral, psychodynamic, body-based, medical, and so on. When ignored or suppressed, they can interfere with and derail even the most rigorously applied techniques.

Therapist's Self-disclosure

Numerous authors have explored the question of self-disclosure in the therapeutic process. Gerson (2001), Mitchell (1998) and Goldstein (1994) have made interesting cases for the significance of the inadvertent self-disclosures on the part of a clinician, including wearing or not wearing a wedding ring, changes in appearance due to aging, illness or life events like pregnancy. Like Wallerstein (2000), they suggest that clients are often quite interested in personal details about their therapists, but boundaries that maintain the professional relationship are crucial for therapeutic work to be done (see also Frank, 2005; Gabbard & Lester, 1995). Wallerstein (2000) suggests that often these inadvertent comments or revelations have far more significance to the outcome of therapy than clinicians generally recognize. Our being human is an important part of our being therapists and helps clients feel understood and recognized by another person. A willingness to listen to and think about clients' reactions to our personalities without always considering such reactions to be manifestations of transference issues is also extremely important (see Bollas, 1989).

It is important to know that a therapist's self-disclosure is not appropriate for every client or in every situation. For example, many clients seem to feel comforted by knowing that their therapist knows first-hand something about their experience—e.g. parents struggling with issues with their children like to know that a clinician has children of his own. In an attempt to overcome an addiction, it can sometimes be helpful to know that a therapist has overcome something similar. On the other hand, many clients feel intruded on by any information about a clinician and cannot tolerate a therapist's self-revelations, even of the most insignificant sort. Basch (1980) makes a case for listening carefully to the needs clients actually communicate to their therapists rather than imposing a theoretically bound or "experience distant" (Kohut, 1971) generalization on every client.

Similarly, Johnson (1999) and Bloomgarden (2000) suggest that therapists who have struggled with eating disorders may be particularly vulnerable in working with clients with these symptoms. He also believes that they can also be powerful role models and that they can sometimes understand some of the struggles more fully than someone who has not suffered themselves. He warns that a clinician needs to be clear, however, that just because something worked for her does not mean that it will work for clients, even those who seem very similar to the clinician in dynamics and symptoms. In such situations, self-disclosure can also be a double-edged sword: while some clients may be comforted to know that their therapist has struggled with and overcome these issues, others may feel that it is a command to them that they be able to follow a similar path. Still others may become frightened that this clinician is too vulnerable to help them. As always, our understanding of a client is one of the most powerful tools for deciding what will be the most useful for a specific individual at a given time (see also Thompson-Brenner, Satir, Franko, & Herzog, 2012). Goldstein (2007) makes a similar comment about therapists who are in mid-life working with clients at the same stage of their lives, noting as well that a clinician's narcissistic vulnerabilities can make it difficult be empathically attuned to a client's needs.

There is a growing body of research on another aspect of this issue, the experience of shared and secondary trauma on a clinician's part. Shared trauma occurs when client and clinician have both experienced the same traumatic event, such as a natural disaster or an act of violence or war occurring in their community. According to Tosone, Nuttman-Schwartz and Stephens (2012) secondary trauma phenomena or collective catastrophic events can have a powerful and often unrecognized impact on mental health professionals living and working in traumatogenic environments. Shared trauma occurs when clinicians are exposed to the same community trauma as their clients. They suggest that clinicians must pay close attention to and put into words their own trauma narrative, and must be assiduous about their self-care in order to provide appropriate help to clients. These shared experiences can be important aspects of a therapeutic relationship, but a clinician must be both alert to and cautious about any changes in boundaries that might result from intentional and unintentional self-disclosure around these experiences. Agencies need to be prepared to offer training, supervision, and support to help clinicians navigate the effects of both shared and secondary trauma. Clinicians in private practice should look for such settings in which they can receive additional assistance processing these experiences.

Understanding, Attachment and Affect Regulation in a Therapeutic Relationship

Silverman (1998) points out that attachments are one of the most important ways that we learn to regulate our affects, which explains one of the reasons that attachment to a clinician can be helpful, no matter what techniques he uses (see also Kohut, 1977). Schore (2003) describes neuropsychological research that underscores the importance of attachment experiences in the development of affect regulation. Thus it seems that it might be useful for clinicians to be as alert as possible to some of the issues that might arise in this area, whether or not we use this information directly in the work with a client.

In order to enhance these processes, a clinician has to manage his own affects and regulate his own self-esteem and attachment needs. This is especially true when work with a particular client triggers strong feelings. Such responses may be related to a clinician's personal history and dynamics or simply be normal reactions to this client's behaviors and emotions. In either case, a clinician's work—or lack thereof—on personal feelings will very likely have an impact on the therapeutic experience.

Some common problematic reactions from therapists include: anxiety, over-identification with a client, denial of the severity of symptoms, over-concern about the symptoms, over-simplification or over-complication of a disorder, frustration, anger, impatience, disgust, confusion, judgment, romantic impulses, and a desire to rescue a client. These feelings are not abnormal and are human responses to another person's vulnerabilities. What is important is how the feelings are handled and incorporated in the work.

Attachment, relational and neuroscience based theorists have for some time now been integrating a clinician's thoughts and feelings into the therapeutic work (see for just a few examples, Aron, 1991, 1996; Bollas, 1989; Bromberg, 2001; Boston Change Process Study Group, 2005, 2010; Davies, 2002, 2006; Fonagy, Gyorgy, Jurist, & Target, 2003; Hoffman, 1998; Stern, 1985, Schore, 2003). A clinician's responses have been found to be especially helpful as clients work through dissociated and/or unformulated material within a therapeutic relationship. Yet how can feelings of anxiety, disgust, and helplessness be useful? According to Kohut (1977), clinicians need to be careful not to use our clients to meet our own needs for self-esteem. Many of us become therapists precisely because of some of our personal and often unconscious needs to "cure" ourselves and our loved ones. How do we balance these different needs and interests in order to provide our clients with the best possible therapeutic experience?

I have found it particularly useful to heed Novick and Novick's (1998) warning that understanding something about our experiences with a given client does not mean that we know precisely what that client is experiencing. Instead, empathic responses offer us tools for beginning to explore what might be happening beneath the surface of an interaction. Attention to the details of these interactions provides an opportunity to sift through and understand a range of emotions and thoughts that a client experiences at a given time, and to differentiate those experiences from our own. Like Novick and Novick (1998), Parish and Eagle (2003) emphasize the difference between transference and the therapeutic alliance. They add that a theme that runs through these and many other aspects of any relationship between clinician and client is the issue of attachment. Using a clinician as a "secure base" (Bowlby, 1988), a client may explore his inner world or may "simply" learn ways to manage affects. Sometimes the therapeutic alliance is background to the ongoing work (see Mitchell, 1999) and should not be examined or otherwise touched. Kohut (1971) describes a phenomenon he calls a "silent idealizing transference" in this way, and suggests that it needs to be allowed to evolve without discussion or even open acknowledgement.

It may seem obvious, but it is well worth noting that one of the most important tools available to any therapeutic dyad is talking. While we have seen that words do not always communicate everything a person is feeling, they are a powerful method for exploring not only what someone else is experiencing, but also what we feel, think, need and want. This is, of course, one of the reasons parents and teachers exhort young children to "use your words." Again, clinicians often have to work hard not to take communications from clients personally. This means that we learn to listen to what a client says, even criticism of our work, as information about that client. Of course, they may also be telling us truths about areas that we need to work on. Like many of my colleagues, I have found that my clients are some of my best teachers. But even when what they have to say about me is a useful insight into my own dynamics, it almost always tells me something useful about them as well. Clients are often uncomfortable telling us things that they worry might make us feel badly. Part of our work is to help them understand that these communications can be useful to both of us.

Deciding when to open up a discussion about a therapeutic relationship or when to allow it to function quietly in the background depends on several factors. An integrative clinician will consider questions such as: Is the relationship working as a silent holding environment in which the therapeutic work is moving forward? Is something happening that is interfering with the work? Is it necessary to the process? A client's needs will help an integrative clinician determine what interventions will be most useful at a particular time. Untangling these needs gets easier with experience, but an understanding of some of the issues involved can improve any clinician's ability to make these distinctions and apply appropriate interventions.

From Understanding to Intervening

Familiarity with a number of different approaches is of course extremely important in an integrative practice. However, since none of us is capable of being an expert in every possible approach, it is also very useful to have a team of colleagues who are available for both consultation and/or referrals of clients when they need interventions that we are not qualified to provide. We will discuss teamwork from this perspective in Chap. 9. For the moment, however, let us focus on how understanding what a client is communicating can help us choose and integrate appropriate interventions.

In my experience, if we listen closely, without a personal investment in immediately changing a client, we can often find clues to the best intervention for that client. For instance, when I began working with anorexic clients many years ago, I was just finishing up my analytic training, where I was taught that to "gratify" either abstract needs for love or attention or concrete needs for physical care would interfere with the analytic process. However, as I listened to my clients, I realized that some of them were literally starving to death with no capacity to feed themselves. I discovered that a starving person cannot engage in any kind of self-exploratory work. I began to keep granola bars, fruit and yogurt in my fridge and found that, contrary to what I had been led to believe, a tremendous amount of exploration went on when I offered food to these young women (and occasionally men) in order, as I often put it, "to help them think." My offer was rejected almost as often as it was accepted, but it was almost always met with surprise, interest, and some curiosity. In many instances the relational meaning of the interchanges was only examined years later, when the symptoms were diminished, but that the action was meaningful from the beginning was apparent in the immediate thoughts and reactions it elicited.

Another example of how listening to what a client asks for, both verbally and nonverbally, can inform a clinician's interventions, can be found in the ongoing work with Hank, the young emergency worker. Months after referring his colleague to his acupuncturist, Hank called and asked if he could come in for a "refresher." He said that his back was just a little "out," and he thought it might be helpful to have a treatment to keep it from getting worse. She told him she thought that was an excellent idea and they set up an appointment. When he came in for the session, she asked him about how things were going since the last time they had met. He replied that everything was pretty good, that his back had been fine, and that work was just its normal stress level these days. As she was setting him up on the treatment table, he thanked her for seeing his buddy and said that he heard she had referred him to a couple's therapist for some problems he and his wife were having. She told him she had been happy to help, and added that she thought couples therapy could be really useful for a lot of people.

When they were finished with the appointment, Hank again thanked her for referring his friend to the other therapist. Since he had rebuffed her first attempt to refer him to a therapist himself, the acupuncturist did not think she should ask him if he wanted a referral, but she had the thought that this might be the underlying message in his repeated reference to this friend. She said again that she thought that couples therapy could be really useful for a lot of couples. She added that she and her husband had done it at one point in their marriage and that they were very glad that they had. Hank said nothing more at that point, but several days later he called and shyly asked her for a referral for his wife and himself. "We've just got a couple of things we need to talk to someone about," he said.

Conclusion

What happened with Hank is a common occurrence in the therapeutic process. A connection to a helping professional can make it feel safe for a client to seek out further help (e.g. Bacal & Herzog, 2003; Frank, 2004, 2005; Leichsenring, 2005; Parish & Eagle, 2003; Roth & Fonagy, 1996; Schore, 2003; Siegel, 1999; Wallerstein, 2000; Wampold & Brown, 2005). It is not simply what a clinician offers, but how it is presented that is significant. Empathy and understanding are extremely important, but so are knowledge, experience, and an ability to recognize both our own and our client's limitations. A therapeutic tool that seldom receives its due is a therapist's tact, but the kind of thoughtful and sensitive response to a client's resistance shown by the acupuncturist working with Hank can go a long way towards building a working alliance, which is key to a therapeutic relationship. Setting limits is also important. Boundaries are not only important to protect a client, but also to protect the therapeutic work. We will discuss this aspect of the work in Chap. 8.

Chapter 8
Small Steps and Manageable Goals

Keywords Clinical interventions • Research • Clinical illustrations • Integrative practice • Rigidity versus flexibility • Individualized approach • Detailed inquiry • Small steps • Integrative social work • Reasonable goals • Manageable goals • Cognitive therapy • Behavioral therapy • Body-mind dynamics • Psychodynamic • Beginnings • Endings • Termination • Developmental process

Not only clients, but clinicians may be overwhelmed by the magnitude of the problems clients bring into therapy. I have noted in various chapters the importance of breaking both problems and goals into smaller, more manageable components. In fact, I see teaching clients how to take small steps towards manageable goals as one of the hallmarks of an integrative practice. In order to do so, clinicians also need to find ways to break down our own goals as well as those of our clients into manageable segments. It is not uncommon for us to want our clients to feel better immediately, but we also hope to help them make changes that will pave the way for happier and more productive lives in the future. In some cases, these goals are achievable; but we have to start at the beginning, which is often helping them manage painful feelings and circumstances in the present. Sometimes what seems to be a small intervention can lead to surprisingly large changes. Perhaps more often than we and our clients like, our task is not to take away painful emotions or change difficult situations, but to help clients learn to live with a degree of unpleasantness in the short term in order to make changes in the long-term.

Utilizing knowledge from a variety of different theories helps a clinician determine how to decide what steps to take at each point in a client's progression. For example, according to research conducted by Hersoug, Hogland, Monsen, and Havik (2001), clients report feeling most helped in the initial stages by a supportive and educative approach. (Interestingly, this study found that a clinician's experience and training can have a negative impact on the development of therapeutic alliance when it leads to a protocol that feels rigid and experience distant to the client). Prochaska, DiClemente, and Norcross (1992) outline a five stage model of change in addictive

F.D. Barth, *Integrative Clinical Social Work Practice: A Contemporary Perspective*, Essential Clinical Social Work Series, DOI 10.1007/978-1-4939-0351-1_8,

behaviors from the perspective of using small steps that is also applicable for other symptom pictures. Their stages are: *precontemplation, contemplation, preparation, action and maintenance*. Precontemplation is the period during which there is often no awareness of a problem and no intent to change. During the contemplation stage, there is an awareness and perhaps desire to change, but no commitment to a plan to create that change. Preparation usually includes a desire to change and some small, but possibly ineffective changes. During the action stage, a commitment to change and significant shifts in behavior are made. And the final stage, maintenance, is the ongoing process of learning to maintain and consolidate the gains. However, describing what they call "spiral patterns of change," these authors remind us that change in addictive behavior does not generally take a straight path. It is not a linear progression, but instead is usually a prolonged pattern of "relapse and recycling through the stages." (Prochaska et al., 1992, p. 1104).

These stages need little alteration to be utilized in an integrative practice with a wide range of clients. Given the extensive research showing that factors such as a client's level of functioning and psychological-mindedness have a significant impact on outcome of *all* therapeutic interventions (Norcross, 2002), I find it helpful to assess a client's state of mind on a regular basis not only at the beginning, but throughout any clinical work. These stages are useful tools for breaking the therapeutic process down into small, manageable steps. For example, these stages help us think about where a client is at any given moment in the work.

Recognizing "Where a Client Is"

Winnicott (1987) suggests that part of a clinician's job is to hold in mind where a client is able to go in the future. However, following the maxim of "starting where a client is" makes it more likely that he will succeed in making initial steps towards change. And as motivational interviewers remind us, feeling successful is a powerful impetus for further change (Rollnick, Butler, & Miller, 2008). Paying attention to where a client is can help a clinician set reasonable goals, recognize small but valuable accomplishments, and help a client begin building "feeling muscles" that will help him move to the next level of his development, even after therapy is finished.

For instance, let us return to Hank, the emergency worker who sought acupuncture and then asked for a referral for couple's therapy for himself and his wife. Hank and his wife Trish explained to George, the couple's therapist to whom they had been referred, that they needed help resolving a conflict about Trish's desire to go back to work now that their youngest child was in school. Although George quickly assessed that Hank was struggling with some latent insecurities and anger, he also accepted that asking for help was not high on Hank's agenda. He took into account not only Hank's characterological reluctance to ask for aid, but also his probable professional and cultural need to seal over some of his more vulnerable emotions. By asking for help with his marriage Hank could be opening a door for working on other issues, but George did not want to scare Hank off by pushing him to work on these issues before he was ready to do so. Thus he accepted the couple's expressed desire to focus on a very specific goal. George knew that establishing a relationship in which he clearly respects a client's agenda, while at times acknowledging other future possibilities, can give a resistant client a positive experience of therapy, which might be the most valuable aid he offers.

In the first session, George helped both Trish and Hank talk about the conflict as openly and clearly as possible. He stopped each of them from interrupting the other, but it soon became clear that the problem was not between them, but between Hank and his father, who believed that women should not work outside of the home. When George shared this conclusion with them, they looked at one another and laughed. He asked them if they minded explaining the shared moment with him. Hank gestured for Trish to speak. "Hank's dad is a wonderful person," she said, "but he has very strong opinions. It's kind of amazing that you picked up on that so fast. We hadn't put it together that it's our fear of telling him about me going back to work that's making this so hard, but it makes total sense."

Over the course of three more sessions, George explored previous times Hank and Trish had struggled to find ways to manage disagreements with Hank's dad. In the course of these sessions, they problem-solved and role-played ideas for letting him know that Trish was going back to work. "It's only part-time, for Pete's sake," Hank said. Trish added, "Big Hank (Hank's father) lets me get away with stuff he doesn't accept in some of the other kids and their spouses. But we're both worried that this will push him over the edge." In the process of working on these issues, even in the course of four sessions, George felt that Hank and Trish strengthened their own relationship. He thought that doing so also might help with some of the ongoing developmental issues around separation, individuation and autonomy that he heard in their descriptions of their relationships with their families of origin and with their own children. However, since his assessment was that the family was functioning well overall, he maintained her focus on their success in taking the small steps that they were interested in taking.

There are times when it can be useful to set an impossible goal with clients—e.g. asking an alcoholic or chronic drug user to be completely abstinent from the beginning of treatment. McMain, Sayrs, Dimeff, and Linehan (2007) discuss the importance of a clinician's working with a client to recognize and manage the tension between the desire to accomplish large goals and the frustration of taking small steps to get there. They sometimes begin with what they call a "door in the face" demand that a client immediately commit to an often unrealistic goal of immediate total abstinence. When a client recognizes the impossibility of achieving this goal, a clinician will introduce a "foot in the door" strategy of finding a smaller, more manageable agreement. For example, they suggest determining with a client what he thinks is the longest period that they can commit to being abstinent at that moment. DBT techniques are used to help him achieve that initial goal and gradually expand the period of abstinence over time until he reaches the goal of total abstinence.

Ongoing Assessment

Small steps work best in conjunction with an ongoing assessment of a client's level of discomfort and also that client's ability to tolerate some degree of unpleasantness in order to achieve a future shift. We can utilize information from a client in almost any session to determine whether an immediate symptom-focused intervention is necessary or whether a client can tolerate some exploration and opening up of dynamics that might be causing the difficulties (see Connors, 2006). However, since it is often necessary to intervene before an assessment is complete, it is useful to remember that a client's reactions to an intervention can often provide additional information about a client's symptoms, strengths and needs (see Mitchell, 1993). A clinician can also engage a client in the decision-making process, discussing whether to focus on direct symptom-relief or gradual uncovering of underlying causes in order to make longer-term change. Not only do these discussions help clarify the therapeutic contract, but they can also empower and enhance a sense of agency in a client.

This is how it went with James and Laurie. In consultation with Ms. Herman (we will discuss this further in Chap. 9), James came to understand that Laurie's impulsive and self-harming behavior was at least in part related to her fear of being hurt and abandoned by important people in her life. He realized that building trust with her would be a slow process and needed to be a long term goal. As a step towards that goal, he began to work with her on building some skills that would give her more control over some of her behaviors and feelings. He also began to put into words his understanding not only of how hard it was for her to tolerate those feelings, but of how her behaviors had been a way of coping with them. "Listen," he said to her at one point when she was putting herself down for not being able to carry through on an assignment, "you did the best you could. These behaviors have been your way of coping for a long time. We're not going to change everything overnight. But you're starting to pay attention to what you're feeling, aren't you?" She nodded. "And you're starting to notice when you're getting ready to act in an impulsive and counterproductive way, right?"

She nodded but added, "Yeah, but I'm still doing the same things that have always gotten me into trouble."

James acknowledged that this was true. "But the first step is to recognize the moments before you start to act," he said. "You can't change anything if you don't know that it's happening. You've taken that step. Let's keep practicing that step for a little while. When you've got it down pat, you'll be ready to take the next one."

While the idea of breaking larger goals into smaller steps is a distinct element of DBT and ACT as well as other contemporary cognitive behavioral techniques (see, for just some examples, McMain et al., 2007; and Raja, 2012), it can also be an important component of psychodynamic and body-based work. For example, Sullivan's (1953) emphasis on small details encourages clinicians to focus not on the greater goal of personality change, but on the small steps that lead to any problematic behavior. Mindfulness techniques that help bring awareness to the specifics of a given moment can also help clients break experience into smaller, more manageable factors rather than overwhelming generalizations.

Clinicians who work in the medical field have found the idea of small steps crucial in work with clients who have to change life habits for medical reasons. There is often tremendous pressure on clients to make these alterations quickly; but often small modifications that can actually be accomplished are better than large changes that never happen. For precisely this reason, the American Diabetes Association (1995–2013) encourages patients who need to reforms their diets to make minimal and manageable dietary shifts with which they gradually become comfortable; then they can attempt other modifications. The Harvard Medical School (2000–2013) advocates a similar approach to lifestyle changes needed to manage heart disease. I am always reminded in this discussion of my own father, whose doctors recommended a heart healthy diet after major coronary surgery. When he arrived home to cabinets stocked with his new foods, he informed his loving and over-zealous family that he would rather starve to death. Unhappily, we restored all of his high fat and salt-loaded favorites, leaving him to slowly make minute alterations to his life style on his own time. He continued with these small shifts until he died at 91. Another protocol of manageable (although far from simple) steps, revisited and reworked over time, is of course offered by Alcoholics Anonymous and the many 12-step programs based on this philosophy (see Kaskutas, 2009; Prochaska et al., 1992). Again, despite internal and external pressure on individuals who struggle with addictions, it seems that making small, sustainable shifts in behavior can lead to larger, more lasting change.

Setting Limits

As we noted in the last chapter, boundaries are extremely important in any therapeutic endeavor, in order to protect not only a client (Gabbard & Lester, 1995) but also the therapeutic process. Boundaries in therapeutic work include the frame—that is, when a session begins and ends, how long a session will last, who will come into the office, and clients' payments for therapy. When a clinician sets and reinforces boundaries firmly and tactfully, she models an important set of behaviors for clients, especially those who have difficulties setting limits themselves. Questions of extra-therapeutic contact, with a client, family members and other professionals involved in a client's life, need to be discussed and boundaries established. However, there are also times when such agreements need to be revisited. For instance, Laurie was often late to her sessions. Although James was working to soften her overly self-critical attitude towards her own imperfections, he also maintained the therapeutic frame by ending her sessions on time and by encouraging her to arrive on time. When she became self-critical, he re-focused her by suggesting that they try to examine some of the reasons she might be having difficulty getting to her sessions. With gentle exploration, it became clear that Laurie often underestimated the amount of time that it would take her to get anywhere. Further discussion led to links between her lateness and her tremendous dislike of being kept waiting. "I'd rather arrive late than have to wait around," she said. She often felt hurt and rejected when someone else was late. Although James thought it was significant that she was not particularly worried about doing the same thing to others, given Laurie's insecurities he decided to leave exploration of that issue for later in their work. He focused instead on what she lost by being late.

When they had established that she did not like missing part of her appointment every week, he opened up the idea that she took it personally when someone was late. "Yes, of course," she said. "It means someone doesn't care enough about me to get there on time." He asked if that was her sense of him. "No. But if I sit outside your office and wait, I'll start to think about it. You never let my sessions go over," she added, "so if you let someone else run over their time, I'll feel hurt—and angry." James encouraged Laurie to talk about these issues with Ms. Herman, who was still working with her on the underlying psychodynamic issues that were feeding into her symptoms. He said, however, that she seemed to want to hold onto these beliefs. She said that she did not want to hold onto them, but that if she arrived and he was late, she would not be able to avoid them. He asked if it would help to have something else to distract her when she arrived, just as a parent might distract a small child while waiting for something. She looked a little taken aback. "You mean, if I bring a book, I won't mind waiting so much. And my mind will be occupied, so I won't be thinking about whether or not you care about me." It was somewhat amazing to James that this had never occurred to her before, but some weeks later she eagerly shared that it was something she had begun to apply in a variety of situations—waiting for a friend, or for a dance teacher to arrive. By setting firm boundaries in a tactful and nonjudgmental manner, James opened up an area for psychodynamic exploration. He also heard and addressed rigidified thoughts (e.g. that if someone kept her waiting, it meant that they did not care about her) and then, when Laurie had more of a sense of what might be creating some of these difficulties, he offered her a specific tool for managing some of the problematic thoughts and associated feelings.

Small Successes, Powerful Motivators

Psychologically, the idea of breaking any goal into smaller steps that can be achieved more quickly makes good sense. In part, this is because success motivates us to move forward, which means that over time, with the help of ongoing small successes, we are more likely to get to the larger goals we have set (Hayes, 2004; Linehan, 1993; Prochaska et al., 1992; Raja, 2012). Similarly, when goals are smaller, failure to achieve them may be easier to deal with. These small disappointments have other benefits as well, including providing an opportunity to work on coping with the feelings attached to them—pain, frustration, disappointment, sadness, sense of inadequacy, self-blame and blame of others—which frequently cannot be addressed as easily when the letdown is too great. I have written about the ways that this process helps clients to strengthen their "feeling muscles" (Barth, 1998, 2003). As with any form of exercise, beginning with small, manageable activities and, as the "muscles" get stronger, gradually progressing to more difficult ones, is often more productive than trying to do tasks that are beyond our capacities. Disappointment is also an opportunity for reviewing goals. Is it a signal that they need to be broken down further? Are they unrealistic? Is it time to move in a different direction or to choose different objectives? One of our most important tasks as clinicians is to help clients feel good about the small steps they are taking. We can do this by keeping in mind the parallel between clinical work and normal development.

Developmental Progression

Working in small steps is also an occasion to engage with a client from a developmental perspective. Children may appear to grow in leaps and bounds, but they actually develop one step at a time. Because it seems inevitable that there will be gaps in any developmental process, most of our clients will have missed out on some component of their psychological and emotional development. As they learn about taking small steps in therapy, clients will hopefully internalize a way of thinking about any learning process, whether it is within their own experience regarding a new job or new relationship, or about their children's developmental paths.

When I think about these ideas, I often find myself thinking of an example I was privileged to observe many years ago. I was visiting friends on a holiday weekend, and we were outside, talking and visiting and watching their young children. Their toddler approached the front stoop and sat looking thoughtfully at it. She was a competent walker who had not yet mastered stair-climbing; but she was at the age where the world was her oyster (Mahler, Pine, & Bergman, 1973) and saw every new obstacle as simply one more opportunity for expansion. As we watched, she stood and started to walk up the stairs. One of her parents dashed over to keep her from tumbling down, but before they arrived, the little girl seemed to realize it was beyond her capacity and quickly solved the problem by crawling up on her hands and knees. With her mother standing nearby, she reached the top, sat for a moment, and then started to crawl back down. Apparently deciding going down the steps face first was not a good idea, she carefully turned around to sit and bump her way down on her bottom. She repeated these steps several times over the course of the first day. The next day, engaging again in her new activity, she stood and slowly made her way up, steadying herself with the aid of the railing. She turned and grinned at her admiring audience, then sat and again bumped down as she had the day before. After 3 days of up and down practice, she decided to try to take the steps in both directions standing on her feet. Angrily rebuffing parental attempts to hold her hand, she regally marched up the steps and slowly, again with the aid of the railing, walked down them. Our applause was totally unnecessary. She was incredibly pleased with her accomplishment; and then, in the next moment, she was ready to move on to other challenges.

This image captures some of the work that James and Laurie were engaged in as well. Explaining to Laurie how important it was to practice each step before she could move on to the next one, James said that he thought she had missed some important developmental steps in her childhood. "You can't go back and undo what has—or hasn't—happened," he said, "but we can strengthen some of the places that are kind of weak. That's what these exercises are about." He added that her intelligence and sense of humor had probably helped her manage despite those areas of vulnerability. "As you get stronger, they'll be even more useful!"

Although clients and clinicians understandably wish that achievements could be made more quickly and in larger chunks, it is often these small steps that are the most significant in the long term (not unlike Sullivan's idea that small details are the most revealing). Focusing on existing strengths can be a great help in building the skills and "muscles" in areas of weakness. While clients often feel pressure, both internal and external, for example, to begin an extensive exercise regimen in order to improve their bodies, I have found that it is often far more useful to help a client start with much smaller goals—even with a single workout a week, or sometimes simply with a 5 min stretch routine 1 day each week. A clinician's personal experience can be useful in supporting our belief that such change can occur. Looking back at my own early experience of taking dance classes at the same time that I was starting therapy, I am impressed with the amount of change that occurred in my life after 6 months of doing each only one time a week!

Raja (2012) similarly encourages clients to see small stages as important in developing an ongoing exercise routine. Although developing such a routine can make a client feel better, sometimes exercise itself can create distress. Raja (2012) further notes that some clients can be overwhelmed or traumatized by the initial bodily experiences that come with exercise, which is another reason that she takes a step by step approach to developing an exercise routine with clients. The struggle is to help clients find an activity that is tolerable, not overly distressing, and that also provides them with a sense of accomplishment. Sometimes this balance is only found by trial and error. A clinician's belief in a small step approach, while empathizing with a client's frustration that change is not occurring more quickly, can provide a holding environment during these initial stages. It can also be an important source of motivation as a client moves slowly forward.

Development of Trust

While we might wish that a client could come in for several sessions a week, it can sometimes be more productive to start slowly, to allow a relationship and sense of trust to grow. This is, of course, not always the case, in particular when a client is extremely anxious or depressed and needs more frequent contact with a clinician. When a client enters our office with overwhelming symptoms, it is part of our work to offer them tools to help them begin to feel better as quickly as possible (for further discussion of this idea from an integrative perspective, see Connors, 2006;

Frank, 2005; Wachtel, 1997). An integrative clinician may decide to recommend a consultation for medication as well as suggesting some specific tools for managing the symptoms immediately (such as breathing, mindfulness, body work, cognitive behavioral interventions, and so on), and offering more frequent contact. I have found that sometimes just the offer of extra contact can be enough for some clients. They do not always need to come in for extra sessions, especially when they are able to begin engaging in some of the other work that a clinician might suggest.

A client's history, personality, social and professional environment and current issues can all influence his capacity to trust his therapist, as can a clinician's personality, style and the setting in which he practices (e.g. see Meissner, 2007a, 2007b). For instance, James had come to understand that Laurie longed to trust him but was afraid of being hurt by him. The idea that the process of change involves small steps is hard for many clients to grasp (it is, in my experience, difficult for most people). A client's struggles to manage the conflict between high expectations and limited capacity can be manifested in their transference to their therapist. Worries that a clinician is either critical and/or dismissive of their abilities may emerge along with unarticulated (at least not directly) criticism and denigration of the therapist. What is often difficult for clients and therapists is that both idealization and denigration of a therapist can exist practically simultaneously. Kohut (1971, 1977) suggests that idealization is a natural part of development and that non-traumatic disappointment in and anger at an idealized object is necessary to healthy human development. While Kohut advocates an empathic, understanding approach to both idealization and disappointment, Kernberg (2000) believes that underlying aggression must be recognized and formulated in order for opposing emotions (like love and hate) to be integrated. I would suggest that at different times both are right, but that the real trick is to find ways for a client to manage whatever emotions are beginning to emerge throughout the therapeutic process. My experience has been reinforced by recent research (see Bateman & Fonagy, 2004; Weinberg, Ronningstam, Goldblatt, Schechter, & Maltsberger, 2010) showing that different treatment techniques directed at managing these emotions all focus on understanding of clients' needs for help regulating affects, behavior and interpersonal interactions (see also Connors, 2006; Frank, 2001; Wachtel, 1997).

Agendas, Hidden and Overt

For any clinician, one of the hardest tasks may be to limit our own goals for our clients. Our goals may be far grander than those of our clients; or we may share their unrealistically high expectations. This is not to say that people cannot change, and change a great deal. It is only to say that sometimes the smallest changes are the most important; and a clinician's task is to recognize and underscore these changes in order to promote further growth—or, as Basch (1980) has pointed out, to allow a client to leave therapy with a feeling of accomplishment.

For example, in his work with Hank and Trish, George recognized that he was going to have to limit his expectations. Although he thought it would be useful for Hank to work on some of the issues he heard in his relationship with his father, Big Hank, he recognized that Hank was not interested in delving into his own psyche in that way. His culture, both personal and professional, was not one in which feelings were discussed or examined, and the accomplishments made in the five marital sessions seemed to be making a difference not only in his relationship with Trish, but also in his sense of anxiety and the physical symptoms which had been distressing him. George knew that to push Hank to do further work would be outside of the therapeutic agreement with him. It would also negate the very real positive accomplishments they had made by suggesting they had not done the "real" work (see Basch, 1980, for a further discussion of this idea). And as a result it would also diminish Hank's and Trish's sense that they could trust George, who might represent a different kind of father figure to Hank, to do what he said he would. He thought it was far better to end the contract as they wanted, supporting the clear gains they had made, and leaving the door open for further contact if they should feel the need for it, either individually or as a couple. Because he knew that therapy was not something they were familiar with, he also made a few suggestions of the types of things that might be signals that they should come back to see her. "Sometimes sleep problems, nightmares, arguments that you feel like you didn't really want to get into, feelings of frustration, changes in appetite, or a return of some of the pain you were feeling; or if the two of you aren't able to keep doing the work we've started. All of those things could come back. It doesn't mean you've failed in anyway. Sometimes it takes a few brush-up times in therapy to completely change habits that we tend to fall into without realizing it."

Not Pushing a Client Out of the Door

Therapists have a reputation for holding onto clients far too long. Perhaps out of a fear of being seen in this way, therapists sometimes end the work prematurely, before a client has accomplished his own goals. It is important to remember that sometimes a client would like to continue to work with us on longer term goals. I have often had supervisees share that they are concerned that they are forcing clients, either directly or indirectly, to stay in therapy for their own (the clinician's) needs. When I have explored this concern, I occasionally hear that a client is communicating, albeit sometimes indirectly or very subtly, a desire to end the work. Often, however, I have heard material that suggests that a client is happy to be coming to therapy. For example, he arrives on time or even early for all of his appointments, brings in material that shows that he has been thinking about or responding to previous sessions, and talks about changes that he or his family and/or friends have noticed since he started coming to therapy. This material may be blended with less overt expressions of anxiety about potential loss of the support of therapy or with behavior that is still problematic or indicates an underlying resistance to the work. Overt compliance can, of course, also disguise resistance. An assessment of a client's actual needs can be colored by a clinician's needs; but it can also be colored by a clinician's worries about imposing those needs on a client.

Many of the clinicians who have discussed fears about "keeping" a client in therapy past the time they should be there have expressed something like, "I am enjoying the work, and I don't want to keep him (a client) in therapy just because I enjoy it." In my experience, it is often (though certainly not always) the case that if a clinician is enjoying the process, a client is getting something out of it as well. Rather than stopping therapy arbitrarily because of an "experience-distant" application of theory, it can be an important part of the process to engage a client in a discussion of his accomplishments thus far, and a reassessment of his goals and expectations. Such a discussion must be engaged in with some care. Clients often attempt to read between the lines of any intervention; and they may experience such an exploration as a clinician's attempts to get them end therapy.

This kind of miscommunication can be alleviated—or turned into further grist for the therapeutic mill—if a clinician shares something of her thought processes with her client, not only in this discussion but also throughout the exploratory process. As noted in Chap. 7, showing how we think is not the same thing as disclosing all of our feelings and wishes. As Renik (2006) explains, it is instead a way of modeling what we hope our clients will learn to do in the course of any integrative therapeutic work: pay attention to the gradual unfolding of their own thoughts and feelings.

Modeling one's thought processes in this way can also help when a client has a hidden agenda (see Barth, 2003).

Conclusion

Frank (1999) reminds us that any psychotherapy is an interactive process between two individuals. Not only does a clinician's theoretical approach impact the work, but a client's personality, style, needs, capacity to understand and ability to act (what Frank, 1999, calls "talent for action") also color how much and what kind of work gets done in therapy. Setting small, realistic goals and recognizing and reinforcing small achievements is extremely useful in managing individual differences in the capacity to accomplish therapeutic change.

Chapter 9
Building and Working with an Integrative Team

Keywords Fragile clients • Interdisciplinary teams • Teamwork • Managing conflict • Splitting • Support • Clinical interventions • Research • Clinical illustrations • Integrative social work practice • Evidence • Cognitive therapy • Behavioral therapy • Body-mind dynamics • Psychodynamic work • Attachment • Secure base

When I was in analytic training, it was generally accepted that working with more than one clinician would be harmful to a client. The belief was that having two therapists would disrupt the development of transference, which was where much of the therapeutic work was supposed to take place. But in the psychiatric hospital where I worked and in the agency where I saw people with eating disorders, many clients were in therapy with several different professionals at the same time, since they might be in any combination of medical, group, family, individual, nutritional and occupational therapy. I discovered that there were actually a number of advantages to a client's being seen by several different therapists. Team members provided different perspectives on dynamics and behaviors, supported one another through difficult situations, and provided backup so that a client was never without the support of a known and trusted therapist. Meissner (1983) and Adler (1985) discuss the importance of such backup for the needs of both client and clinician, especially when working with fragile or difficult clients who need extra support or tend to fragment or de-stabilize when their primary therapist is unavailable. What I learned during those years was that when a team worked together to help a client manage difficulties and explore conflicts, the therapeutic process seemed enhanced rather than diluted by the involvement of more than one professional, and even, when appropriate, more than one therapist.

Teamwork, or "work done by several associates with each doing a part but all subordinating personal prominence to the efficiency of the whole" (Merriam Webster Online Dictionary, 2013), has become increasingly popular in fields ranging from business to medicine to education. Research shows that teamwork can improve productivity in business to a significant degree (Ezzamel & Willmott, 1998)

F.D. Barth, *Integrative Clinical Social Work Practice: A Contemporary Perspective*, Essential Clinical Social Work Series, DOI 10.1007/978-1-4939-0351-1_9,

and, in medical settings, can significantly reduce accidental patient death (Lerner, Magrane, & Friedman, 2009). Although the data to date on the impact of teamwork on mental health is somewhat limited, what has been done suggests that teamwork in this field can improve client care as well (Brown, Crawford, & Darongkamas, 2000; Dorahy & Hamilton, 2009).

Teamwork also seems to be a natural component of an integrative approach. Given that a single practitioner cannot know every possible way of working with every possible combination of difficulties presented by clients, and given the idea that an integrative approach can often enhance our clinical work, it seems natural that at some point a team might be a useful way of working with certain clients. However, how does this work? When do we decide to utilize a team approach? What are some of the potential pitfalls, and how can an integrative clinician avoid them?

Throughout this book we have seen examples of teamwork, some formally and others more loosely organized. In the mental health field, teams may be formally organized, in an agency or hospital or college counseling office, or informal, for instance when a psychotherapist in private practice refers a client for adjunct work such as medical intervention, family or group therapy, nutritional or job coaching, and so on. They may be well-planned or ad hoc; they may be instigated at the suggestion of a clinician, physician or client. They may involve different forms of psychotherapy, different professions and/or different modalities. Sometimes a team may even be composed of two therapists doing basically the same work, but in different settings. September 25, 2013.

When I began working with college students struggling with eating disorders, I discovered that they were often struggling with what we then called separation-individuation issues, and also with what, as I explained in Chap. 3, I would now call attachment-individuation issues (Barth, 2003; Lyons-Ruth, 1991). Often these difficulties were linked not only to their current developmental stage of development, but also to earlier difficulties negotiating the difficult process of individuating from and remaining attached to their parents. And equally often, the separation difficulties were also linked to problems they had with self-soothing and self-regulation, for which they still needed parental assistance, but for any number of reasons were either unable to obtain or accept from their parents. Sometimes lack of ability to self-soothe was related to parental management of the complex process of separating from, yet still maintaining a connection to, their maturing child. At other times, it was related to the child's physiological and personality characteristics. Many times incapacity to soothe and regulate the self was simply a result of an adolescent and family having a particularly hard time with some of the developmental demands of this stage of life.

What I learned was that it was often useful to take a team approach to this work. For example, it could be important to coordinate with a physician and/or nurse who would supervise medical issues related to a client's weight loss and physical condition. Since we were discovering that anti-depressant medication helped many of these young women, it was also important to stay in touch with the prescribing psychopharmacologist in order to monitor the effectiveness of the drugs and their potentially serious side effect. n. My regular contact with the psychiatrist helped us address resistance and minimize acting out with medication. For many of our clients with eating disorders, a mixture of family, group and individual work was often more beneficial than a single therapeutic approach (see also Brown et al., 2000; Stewart & Williamson, 2004). Expediency, experience and training meant that sometimes the same clinician worked in several modalities and sometimes the involvement of several different professionals was needed.

I also found that while it might complicate the transference to one therapist or the other, it could also be extremely helpful for some of these young women to have two different therapists—one at school and the other when they were home for holidays and summer vacation. One advantage to this system was an "in-person" relationship with two supportive professionals. Although splitting was sometimes a problem, as we will discuss shortly, this arrangement actually seemed to help clients build a strong alliance with both clinicians, which was particularly useful in terms of dealing with separation issues and developing a greater capacity for self-soothing and managing affects. I have written about the idea that eating disorders in college students are often related to developmental struggles in the arena of separation and attachment (Barth, 1989, 2003). Issues of object constancy and affect regulation can be overwhelming during this period. Having a face-to-face relationship with a therapist both at school and at home provided a secure base in each place when a client had a tendency to over-exercise, restrict food intake, withdraw, and/or lose a dangerous amount of weight in a short period of time. Although phone sessions were sometimes useful, we discovered that it was important to have a professional who could see any physical changes that a client might not report herself.

Similarly, despite traditional ideas about separating parents from their adolescent children's therapy and therapist in order to protect their nascent identities, I have found that it is often extremely important for the parents' and individual therapists to work closely together in many of these cases. Issues of confidentiality and privacy are relatively simple to manage when both clinicians focus on the common goal of helping a youngster and her family move away from problematic patterns of behavior. Team work also can help both therapists recognize that there are two sides (at least) to most difficulties. Splitting, victimization and parent-blaming, which are all common complications in this work, can be ameliorated by ongoing team contact.

Group work, family therapy and medical supervision also often provide a sense of safety, a secure base from which these clients can begin to integrate a healthy and functional sense of self as they move into the adult world. Knowing that the professionals involved are pulling together to help her get better can be a powerful factor in a client's investment in her own therapeutic development. Recognizing that symptoms are often the result of an interaction of a number of complex dynamics can also help eliminate blame and criticism not only within the family, but also between professionals. This is particularly useful in dealing with families in conflict, where interpersonal antagonism can derail the therapeutic work. Open communication and a respectful stance can also help clinicians manage the splitting that often occurs when there is more than one therapist involved.

Clearly, one of the potential pitfalls of such an approach is that for some clients such information-sharing feels like an invasion of privacy or a crossing of personal boundaries. In order to make decisions about how a team will proceed with each client, therefore, a thorough assessment of a client's needs, dynamics and goals must be made.

Tools for Working in a Team

Working with a team can sometimes be complicated and requires specific tools, but an integrative practitioner already has many of these tools in her repertoire. Three important tools that we have actually already discussed in other contexts make teamwork viable. They are (1) establishment of mutually agreed-upon goals; (2) mutual respect; and (3) open communication. As these three aspects of a team are operationalized, they enhance and strengthen all therapeutic alliances and a client's sense of agency.

Establishing Goals

As we talked about in the chapter on the therapeutic relationship, it is extremely important for a clinician to engage with a client around establishing goals for the work. Often this means both helping a client articulate previously unformulated desires as well as both short-term and long-term goals. A clinician must also be clear with a client about what he is able to provide, and how he will provide it. This brings the question of information-sharing into the work early in therapy. This is one of the times when the myriad of unpleasant paper-work that is part of our professional lives today actually serves an important therapeutic function. When we ask clients to sign releases for us to share and/or gather information, we have an opportunity to explore their feelings about our talking to others concerning them, and to establish boundaries for those discussion.

For example, when Laurie, the young dancer, began working with both her individual therapist, Ms. Herman, and the team at the drug treatment center, there was a great deal of discussion about what Ms. Herman would and would not share with James, who headed up Laurie's team. From the perspective of the treatment center, Ms. Herman was being brought onto the team and therefore expected to share everything Laurie told her. From Ms. Herman's perspective, such an expectation could be potentially damaging to her work with Laurie. As she and Laurie explored this issue, they opened up a number of extremely important aspects of Laurie's dynamics centering on boundaries. For example, it turned out that Laurie was extremely close with her mother, with whom she shared everything about herself and her life. Her mother then told everything to her father. "I know she's going to tell him," Laurie said, "which means I don't ever have a real conversation with him." Ms. Herman asked her to talk about how that worked. "Well, sometimes it's fine. But other times it feels like I don't have a real relationship with him, either."

One way of thinking about therapy is that it gives clients an opportunity to tell someone else their personal stories, and in the process, to hear some of the contradictions and/or unformulated meanings contained in ideas they have always simply taken for granted. As Laurie and Ms. Herman focused on the ways in which Laurie and her parents had traditionally interacted, Laurie began to wonder if she could have a different kind of relationship with each of her parents. The work with Ms. Herman and James became a kind of testing ground for some of the changes she gradually began to put in place with her family, and eventually with friends, colleagues and her boyfriend.

Communication

Communication between team members is probably the single most important means of keeping a team running smoothly. A formal, structured team generally has built-in regular meetings which often provide an opportunity for working through issues related to clients' needs and team conflicts. Thus it is important for a team leader to set the stage for open, nonjudgmental exchanges of information and ideas. When I worked on a locked inpatient unit of a psychiatric hospital many years ago, I learned the importance of such leadership very quickly. The psychiatrist and head nurse had worked together for many years and encouraged team members to talk openly about a variety of issues related to patient care. When the team began to uncharacteristically argue about applying standard rules to a recent admission, the nurse grinned at the psychiatrist and said, "Guess we've got a borderline on the unit." They explained that in their experience, clients with Borderline Personality Disorder frequently seemed to unintentionally but dynamically stir up conflict in an otherwise cohesive unit. Besides offering helpful lessons in assessment and splitting, these two pros helped the team begin to sort out the conflict and understand the ways that certain interactions from the client had divided and stirred up conflict among the team members. Working with this client in both family and group therapy, I found that understanding the dynamics within the context of the team helped me begin to recognize and address splitting that appeared in both therapeutic settings.

Communication among members of an informal team often requires more effort on the part of the members, since there is not a built-in structure of regular meetings available. However, it is worth the energy, since maintaining some sort of ongoing interactive contact is often crucial to the smooth flow of the different aspects of the therapy. Assessing a client's needs and negotiating with client and all collaterals over confidentiality, loyalty and goals are important. Recognizing that team members have different but not mutually exclusive techniques is part of the process. Similarly, goals of an identified client may need clarification when the client base also expands to family and group members.

Mutual Respect

Clearly, there are ways in which each of these factors interacts with the others. According to researchers, one important key to successful teamwork lies in mutual respect and trust between team members (Ezzamel & Willmott, 1998; West et al., 2012). Mutual respect involves both acknowledgement of one another's strengths and open but courteous communication about conflicts or disagreements. By definition an integrative perspective recognizes the importance of different types of interventions, different skill sets and different views of the same client's dynamics. However, even these firmly held beliefs cannot always provide an adequate buffer against feelings of frustration and devaluation when a client chooses one form of therapy over another, or prefers one clinician to another. One important antidote to such conflicts is open and mutually respectful discussion between team members when such conflicts arise.

Part of the work for an integrative clinician, whether or not she is in the role of team leader, is to help a client make the best use of the team experience. This may mean running interference for a client when there is conflict among team members, or helping a client negotiate different aspects of the team experience. It also may mean accepting and working with some negative transference from a client and/or from other members of a team.

For example, in the drug treatment facility where James worked with Laurie, there were daily team conferences to discuss each client's progress and difficulties. Ms. Herman became an informal adjunct to the team, although there was some concern about this "bump" in their system among the staff at the agency, and Ms. Herman felt that there was also some resentment from staff both because she did not join the daily meetings, and also about her "special" relationship with Laurie. Laurie seemed to be sensing this conflict but was unable to put it into words until she complained that she was starting to binge again. "How can this be?" she demanded. "I've been doing so well!"

Ms. Herman asked her to talk about what had been happening in the days before she started bingeing, and Laurie said that some of the staff was making comments about her being given special treatment. "And that made you uncomfortable?"

Laurie nodded. Based on the material that she and Laurie were opening up, she hypothesized that some of these feelings mirrored some of Laurie's dynamics within her family. She said to Laurie, "It's sort of like you and your mom isn't it? You tell me everything, and then I'm supposed to share it with James and the folks at the center. But I think they may feel like you and I are both getting special treatment. Maybe they're a little envious?"

Laurie said that she hated that idea. "I don't want anyone ever to envy me." Ms. Herman asked her to talk about that concern, and Laurie spoke about how much she hated people she envied, and how she did not want anyone to feel that way about her. I have written about how envy is often viewed as all-bad, and the importance of helping clients begin to see some other aspects of this so-called negative emotion

(Barth, under consideration for publication). Ms. Herman was working to help Laurie begin to manage some of the contradictory aspects of her feelings, and also to put the feelings into the context of some of her personal stories. She therefore offered Laurie an explanation of why these feelings distressed her so much. "I think maybe they feel like they disrupt all of the good feelings you have about someone or that someone might have about you," she said. Laurie agreed. "I don't think they have to do that," Ms. Herman said. "Maybe we can find some ways for you to feel special and maybe even be envied, but also to help the staff and the other members of your group feel that they're special too?"

Laurie was intrigued by the idea but wondered if it was being manipulative. Ms. Herman asked her to talk about that concern, which opened up more of Laurie's feelings and more of her personal story. It turned out that she felt that to talk directly to her father would in some way be manipulative. "It's like I want him to pay attention to me, and that's how I get him to do it." Ms. Herman said she had a slightly different perspective, and asked Laurie if she would like to hear it. When Laurie nodded, she said, "I think people don't always know when they are loved or cared about. I wonder if both James and your dad feel like you don't talk to them because you don't like them." Laurie did not think this could possibly be true, because she adored her father and had a huge crush on James, but she was willing to try an experiment suggested by Ms. Herman. "Let's take me out of the equation with James and the other team members about one thing," she said. "You choose what, but why don't you try talking to James about something you haven't shared with him before now? And if that seems to work out, maybe you can try the same thing with your dad."

Basch (1980) writes about the stories that we tell ourselves about our parents and how these stories are often based on childhood explanations of parental behavior. Since children have limited explanations for complex behavior, it can be powerful to re-examine the stories from an adult perspective and sometimes, as Basch beautifully illustrates, can lead to significant changes not only in parent-child relationships, but in how that individual experiences other aspects of her life as a result. In Laurie's case, beginning to speak directly to James was not easy, but it was both freeing and empowering. She then spoke to her father and found that he responded with such gentleness and pleasure that she could not imagine why she had never done so before. "It just wasn't part of the story," Ms. Herman said. "You're writing the next chapter now."

In this discussion Ms. Herman directly addressed both the team issues and goals and the dynamics that she and Laurie were working on. She also encouraged Laurie to be an active part of her own team. In doing so she was also helping promote her client's sense of agency, and offering an opportunity to talk about, explore and hopefully work through long-term sibling rivalry and problematic interactional issues with parental figures within the context of an in vivo experience. And she was engaging with Laurie in negotiating and setting a contract and boundaries for their therapeutic relationship both individually and as part of a team.

A More Complex Therapeutic Alliance

An umbrella over all of these concepts is the therapeutic alliance. Adler (1985) notes that mutuality and collaboration are important components of any therapeutic alliance. As we have also discussed throughout this book, significant amounts of research (e.g. Meissner, 2007a, 2007b) show that a strong working alliance with a professional improves a client's chances of recovery from a wide variety of ailments, both physical and psychological. Mutually agreed upon goals, mutual respect, and communication are components of a strong therapeutic alliance. When the therapeutic alliances are with more than one clinician, there is a possibility of splintering and disintegration that can disrupt the positive outcome. Mutual support and respect among team members, even in the face of disagreement with one another, can help clients manage splitting and other forms of internal conflict that may be manifested in their relationships with team members. Division of labor can also help both clients and clinicians manage the multiple transferences. One of the ways that this approach can be helpful is when a resistant client is able to transfer positive feelings about one clinician or form of therapy onto another, which he may be more reluctant to try.

For instance, at the agency where Hank, the emergency worker went first for acupuncture and then for couple's therapy, team members met weekly to discuss any problems that might arise with clients, but they did not formally discuss shared clients on a regular basis. However, the sense that all of the members worked together as a team was very strong, and was communicated both directly and indirectly to clients. When his acupuncturist referred Hank to a couples' therapist, it was done seamlessly because they were both part of the same team. Hank said that he trusted his acupuncturist to send him to a good guy. After they had developed a positive relationship with George, their couple's therapist, Trish, Hank's wife, told George that she was worried about Hank.

"She always worries," Hank said. But when George gently probed, it turned out that Hank was having nightmares again and that he was often irritable. George recommended that he see one of the individual therapists on staff. "He's part of our team," he said, "so if you'd like, I can tell him some of what we've been working on." This information-sharing, which for some clients feels like an invasion of privacy, was perfect for Hank who had difficulty talking about himself and his feelings. George went on to say, "I think this is something you can get under control pretty easily. He has some tools that will help you deal with whatever's triggering the nightmares. You should feel better after that." Because Hank had already come to trust two members of the team—the acupuncturist and George—and also because he knew that some of his older and respected colleagues had also utilized the agency, Hank accepted the referral to the individual therapist this time. Thus in some situations a team approach can not only make a client feel safer, but it can sometimes also help some clients overcome resistance to the therapeutic process itself.

Trust is also an important factor, but it does not come automatically. As we have discussed, trust is something that must be earned by a clinician. Clients bring different degrees of trust to their therapy. A capacity for trust is built by life experiences and personality; but a client's reasons for seeking help and the setting in which they are being seen will also color their feelings about any new clinician. Clients also put their therapists through conscious and unconscious tests to help them decide whether or not they can trust both the clinician and the clinic (see Weiss & Sampson, 1986). The same is true about developing a positive relationship with a team.

Transference to a Team or to a Setting

When I was in college, I worked as an aide in a residential treatment facility with young children who for various reasons could not live at home or even in a foster home. While these youngsters became attached to individual members of the treatment team, they were often more significantly attached to the residence itself. When sent home for an overnight, they would show evidence of separation anxiety; and when they returned in an agitated state to the building after a visit with a parent, they could be calmed by sitting in a familiar and comfortable chair and watching television, or sitting at their regular spot at the table and having a snack. Interestingly, many of the children had a parent and often a sibling who had grown up either at that residence or within the umbrella of the larger agency that managed it. One of the long-term staff members, who had worked with several of these multigenerational clients, told me that the parents brought their children to the facility "the way you and I would take our little ones to stay with our parents when we needed help managing them." Transference, then, was to the institution and not necessarily to an individual. In attachment language, the institution was the secure base for the parents and became a secure base for their children.

Although Winnicott is known for his contributions to individual psychoanalysis, he has also left us a lovely description of his own discovery of the importance of the setting, not just as a transference object, but also as a soothing and containing other. His comments are, like so much of his writing, poetic and inspirational. Part of his war-time work was at a residence for boys separated from their families in England during World War II. The youngsters at what he calls a "wartime hostel for evacuation failures" were acting out, having difficulties with the separation that was supposed to protect them from the trauma and danger of the bombings in the cities. As we know today, this well-intentioned separation was actually far more traumatic than anyone had imagined, so from a contemporary perspective it is not surprising that Winnicott's exploratory approach and focus on intrapsychic conflict did not have the impact that he had hoped. He describes something else that was far more useful in helping the boys deal with their emotional pain. As he puts it, "the therapy was being done in the institution, by the walls and the room, by the glass conservatory which provided a target for bricks, by the absurdly large baths…by the cook, by the regularity of the arrival of food on the table, by the warm enough… bedspreads, by the efforts of David [the director] to maintain order in spite of shortage of staff and a constant sense of futility of it all…" (Winnicott, 2011, material in brackets added by this author).

Some Difficulties for a Team Therapist

Winnicott touches on an important aspect of teamwork in this brief but beautiful paper. Gently laughing at himself and his own grandiosity, he describes "growing downward," the phrase with which he characterizes learning that his psychoanalytic skills were only a tiny part of the therapeutic community that was healing these boys. Although we recognize the importance of a therapeutic relationship to the successful outcome of the work we do, in some cases a successful transference is to a setting or an institution instead of an individual. As Kohut (1971) points out, a clinician needs to have a good handle on his own narcissistic needs in order to work well with clients who cannot view him as a separate entity. Humility and team spirit can be important tools when working with clients whose transference is to a group rather than to an individual therapist. The three tools described above are useful in helping team members negotiate the narcissistic injuries that may occur when we find ourselves less significant as individuals and important only in the context of the team.

Agreeing on Goals

Different professionals may have widely differing goals for a client, not only in terms of what is to be accomplished, but also in terms of how the goals will be achieved. A psychopharmacologist, for example, may focus on immediate symptom-relief while a psychoanalyst or psychodynamically-oriented psychotherapist may see symptoms as signals of underlying issues that need to be addressed. Family members, friends and clients themselves also often have varying expectations. For example, a man who complains incessantly about his girlfriend will perhaps be encouraged by friends and family to seek a solution—either to go for couple's therapy or to consider ending the relationship. Yet there may be psychodynamic reasons that he stays with this woman, for instance that he is uncomfortable acknowledging how much he depends on her, or that he doubts his ability to meet another woman. However, he may not be consciously aware of these issues and may not be able to articulate them even if he is aware. This can make an assessment of the dynamics and the goals toward which he wants and needs to be working difficult. One of the benefits of a team is that a clinician can consult with other professionals who know a client to help make such an assessment.

Splitting, which is generally viewed as problematic, and which can certainly create difficulties in teamwork, can also paradoxically sometimes be worked with more easily in a team than in individual therapy. When a client views one member of a team as helpful and kind and another as potentially critical and unkind, if the team members can remain united during the process, they can provide an opportunity to work through some of the difficulties this client has in interpersonal relationships. The process often involves both clinicians accepting and being curious about that client's feelings about both of them without judgment or defensiveness. Eventually, some of the "other side" of these feelings may begin to emerge in a client's conscious awareness. It is important for both clinicians to listen carefully to these tiny shifts, but without insisting that a client acknowledge the feelings or accept their presence until he has tools for coping with these emotions. Sometimes exploring how a client would like to handle team-related issues can provide an opportunity for developing some of these tools and building skills for using them.

For example, with Laurie's permission, Ms. Herman reached out to James to find out more about his team's concerns and goals for Laurie and to explain any dynamics that she saw and thought might be useful for the team to work with. She was careful, however, to protect Laurie's confidentiality at the same time. As she explained to Laurie, "Unless there is something that I think is putting you in danger, or something specific that they need to know—which I will try to discuss with you before I share it with them—I will talk to James more about dynamics than about specific things you tell me." Laurie wanted to know what that meant, so Ms. Herman gave her an example that actually reflected on some of the transference issues that were beginning to emerge in their work.

"You've told me you have a crush on James, right?" Laurie nodded. "So I wouldn't tell him that, of course." Laurie sighed with relief. "But you told me the other day that you feel angry that he gives some of the other group members more attention than he does to you. I might ask if he has noticed that you are more withdrawn in the group and ask him what he thinks that's about. And I might ask how they approach group dynamics. Once I hear what he says, I might say that I think that you're feeling something that's like what you feel in your family—a little sibling rivalry—and ask if he has any thoughts about how you might deal with that." Laurie was both fascinated and uncomfortable with the idea that Ms. Herman would share this information about her with James.

"Does it feel like I would be exposing you in some way?" Ms. Herman asked.

Laurie nodded and said, "I know that doesn't make sense, because I've talked to him about those things, but somehow it still feels like you're going behind my back and opening up something I'm not ready to open up."

Ms. Herman said, "We've been working on boundaries—how you can pay more attention to them, and set and maintain them even with people you're close to. This sounds like it's somehow connected to that theme. Let's keep talking about it for a while and see where it takes us. So for the moment I won't say anything to James about this issue, then, unless he brings it up himself. And if he does, I'll tell him you and I have discussed it and ask him to talk with you about it. Does that feel okay to you?"

Laurie nodded. "I can't believe that you actually will do what feels right to me," she said. "What if I'm wrong? You're the professional. How can I tell you what to do?"

This discussion opened up many different aspects not only of Laurie's therapy, but also of her dynamics in the world at large. Ongoing conversation about her own ideas about what she needed led to a further elaboration of the idea that feelings and thoughts are not static. They are part of a process, and they develop and become clarified in interaction with another person.

Conclusion

Teams provide a number of supports for clients, including back-up in time of crisis and different perspectives on a client's dynamics. They can also create difficulties, of course, including splitting and conflict within a team, which can then interfere with a client's therapeutic progress. Mutual respect and mutually established goals among team members and client(s) can help ameliorate such conflict. Recognizing that therapy is a process and maintaining open and honest communication about that process can be key not only to teamwork, but to the therapeutic work itself.

Chapter 10
Working On and Working Through

Keywords Research • Clinical examples • Evidence • Integrative social work practice • Research • Phases of therapy • Beginning • Middle • End • Small steps • Process • Detailed inquiry • Cognitive therapy • Behavioral therapy • Mindfulness • Psychodynamic therapy • Body-mind • Development • Long-term therapy • Short-term therapy • Termination • Ending

In this final chapter, we will look more closely at how an integrative clinician works. By now it should be clear that an integrative practice begins with the first contact with a client, whether it is a phone call to arrange a consultation or an initial meeting in an agency waiting room, and continues throughout the therapeutic work, until and even beyond the termination process. The two organizing principles of (1) a detailed inquiry, or nonjudgmental curiosity about the small particulars of a person's life, and (2) an awareness of the significance of process, both in life and in therapy, can help a clinician make an empathic and professional assessment of a client's needs at any point in their work together. Such an assessment is crucial in determining what interventions will be probably most helpful to that client at that time. As we have seen, a client's response to any intervention is part of any process and provides invaluable data that can help determine the next therapeutic steps. Before turning to this more detailed clinical material, I would simply like to remind readers that these examples are amalgams created from clinical material I have gathered from many sources over the course of a long professional career. Therefore, while they represent situations I have encountered as a clinician, supervisor and consultant, they are not descriptive of any actual clients or clinicians.

As I was working on this chapter, I asked myself why I was returning to this point at the end of this book. Confidentiality needs to always be recognized and respected, whether a therapist is writing process notes for supervision, progress notes and information for records and for insurance purposes, or, as in this case, for clinical discussion. Yet I believe I felt the need to reiterate the way that I write illustrative material at this juncture in the book because of the topic I am about to

F.D. Barth, *Integrative Clinical Social Work Practice: A Contemporary Perspective*, Essential Clinical Social Work Series, DOI 10.1007/978-1-4939-0351-1_10,

discuss: the issue of trust in a therapeutic relationship. Many individuals who seek professional assistance have multiple difficulties feeling safe with others. Some are unwilling or unable to open up to another person for fear of being hurt, rejected, abandoned or worse. Others cannot let go of give up control to another, even for a therapeutic purpose. And still others trust too easily, sometimes indiscriminately, thereby leaving themselves open to boundary violation and loss of self.

While some of these fears may be the result of problematic and/or traumatic experiences with some of the people they should have been able to feel safe with, some are also linked to an inability to trust themselves. As one young man who was speaking to me about his fear that his wife might be unfaithful put it, "I don't know if I would be able to stop myself from doing something I shouldn't with another woman, if the opportunity arose. So how can I believe she won't do the same thing?" This is one of the places in which process is central, since genuine confidence in both self and other can be built only through an ongoing process over time. Unfortunately, in the current climate of health care makes it difficult to engage in the time-consuming progression of rupture and repair that Kohut (1971, 1984) says is the path to such assurance. Still, even in the short term, a therapist's understanding of and nonjudgmental curiosity about inevitable empathic failures can be a therapeutic building block for developing confidence in self and other.

Working On and Working Through

When I turned fifty, I decided to learn Spanish. It was something that I had wanted to do for a long time, and I had even taken a short course in it one summer, but I never seemed to have the time that I needed to truly begin to learn the language. Now I decided that whatever it took, I was going to become conversant in the language. It was a far more difficult task than I had imagined, but I was very lucky to find an incredibly talented, patient and often funny teacher Painstakingly going over material numerous times, repeating vocabulary I "should" have known, he helped me gradually, bit by bit, learn to speak Spanish. And he reminded me of another lesson, one that I had learned in social work graduate school and again in psychoanalytic training: that learning does not happen all at once and is never complete. It is an ongoing process. Loewald (1989) writes about this phenomenon, suggesting that understanding the learning process is a key to doing psychotherapy.

I like to keep this experience in mind when, as sometimes happens, clinicians consult with me because they feel that their work with a particular client is stale or stuck. Although a client is sometimes genuinely not moving forward, often there is deep but quiet work happening. Both members of a therapeutic dyad may feel that they are simply repeating themselves; but sometimes important learning is happening in these repetitions. This is what makes the so-called middle phase of therapy perhaps one of the hardest parts of the clinical process. Whether it lasts a month or a year, whether the interventions are cognitive, psychodynamic, developmental, or bodily, it is often a time when work is progressing, and yet it may seem that it is not going anywhere.

Patience, thoughtfulness and a sense of humor can help us get through this period, as can an understanding that sometimes while in the center of the process, we cannot see or feel how much is actually happening. In the early phase of therapy, client and clinician are getting to know one another. As time goes on, however, and the pair gets more comfortable with one another, the work can seem to slow down. Patterns have become clear, but they continue to be repeated despite both client's and therapist's best efforts. Resistances emerge. Now is when an integrative approach can be particularly useful.

For example, if a clinician is using a cognitive framework to help a client change patterns of behavior, and some patterns simply are not responding, it can be useful to take a few sessions to work on understanding what might be interfering with the work. What anxieties, fears or discomforts is a client avoiding? What would it actually mean to change? What might be the dangers of living without the old symptoms?

Recognizing Patterns and Themes

While most approaches look for repetitive patterns of problematic behavior, there is a wide range of positions on how these patterns should be dealt with. Novick (1982) calls this middle period an "incubation period" during which an idea can develop and take form. In my experience, there are a number of such phases in any therapeutic work. One part of a clinician's task is to provide a setting that feels safe and comfortable for the incubating work to go on. Recognizing patterns, helping clients see continuity from session to session and within their own experience can be part of the incubating work. "Here it is again," or "I'm doing it again," is often said with shame and embarrassment. Yet patterns are part of what makes us human. Beginning to see them when they happen is the first step in being able to change. Reinforcing a client's successful recognition of a pattern, or what Bollas (1989) describes as celebrating the arrival of an emotion, can be a powerful therapeutic intervention.

This is how it happened with Tricia and Hank. Hank was feeling better, and he and Tricia were getting along much better. They were discussing the possibility of ending their work with George in one session, and then they came into the next session quite distraught. George looked at each of them and waited for one of them to start to talk, as they usually did. But neither one said a word. "You look pretty upset," he said. "Are you having troubles talking about it?" They both nodded. "Okay, so why don't we go back to the way we used to start. Would that be okay?" Again they nodded. George reminded them that one of them would tell the story in their own words, without being interrupted by the other, and then they would switch, with the other talking without interruption, even if they did not agree with each other's interpretation of events. They nodded again, but neither was willing, or perhaps able, to start, so George suggested that Tricia, who he knew was the most talkative in general, start the ball rolling.

Not looking at Hank, Tricia said that he was having nightmares again.

"It's just been a couple of times, for pity's sake," Hank said. George knew that Hank saw any psychological distress as a sign of weakness; George responded that he realized it probably was not a huge deal, but that at the same time, he knew that Hank needed his sleep in order to be up to the demands of his job. "Yeah, well, if it gets worse I'll get some sleeping pills," Hank replied.

"What about going back to the acupuncturist?" George asked.

Hank was surprisingly unenthusiastic about the idea. "I thought you found her really helpful," George said. "Can you talk about what has changed your mind?"

Hank was not happy talking about it, but Tricia said that he had told her that he did not like lying on the table with the little needles in his back. George turned to Hank and asked if Tricia had gotten it right.

"Yeah," he said. "I didn't mind it so much at first. And it did help. But I just can't get myself to go back and do it again."

George could have tried to explore Hank's resistance further, but he was concerned about undermining Hank's sense of self-confidence, which was crucial to his work and had already been compromised by the very fact of his asking for help and by his continuing to come to couples therapy. Instead of digging into the material, George opted to share something of his own experience, knowing that Hank identified with and admired him. He said that he understood Hank's feelings about the needles, that he occasionally went for acupuncture and although he found it helpful, he was not particularly fond of the procedure either; and then he added, "But let's see if we can find some other ways to get these nightmares under control."

As we discussed in Chap. 7, much has been written about the pros and cons of self-disclosure (e.g. Gerson, 2001; Goldstein, 1994; Johnson, 1999; Mitchell, 1998). Sharing personal information can be both a powerful tool and disruptive to therapy and needs to be considered carefully. In this instance George believed a limited disclosure would help diminish Hank's feelings of shame and would move the work forward. Mitchell (1999) points out that a clinician does not always know until after the fact why a certain intervention seemed to make sense; but it is extremely important that we try to understand it after the fact, even if we could not explain it to ourselves at the moment. Only in this way can we determine whether our actions are based on a client's needs or our own countertransference enactments. Loewald (1989) writes that confusion and disorganization are necessary parts of learning. Bromberg (1994) suggests that by asking clients to put experience into words, a therapist is not only asking what that experience means, but is also establishing a relational interaction that allows us to understand that meaning. The same is true when a clinician attempts to understand his own unarticulated reasons for any action.

While it is not unusual for either a client or a clinician to feel frustrated at the reappearance of symptoms that seemed to be under control, it is important to recognize that this is a normal part of the working on and working through of therapy. Rather than a sign of failure, it is actually an opportunity to re-visit and re-work issues that are part of a client's dynamics (e.g. Barth, 2008). Recognizing that this was true of the return of Hank's nightmares, George did not feel irritated but instead patiently re-focused the couple on the symptoms. Using something similar to Connors' (2006) two-pronged approach, George reviewed techniques that they had learned for managing the techniques that they had learned to manage the nightmares and also gently probed to see if they could put into words some of the feelings and thoughts that might have triggered them. He reiterated that his goal was to get the nightmares under control. Knowing that Hank would resist any overt sympathy about either the dreams or the lack of sleep, he took a firm, but supportive position as Hank's ally in fighting this problem. He had previously referred Hank for individual therapy, but the couple had reported back that Hank had not gone to see the other therapist. Reluctance to go into individual therapy was not unusual in the population of first responders and emergency workers who were seen at this agency, but George brought the question up again. Hank immediately bridled.

"There's nothing wrong with me. I don't need a head shrinker, thank you very much."

George nodded. He had come to believe that for many of his clients, couples therapy was actually more effective than individual, in part because it was more acceptable within their culture ("oh, you know, the wife made me go with her to talk to somebody" was how one of his clients jokingly said he put it to a buddy) and in part because, if therapy was successful, a spouse could sometimes provide functions that an individual could not provide for him or herself (e.g. see Kohut, 1971; Lapides, 2011). He therefore said that if Hank would like, they could try to deal with what might be stirring up the nightmares and get him back to sleep at night. Hank agreed, although still sounding a little reluctant. George asked if he and Tricia could remember when the first recent set of nightmares had begun.

Hank had no idea, but Tricia said, "Oh yes, it was the night we got back from the beach, honey. You remember? We'd been with the family. I remember, because you'd been out on the dock fishing with little Henry (his nephew), and I thought that was what you were dreaming about. I can't remember why I thought that, though."

Because George had decided to work with the couple as two parts of one whole, using a systems approach, he engaged with Tricia's difficulty remembering as a signal of the couple's difficulties with whatever might be causing Hank's nightmares. They might both be resistant to opening up whatever the underlying issues were; but by exploring the material together, they could be support to one another and perhaps get to some of the material that either one of them might have difficulty addressing alone. George was not trying to help Hank move into psychoanalytic exploration of his underlying conflicts. But since Hank was having troubles using some of the soothing tools he had learned previously, George thought he thought that understanding what might have set off the nightmares could help Hank make use of some of the techniques that had worked before. He therefore worked with the couple as he would have with a resistant client in individual therapy—not pushing for the content of the forgotten memory, but gently asking both of them to try to remember details about the day that Tricia had earmarked as preceding the first nightmare.

Hank looked at Tricia, who said, "Nothing happened that I can think of that might have made Hank have a nightmare."

"Oh, that's okay," said George. "Just take me through the day, step-by-step. What happened, what you did, who you saw, what you were thinking about. It doesn't even have to be in any kind of order." He looked at Hank. "And both of you just jump in and say what you remember."

Tricia began by saying that Hank had gotten up, had a cup of coffee, and then had breakfast. George interrupted her gently. "Actually, Tricia, even though you aren't the one who had the nightmares, I'd like to hear about what you did as well. It will give me a fuller picture of the day."

Together they gradually presented a picture of an idyllic day with Hank's large extended family. George did not try to puncture what he believed might have been an idealized memory, but he believed that something might have gone on that they were not aware of. Since Tricia had said that she somehow thought that first nightmare was related to fishing with Hank's nephew, George decided to see if he could get more details about what had happened down at the dock. Hank answered, since Tricia had not been with them.

"We sat and fished. I had a smoke. Henry's a good kid. Reminds me of myself at that age. He was telling me that he wanted to grow up and be like his dad and me—do the same kind of work."

George noticed a slight shift in Hank's body movement. "Can you use that mindfulness technique we worked on before right now?" he asked. Hank looked surprised. In order not to make Hank feel singled out, he said, "Actually, both of you. Can you close your eyes and just pay attention to what you're feeling physically? What does it feel like in your body? What does your back feel like? Your neck? Your legs? You know the drill, right?"

They both nodded, sat up a little straighter, put their feet flat on the floor, and closed their eyes. They were silent for a few breaths, then Hank looked at George. "So, what did you notice?" George asked.

"I don't know why, but I was feeling tense," Hank said. "My back was tight. I couldn't tell you why. Maybe just because I didn't sleep too well last night."

George nodded. "Were you aware that it was feeling tense earlier today?" he asked. Hank said he had not noticed.

To keep the pressure off of Hank, and because he was working with the couple as a system and thought Tricia's response might help shed some light on the subject, he also asked Tricia about what she had discovered. "I was a little tense, too," she said. "I think it was about Henry. Some of the girls (referring to her mother-in-law and sisters-in-law) and I were talking about how smart he is. We were saying how much we'd like for him to break out of the family tradition and go into another profession. But he thinks Hank walks on water, and wants to be just like him."

"Yeah," Hank said. "We'd all really like him to do something else. Even my dad, whose heart would have broken if I'd followed a different path, wants Henry to make something of himself."

"Hmmm." George said. "Does that mean that your dad doesn't think you made something of yourself?"

Hank looked surprised again. "Nah, he's proud of me. It just means he's seen what the work's done to me and my brothers. It's a lot harder these days than when he started out."

Hank's diagnosis was not PTSD, but George believed that he nonetheless suffered from both direct and secondary trauma (see Tosone, Nuttman-Schwartz, & Stephens, 2012) as a result of his job. Within the context of the couples' work George had taught Tricia and Hank techniques for managing the difficult feelings. These included some simple breath work, mindfulness practice, and some ideas drawn from ACT and DBT workbooks (see Hayes, 2004; Linehan, 1993; Nhat Hanh, 1992). In conjunction with some tools the acupuncturist had also provided, Hank's nightmares and sleep difficulties had receded. Both clinicians had agreed not to label these experiences as trauma-related, because Hank and many of his colleagues viewed the very idea of trauma as a weakness. Therefore it was impressive that Hank's dad, a died-in-the-wool old-schooler, had acknowledged that his sons were being negatively affected by the work they were doing without criticizing them for it.

After obtaining some more details about the day and the evening before the first nightmare, George thought he had an idea about some of the psychological factors that had contributed to the reappearance of Hank's nightmares. He suspected that Hank was feeling some conflicting emotions about his nephew Henry, of whom he was very fond. He was probably worried that he might suffer some of the same (unacknowledged) anxiety and other emotional pain with which Hank struggled; yet at the same time he might also enjoy the boy's admiration and envy his freedom to choose, something Hank and his brothers had not been given. However, rather than point these conflicts out to Hank and Tricia, George asked the couple to both again pay attention to how they were feeling physically and emotionally. Tricia replied that she noticed that she was shredding a tissue in her hands. Hank said that he could feel his legs tensing up.

George reinforced their observations, and asked if they could say what they were feeling emotionally. Tricia said she thought they were both tense. Hank looked at her and then nodded in agreement. George asked if they had any idea why.

Tricia said, "I think Hank worries about Henry." Hank started to deny that he worried, but George said, "Let's hear what Tricia has to say. I think she might be onto something." Tricia said that Henry was like Hank's own kid, and that he wanted him to be happy. "Maybe that conversation that day made us both kind of uncomfortable." George looked at Hank then, and asked if Hank thought that was possible. Hank acknowledged that Tricia might have a point.

It was time for the session to end, so George suggested that they both try to pay attention to any signs that they might be getting worried or tense over the next week, and see if they could try putting some of their concerns into words to each other. "And maybe just for caution's sake, you could try going back to some of those exercises I showed you when you first started coming to see me," George said. He reviewed some of the self-calming exercises he had taught them both, and added a reminder that it might help to do some stretches in the early evening while they were unwinding, before they went to bed. They agreed, and left seeming calmer than when they had come into his office. George was struck by the difference between this session and some of the early meetings with this couple.

Trust in the Therapeutic Relationship

We have looked at the issue of trust previously in the chapters on assessment, the therapeutic relationship, and small steps. Over the years, as I have worked with a wide range of clients and clinicians, I have come to believe that the issue of trust is one of the threads that are woven through, although often not discussed, many different types of psychotherapy. Worked and re-worked in any therapeutic process, I believe that questions about trust of another person link to questions about trusting oneself, and that these questions can be at the heart of an integrative practice. For one thing, in an integrative practice a clinician attempts to understand what a client actually needs rather than to impose a particular type of therapy based on external or, as Kohut (1971) calls it, "experience distant" formulations. For another, as I have pointed out in other chapters, the unconscious testing of another person to ensure that they are trustworthy is both normal and adaptive, even if sometimes frustrating (see Weiss & Sampson, 1986). I have found that a clinician's nonjudgmental acceptance of and interest in a client's doubts and concerns can be an extremely important part of any therapeutic process. In this final chapter, then, let us look at some of the ways that this process can help an integrative clinician practice effectively.

Kohut (1971, 1984) tells us that an ability to tolerate a client's idealization and denigration is necessary for any true therapeutic work to be done. Bollas (1989) similarly notes that both anger and love are part of any therapeutic process, but that one or the other may be too uncomfortable for one or both members of a therapeutic pair to manage. A clinician's capacity to not only endure these difficult emotions, but to be both empathic and interested in what they mean, helps clients work through issues of self-doubt and fear of trusting others—even when these concepts are never verbalized in the therapeutic work, as we saw above. Like many clients, Hank and Tricia did not immediately feel confident that George could help them. In the early days of therapy, in fact, Hank had been quite resistant to most of George's suggestions. But gradually they came to feel that rather than imposing some sort of cold professional techniques on them, George made suggestions that grew directly out of a genuine comprehension of what was troubling them. Over time even Hank's suspicions diminished, so that when George suggested that he go back to some of the old techniques that they had worked on previously, he was willing to comply. The next week he reported that he had forgotten, but Tricia brought up the assignment each night and together they did some stretching, breathing exercises, and mindfulness work. And he had been free of nightmares all week.

Ending

Although a great deal of important psychodynamic work often goes on in the final phase of therapy (e.g. McWilliams,), demands of insurance companies as well as contemporary expectations and life styles do not allow for much exploration of these issues.

However, recently a number of short-term approaches have begun to include discussions of how the termination process can be utilized to enhance or amplify the central themes of any therapeutic work (e.g. Fosha, 2000; Grand, 2009; Miller, Rathus, & Linehan 2006, Selva & Malan, 2004).

Yet even planned terminations cannot change the fact that ending therapy can be difficult for clients and clinicians for a variety of reasons. Not only do old symptoms often re-emerge as clients begin the final phase of the work, but both members of the therapeutic dyad may have to struggle with a re-awakening of their own separation issues as they begin to say goodbye. An integrative approach offers a clinician an opportunity to look at any ending from a several different perspectives, with a goal of finding a way of addressing issues that are most pertinent to a specific client at that specific time.

Hard to Say Goodbye

I have never liked the word "termination" for this part of a clinical experience and was therefore happy to read Davies (2005) comment that it is a cold and clinical term that does not do justice to the deep emotional meaning of the phase. (It is also a little too reminiscent of the popular and violent movie about hired murderers to be a comfortable clinical concept.) Significantly, however, the concept of termination does not resonate with one extremely important component of this part of therapy—the ongoing aspect of the work which a client will be doing now that the clinical process is over. In other words, the last phase of a clinical encounter is both an ending and a beginning—the closing down of an active working alliance and the opening up of a client's ongoing personal practice and integration of what he has learned in the context of this relationship.

Even for individuals without separation difficulties, it can be hard to close down the intense and meaningful relationship that often evolves between client and clinician, sometimes in a surprisingly short period of time. Therapists are sometimes surprised by their sadness and sense of loss when a client they have enjoyed working with leaves therapy, but such feelings seem both normal and appropriate from a perspective that includes both attachment and relational conceptualizations of the relationship. Clients also frequently describe some concern that they have become so attached to a professional who they do not even know very well, but a sense of grief at loss of a supportive and caring person in their lives is a common and normal response to the end of the work.

An integrative perspective can be particularly useful in this phase of a clinical encounter. Different clients have different needs during the ending phase of therapy; and most clients also have needs and capabilities at the end of a clinical experience that are changed from those they had at the beginning, even when old symptoms return for a final farewell. Based on an assessment of a specific client's needs and abilities at this point in time, as well as the goals he and his clinician established, that clinician's personality and professional style, agency policies, and other specifics that color each therapeutic relationship, a clinician can work with a client to choose a way of ending that is both appropriate for and meaningful to her.

Trying to find ways to bring "unthought" feelings into the therapeutic space can be an important part of the work at any stage, but it is not always recognized as part of the ending process. However, since this is often one of the times that both clinician and client's feelings and thoughts are not completely clear, it can frequently be helpful for a clinician to model the process of trying to think and talk about them (Davies, 2005; Renik, 2006) with a client.

Yet it is also important for a clinician to be alert to how a client will experience the feelings he wants to talk about. Who decides when to end?

Most often, a client makes a decision to leave therapy, either because the work is done or because life circumstances make it necessary for him to leave. There are also times, of course, when a client leaves because the work is too hard or the material being opened up is too painful for him to deal with. There are also times when a client is not happy with either his therapist and/or the way his therapist is working. This is one of the times when both an ongoing assessment and an open discussion of goals can aid the therapeutic process. If there has been a clear and honest ongoing discussion, it can be easier for a clinician to express any concerns she might have about a client's decision, and for a client to clarify why she feels that it is time to leave. Such discussions also open the door to discussing the therapeutic relationship, a client's future goals, work he will continue to do outside of the therapist's office, and they clear the way for potential return to therapy at some time in the future.

If a client who is not happy with the direction therapy is taking is willing and able to talk about areas of disappointment, it is also sometimes an opportunity to explore a larger picture of what happens when he is disappointed in others. In some cases, a clinician's willingness to listen and take a client's complaints seriously can actually open up the work in new ways.

This is what happened with Connie, who we met earlier in this book. Her therapist, Dr. Aikens attempted to refer to another clinician when she refused to do any of her assigned DBT tasks. Connie was distressed because she felt that she had disappointed Dr. Aikens. After a consultation with a psychodynamically-oriented clinician, Dr. Aikens was able to shift gears with Connie. Hearing that she was afraid of disappointing him in almost every session, he began to ask her to talk more about this concern and to make some links to these fears in other facets of her life. After exploring this fear in a number of different situations, he also began to hear that she became disappointed in many of the same people she worried about letting down. He asked if this might be a possibility with him. Could she be feeling that he was not giving her what she had wanted or expected from him?

At first Connie denied that she could possibly find anything wrong with his work, but over time, she began to speak of some areas in which she was not completely happy with his suggestions and assignments. Dr. Aikens listened carefully to her complaints and attempted to respond with understanding. In some cases, when appropriate, he even adjusted some of the assignments, so that they better fit Connie's specific needs and lifestyle. Because he was practicing an integrative approach with Connie, he did not have a planned end date with her, but as Connie described feeling more in control and in charge of her own life, he wondered if it was time to move towards ending the work.

As soon as he brought up the question ending, many of Connie's symptoms re-appeared. Dr. Aikens consulted with the therapist to whom he had initially attempted to refer Connie, and she said that she wondered if fear of separation was one of the underlying issues in Connie's initial development of the symptoms. With this dynamic in mind, Dr. Aikens suggested that they not terminate immediately, but spend some time exploring Connie's fears of separation and her difficulties managing the feelings that went along with it. After they had discussed it and explored it for an extended period of time, they agreed to gradually cut back on their meetings. Slowly going from once a week to twice a month and then to once a month allowed Connie time to both get used to managing without the weekly support of Dr. Aikens and also to talk about her struggles with separation in a wide range of situations. They continued to meet more than a year on a once-monthly basis, and then cut back even further. "I just want to know that I can check in with you," said Connie, who had become aware of her need, like a rapprochement aged child, to "check back" with a parental figure. (See Pine, 1985, pp. 143–147, for a wonderful clinical example and discussion of a linked process with a client who almost never came to her sessions.) "I can keep a picture of you in my mind," she said, referring to an ongoing discussion of object constancy. "Is it okay if I call your answering machine from time to time just to hear your voice?"

Dr. Aikens told her she was welcome to do so, and to leave a message for him whenever she liked. He suggested that she let him know if she needed him to call her back or if she simply wanted him to listen to any messages she left. "Would you really do that?" she asked. The question opened up her sense that he might be bored by her, or that it would be a burden for him to listen to her messages. They spent a fair amount of time exploring what this fear was about, which Dr. Aikens found particularly interesting since he had been frustrated, irritated and moved by Connie, but never bored. Eventually she said that this discussion had helped her tremendously. Her fear, she said, had always been that she would disappear from his thoughts and even from his memory when she left therapy. "Out of sight/out of mind," she said. "I like the idea that you will be listening to my voice too."

Unprompted, she also said that she would leave short messages. "I don't want to take up too much of your tape," she said. "I don't need you so much anymore—I can leave space for some of your other clients." She grinned, knowing that he knew that she had once not been able to tolerate the idea that he had other clients.

Not everyone needs a slow weaning from therapy. In other words, as has been true throughout our discussion of an integrative approach, it is very important for a client and clinician to work together to develop an agreement or a contract about how they will proceed in the concluding phase. Once again it is useful to discuss and attempt to establish mutually agreed upon goals and then to move forward based on this agreement. Ideally, client and clinician arrive at a mutual agreement that their work is done, but this ideal is also not always achieved. Clients may leave before a therapist believes they are ready, both with and without alerting their clinician to their planned departure.

Problems of course arise when there is open disagreement, for example, when a client wants to leave therapy and a clinician does not think the time is right. In such cases, it can be extremely important for a clinician to examine his reasons for keeping a client. If the reasons are that he likes working with this client and does not want to lose him, obviously this is something he will need to work out in his own therapy. He may also have goals for the work that his client does not share, and this is something that needs to be explored in supervision. Basch (1980) suggests that when this conflict in goals occurs, if there is no danger to a client, it can be far better to support his gains in therapy and work towards a mutually agreed upon ending than to focus on remaining problems. Acknowledging his strengths and newly learned skills can allow him to leave feeling pleased with the experience, which leaves the door open for a return to the work in the future. Pushing him to see areas of weakness can leave him with both a sense of failure and a bad feeling about therapy itself, which may close the door on future work.

When a Therapist Ends the Work

As I noted earlier, some therapies include a built-in concluding date from the beginning of the work. In such cases there is also sometimes a formal recognition of a client's accomplishments in therapy. Miller et al. (2006), for example, offer a detailed DBT approach to helping vulnerable clients with the ending process when contracted goals have been achieved, including a formalized "graduation" ceremony with certificates and, at times, gifts that have specific meaning to a client and to the work she has done with her DBT therapists. However, there are times when a clinician ends the work without a mutual agreement with a client. Sometimes, however, a therapist ends therapy before a client seems ready. Changes in a clinician's life, including illness or psychological problems (his own or a family member's), marriage, pregnancy and/or birth of a child, professional move (e.g. going back for further training, graduation, and/or a new job), retirement, and so on can all create the need to end a therapeutic relationship before a client is clinically ready. In other cases, a clinician may feel that she has reached the end of her capacity to help a particular client, or may feel that she does not have the ability to deal with the issues a client is bringing into the work.

In some cases, setting a time to end may be utilized as an attempt to force a client to do work he has been avoiding; however, this approach can backfire on both client and clinician. Freud's famous decision to set an arbitrary final date with his client the Wolfman, for example, has been the subject of much discussion over the years (see Couch, 1999; Tosone, 1997) including his own review near the end of his career, in which he notes that setting the time limit was little more than a misguided attempt to coerce his client into changing (Freud, 1937). Novick (1997) points out that no matter what the reason, when a clinician initiates the end of therapy, a client will almost inevitably feel rejected and hurt. Oddly, even when a client is being difficult and almost appears to be asking to have a clinician end their work together, his feelings can be hurt when it actually happens. In some cases, paying attention to and even putting this conundrum into words can be enough to get the work back on track with an acting out client. Something like "I think you want me to kick you out, but I'm not really interested in doing that," can reassure a client that her therapist both understands something about her internal conflicts and can tolerate her confusion. Sometimes it can also be important for a clinician to share that she thinks a client is ending therapy too soon. Directly explaining some of the reasons for a clinician's thoughts, including concerns about such issues as self-destructive behavior and depressive symptoms, can lead to a client's ability to talk about fears of addressing important or disturbing material. It can also be yet one more way to model the process of thinking about how we think to a client (see Renik, 2006). Paradoxically, clinicians also sometimes err on the side of ending therapy prematurely in order to avoid being seen as holding onto a client too long.

This is how it worked for Ms. Robinson, who began working with Mr. Andrews when her son was hospitalized for medical reasons. After an initially rocky start, Ms. Robinson clearly made good use of her meetings with the clinician and showed significant evidence that their work together was helping her. When her son was discharged from the hospital, she asked if she could continue to work with Mr. Andrews. Although it was not general policy for a clinician to continue with a family when a child was no longer an inpatient, Ms. Robinson was part of a new project which would have allowed her to continue her work with her social worker. However, Mr. Andrews was concerned that he was holding onto her inappropriately because he enjoyed working with her so much. "I don't want to keep her in longer-term work to satisfy my own needs," he told his supervisor. "And I don't want to make her dependent on me." Mr. Andrews' supervisor asked if there was evidence that Ms. Robinson was becoming dependent on him. "No, actually she talks about feeling like she has more agency—well, she doesn't use that word, but that's what she describes," was the answer.

One of the great benefits of an integrative perspective is that it allows a clinician to look at a client from a broad perspective. Mr. Andrews was caught up in a particular vision of clinical process, one in which he felt that clients could be "bamboozled" (in his words) into staying with a therapist longer than necessary. His supervisor helped him see that sometimes clients stay because they are still getting something out of the work. "When she has accomplished all of her goals, or when she is feeling like she's no longer getting anything of value from therapy, if you try to hold onto her then, we can re-visit this question. But for the moment," his supervisor said, "it seems like she's getting something very valuable from the process." His supervisor added that it might be useful to think about what it would mean to Ms. Robinson if her therapist told her she should not continue with therapy. Mr. Andrews spontaneously answered, "Oh, I think she would feel hurt. It actually would probably undo some of her new-found sense of self-confidence."

A Positive Ending

Providing a positive experience at the end of the work, celebrating a client's accomplishments, and discussing tools he now has for coping with the difficulties that brought him into therapy can all help clients make a successful and positive transition out of therapy (e.g. Basch, 1980). Mirroring and empathizing with painful feelings that are evoked at the end of the work, and exploring both what these feelings mean and the ways a client has learned to cope with them over the course of therapy can be helpful to some clients.

A clinician must attempt to recognize and be attuned to a client's needs and capacities for managing certain kinds of feelings. Although we might want to share our own sense of connection to a client, sometimes a direct expression of caring can create more discomfort than pleasure. At other times, discussing what a client might continue to work on when therapy is done, exploring the possibility (when a clinician believes it to be the case) that it would be better to continue in the work until a particular goal is reached, or establishing an agreement about how the work will continue can also be ways of expressing caring. These discussions, which may begin as early as the first session or as late as the last one can also be a way of addressing the idea of ending, like therapy itself, as a process.

When a Therapist Disagrees with a Client's Decision

While I agree with that it is important to reinforce a client's accomplishments at the end of any therapeutic experience, I also believe that there are times when it is appropriate for a clinician to take a stand against a client's leaving therapy at a given time. This can include when a client is overtly acting out and/or resisting therapy, when there is danger to a client or to members of his personal support group if he leaves, when there has been a rupture between client and clinician, and when a client feels conflicted about deepening the work at a specific time. This does not mean that a client must be forced to remain in therapy with a specific clinician. Sometimes referral to another professional, either within or outside of the therapeutic community in which the clinician works, can be the most productive approach. This is yet one more of the many benefits of having a team already in place when working with any client. Another team member may step in and take over the work in a seamless manner when there is a need.

I have worked with a fair number of clients who I helped make a transition to another therapist or to a clinic or agency that seemed to be able to meet their needs in ways that I could not. I have sometimes been pleasantly surprised to receive a phone call from some of these clients, sometimes years later, saying that there are some aspects of the work with me that they now would like to pursue. An integrative perspective takes into account that clients have different needs and therefore need different interventions at different times in their lives.

Conflict and Contradiction

Accepting that endings, like many other aspects of life, are often filled with contradictions can be part of the work that leads to some kind of closure. In a wonderful discussion of the conclusion of a therapy filled with conflict and contradiction, Davies (2006) describes how finding ways to tolerate and manage paradox can be part of the therapeutic work for both client and clinician. Even in straightforward work, there is also often a sense of sorrow and frustration that the relationship cannot go on. Sometimes a clinician is distressed by not knowing what will happen next in a client's life, or how his story will unfold in the future. Clients often express pain that no one in their daily lives can understand them the way their therapist does. Thcsc fcclings can bc titratcd by a scnsc of accomplishmcnt and plcasurc at what has been done, and by recognizing the importance of the relationship and the work to both members of the therapeutic dyad.

When the outcome is less than successful, there are other dynamics for both client and clinician to deal with, including mourning the unachieved goals of the therapeutic work and managing feelings of disappointment and dissatisfaction both in each other, in the therapeutic work, and in ourselves. Awareness of what has not been done and articulating and managing disappointment in unmet expectations can also be an extremely important part of the therapeutic work (Kohut, 1971). What is perhaps most important of all, in this process, is a clinician's struggle not to take the content of a client's communications or his behavior personally.

Not Taking It Personally

When I was a young therapist, I worked with a woman who started every session with a criticism of something I was wearing or something about my office. Since I was just starting out, I was very sensitive about how I appeared. Did I look professional enough? Did my office? She always prefaced her remarks with, "I never say these things to anyone else, but I'm supposed to say everything I think in therapy, aren't I?" I did not know how to respond to these digs. I felt both hurt and irritated, but I did not think it would be therapeutic to tell her as much. In fact, since I believed that therapists were not supposed to get upset with their clients, both my sensitivity and my irritation seemed to me to indicate a major inadequacy on my part.

I discussed my concerns with my supervisor, who did not seem to share my fear that I was too self-involved to be helpful to her, but who suggested that rather than take her comments personally, I try to understand what they meant to her. He asked how I would think about her comments if I did not take them personally. I had troubles getting my mind around the idea at first. The words were directed at me, so how could they not be personal? But as I thought about it, I remembered something else this young woman frequently said. She had always been a "good girl," never arguing with her mother or older sister. Could she possibly be practicing being a little less good with me? And at the same time, could she be checking to see how I reacted when she said these things to me? Without knowing that she was doing it, could she be hoping that I would show her a better way to handle the kind of criticism she often heard at home? Just putting these ideas into words for myself changed my feelings from hurt and irritation to empathy for her.

The next time she put me down I asked her if she was being intentionally critical. She said, "No, of course not!" After a brief silence she added quietly that she hadn't realized it, but she could see that what she said could have sounded mean. She was extremely upset by the idea that I could possibly have thought that she was trying to hurt me. It took some time to soothe her, but over the next months and years we talked a great deal about the "unthought" or unformulated ideas and feelings that she had been expressing without realizing she was doing so.

When she was ready to leave therapy, she spoke of that early incident as one of the most powerful components of our work. "I was so hurt that you could think I would try to be mean to you," she said. "But you just kept trying to understand what might be behind those words. You weren't mad at me. You didn't hate me." She said that that was the moment when she started learning that she could be honest with me. "I didn't have to hide what I was feeling. You would be there if I was nasty, even if it was unintentional, just as much as when I was nice." The idea broadened over time. "I think you'll always be here for me, in my heart, even if I leave you."

Separation was also a struggle for this young woman. She left therapy and came back to see me any number of times over the subsequent years. We talked about her fear that leaving someone would feel like a rejection to them, and her need, like a rapprochement aged child, to make sure that I would still be here and would be glad to see her if she needed to come back. From a developmental perspective, it is easy to understand why we take things personally. During infancy and early childhood, we experience the world as revolving around us. Piaget (1952) found that a young child looking at a picture believes that an adult on the other side of the table sees exactly what he sees (even though the adult actually sees the picture upside down). When the picture is turned so that it is right side up for the adult and upside down for him, the youngster continues to believe that they are both seeing the same image.

Obviously, part of our intellectual and psychological growth includes the gradual understanding that we do not always see the same thing as someone else. Yet sometimes we confuse this understanding with experiences of empathy. Very early in life, long before we learn to differentiate perspectives, we see our own emotions mirrored in the eyes of others—and we are mirroring emotions back to loved ones (Fonagy, Gyorgy, Jurist, & Target, 2003; Schore, 2003; Siegel, 1999). In adulthood, empathy and perspective sometimes get tangled up. Even professionals who are trained to be aware of our own feelings can have difficulty separating our own feelings from those of others, particularly those who we think we understand or who understand us. In other words, it can be hard to sort out what is about or inside us and what is about or inside the other person. Especially in moments of vulnerability, this distinction can get lost. This struggle can be particularly true in any highly charged period of psychotherapy, and the ending phase is often one of those times.

The Work of Therapy Goes On

It is also important to remember that endings come in many different forms. As noted above, even some structured and time-limited approaches make room for a client to "re-contract" for further work, either in a group or individual setting. Yet the time eventually comes for therapy to end. Because the work is never really completely done, even the best-planned ending must leave some things unaccomplished, which may mean that one or both participants feel like failures. Making space for a client to talk about painful feelings like disappointment and sadness about loss not only of a clinician's support and understanding, but also of hope for a "new" self can be an extremely important part of the therapeutic process. In many instances, I have found that clients learn to embrace not only an imperfect self, but also an imperfect world in the final stage of the work.

However, I do not wish to communicate that there is a way to tie clinical work up in a nice, neat package. The end of any therapeutic engagement is never the end of the therapeutic process. One hopes that in any clinical work a client has developed new tools for living a healthier and more productive life and has gained an expanded vision of himself and the world in which he lives. But perhaps more than anything, the goal of all therapy is that a client will use these tools and this widened perspective in order continue to grow and develop as much as he is able to. For many of us in clinical work, we frequently do not get to see our clients engaged in this ongoing development. One of the great pleasures of having practiced for as long as I have is that I have also had the joy of hearing from many of my previous clients over the years. Some have returned to work further on issues that we began dealing with in our first engagement. Others have returned to deal with painful life experiences that I would have preferred they had not had to face, but that I am glad that I am available to support them through. And still others have simply contacted me to let me know that they are continuing to move forward in life—sometime in ways we had hoped, and sometimes in directions we could not have even imagined when we ended our work together.

Conclusion

We have reviewed a wide range of research in the course of this book. As we have seen, there is significant evidence (Connors, 2006; Johnson, 1999; Kaplan and Garfinkel, 1999; Novick & Novick, 1998; Roth & Fonagy, 1996; Zerbe, 2008) a mixture of symptom-focused, cognitive behavioral, supportive, insight-oriented, affect-regulatory, medical and psychopharmacological interventions is often more helpful with a variety of clients than a single, linear approach. Much of this same research has shown that work with a team in which different specialties are provided by different therapists—e.g. family, group and individual, medical and psychopharmacological, cognitive behavioral and insight-oriented—can also be beneficial (see also Novick & Novick, 2005). In this book we have considered two distinct but often intercepting concepts of integrative work: the use of multiple theories and techniques by a single clinician and also the use of a structured (whether formally or informally) group of professionals with different specialties working together as an integrative team in the therapy.

While psychodynamic exploration alone is seldom enough to produce significant change in some clients (e.g. Barth, 1998, 2008; Connors, 2006; Johnson, 1999; Kaplan and Garfinkel, 1999; Zerbe, 2008), it can still be a powerful tool for helping a clinician choose appropriate interventions, and for enhancing the effectiveness of other approaches with a range of symptoms, personality styles and family dynamics that manifest with these symptoms (Bromberg, 2001; Connors, 2006; Frank, 1999; Leichsenring & Rabung, 2008; Wachtel, 1997). On the other hand, a two pronged approach, such as that described by Connors (2006, 2011) focusing on self-regulation and self-initiated behavior change, can help a client manage emotions stirred up by psychodynamic exploration. Thus in my own work as both a social worker and a psychoanalyst, I have learned that it is not only not antithetical to provide concrete services and focus on psychodynamics at the same time, but that these two different aspects of the human experience are deeply and inextricably linked with each other. They inform one another, enhance one another and simultaneously explain one another. An integrative perspective is extremely useful in that it expands both available tools for working with different aspects of any client's struggles, and provides a larger therapeutic pool upon which a client can draw for assistance.

Years of clinical work have led me to believe that many, if not most clinicians bring integrative practices into the work on a daily basis. This book has been an attempt to help professionals find a way to talk and think about these practices. Further, I would suggest that today almost any intervention, whether a psychoanalytic interpretation, a cognitive behavioral exercise, a mindfulness technique, a self-soothing strategy or a prescription for medication—or anything else in our deep basket of contemporary psychotherapeutic possibilities—is, in and of itself, an integration. The concepts of "detailed inquiry," "process" and "small steps," which I have discussed throughout this book, can be stepping stones for both clinician and client in this process.

One of the great contributions of an integrative perspective is the recognition that endings, like therapy itself, and indeed like human beings, come in many different forms. The work of finishing therapy, like that of every other aspect of the process, from an integrative perspective is to help clients find ways to end that are appropriately growth-promoting and directed specifically at their needs at a given time. Recognizing and reflecting feelings that emerge during and handling tasks specific to this phase can enhance work that has already been done and make it possible for a client to continue to grow on his own, without the supportive presence of his therapist. Paying attention to a client's goals and finding ways to help him both articulate and work towards these goals can help a clinician find the most meaningful way to end a therapeutic encounter, whatever the reason for the ending. Perhaps what is most important is that we have provided a client with new tools for coping with situations and emotions that have previously been problematic, and that we have helped them recognize that neither we nor they will always have the perfect solution to any problem. But that a good enough solution is, as Winnicott (1965) says, often better than perfect.

References

Adler, G. (1985). *Borderline psychopathology and its treatment*. Hillsdale, NJ: Jason Aronson, Inc.

American Diabetes Association. (1995–2013). *Small steps for your health*. Retrieved June 19, 2013, from http://www.diabetes.org/ diabetes-basics/prevention/checkup-america/small-steps.html

Amundson, N., Borgen, W. & Tench, E. (1995). Counseling and the role of personality and intelligence. In D. Saklofske and M. Zeidner (Eds.). International handbook of personality and intelligence. New York, NY: Plenum Press.

Anderson, F. S. (1998). Psychic elaboration of musculoskeletal back pain: Ellen's story. In L. Aron & F. S. Anderson (Eds.), *Relational perspectives on the body* (pp. 287–322). Hillsdale, NJ: The Analytic Press.

Aron, L. (1991). The patient's experience of the analyst's subjectivity. *Psychoanalytic Dialogues, 1*, 29–51.

Aron, L. (1996). *A meeting of the minds: Mutuality in psychoanalysis*. Hillsdale, NJ: Analytic Press.

Aron, L., & Anderson, F. S. (Eds.). (2000). *Relational perspectives on the body (relational perspectives book series)*. London: Routledge.

Astin, J., Shapiro, S., Eisenberg, D., & Forys, K. (2003). Mind-body medicine: State of the science, implications for practice. *Journal of the American Board of Family Medicine, 16*, 131–147. doi:10.3122/jabfm.16.2.131.

Austrian, S. (2008). *Developmental theories through the life cycle*. New York: Columbia University Press.

Babyack, M., Blumenthal, J., Herman, S., Khatri, P., Doraiswamy, M., Moore, K., et al. (2000). Exercise treatment for major depression: Maintenance of therapeutic benefit at 10 months. *Psychosomatic Medicine, 62*, 633–638.

Bacal, H., & Herzog, B. (2003). Specificity theory and optimal responsiveness: An outline. *Psychoanalytic Psychology, 20*, 635–648.

Bandura, A. (1986). *Social foundations of thought and action: A social cognitive theory*. Englewood Cliffs, NJ: Prentice Hall.

Barnes, M., Bloom, B., and Nahin, R. (2008). Complementary and alternative medicine use among adults and children: United States, 2007. *National Health Statistics Report, 12*, 1–24.

Barth, F. D. (1989). Separation-individuation, sense of self, and bulimia in college students. In L. Whitaker & W. N. Davis (Eds.), *The bulimic college student: Evaluation, treatment and prevention*. New York: The Haworth Press.

F.D. Barth, *Integrative Clinical Social Work Practice: A Contemporary Perspective*, Essential Clinical Social Work Series, DOI 10.1007/978-1-4939-0351-1,

Barth, F. D. (1998). Speaking of feelings: Affects, language, and psychoanalysis. *Psychoanalytic Dialogues, 8*, 685–705.

Barth, F. D. (2003). Separate but not alone: Separation-individuation issues in college students with eating disorders. *Clinical Social Work Journal, 31*, 139–153.

Barth, F. D. (2008). Hidden eating disorders: Attachment and affect regulation. *Clinical Social Work Journal, 36*, 355–365.

Basch, M. F. (1980). *Doing psychotherapy*. New York: Basic Books.

Bateman, A. W., & Fonagy, P. (2004). *Psychotherapy for borderline personality disorder: Mentalization-based treatment*. London: Oxford University Press.

Beck, A. T. (1976). *Cognitive therapy and the emotional disorders*. New York: International Universities Press.

Beck, A. T., Rush, A. J., Shaw, B. F., & Emery, G. (1979). *Cognitive therapy of depression*. New York: The Guilford Press.

Beebe, B., & Lachmann, F. (2005). *Infant research and adult treatment: Co-constructing interactions*. London: Routledge.

Bjornsson, A. S., Didie, E. R., & Phillips, K. A. (2010). Body dysmorphic disorder. *Dialogues in Clinical Neuroscience, 12*, 221–232.

Bloomgarden, A. (2000). Therapist's self disclosure and genuine caring: Where do they belong in the therapeutic relationship? *Eating Disorders: The Journal of Treatment and Prevention, 8*, 347–352.

Blos, P. (1967). The second individuation process of adolescence. *Psychoanalytic Study of the Child, 22*, 162–186.

Bollas, C. (1989). *The shadow of the object*. New York: Columbia University Press.

Boston Change Process Study Group. (2005). The "something more" than interpretation revisited: Sloppiness and co-creativity in the psychoanalytic encounter. *Journal of the American Psychoanalytic Association, 53*, 693–729.

Boulanger, G. (2007). *Wounded by reality*. London: Routledge.

Boulanger, G. (2011). Arguing with myself: Thoughts on taking an integrative approach. *Clinical Social Work Journal, 39*, 201–203.

Bowlby, J. (1973). *Attachment and loss* (Separation, Vol. 2). New York: Basic Books.

Bowlby, J. (1988). *A secure base: Clinical applications of attachment theory*. London: Routledge.

Brandell, J., & Ringel, S. (2011). *Trauma: Contemporary directions in theory, practice, and research*. Thousand Oaks, CA: Sage.

Breuer, J., & Freud, S. (1957). *Studies on hysteria* (J. Strachey, Ed. & Trans.). London: Hogarth. (Original work published 1895)

Bromberg, P. (2001). *Standing in the spaces: Essays on clinical process, trauma and dissociation*. London: Routledge.

Brown, B., Crawford, P., & Darongkamas, J. (2000). Blurred roles and permeable boundaries: The experience of multidisciplinary working in community mental health. *Health and Social Care in the Community, 8*, 425–435.

Brown, R., & Gerbarg, P. (2012). *The healing power of the breath: Simple techniques to reduce stress and anxiety, enhance concentration, and balance your emotions*. Boston, MA: Shambhala.

Buchheim, A., Viviani, R., Kessler, H., Kächele, H., Cierpka, M., Roth, G., et al. (2012). Changes in prefrontal-limbic function in major depression after 15 months of long-term psychotherapy. *PLoS ONE, 7*, e33745. doi:10.1371/journal.pone.0033745.

Burch, B. (1993). Heterosexuality, bisexuality, and lesbianism: Rethinking psychoanalytic views of women's object choice. *The Psychoanalytic Review, 80*, 83–99.

Burks, R., & Keeley, S. (1989). Exercise and diet therapy: Psychotherapists' beliefs and practices. *Professional Psychology: Research and Practice, 20*, 62–64.

Burns, D. (1999). *The feeling good handbook*. New York: PLUME/Penguin Group.

Busch, F., & Sandberg, L. (2007). *Psychotherapy and medication: The challenge of integration*. London: Routledge.

Campbell, M., & Morrison, A. (2007). The subjective experience of paranoia: Comparing the experiences of patients with psychosis and individuals with no psychiatric history. *Psychology and Psychotherapy, 14*, 63–77.

Cancer.org. (2008). *Mind, body and spirit in cancer care*. Retrieved September 7, 2013, from http://www.cancer.org/treatment/treatmentsandsideeffects/complementaryandalternativemedicine/mindbodyandspirit/index

Cancer.org. (2011). *Therapeutic touch*. Retrieved September 7, 2013, from http://www.cancer.org/treatment/treatmentsandsideeffects/complementaryandalternativemedicine/manualhealingandphysicaltouch/therapeutic-touch

Carr, G. (2011). Psychotherapy research: Implications for practice. *Psychiatric Times, 28*. Retrieved from http://www.psychiatrictimes.com/display/article/10168/1926944

Cassidy, J. & Shaver, P. (Eds.) (2008). *Handbook of attachment: Theory, research, and clinical applications* (2nd ed.). New York: The Guilford Press.

Castonguay, L., Schut, A., Aikins, D., & Constantino, M. (2004). Integrative cognitive therapy for depression: A preliminary Investigation. *Journal of Psychotherapy Integration, 14*, 4–20.

Chodorow, N. (1999). *The reproduction of mothering: Psychoanalysis and the sociology of gender*. Berkeley: University of California Press.

Christenson, G. A., Faber, R. J., de Zwaan, M., Raymond, N. C., Specker, S. M., Ekern, M. D., et al. (1994). Compulsive buying: Descriptive characteristics and psychiatric comorbidity. *The Journal of Clinical Psychiatry, 55*, 5–11.

Connors, M. (2006). *Symptom-focused dynamic psychotherapy*. Hillsdale, NJ: Analytic Press.

Connors, M. (2011). Integrative symptom-focused dynamic psychotherapy. *The Clinical Social Work Journal, 39*, 122–131.

Couch, A. S. (1999). Therapeutic functions of the real relationship in psychoanalysis. *Psychoanalytic Study of the Child, 54*, 130–168.

Cowger, C. D. (1994). Assessing client strengths: Clinical assessment for client empowerment. *Social Work, 39*, 262–280.

Craige, H. (2013). EMDR presentation. Panel discussion: Under one tent, really? In *AAPCSW conference*, March 22, 2013, Durham, NC.

Crits-Christoph, P. (1996). The dissemination of efficacious psychological treatments. *Clinical Psychology: Science and Practice, 3*, 260–263.

Damasio, A. (1999). *The feeling of what happens*. New York: Harcourt, Brace.

Davies, J. M. (1998). Repression and dissociation—Freud and Janet: Fairbairn's new model of unconscious process. In N. Skolnick & D. Scharff (Eds.), *Fairbairn, then and now* (pp. 53–69). Hillsdale, NJ: The Analytic Press.

Davies, J. M. (2002). *Whose bad objects are these anyway? Repetition and our elusive love affair with evil*. Presented at meeting of international association for relational psychoanalysis and psychotherapy, January, New York.

Davies, J. M. (2005). Transformations of desire and despair: Reflections on the termination process from a relational perspective. *Psychoanalytic Dialogues, 15*, 779–805.

Davies, J. M. (2006). The times we sizzle, and the times we sigh: The multiple erotics of arousal, anticipation and release. *Psychoanalytic Dialogues, 16*, 665–686.

DiClemente, C. (2006). *Addiction and change: How addictions develop and addicted people recover*. New York: The Guilford Press.

Dobson, K., Hollon, S., Dimidjian, S., Schmaling, K., Kohlenberg, R., Gallop, R., et al. (2008). Randomized trial of behavioral activation, cognitive therapy, and antidepressant medication in the prevention of relapse and recurrence in major depression. *Journal of Consulting Clinical Psychology, 76*, 468–477.

Dorahy, M., & Hamilton, G. (2009). The 'Narcissistic-We' model: A conceptual framework for multidisciplinary team working, researching and decision-making with traumatised individuals. *Counseling and Psychotherapy Research, 9*, 57–64.

Dozier, M., Stovall-McClough, K., & Albus, K. (2008). Attachment and psychopathology in adulthood. In J. Cassidy & P. Shaver (Eds.), *Handbook of attachment: Theory, research, and clinical applications* (2nd ed., pp. 718–744). New York: The Guilford Press.

Dozois, D., & Beck, A. (2010). Cognitive therapy. In J. D. Herbert & E. M. Forman (Eds.), *Acceptance and mindfulness in cognitive behavior therapy: Understanding and applying the new therapies* (pp. 26–57). Hoboken, NJ: Wiley.

Eagle, M. (1989). *Recent developments in psychoanalysis: A critical evaluation*. Boston, MA: Harvard University Press.

Eagle, M. (1995). The developmental perspectives of attachment and psychoanalytic theory. In S. Goldberg, R. Muir, & J. Kerr (Eds.), *Attachment theory: Social, developmental, and clinical perspectives* (pp. 123–150). Hillsdale, NJ: Analytic Press.

Eagle, M. N. (2000). A critical evaluation of current conceptions of transference and countertransference. *Psychoanalytic Psychology, 17*, 24–37.

Eccleston, C. (2001). Role of psychology in pain management. *British Journal of Anaesthesia, 87*, 144–152.

Eden, D., & Feinstein, D. (2008). *Energy medicine: Balancing your body's energies for optimal health, joy, and vitality*. New York: Jeremy Tarcher (Penguin Books).

Ekblad, A., Chapman, A., & Lynch, T. (2010). Borderline personality disorder and co-occurring substance use disorders: Conceptualization & treatment. In E. Nunes (Ed.), *Substance dependence and co-occurring psychiatric disorders: Best practices for diagnosis and treatment* (pp. 2–26). Kingston: Civic Research Institute.

Ellis, A. (1961). *A guide to rational living*. Englewood Cliffs, NJ: Prentice-Hall.

Epstein, M. (2004). *Thoughts without a thinker: Psychotherapy from a Buddhist perspective*. New York: Basic Books.

Erikson, E. (1980). *Identity and the life cycle*. New York: W.W. Norton. (Original work published 1959)

Ezzamel, M., & Willmott, H. (1998). Accounting for teamwork: A critical study of group-based systems of organizational control. *Administrative Science Quarterly, 43*, 358–396.

Farmer, E. M. (2009). What's the relationship got to do with it? Understanding the therapeutic relationship in therapeutic foster care. *Child & Adolescent Social Work Journal, 26*, 49–63.

Fawcett, J. (1997). Psychopharmacotherapy and psychotherapy: Treating target symptoms and learning. *Annual of Psychoanalysis, 25*, 17–25.

Fawcett, L., & Hurrell, A. (2000). *Regionalism in world politics: Regional organization and international order*. New York: Oxford University Press.

Fehmi, L., & Robbins, J. (2008). *The open-focus brain: Harnessing the power of attention to heal mind and body*. Boston, MA: Trumpeter Publisher.

Feiner, A., & Epstein, L. (1993). *Countertransference: The therapists's contribution to the therapeutic situation*. Hillsdale, NJ: Jason Aronson, Inc.

Fonagy, P. (2002). The history and current status of outcome research at the Anna Freud Centre. *Psychoanalytic Study of the Child, 57*, 27–60.

Fonagy, P. (2005). *Affect regulation, mentalization, and the development of self*. New York: Other Press.

Fonagy, P., Gyorgy, G., Jurist, E., & Target, M. (2003). *Affect regulation, mentalization and the development of the self*. London: Karnac Books.

Fosha, D. (2000). *The transforming power of affect: A model for accelerated change*. New York: Basic Books.

Frank, K. A. (1999). *Psychoanalytic participation: Action, interaction, and integration*. London: Routledge.

Frank, K. A. (2004). The analyst's trust and therapeutic action. *Psychoanalytic Quarterly, LXXIII*, 335–378.

Frank, K. A. (2005). Toward conceptualizing the personal relationship in therapeutic action: Beyond the "real" relationship. *Psychoanalytic Perspectives, 3*(1), 15–56.

Freedman, N., Hoffenberg, J. D., Vorus, N., & Frosch, A. (1999). The effectiveness of psychoanalytic psychotherapy: The role of treatment duration, frequency of sessions, and the therapeutic relationship. *Journal of the American Psychoanalytic Association, 47*, 741–772.

Freis, E. (2012). Perchance to sleep: Minding the unworded body in psychoanalysis. *Psychoanalytic Dialogues, 22*, 586–605.

Freud, S. (1893–1895). Studies on hysteria. (J. Strachey, Trans.) In *The standard edition of the complete psychological works of Sigmund Freud* (vol. 2, pp. 106–181). London: Hogarth.
Freud, S. (1914). Remembering, repeating and working through (J. Strachey, trans.). In *The standard edition of the complete psychological works of Sigmund Freud* (vol. 12, pp. 146–156). London: Hogarth.
Freud, S. (1937). Analysis terminable and interminable (J. Strachey, Trans.). In *The standard edition of the complete psychological works of Sigmund Freud* (vol. 23, pp. 211–255). London: Hogarth.
Gabbard, G. O. (1991). Technical approaches to transference hate in the analysis of borderline patients. *International Journal of Psycho-Analysis, 72*, 625–636.
Gabbard, G. O., & Lester, E. (1995). *Boundaries and boundary violations in psychoanalysis*. New York: Basic Books.
Gabbidon, S. (2003). Racial profiling by store clerks and security personnel in retail establishments: An exploration of "shopping while black". *Journal of Contemporary Criminal Justice, 19*, 345–364.
Ganzer, C., & Ornstein, E. D. (2002). A sea of trouble: A relational approach to the culturally sensitive treatment of a severely disturbed client. *Clinical Social Work Journal, 30*, 127–144.
Gaudiano, B., & Herbert, J. (2000). Can we really tap away our problems? A critical analysis of thought field therapy. *Skeptical Inquirer, 24*, 29–33.
Gay, P. (2006). *Freud: A life for our time*. London: W.W. Norton.
Gedo, J. (1991). *The biology of clinical encounters: Psychoanalysis as a science of mind*. London: Routledge.
Gedo, J. (1997). The primitive psyche, communication, and the language of the body. *Psychoanalytic Inquiry, 17*, 192–203.
Gerson, B. (2001). *The therapist as a person: Life crises, life choices, life experiences, and their effects on treatment*. London: Routledge.
Gilligan, C., & Machoian, L. (2002). Learning to speak the language: a relational interpretation of an adolescent girl's suicidality. *Studies in Gender and Sexuality, 3*, 321–341.
Girard, J., Cohn, J., Mahoor, M., Mavadati, S., Rosenwald, D., & Torre, F. (2013). Manual and automatic analysis of facial affective reactivity in major depressive disorder. In *IEEE international conference on automatic face and gesture recognition*, Shanghai, China.
Gitterman, A. (2014). *Handbook of social work practice with vulnerable and resilient populations*. New York, NY: Columbia University Press.
Gitterman, A., & Germain, C. (2008). *The life model of social work practice: Advances in theory and practice*. New York: Columbia University Press.
Goldberg, A., & Gedo, J. (1973). *Models of the mind*. Chicago: University of Chicago Press.
Goldberg, S., Muir, R. & Kerr, J. (Eds.) (1995). *Attachment theory: Social, developmental, and clinical perspectives*. Hillsdale, NJ: Analytic Press.
Goldstein, E. (1994). Self-disclosure in treatment: What therapists do and don't talk about. *Clinical Social Work Journal, 22*, 417–433.
Goldstein, E. (1999). Chapter 3: Integrative short-term treatment of the borderline patient. *Psychoanalytic Social Work, 6*, 87–111.
Goldstein, E. (2007). When midlife therapists treat midlife patients: Challenges to empathic attunement. *Psychoanalytic Social Work, 14*, 3–14.
Goodman, G. (2013). Is mentalization a common process factor in transference-focused psychotherapy and dialectical behavior therapy sessions? *Journal of Psychotherapy Integration, 25*, 179–192.
Gordon, J., Staples, J., Blyta, A., Bytyqi, M., & Wilson, A. (2008). Treatment of posttraumatic stress disorder in postwar Kosovar adolescents using mind-body skills groups: A randomized controlled trial. *Journal of Clinical Psychiatry, 69*, 1469–1476.
Grand, S. (2009). Termination as necessary madness. *Psychoanalytic Dialogues, 19*, 723–733.
Greenberg, J. (1991). *Oedipus and beyond: A clinical theory*. Cambridge, MA: Harvard University Press.
Greenberg, T. M. (2009). *Psychodynamic perspectives on aging and illness*. London: Springer.

Greenson, R. (1967). *The technique and practice of psychoanalysis*. New York: International Universities Press.
Grzesiak, R. C. (1994). The matrix of vulnerability. In R. C. Grzesiak & D. S. Ciccone (Eds.), *Psychological vulnerability to chronic pain* (pp. 1–27). London: Springer.
Hansell, J., & Damour, L. (2008). *Abnormal psychology*. New York: Wiley.
Hartmann, H. (1939). *Ego psychology and the problem of adaptation*. New York, NY: International Universities Press, Inc.
Harvard Medical School. (2013). *Healthy eating for a healthy heart*. Retrieved June 19, 2013, from http://www.health.harvard.edu/special_health_reports/healthy-heart-diet
Hausner, R. (2000). The therapeutic and working alliances. *Journal of the American Psychoanalytic Association, 48*, 155–187.
Hayes, S. (2004). Acceptance and commitment therapy, relational frame theory, and the third wave of behavioral and cognitive therapies. *Behavior Therapy, 35*, 639–665.
Hayes, S., Strosahl, K., & Wilson, K. (1999). *Acceptance and commitment therapy: An experiential approach to behavior change*. New York: The Guilford Press.
Hersoug, A., Hogland, P., Monsen, J., & Havik, O. (2001). Quality of working alliance in psychotherapy: Therapist variables and patient/therapist similarity as predictors. *Journal of Psychotherapy Practice Research, 10*, 205–216.
Hirsch, I. (2002). Beyond interpretation: Analytic interaction in the interpersonal tradition. *Contemporary Psychoanalysis, 38*, 573–587.
Hoffman, I. (1996). Merton M. Gill: A study in theory development in psychoanalysis. *Psychoanalytic Dialogues, 6*, 5–53.
Hoffman, I. (1998). *Ritual and spontaneity in the psychoanalytic process: A dialectical constructivist perspective*. London: Routledge.
Holmes, J. (1996). *Attachment, intimacy, autonomy: Using attachment theory in adult psychotherapy*. Hillsdale, NJ: Jason Aronson.
Holmes, J. (1998). The changing aims of psychoanalytic psychotherapy: An integrative perspective. *International Journal of Psycho-Analysis, 79*, 227–240.
Horvath, A. O., & Greenberg, L. S. (1994). *The working alliance: Theory, research and practice*. New York: Wiley.
Jakubovski, E., Pittenger, C., Torres, A., Fontenelle, L., do Rosario, N., Ferrao, Y., et al. (2011). Dimensional correlates of poor insight in obsessive-compulsive disorder. *Progress in Neuro-Psychopharmacology & Biological Psychiatry, 35*, 1677–1681.
Johnson, C. (1999). *Been there—done that: The use of clinicians with personal recovery in the treatment of eating disorders*. Presented at the annual meeting of the academy of eating disorders, San Diego, CA.
Kabat-Zinn, J. (1990). *Full catastrophe living: Using the wisdom of your body and mind to face stress, pain, and illness*. Knoxville, TN: Delta Publishing.
Kanter, J. (2013). Helping, healing and interpreting: Sullivan, the Interpersonal School and Clinical Social Work. *Journal of Social Work Practice, 27*, 273–287.
Kaplan, A.S. and Garfinkel, P.E. (1999). Difficulties in treating patients with eating disorders: A review of patient and clinician variables. *Canadian Journal of Psychiatry*, 44.
Kaskutas, L. (2009). Alcoholics anonymous effectiveness: Faith meets science. *Journal of Addictive Disorders, 28*, 145–157.
Kernberg, O. (2000). *Borderline conditions and pathological narcissism*. Hillsdale, NJ: Jason Aronson, Inc.
Kohut, H. (1971). *Analysis of the self: Systematic approach to treatment of narcissistic personality disorders*. New York: International Universities Press.
Kohut, H. (1977). *The restoration of the self*. New York: International Universities Press.
Kohut, H. (1984). *How does analysis cure?* Chicago: Chicago University Press.
Krystal, H. (1988). *Integration and self-healing: Affect, trauma, and alexithymia*. Hillsdale, NJ: The Analytic Press.
Lachmann, F. (2001). Some contributions of empirical infant research to adult psychoanalysis. *Psychoanalytic Dialogues, 11*, 1677–1685.

Lacy, T., & Hughes, J. (2006). A systems approach to behavioral neurobiology: Integrating psychodynamics and neuroscience in a psychiatric curriculum. *Journal of the American Academy of Psychoanalysis and Dynamic Psychiatry, 34*, 43–74.

Langs, R. (1981). *The technique of psychoanalytic psychotherapy* (Initial contact, theoretical framework, understanding the patient's communications, the therapist's interventions, Vol. 1). Lanham, MD: Rowman & Littlefield Publishers.

Lapides, F. (2011). The implicit realm in couples therapy: Improving right hemisphere affect-regulating capabilities. *Clinical Social Work Journal, 39*, 161–169.

Leichsenring, F. (2005). Are psychodynamic and psychoanalytic therapies effective? A review of empirical data. *International Journal of Psycho-Analysis, 86*, 841–868.

Leichsenring, F., & Rabung, S. (2008). Effectiveness of long-term psychodynamic psychotherapy. A meta-analysis. *Journal of the American Medical Association, 300*, 1551–1565.

Lerner, S., Magrane, D., & Friedman, E. (2009). Teaching teamwork in medical education. *Mount Sinai Journal of Medicine, 76*, 318–329.

Levenson, E. (1989). Whatever happened to the cat? Interpersonal perspectives on the self. *Contemporary Psychoanalysis, 25*, 537–553.

Levine, P. (1997). *Waking the tiger: Healing trauma: The innate capacity to transform overwhelming experiences*. Berkeley, CA: North Atlantic Books, Inc.

Linehan, M. (1993). *Cognitive-behavioral treatment of borderline personality disorder*. New York: The Guilford Press.

Loewald, H. (1989). *Papers on psychoanalysis*. New Haven, CT: Yale University Press.

Lukas, S. (1993). *Where to start and what to ask: An assessment handbook*. New York: W.W. Norton.

Lyons-Ruth, K. (1991). Rapprochement or approchement: Mahler's theory reconsidered from the vantage point of recent research on early attachment relationships. *Psychoanalytic Psychology, 8*, 1–23.

Mahler, M., Pine, F., & Bergman, A. (1973). *The psychological birth of the human infant*. New York: Basic Books.

Main, M. (1999). Mary D. Salter Ainsworth: Tribute and portrait. *Psychoanalytic Inquiry, 19*, 682–736.

Martin, D. C. (1990). The mental status examination. In H. K. Walker, W. D. Hall, & J. W. Hurst (Eds.), *Clinical methods: The history, physical, and laboratory examinations* (3rd ed., Chap. 207). Boston: Butterworths. Retrieved from http://www.ncbi.nlm.nih.gov/books/NBK320/

Martin, D., Garske, J., & Davis, M. (2000). Relation of the therapeutic alliance with outcome and other variables: A meta-analytic review. *Journal of Consulting and Clinical Psychology, 68*, 438–450.

McDougall, J. (1989). *Theaters of the body: A psychoanalytic approach to psychosomatic illness*. New York: W.W. Norton.

McElroy, S., Keck, P., & Phillips, K. (1995). Kleptomania, compulsive buying, and binge-eating disorder. *Journal of Clinical Psychiatry, 56*, 14–26.

McElroy, S., Soutullo, C., Beckman, D., Taylor, P., Jr., & Keck, P., Jr. (1998). DSM-IV intermittent explosive disorder: A report of 27 cases. *Journal of Clinical Psychiatry, 59*, 203–210.

McMain, S., Sayrs, J., Dimeff, L., & Linehan, M. (2007). Dialectical behavior therapy for individuals with borderline personality disorder and substance dependence. In L. Dimeff & K. Koerner (Eds.), *Dialectical behavior therapy in clinical practice: Applications across disorders and settings* (pp. 145–173). New York: The Guilford Press.

McWilliams, N. (2004). *Psychoanalytic psychotherapy: A practitioner's guide*. New York: The Guilford Press.

Meissner, W. (1983). Notes on the levels of differentiation within borderline conditions. *Psychoanalytic Review, 70*, 179–209.

Meissner, W. (2007a). Mind, brain, and self in psychoanalysis: Therapeutic implications of the mind-body relation. *Psychoanalytic Psychology, 24*, 333–354.

Meissner, W. (2007b). Therapeutic alliance. *Psychoanalytic Psychology, 24*, 231–254.

Merriam Webster Online Dictionary. (2013). Retrieved July 3, 2013, from http://www.merriam-webster.com/dictionary/teamwork

Miller, A., Rathus, J., & Linehan, M. (2006). *Dialectical behavior therapy with suicidal adolescents*. New York: The Guilford Press.

Milrod, B., Leon, A., Busch, F., Rudden, M., Schwalberg, M., Clarkin, J., et al. (2007). A randomized controlled clinical trial of psychoanalytic psychotherapy for panic disorder. *American Journal of Psychiatry, 164*, 265–272.

Mischel, W. (2009) Connecting clinical practice to scientific progress. *Psychological Science in the Public Interest, 9*. Retrieved from www3.interscience.wiley.com/

Mishna, F., Van Wert, M., & Asakura, K. (2013). The best kept secret in social work: Empirical support for contemporary psychodynamic social work practice. *Journal of Social Work Practice: Psychotherapeutic Approaches in Health, Welfare and the Community* http://dx.doi.org/10.1080/02650533.2013.818944.

Mitchell, S. (1988). *Relational concepts in psychoanalysis*. Cambridge, MA: Harvard University Press.

Mitchell, S. (1993). *Hope and dread in psychoanalysis*. New York: Basic Books.

Mitchell, S. (1999). Attachment theory and the psychoanalytic tradition: Reflections on human relationality. *Psychoanalytic Dialogues, 9*, 85–107.

Mitchell, S., & Black, M. (1995). *Freud and beyond: a history of modern psychoanalytic thought*. New York: Basic Books.

Monti, D., & Beitman, B. (2009). *Integrative psychiatry (Weil Integrative Medicine Library)*. London: Oxford.

National Institute of Mental Health. (2013). *What is psychotherapy?* Retrieved November 13, 2012, from http://www.nimh.nih.gov/health/topics/psychotherapies/index.shtm

National Institutes of Health. (2008). *Complementary, alternative, or integrative health: What's in a name?* Retrieved August 6, 2013, from http://nccam.nih.gov/sites/nccam.nih.gov/files/CAM_Basics_What_Are_CAIHA.pdf

National Institutes of Health. (2013). *Ayurvedic medicine: An introduction*. Retrieved September 14, 2013, from http://nccam.nih.gov/health/ayurveda/introduction.htm

Newhill, C. (2004). *Client violence in social work practice: Prevention, intervention, and research*. New York: The Guilford Press.

Nhat Hanh, T. (1992). *Peace is every step: The path of mindfulness in everyday life*. New York: Bantam Books.

Norcross, J. (2002). *Psychotherapy relationships that work: Therapist contributions and responsiveness to patients*. London: Oxford University Press.

Novick, J. (1982). Termination: Themes and issues. *Psychoanalytic Inquiry, 2*, 329–365.

Novick, J. (1997). Termination conceivable and inconceivable. *Psychoanalytic Psychology, 14*, 145–162.

Novick, K., & Novick, J. (1998). An application of the concept of the therapeutic alliance to sadomasochistic pathology. *Journal of the American Psychoanalytic Association, 46*, 813–846.

Novick, K., & Novick, J. (2005). *Working with parents makes therapy work*. New York: Jason Aronson, Inc.

Novick, J., & Novick, K. (2006). *Good goodbyes: Knowing how to end in psychotherapy and psychoanalysis*. Hillsdale, NJ: Jason Aronson, Inc.

Ogden, P., Minton, K., & Siegel, D. (2006). *Trauma and the body: A sensorimotor approach to psychotherapy (Norton Series on Interpersonal Neurobiology)*. New York: W.W. Norton.

Parish, M., & Eagle, M. N. (2003). Attachment to the therapist. *Psychoanalytic Psychology, 20*, 271–286.

Piaget, J. (1952). *The origins of intelligence in children*. New York: International Universities Press.

Pine, F. (1985). *Developmental theory and clinical process*. New Haven, CT: Yale University Press.

Pine, F. (1990). *Drive, ego, object, and self: A synthesis for clinical work*. New York: Basic Books.

Pine, F. (2006). If I knew then what I know now: Theme and variations. *Psychoanalytic Psychology, 23*, 1–7.
Pizer, B. (1997). When the analyst is ill: Dimensions of self-disclosure. *Psychoanalytic Quarterly, 66*, 450–469.
Prochaska, J., DiClemente, C., & Norcross, J. (1992). In search of how people change: Applications to addictive behaviors. *American Psychologist, 47*, 1102–1114.
Racker, H. (1957). The meaning and uses of countertransference. *Psychoanalytic Quarterly, 26*, 303–357.
Raja, S. (2012). *Overcoming trauma and PTSD: A workbook integrating skills from ACT, DBT, and CBT*. Oakland, CA: New Harbinger Press.
Reich, W. (2013). *Character analysis* (Vincent Carfagno, Trans.). New York: Farrar, Straus and Giroux.
Reichstein, G. (1998). *Wood becomes water: Chinese medicine in everyday life*. New York: Kodansha USA.
Renik, O. (2006). *Practical psychoanalysis for therapists and patients*. New York: Other Press.
Rollnick, S., Butler, W., & Miller, C. (2008). *Motivational interviewing in health care: Helping patients change behavior*. New York: The Guilford Press.
Roth, A., & Fonagy, P. (1996). *What works for whom: A critical review of psychotherapy research*. New York: The Guilford Press.
Rustin, J. (2012). *Infant research and neuroscience at work in psychotherapy: Expanding the clinical repertoire*. New York: W.W. Norton.
Samuels, A. (1985). Countertransference, the 'Mundus Imaginalis' and a research project. *Journal of Analytic Psycholology, 30*, 47–71.
Schachter, J., & Kächele, H. (2007). The analyst's role in healing: Psychoanalysis-plus. *Psychoanalytic Psychology, 24*, 429–444.
Schafer, R. (1994). *Retelling a life: Narration and dialogue in psychoanalysis*. New York: Basic Books.
Schore, A. (2003). *Affect regulation and repair of the self*. New York: W.W. Norton.
Segal, Z., Williams, M., & Teasdale, J. (2012). *Mindfulness-based cognitive therapy for depression* (2nd ed.). New York: The Guilford Press.
Seligman, M. (1995). The effectiveness of psychotherapy: The Consumer Reports study. *American Psychologist, 50*, 965–974.
Seligman, S., & Shanok, R. (1996). Erikson, our contemporary. *Psychoanalysis of Contemporary Thought, 19*, 339–365.
Selva, P. & Malan, D. (2004). *Intensive short term dynamic psychotherapy: Theory and technique synopsis*. London: Karnac.
Shapiro, F. (1998). *EMDR: The breakthrough "eye movement" therapy for overcoming anxiety, stress, and trauma*. New York: Basic Books.
Shedler, J. (2010). The efficacy of psychodynamic psychotherapy. *American Psychologist, 65*, 98–109.
Siegel, D. (1999). *The developing mind: Toward a neurobiology of interpersonal experience*. New York: The Guilford Books.
Sifneos, P. (1996). Alexithymia: Past and present. *American Journal of Psychiatry, 153*, 137–142.
Silverman, D. (1998). The tie that binds: Affect regulation, attachment, and psychoanalysis. *Psychoanalytic Psychology, 15*, 187–212.
Skinner, B. (1957). *Verbal behavior*. New York: Appelton-Century-Crofts.
Slade, A. (2006). Reflective parenting programs: Theory and development. *Psychoanalytic Inquiry, 26*, 640–657.
Smith, B. (2008) *The examined life: Personal therapy and the social worker's ethical obligations to self*. Thesis in partial fulfillment of requirements for the Master of Social Work degree in the Graduate College of The University of Iowa.
Sonne, S., & Brady, K. (2002). *Bipolar disorder and alcoholism*. Retrieved June 1, 2013, from http://pubs.niaaa.nih.gov/publications/arh26-2/103-108.htm

Spence, D. (1984). *Narrative truth and historical truth: Meaning and interpretation in psychoanalysis*. New York: W.W. Norton.

Steele, H. (2008). Attachment and day care revisited. *Attachment & Human Development, 10*, 223.

Stern, D. N. (1985). *The interpersonal world of the human infant: A view from psychoanalysis and developmental psychology*. New York: Basic Books.

Stern, D. B. (1997). *Unformulated experience: From dissociation to imagination in psychoanalysis*. Hillsdale, NJ: The Analytic Press.

Stern, D. B. (2013). Psychotherapy is an emergent process: In favor of acknowledging hermeneutics and against the privileging of systematic empirical research. *Psychoanalytic Dialogues, 23*, 102–115.

Stewart, T., & Williamson, D. (2004). Multidisciplinary treatment of eating disorders—Part 1 structure and costs of treatment. *Behavior Modification, 28*, 812–830.

Stolorow, R. (1975). The narcissistic function of masochism (and sadism). *International Journal of Psycho-Analysis, 56*, 441–448.

Straker, G. (2006). Signing with a scar: Understanding self-harm. *Psychoanalytic Dialogues, 16*, 93–112.

Ströhle, A. (2009). Physical activity, exercise, depression and anxiety disorders. *Journal of Neural Transmission, 116*, 777–784.

Sullivan, H. (1953). *The interpersonal theory of psychiatry*. New York: W.W. Norton.

Sulloway, F. (1979). *Freud, biologist of the mind: Beyond the psychoanalytic legend*. New York: Basic Books.

The Boston Change Process Study Group. (2010). *Change in psychotherapy: A unifying paradigm*. New York: W.W. Norton.

Thompson-Brenner, H., Satir, D., Franko, D., & Herzog, D. (2012). Clinician reactions to patients with eating disorders: A review of the literature. *Psychiatric Services, 63*, 73–78. doi:10.1176/appi.ps.201100050.

Tosone, C. (1997). Sándor Ferenczi: Forerunner of modern short-term psychotherapy. *Psychoanalytic Social Work, 4*, 23–41.

Tosone, C., Nuttman-Schwartz, O., & Stephens, T. (2012). Shared trauma: When the professional is personal. *The Clinical Social Work Journal, 40*, 231–239.

Van der Kolk, B. (1987). *Psychological trauma*. Arlington, VA: American Psychiatric Publishing.

Wachtel, P. (1997). *Psychoanalysis, behavior therapy and the relational world*. Washington, DC: American Psychological Association.

Wachtel, P. (2010). Beyond "ESTs": Problematic assumptions in the pursuit of evidence-based practice. *Psychoanalytic Psychology, 27*, 251–272.

Wahbeh, H., Elsas, S., & Oken, B. (2008). Mind–body interventions: Applications in neurology. *Neurology, 70*, 2321–2328.

Waldinger, R., & Jacobson, A. (2001). The initial psychiatric interview. In J. L. Jacobson & A. M. Jacobson (Eds.), *Psychiatric secrets* (2nd ed.). Philadelphia: Hanley & Belfus, Inc.

Wallerstein, R. (2000). *Forty-two lives in treatment: A study of psychoanalysis and psychotherapy*. New York: Other Press.

Wallerstein, R., & Sampson, H. (1971). Issues in research in the psychoanalytic process. *International Journal of Psycho-Analysis, 52*, 11–50.

Wampold, B. (2001). *The great psychotherapy debate: Models, methods and findings*. Mahwah, NJ: Lawrence Erlbaum.

Wampold, B., & Brown, G. (2005). Estimating variability in out-comes attributable to therapists: A naturalistic study of outcomes in managed care. *Journal of Consulting and Clinical Psychology, 73*, 911–923.

Watzke, B., Rüddel, H., Jürgensen, R., Koch, U., Kriston, L., Grothgar, B., et al. (2010). Effectiveness of systematic treatment selection for psychodynamic and cognitive–behavioural therapy: Randomised controlled trial in routine mental healthcare. *The British Journal of Psychiatry, 197*, 96–105.

Weinberg, I., Ronningstam, L., Goldblatt, M., Schechter, M., & Maltsberger, J. (2010). Common factors in empirically supported treatments of borderline personality disorder. *Current Psychiatry Report, 13*, 60–68. doi:10.1007/s11920-010-0167-x.

Weiss, R., Kolodziej, M., Najavits, L., Greenfield, S. F., & Fucito, L. M. (2000). Utilization of psychosocial treatments by patients diagnosed with bipolar disorder and substance abuse. *American Journal on Addictions, 9*, 314–320.

Weiss, J., & Sampson, H. (1986). *The psychoanalytic process*. New York: The Guilford Press.

West, M., Alimo-Metcalfe, B., Dawson, J., el Ansari, W., Glasby, J., Hardy, G., et al. (2012). *Effectiveness of Multi-Professional Team Working (MPTW) in mental health care*. National Institute for Health Research Service Delivery and Organisation programme. Retrieved from http://www.onyett.org/wp-content/uploads/2012/09/MPTW_Final_report.pdf

Westen, D., & Morrison, K. (2001). A multidimensional meta-analysis of treatments for depression, panic, and generalized anxiety disorder: An empirical examination of the status of empirically supported therapies. *Journal of Consulting and Clinical Psychology, 69*, 875–899.

Westra, H., Aviram, A., Barnes, M., & Angus, L. (2010). Therapy was not what I expected: A preliminary qualitative analysis of concordance between client expectations and experience of cognitive-behavioural therapy. *Psychotherapy Research, 20*, 436–446.

Williams, P., & Schaefer, M. (2005). On confidentiality. *Fort Da, 11*, 74–87.

Winnicott, D. (1965). *The maturational processes and the facilitating environment*. New York: International Universities Press.

Winnicott, D. (1987). *Holding and interpretation: Fragment of an analysis*. New York: Grove Press.

Winnicott, D. (2011). *Deprivation and delinquency*. London: Routledge.

Wolsko, P., Eisenberg, D., Davis, R., & Phillips, R. (2004). Use of mind–body medical therapies: Results of a national survey. *Journal of General Internal Medicine, 19*, 43–50.

Zerbe, K. (2008). *Integrated treatment of eating disorders: Beyond the body betrayed*. New York: W.W. Norton.

Index

F.D. Barth, *Integrative Clinical Social Work Practice: A Contemporary Perspective*, Essential Clinical Social Work Series, DOI 10.1007/978-1-4939-0351-1,

T